HEPATITIS C

Biomedical Research Reports

Biomedical Research Reports

Series Editors

John I. Gallin
Warren G. Magnuson Clinical Center
National Institutes of Health
Bethesda, Maryland

Anthony S. Fauci
National Institute of Allergy and Infectious Diseases
National Institutes of Health
Bethesda, Maryland

HEPATITIS C

Biomedical Research Reports

Volume Editor

T. Jake Liang

Jay H. Hoofnagle

National Institute of Diabetes and Digestive and Kidney Diseases
National Institutes of Health
Bethesda, Maryland

ACADEMIC PRESS

San Diego   London   Boston   New York   Sydney   Tokyo   Toronto

Academic Press
A Harcourt Science and Technology Company
525 B Street, Suite 1900, San Diego, California 92101-4495, USA
http://www.academicpress.com

Academic Press
Harcourt Place, 32 Jamestown Road, London NW1 7BY, UK
http://www.academicpress.com

Library of Congress Catalog Card Number: 00-102552
International Standard Book Number: 0-12-447870-0

PRINTED IN THE UNITED STATES OF AMERICA
00 01 02 03 04 05 MM 9 8 7 6 5 4 3 2 1

We dedicate this book to our wives
Velma and Cheryl
and our families
Samantha, Sydney and Spencer,
and
Holden, Chris and Mark
without whom all this effort is not worth much.

CONTENTS

1 Molecular Biology of Hepatitis C Virus   1

MICHAEL THOMSON AND T. JAKE LIANG

2 Hepatitis C: Viral Markers and Quasispecies   25

JEAN-MICHEL PAWLOTSKY

3 Hepatitis C Virus Genotypes   53

PETER SIMMONDS

4 Acute Hepatitis C   71

JAY H. HOOFNAGLE

5 Natural History of Hepatitis C   85

LEONARD B. SEEFF

6 Pathology of Hepatitis C   107

DAVID E. KLEINER

7 Humoral Response to Hepatitis C Virus   125

AMY J. WEINER, DAVID CHIEN, QUI-LIM CHOO, STEPHEN COATES,
GEORGE KUO, AND MICHAEL HOUGHTON

8 **Immunopathogenesis of Hepatitis C** **147**
BARBARA REHERMANN

9 **Epidemiology of Hepatitis C** **169**
MIRIAM J. ALTER, YVAN J. F. HUTIN, AND GREGORY L. ARMSTRONG

10 **Worldwide Prevalence and Prevention
of Hepatitis C** **185**
DANIEL LAVANCHY AND BRIAN MCMAHON

11 **Therapy of Chronic Hepatitis C** **203**
JOHN G. MCHUTCHINSON AND JAY H. HOOFNAGLE

12 **Hepatitis C and Cirrhosis** **241**
GIOVANNA FATTOVICH AND SOLKO W. SCHALM

13 **Hepatitis C and Hepatocellular Carcinoma** **265**
ADRIAN M. DI BISCEGLIE

14 **Hepatitis C and Liver Transplantation** **277**
MARINA BERENGUER AND TERESA L. WRIGHT

15 **Mixed Cryoglobulinemia and Other Extrahepatic
Manifestations of Hepatitis C Virus Infection** **295**
VINCENT AGNELLO

16 **Hepatitis C Virus and Human Immunodeficiency Virus
Coinfection** **315**
MARC GHANY AND DARYL T.-Y LAU

17 **Hepatitis C and Renal Disease** **329**
STEVEN ZACKS AND MICHAEL W. FRIED

18 **Chronic Hepatitis C and Porphyria Cutanea Tarda** **351**
JOSEPH R. BLOOMER

19 **Hepatitis C Virus Infection and Alcohol** **363**
JAMES EVERHART AND DAVID HERION

20 **Hepatitis C in Children** **389**
MAUREEN M. JONAS

21 **Hepatitis C and Pregnancy** **405**
AUGUSTO E. SEMPRINI AND ALESSANDRO R. ZANETTI

22 **Hepatitis C and Iron**   **415**

JOHN K. OLYNYK AND BRUCE R. BACON

23 **Complementary and Alternative Medicine in Hepatitis C**   **427**

DORIS B. STRADER AND HYMAN J. ZIMMERMAN

24 **Development of Novel Therapies for Hepatitis C**   **453**

JOHNSON Y. N. LAU AND DAVID N. STANDRING

25 **Hepatitis C Vaccines**   **469**

SARA GAGNETEN AND STEPHEN M. FEINSTONE

INDEX   **487**

CONTRIBUTORS

Vincent Agnello (295) Lahey Clinic, Burlington, and The Edith Norse Rogers Memorial Veterans Affairs Hospital, Bedford, Massachusetts 01805

Miriam J. Alter (169) Hepatitis Branch, National Center for Infectious Diseases, Centers for Disease Control and Prevention, Atlanta, Georgia 30333

Gregory L. Armstrong (169) Hepatitis Branch, National Center for Infectious Diseases, Centers for Disease Control and Prevention, Atlanta, Georgia 30333

Bruce R. Bacon (415) Division of Gastroenterology and Hepatology, Department of Internal Medicine, Saint Louis University School of Medicine, St. Louis, Missouri 63110

Marina Berenguer (277) Department of Veterans Affairs Medical Center, University of California, San Francisco, California 94121

Joseph R. Bloomer (351) The Liver Center, University of Alabama at Birmingham, Birmingham, Alabama 35294

David Chien (125) Chiron Corporation, Emeryville, California 94608

Qui-Lim Choo (125) Chiron Corporation, Emeryville, California 94608

Stephen Coates (125) Chiron Corporation, Emeryville, California 94608

Adrian M. Di Bisceglie (265) Department of Internal Medicine, Saint Louis University School of Medicine, St. Louis, Missouri 63104

James Everhart (363) Epidemiology and Clinical Trials Branch, Division of Digestive Diseases and Nutrition, National Institute of Diabetes and Digestive and Kidney Diseases, National Institutes of Health, Bethesda, Maryland 20892

Giovanna Fattovich (241) Servizio Autonomo Clinicizzato di Gastroentero-logia, Dipartimento di Scienze Chirurgiche e Gastroenterologiche, Università di Verona, 37134, Verona, Italy

Stephen M. Feinstone (469) Laboratory of Hepatitis Viruses, Center for Bio-logic Evaluation and Research, Food and Drug Administration, Bethesda, Maryland 20892

Michael W. Fried (329) Division of Digestive Diseases and Nutrition, University of North Carolina, School of Medicine, Chapel Hill, North Carolina 27599

Sara Gagneten (469), Laboratory of Hepatitis Viruses, Center for Biologics and Evaluation and Research, Food and Drug Administration, Bethesda, Maryland 20892

Marc Ghany (315) Liver Diseases Section, Digestive Diseases Branch, National Institute of Diabetes and Digestive and Kidney Diseases, National Institutes of Health, Bethesda, Maryland 20892

David Herion (363) Liver Diseases Section, National Institute of Diabetes and Digestive and Kidney Diseases, National Institutes of Health, Bethesda, Maryland

Jay H. Hoofnagle (71) Division of Digestive Diseases and Nutrition, National Institute of Diabetes and Digestive and Kidney Diseases, National Institutes of Health, Bethesda, Maryland 20892

Michael Houghton (125) Chiron Corporation, Emeryville, California 94608

Yvan J. F. Hutin (169) Safe Injection Global Network, World Health Organi-zation, Geneva, Switzerland

John K. Olynyk (415) Division of Gastroenterology and Hepatology, De-partment of Internal Medicine, Saint Louis University School of Medicine, St. Louis, Missouri 63110

Maureen M. Jonas (389) Division of Gastroenterology, Children's Hospital, and Harvard Medical School, Boston, Massachusetts 02115

David E. Kleiner (107) Laboratory of Pathology, National Cancer Institute, National Institutes of Health, Bethesda, Maryland 20892

George Kuo (125) Chiron Corporation, Emeryville, California 94608

Daryl T.-Y. Lau (315) Division of Gastroenterology and Hepatology, University of Texas, Galveston, Texas 77555

Johnson Y.N. Lau (453) Department of Research and Development, ICN Pharmaceuticals, Costa Mesa, California 92626

Daniel Lavanchy (185) World Health Organization (WHO), Communicable Diseases Surveillance and Response, Geneva, Switzerland

T. Jake Liang (1) Liver Diseases Section, National Institute of Diabetes and Di-gestive and Kidney Diseases, National Institutes of Health, Bethesda, Mary-land 20892

John G. McHutchison (203) Division of Gastroenterology/Hepatology, Scripps Clinic and Research Foundation, La Jolla, California 92037

Brian McMahon (185) Alaska Native Medical Center and Arctic Investigations Program, Centers for Disease Control and Prevention, Anchorage, Alaska 99508

Jean-Michel Pawlotsky (25) Department of Bacteriology and Virology and INSERM U99, Hôpital Henri Mondor, Université Paris XII, Créteil, 94010 France

Barbara Rehermann (147) Liver Diseases Section, National Institute of Diabetes and Digestive and Kidney Diseases, National Institutes of Health, Bethesda, Maryland 20892

Solko W. Schalm (241) Hepatogastroenterology, Erasmus University Hospital Dijkzigt, Rotterdam, The Netherlands

Leonard B. Seeff (85) Division of Digestive Diseases and Nutrition, National Institute of Diabetes and Digestive and Kidney Diseases, National Institutes of Health, Bethesda, Maryland 20892

Augusto E. Semprini (405) Department of Obstetrics and Gynecology, University of Milan, 8-20142, Milano, Italy

Peter Simmonds (53) Laboratory for Clinical and Molecular Virology, University of Edinburgh, Edinburgh, EH8 9aG, United Kingdom

David N. Standring (453) Department of Antiviral Therapy, Schering-Plough Research Institute, Kenilworth, New Jersey 07033

Doris B. Strader (427) Veterans Affairs Medical Center, and Georgetown University School of Medicine, Washington, DC 20422

Michael Thomson (1) Liver Diseases Section, National Institute of Diabetes and Digestive and Kidney Diseases, National Institutes of Health, Bethesda, Maryland 20892

Amy J. Weiner (125) Chiron Corporation, Emeryville, California 94608

Teresa L. Wright (277) Department of Veterans Affairs Medical Center, University of California, San Francisco, California 94121

Steven Zacks (329) Division of Digestive Diseases and Nutrition, University of North Carolina School of Medicine, Chapel Hill, North Carolina 27599

Alessandro R. Zanetti (405) Institute of Virology, University of Milan Medical School, 38-20133, Milano, Italy

Hyman J. Zimmerman (427) Armed Forces Institute of Pathology, WRAMC, Washington, DC 20422

■ FOREWORD

In the United States, as of the year 2000, hepatitis C has become the most common cause of chronic hepatitis and cirrhosis and is the single major reason for liver transplantation. The current public health impact of the hepatitis C virus (HCV) stands in striking contrast to the lack of its recognition only a few decades ago. In the initial studies on viral hepatitis conducted from 1940 to 1960, investigators identified two distinct forms of viral hepatitis: infectious hepatitis, which was designated as hepatitis A, and serum hepatitis, which was designated as hepatitis B. There was little or no suggestion of a third form of viral hepatitis.

The dual nature of viral hepatitis was strengthened and confirmed by the discovery of the Australia antigen by Baruch Blumberg and coworkers in 1964, and the later association of this antigen with serum hepatitis by multiple investigators. By 1973 the Australia antigen was officially named the hepatitis B surface antigen (HBsAg), and application of tests for HBsAg in blood banks led to an important decrease in posttransfusion hepatitis B. Cases of posttransfusion hepatitis, however, still occurred despite the screening of blood using sensitive methods for HBsAg detection. The continued transmission was attributed to a lack of sensitivity in tests for HBsAg and perhaps to the spread of hepatitis A by blood transfusion. At this point, on the basis of epidemiological features alone, several investigators had raised the question of a third form of viral hepatitis. The existence of this third hepatitis type was convincingly and elegantly demonstrated in 1974 by Stephen Feinstone and coworkers, as well as independently by Alfred Prince and his colleagues, who showed that the residual cases of HBsAg–negative posttransfusion hepatitis were not due to hepatitis A. This disease was thus named "non-A, non-B hepatitis" in deference to previous errors in separating hepatitis into only two forms and in acknowledgment that this diagnosis was one of exclusion.

The description of non-A, non-B hepatitis led to a readjustment of concepts in viral hepatitis and an outpouring of effort by investigators throughout the world to identify the agent of non-A, non-B hepatitis. The methodologies used to discover and define the hepatitis A and B viruses were applied to serum samples and tissues believed to harbor the non-A, non-B agent, but with little success. A number of candidate assays and viral particles were reported to be associated with non-A, non-B hepatitis, but none withstood scrutiny. For many years the identity of non-A, non-B hepatitis remained a difficult nut to crack for the scientific community.

The seminal breakthrough in non-A, non-B hepatitis research occurred when concurrent advances in modern molecular technology afforded Michael Houghton and his colleagues the molecular tools to identify and characterize the causative agent of hepatitis C. This technical tour de force, initially reported in 1989, also represented a changing paradigm in the field of infectious diseases, that is, the identification of an important human pathogen without the ability to grow, visualize, or detect the organism.

During the last decade substantial progress has been made in defining the epidemiology and natural history of HCV infection. These studies firmly established the magnitude of this infection as a major public health problem and underscored the global disease burden associated with hepatitis C. For the first time, hepatitis C, whether justifiably or not, reached the level of public sensationalism rivaling that of the HIV pandemic. While there are many public misconceptions about HCV, it remains true that the disease is common and that it can cause devastating consequences. In the same vein, therapy of hepatitis C, while continually evolving, has improved substantially, so that many patients can now be treated successfully. In the arena of laboratory investigations, the scientific community has made significant strides in characterizing the virus, defining the functions of viral gene products, and unraveling the replication pathway. Scientists are also beginning to understand the molecular and immunologic mechanisms of liver injury associated with HCV infection.

Have advances in the understanding of hepatitis C been such that a book dedicated solely to the virus and its disease is needed? We believe the answer is a resounding yes, and we offer the readers the opportunity to agree or disagree based on the twenty-five chapters of this book. To highlight all the advances in the field of hepatitis C in the last decade, we have assembled a cadre of outstanding contributors. This book covers such diverse topics as viral diagnostics, epidemiology, natural history, disease manifestations and treatments, basic virology, immunopathogenesis, vaccine development, and molecular approaches to novel therapy. We thank all of the contributing authors for the long hours and efforts that they put into this book.

No human effort is totally without its regrets or totally without its consolations. While this book has had its consolations for us, we realize that many topics covered in this book are continuously evolving. We hope this volume will serve as a useful reference book devoted solely to the clinical and basic science of hepatitis C. Aside from the state-of-the-art summaries of various topics on hepatitis C, each chapter also highlights the important questions yet to be resolved in the next decade. In this book we hope to illustrate that the marriage between basic science and clinical medicine is paramount in our ultimate success of controlling this global health problem. The first decade of research on hepatitis C has focused on the fundamentals of the virus and the disease. The next decade, as the beginning of the "postgenomic era," promises greater opportunities with unprecedented molecular, immunologic, and genetic technologies as well as with powerful computational bioinformatics and structural resolution of biomolecules. In the second decade of hepatitis C research, these techniques must be parlayed with clinical medicine as translational research to provide more reliable and practical means of diagnosis, evaluation, treatment, and prevention of hepatitis C.

T. Jake Liang
Jay H. Hoofnagle

■ PREFACE

"Hepatitis C" was selected as the subject for the second volume of *Biomedical Research Reports* because it is timely, challenging and has broad scientific, clinical, and social interest. We are fortunate that T. Jake Liang, M.D. and Jay H. Hoofnagle, M.D. agreed to edit this volume. These investigators bring a balanced perspective to this subject. It has been estimated that 3.8 million Americans, about 2% of the population, are seropositive for hepatitis C. Infection with hepatitis C can be indolent and results in chronic infection in 70–80% of patients. Chronic infection with hepatitis C has been shown to cause almost 60% of the cases of chronic liver disease and results in about 10,000 deaths each year from end-stage liver disease and its complications, including hepatocellular carcinoma in the United States. As a consequence, hepatitis C is both a devastating problem for individual patients and a huge burden on society. It is an ideal subject for *Biomedical Research Reports*. The progress in understanding the pathophysiology and treatment of hepatitis C in recent years has been remarkable. This volume provides a forum for the leaders in the field to present an outstanding perspective of the history and to identify future opportunities for progress. We welcome comments from our readers about this volume and opportunities for future volumes in the series.

John I. Gallin, M.D.
Anthony S. Fauci, M.D.

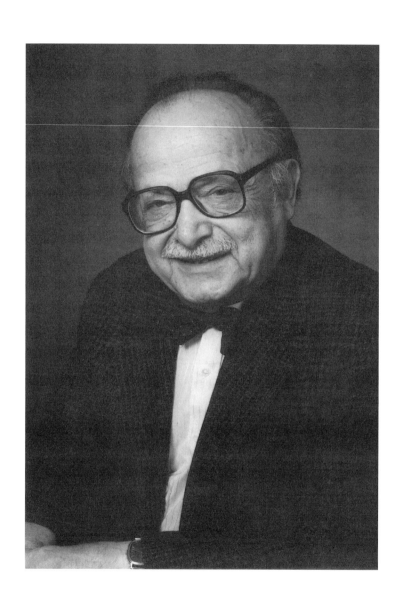

■ IN MEMORIAM

Hyman J. Zimmerman, a contributor to this book and a giant in the field of liver disease research, died on July 12, 1999, in Bethesda, Maryland, just a week before his eighty-fifth birthday and two months before the publication of his long-awaited, invaluable, single-authored textbook, *Hepatotoxicity*. Hy was a special mentor and father figure for many young hepatologists and liver disease investigators, including the editors and many of the authors of this book. For three decades, he served as the focal point of hepatology and liver disease research in Washington, DC.

Hy was born in upstate New York in 1914. He graduated from the University of Rochester and received his medical degree from Stanford. He made his initial contributions to the field of liver disease when he served in the U.S. Army from 1943 to 1946 as the chief of a military hospital in France, where he systematically collected data on patients and wrote what is still today the best clinical description of acute viral hepatitis. After the war Hy worked in the Veterans Administration (VA) medical system, and in 1950, he became the first chief of medicine at the VA Medical Center in Omaha, Nebraska. Later he served as the chairman of medicine at the University of Chicago, at the Boston VA Medicine Center, and the Washington, DC, VA Medical Center.

Throughout his career Hy wrote the classical descriptions of hepatotoxicity for many of the drugs that cause liver injury and made seminal contributions in laboratory research to the elucidation of the mechanisms of liver injury. He was an invaluable resource of knowledge and expertise in drug-induced liver injury and served as lead adviser to both the National Institutes of Health and the Food and Drug Administration, continuing in these capacities until just days before his death. He was a brilliant and beloved physician, a man of great knowledge, great integrity, and great heart. The authors and editors of this book salute his career and his contributions to medicine and wish to express our great sorrow over his loss.

1
MOLECULAR BIOLOGY OF HEPATITIS C VIRUS

MICHAEL THOMSON AND T. JAKE LIANG

Liver Diseases Section
National Institute of Diabetes and Digestive and Kidney Diseases, National Institutes of Health
Bethesda, Maryland

INTRODUCTION

Early studies on the etiology of non-A, non-B hepatitis described a blood-borne agent that could be transmitted to chimpanzees and caused ultrastructural alterations within infected hepatocytes. The agent was rendered inactive by treatment with organic solvents and could pass through an 80-nm filter. These observations led to the conclusion that the infectious agent was a small, enveloped virus, but there was no immunological or molecular evidence to support this conclusion. The term hepatitis C virus (HCV) was first adopted in 1989 following the identification of an RNA viral genome in a random-primed cDNA library derived from a human plasma sample containing the putative non-A, non-B hepatitis agent. (1) This RNA was approximately 10 kb in length and shared similarities with the genomes of flaviviruses and pestiviruses. The complete infectious HCV genomes from several genotypes have now been defined through the demonstration that RNA transcribed from cDNA clones caused hepatitis following intrahepatic inoculation into chimpanzees. (2–6)

Substantial progress has been made in the characterization of the HCV genome and its gene products, despite a lack of a tissue culture system or small animal model for efficient propagation of the virus. Much of the speculation on HCV pathogenesis and replication is either derived from limited studies of infected humans or inferred from studies of similar viruses, particularly the flaviviruses and pestiviruses, for which cell culture and animal models are available. Investigations into the molecular biology of HCV have, for the most part, relied on artificial expression systems, with the obvious disadvantage that data from such studies may not accurately reflect how the virus behaves *in vivo*. To overcome this disadvantage, much effort is being devoted to establishing alternative ways of studying the virus in the laboratory, including the development of novel expression systems, the production of stably transfected cell lines, and the use of transgenic animal models.

This chapter describes current understanding of the molecular virology of hepatitis C, including the known physical properties of the infectious particle and its RNA genome, the proposed functions of the virally encoded proteins, and the postulated pathway of virus replication.

PHYSICAL PROPERTIES

Particle Structure

Efforts to visualize the infectious HCV particle in blood and tissue specimens have been largely unsuccessful, presumably because the virus is present only in very low numbers. Most of the early evidence for the physical nature of the virus particle derived from transmission studies in chimpanzees. The infectivity of various human-derived inocula was inactivated by chloroform, suggesting that the virus was associated with lipids and thus enveloped. Filtration studies estimated the particle size as 30–60 nm in diameter, similar to flaviviruses and pestiviruses. (7)

A few groups have reported observing HCV particles in various specimens and cell lines using electron microscopy (EM). These include infected chimpanzee liver, human T- and B-cell lines. (8) Virus grown in Daudi cells was subsequently shown to be infectious in chimpanzees. (9) Particles observed in these studies resided in cytoplasmic vesicles and were approximately 50 nm in diameter (Fig. 1A). Generally only a few particles per cell were visualized, which contrasts with EM studies using the baculovirus expression system (Fig. 1B). (10) Following expression in insect cells of the HCV structural proteins from genotype 1b, abundant viruslike particles of 40 to 60 nm in diameter were visualized by EM. The particles resided in cytoplasmic vacuoles and possessed lipid-bilayer envelopes. Molecular and immunological analyses confirmed that they contained HCV structural proteins. They also exhibited a similar buoyant density and sedimentation coefficient as described for putative infectious HCV particles. (11)

It has proven difficult to generate large quantities of HCV particles in mammalian cells and the reason for this is not apparent at present. Using recombinant vaccinia virus to express HCV structural proteins, viruslike particle formation was not observed, despite a high level of protein expression. (12) This suggests that virion formation is somehow restricted at the level of assembly rather than as a consequence of limiting concentrations of component structural proteins. One would suspect that this unique aspect of HCV may be a means by which the virus maintains a low level in chronic infection and may serve an important advantage to the virus for evading host defenses.

Genome Organization

The HCV genome is a single-stranded RNA molecule of positive polarity approximately 9.6 kb in length. It contains a single open reading frame (ORF) of ~9 kb that encodes a polyprotein of ~3000 amino acids. The ORF is flanked at both ends by untranslated regions (UTR), which are the most conserved regions of the genome. The genome organization of HCV is similar to that of the flaviviruses and pestiviruses, indicating that these viruses are distantly related. In particular, there is a considerable sequence homology between the 5'UTR and its equivalent in pestiviral genomes. (13) The HCV polyprotein also contains regions that are homologous to parts of pestiviral polyproteins and, to a lesser extent, those of flaviviruses. Overall, there is not much primary sequence homology between these viruses, but their hydrophobicity profiles are similar.

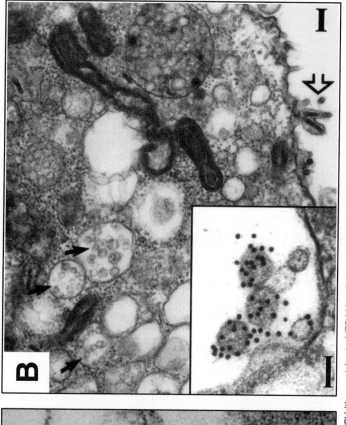

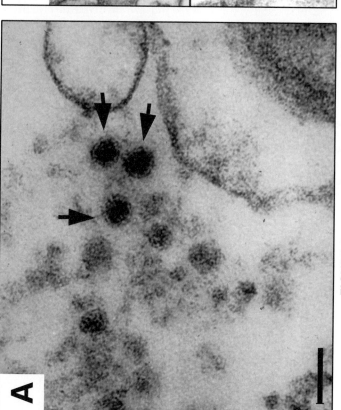

FIGURE 1 (A) Thin-section electron microscopy of HCV-like particles in HPBALL cells harvested 25 days postinoculation. Arrows indicate electron-dense viruslike particles in a cytoplasmic vesicle. Bar: 100 nm. Adapted from Shimizu et al., (8) with permission. (B) Electron microscopy of viruslike particles in insect cells infected with a recombinant baculovirus expressing HCV (J strain) structural proteins. (10) Closed arrows indicate numerous viruslike particles of 40–60 nm in cytoplasmic vacuoles. Open arrow indicates baculovirus particle. Bar: 120 nm. (Inset) Immunogold labeling of viruslike particles with an anti-E2 antibody. Bar: 50 nm.

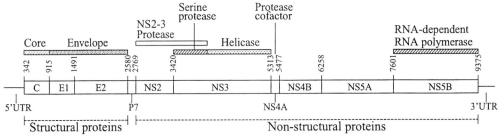

FIGURE 2 Schematic diagram of HCV genome organization showing the location of HCV genes and proposed functions of gene products. 5′- and 3′-untranslated regions (UTR) are indicated. Numbering refers to nucleotide positions of genes, based on the sequence of the HCV genotype 1a infectious clone. (2)

This suggests that these polyproteins are processed similarly and that their cleavage products have comparable functions. Indeed, much of the information about the nature and function of mature viral proteins derives from comparative studies with flaviviruses and pestiviruses. (14)

The HCV polyprotein is cleaved co- and posttranslationally by cellular and viral proteases to yield functional proteins. Figure 2 shows a diagram of the HCV genome and the polyprotein cleavage products, including known functions of the mature viral proteins. The structural proteins, thought to comprise the mature virion, are encoded by the 5′ quarter of the ORF, in the order C-E1-E2. Nonstructural proteins are encoded by the 3′ three-quarters of the ORF in the order NS2-NS3-NS4A/B-NS5A/B and are involved in polyprotein processing and replicative functions of the virus. It is not yet known if the p7 cleavage product is part of the structural proteins forming the virion.

CELL CULTURE AND ANIMAL MODELS

Tissue Culture Systems

Considerable information on HCV protein structure and function has been obtained from the use of a variety of cell culture and *in vitro* expression systems. Despite the fact that infectious HCV RNA can be generated by *in vitro* transcription from cDNA clones, to date it has not been possible to propagate to high levels or artificially generate infectious HCV particles in tissue culture. A number of reports have described the propagation of HCV particles in tissue culture, including one in which the propagated virus was subsequently shown to be infectious in chimpanzees. (9) However in all these reports the levels of propagation were very low, preventing a detailed analysis of the viral replication cycle. Typically polymerase chain reaction (PCR) was used to detect negative strand HCV RNA in cell extracts as an indication of genome replication. Unfortunately, this method is prone to giving false-positive results and is not a true measure of infectivity. A novel approach that may prove invaluable for studying HCV replication in tissue culture has been described. Constructs were produced containing HCV nonstructural genes placed downstream of the neomycin phosphotransferase gene. Following transfection of RNA transcribed from these constructs into a human hepatoma cell line, G418-resistant cells were obtained in which the subgenomic RNA replicated autonomously to high levels. (15)

Strong viral promoters are often used to overexpress foreign genes in tissue culture. The gene of interest is placed downstream of the desired promoter and is either introduced into a particular cell line by transfection or used to make a recombinant virus, which can then enter the cell by infection. In mammalian cells, the vaccinia virus late gene promoter and the cytomegalovirus early promoter have been used widely for expressing HCV proteins. The vaccinia-T7 infection/transfection system in particular has been used extensively because it forgoes the need to generate a recombinant virus; however, expression levels are not so high and translation must be mediated through an internal ribosome entry site (IRES). This system was employed in initial studies of HCV polyprotein processing (16) and has been used for generating infectious RNA from cDNA clones of many negative-stranded RNA viruses.

A drawback of using vaccinia virus expression systems is that the vaccinia virus rapidly causes extensive cytopathic effects and prevents long-term analysis of expressed proteins. A replication-deficient adenovirus expressing the T7 RNA polymerase has been used to express a reporter gene driven by the HCV IRES. (17) This alternative viral vector is not cytopathic and may prove useful for studying molecular aspects of HCV replication.

The baculovirus expression system has been used widely for the high-level expression of recombinant HCV proteins in insect cells. This system also suffers from the problem of a virus-induced cytopathic effect, leading ultimately to cell lysis, and has a different glycosylation pathway from higher eukaryotic systems. However, the high expression levels allow for the purification of large quantities of recombinant proteins for functional analyses. Unlike prokaryotic systems, insect cells permit correct folding and processing of the HCV polyprotein and can thus be used for investigating the assembly and biological activities of macromolecular complexes.

Animal Models

The chimpanzee has been used as a model for HCV infection in humans. Because of their scarcity and expense, much effort has been devoted to finding a suitable alternative. However, with the possible exception of the Tupaia belangeri chinensis, a tree shrew related to primates, (18) no small animal models have been identified to date that are susceptible to HCV infection. Obviously a convenient animal model is necessary for testing potential antiviral agents and studying HCV pathogenesis. Thus, many investigators have turned to the development of transgenic animals.

Transgenic mouse models have been successfully generated in the study of hepatitis B and delta viruses. Such studies have provided useful information on viral pathogenesis. Several groups have now produced transgenic mice containing various parts of the HCV genome, including the HCV core gene, (19) envelope E1 and E2 genes, (20) the structural genes, (21) and the entire polyprotein coding region. (22) Expression levels vary according to the promoter and enhancer elements used and may also depend on methylation of the transgene, which has been shown to inactivate expression. (23) Although most of the transgenic mice expressing part or all of the structural proteins did not exhibit any phenotypic changes, one model demonstrated hepatic steatosis and subsequent development of hepatocellular carcinoma associated with transgenic

expression of core in the liver. (19) There is much interest in developing transgenic models conditionally expressing transgenes as this facilitates functional
studies of particular gene products. To this end, the Cre/loxP system has been
used to express HCV structural proteins in a transgenic mouse. (24) In this
study, the transgenic mice developed acute hepatitis following induction of HCV
genes with adenovirus expressing the Cre DNA recombinase, and histopathological changes were not observed in CD4/CD8-depleted mice. This observation supports the concept that HCV infection is not directly cytopathic but
rather induces immunologic responses leading to cell injury.

TRANSLATION

The 5′-Untranslated Region

The 5′-untranslated region (UTR) of HCV is a 341 nucleotide sequence closely
resembling the 5′ UTR of pestiviruses in terms of length and putative secondary structure. (25) Unlike other flaviviruses, which have relatively short 5′UTR
regions, it functions via an IRES to direct cap-independent translation of the
genome. This region of the genome is highly conserved in terms of nucleotide
sequence and secondary structure, although there are a number of genotype-
specific variations. This feature has facilitated the development of PCR-based
genotyping methods.

Similar to the UTR of picornaviruses, the HCV 5′ UTR region is predicted
to form extensive secondary structures and possesses three to five noninitiating
AUG triplets (Fig. 3). Replacement of the 5′UTR of bovine viral diarrhea virus
(BVDV), a pestivirus, with that of HCV or encephalomyocarditis virus (EMC)
impaired BVDV translation and replication severely, demonstrating that these
viruses require their own 5′UTR for efficient function. (26) In order to achieve
this specificity it is thought that the 5′UTR may interact with other regions of
the genome or with viral proteins.

While it is not known to date whether the HCV genome is capped, there
is now compelling evidence that the 5′UTR functions as an IRES. This evidence was based initially on secondary structure similarities with known IRES
elements and subsequently supported by experiments using reporter gene constructs, the expression of which was dependent on an IRES. (27) The precise
region of the HCV genome comprising the IRES has been the subject of some
debate. (28) Conflicting data have emerged from studies using IRES-driven
reporter genes, perhaps because the reporter gene itself interacts with IRES
structural elements. This influence is likely to vary according to the reporter
gene used.

Mutational analyses of the IRES in the context of a near full-length HCV
genome have provided further insights into the structural elements involved in
internal initiation of translation. (28–30) These studies were performed *in vitro*, using rabbit reticulocyte lysates and cell transfection. The IRES was shown
to encompass most of the 5′UTR, with the 5′ end residing between nucleotides
28 and 69. Deletion of most of the 5′-terminal hairpin (stem–loop I) increased
translational efficiency of the IRES *in vitro*, suggesting that this structure functions to suppress translation. Domains II and III of the 5′ UTR were essential

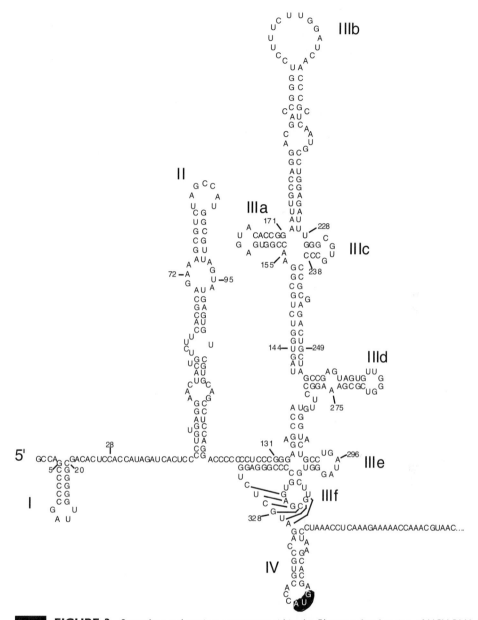

FIGURE 3 Secondary and tertiary structures within the 5'-untranslated region of HCV RNA (H strain). Roman numerals indicate major domains and letters denote individual stem–loop structures within each domain. The initiating codon within domain IV is highlighted. Reproduced from Honda et al., (30) with permission.

for IRES activity. In addition, the region just downstream of the initiator AUG codon was shown to be essential for efficient translation. Thus the 3' limit of the IRES probably resides within the core protein-coding region. The initiator AUG codon is located within a stem–loop structure (stem–loop IV), the stability of which is inversely correlated with the efficiency of translation. The low stability of stem–loop IV may allow it to dissociate readily and permit direct binding to the 40S ribosome subunit. In addition, this domain may be stabilized by association with viral proteins, providing a feedback mechanism for translation. Sequences outside the IRES structure may also be important for translational activity. Mutational studies using an *in vitro* translation system showed that changes in the dinucleotide at position 34 alters translational efficiency. (31) This effect was only observed if a region of the capsid coding sequence downstream of the IRES was present in the construct, suggesting that an RNA–RNA interaction occurs between these two regions flanking the IRES.

Internal initiation of translation is likely to involve host cell factors. Several groups have identified proteins that bind to and alter the activity of the IRES. These include a HeLa cell-derived 25-kDa protein, (32) liver cell-derived La antigen, (33) and heterogeneous nuclear ribonucleoprotein L. (34) It is not known whether these interactions occur *in vivo*. However, characterization of these cellular binding proteins required for viral translation may be important in the discovery of novel antiviral agents.

The 3′-Untranslated Region

The 3′ terminus of the HCV genome contains an untranslated region of approximately 30 nucleotides downstream of the 3′ terminus of the polyprotein-coding region followed by a poly U-C stretch of variable length. The extreme 3′ terminus is a highly conserved region of 98 nucleotides, known as the X region, predicted to form three stem–loop structures (Fig. 4). (35, 36) Analyses of the X region by chemical and enzymatic methods suggest a stable stem–loop structure within the 3′-terminal 48 nucleotides and a less ordered 5′ half, which may exist in multiple conformations. (37) The X region has been shown by UV cross-linking studies to bind a polypyrimidine tract-binding protein (PTB). (38) This protein has been implicated in the cap-independent initiation of translation. The X region has been demonstrated to specifically enhance IRES-driven translation from the HCV 5′UTR. (39, 40) This activity occurred only in *cis* and was possibly mediated through PTB binding or other factors. The X region was also able to enhance translation from an unrelated IRES derived from encephalomyocarditis virus. These studies suggest that the X region is involved in the regulation of translation, probably by interacting directly or indirectly with the IRES element.

Polyprotein Translation and Processing

Concurrent with and following translation, the HCV polyprotein undergoes a series of cleavages to form functional viral proteins. The structural proteins are cleaved from the polyprotein by cellular signal peptidases within the endoplasmic reticulum and nonstructural proteins by virally encoded proteases. Figure 5 shows the various cleavage sites in the polyprotein and the final products of digestion.

All the structural proteins have hydrophobic C termini. This feature is thought to be important for membrane association and cleavage from the polyprotein by host signal peptidases. The C-terminal region of the core domain is a signal sequence that directs E1 and E2 to the lumen of the endoplasmic reticulum (ER). The core protein remains on the cytoplasmic side of the ER and is

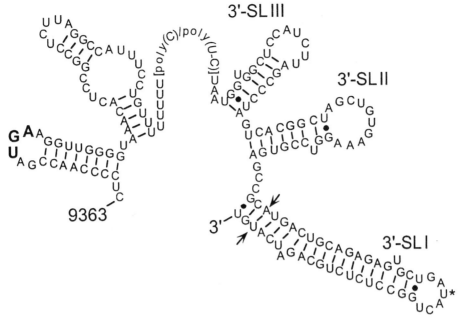

FIGURE 4 Computer-generated secondary structure prediction of HCV (H-strain) 3′-untranslated region. Stem–loop structures (SLI–III) within the 3′-terminal 98 nucleotide X region are indicated. Bold-type UGA denotes the termination codon of HCV ORF. Arrows indicate variable base pairs in the stem of SLI and the asterisk denotes the variable nucleotide in the loop of SLI. Reproduced from Kolykhalov et al., (35) with permission.

cleaved from E1 and E2. (41) Within the ER, E1 and E2 are modified by N-linked glycosylation and are thought to form the HCV envelope proteins. The folding and assembly of the envelope proteins within the ER are likely assisted by cellular chaperones. (42)

Nonstructural proteins are cleaved by two virally encoded proteases. The junction of NS2 and NS3 is cleaved autoproteolytically by a protease activity that spans NS2 and the serine protease domain of NS3 (the NS2-3 protease). The remaining four junctions of the polyprotein are cleaved by the NS3 serine protease, which resides in the N-terminal third of NS3. The cleaved NS5A and NS5B are modified further by phosphorylation.

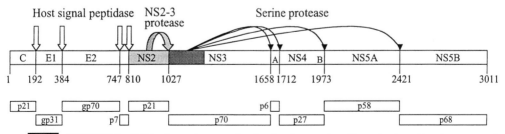

FIGURE 5 HCV polyprotein processing showing cleavage sites of host signal peptidase (open arrows), NS2-3 protease (gray arrow), and NS3 serine protease (thin arrows). Numbering denotes amino acid position upstream of cleavage sites (position P1). Processed HCV proteins and their approximate size by sodium dodecyl sulfate–polyacrylamide gel electrophoresis are shown.

To date, relatively little is known about the precise functions of nonstructural proteins in the HCV replication cycle. The protease activities of NS2 and NS3 and the polymerase activity of NS5B have been studied in great detail because of their importance as targets for antiviral therapy. However, the functions of NS4B and NS5A are not known. The following sections describe current understanding of the nature and function of each of the HCV proteins and provide a model summarizing what is known about the replicative strategy and possible pleiotropic effect of the virus within the infected cell.

PROTEIN STRUCTURE AND FUNCTION

Structural Proteins

Core

The core protein of HCV is located at the amino terminus of the polyprotein and is believed to be the main structural component of the viral capsid. The protein contains a hydrophobic C terminus that functions as a signal peptide, the cleavage of which from the polyprotein by a cellular signal peptidase yields a 21-kDa protein. The core protein is highly conserved among all HCV genotypes. Because of the high prevalence of anticore antibodies in infected individuals, the protein or its derivative has been used extensively in serologic assays for detecting HCV infection. Protein expression studies have identified different forms of the core protein. The full-length form of 21 kDa is derived from the first 191 amino acids of the polyprotein and is highly basic with a hydrophobic C terminus. It has been expressed in various mammalian cell lines, insect cells, and cell-free translation systems. An alternative 19-kDa form, produced by cleavage within the hydrophobic region at Leu-179 or Leu-182, has also been observed. (43) Several studies have demonstrated that the 21-kDa form of core localizes to the cytoplasm and the 19-kDa processed core is targeted to the nucleus. (41, 44, 45) Nuclear translocation may be mediated by a putative nuclear localization signal in the N-terminal region of core. (46) The N-terminal region of core has been shown to bind nonspecifically to RNA, but a specific interaction of core protein with HCV RNA has not yet been demonstrated. (47)

In addition to being a structural component of the HCV virion, the core protein has been implicated in a variety of other functions. These include inhibition or stimulation of apoptosis (depending on the cell type), regulation of cellular and viral promoters, and activation of transcriptional factors. Core protein has also been shown to cooperate with oncogenes to transform primary rat embryo fibroblasts *in vitro*. (48) Furthermore, the transgenic expression of core protein has been shown to result in hepatic steatosis and subsequent hepatocellular carcinoma in a transgenic mouse model. (19) However, this phenotype has not been observed in other core transgenic mice. (49) Several studies have demonstrated a physical association of core with various cellular proteins, including the lymphotoxin-β receptor of the tumor necrosis factor (TNF) receptor family, (50) heterogeneous nuclear ribonucleoprotein K (a transcriptional regulator), (51) apolipoprotein II, (44) and an RNA helicase. (52) Association with the lymphotoxin-β receptor is thought to potentiate NF-κB activation and may be important in the development of HCV chronicity. (53)

Envelope Proteins

The HCV proteins E1 (gp31) and E2 (gp70) are membrane-associated glyco-proteins, forming an integral part of the HCV virion envelope. The proteins are targeted to the ER where they are cleaved from the viral polyprotein. Additional cleavage in the C terminus of E2 yields a small 7-kDa hydrophobic polypeptide (p7). E1 and E2 are retained in the ER and ER-like structures and interact with ER chaperones. (42) The transmembrane domains of E1 and E2 are thought to be important for ER retention. (54) The proteins are modified by N-linked gly-cosylation but lack complex carbohydrate additions that are characteristic of protein trafficking through the Golgi. (55)

E1 and E2 are thought to interact to form a heterodimeric noncovalent E1–E2 complex that ultimately constitutes the virion envelope. The formation of E1–E2 complexes has been studied using monoclonal antibodies that only rec-ognize correctly folded E1–E2 heterodimers. (56, 57) These studies suggest that the assembly process is slow and inefficient, requiring cellular chaperones, and the E1 and E2 proteins have the tendency to form misfolded, disulfide-linked ag-gregates when highly expressed in mammalian cells.

The C-terminally truncated E2 protein has been shown to bind specifically to human CD81, but not to other members of the tetraspanin family. (58, 59) This interaction suggests that CD81 is a receptor for HCV and may thus be im-portant for the tissue tropism of the virus and for virion uptake by the host cell. The E2 protein possesses hyervariable regions (HVR) that may be important for the establishment of a persistent infection by HCV. Two such regions, HVR-1 and HVR-2, have been identified in the N-terminal portion of the protein. (60) HVR-1 comprises the first 27 amino acids of E2 and varies considerably among and within genotypes as well as within the same infected individual. Variation in this region accelerates as disease progresses, perhaps enabling the virus to es-cape immune surveillance. (61–63) *In vitro* binding assays suggest that E2 con-tains various neutralizing epitopes, with the principal one residing in the HVR-1 region. (64, 65)

Together with the core protein, envelope proteins play an important role in various stages of the viral life cycle, including cell entry, uncoating, and virion as-sembly. The function of the p7 protein has not been determined. Evidence from studies with pestiviruses (66) and baculovirus expression of HCV-like particles (10) suggests that p7 is probably not necessary for viral assembly.

Nonstructural Proteins

NS2

The NS2 protein, together with the N-terminal domain of NS3, forms an NS2-NS3 protease. It is cleaved from the HCV polypeptide by a host signal pep-tidase acting on the C terminus of E2 and by autoproteolytic action of the NS2-3 protease on the NS2/3 junction. The autocatalytic reaction probably occurs in a membrane compartment because NS2 has been shown to be a transmembrane protein. (67) The NS2-3 protease can also act in *trans,* albeit less efficiently. (68) Studies on the biochemical properties of NS2-3 have been hampered by the dif-ficulty in expressing and purifying the protein in active form. However, genetic analysis has provided evidence for possible mechanisms of autoproteolysis of

NS2-3. (69) One hypothesis is that NS2-3 is a zinc protease. This is supported by observations that proteolytic activity is inhibited by EDTA and stimulated by $ZnCl_2$. The proteolytic activity is also reduced or abolished by the deletion of amino acid residues near the proposed zinc-binding site of the NS3 protein. A second model suggests that NS2-3 is a cysteine protease. Mutation of His-952 and Cys-993 residues in the NS2 domain, which potentially form a catalytic dyad of a cysteine protease, abolished proteolytic activity of the NS2-3 protein. (70)

NS3

The NS3 protein possesses multiple enzyme activities. (71) The N-terminal one-third (180 amino acids) of the protein has serine protease activity and requires NS4A as a cofactor for efficient proteolytic cleavage. The C-terminal region of NS3 possesses RNA helicase and nucleotide triphosphatase activites. By virtue of its protease function, NS3 is an attractive target for antiviral compounds and has been studied in great detail as a consequence.

The three-dimensional structures of the serine protease domain, alone and in complex with NS4A peptides, have been determined by X-ray crystallography and reveal a zinc-binding site and a chymotrypsin-like fold (Fig. 6A). (72, 73) The zinc-binding site is thought to have a structural rather than catalytic function because it lies on the opposite side to the active site of the molecule. The crystal structure of the C-terminal helicase domain has also been elucidated (Fig. 6B). The helicase consists of three domains that form a Y-shaped molecule: an NTPase domain, an RNA-binding domain, and a helicase domain. Single-stranded RNA can be modeled to fit into an interdomain cleft formed between the RNA-binding domain and the rest of the molecule. (74)

The mature form of NS3 (67 kDa) is generated from the HCV polypeptide by cleavage at the N terminus by NS2-3 protease and at the C terminus by the serine protease activity of NS3. NS3 expressed in mammalian and insect cells has also been shown to be cleaved internally within the helicase region, but not by virally encoded proteases. (75) Three conserved amino acid residues within the serine protease domain, His-1083, Asp-1107, and Ser-1165, form the catalytic triad. The first processing event by the NS3 protease is the cleavage in *cis* of the NS3/NS4A junction. This is followed by cleavage in *trans* sequentially at NS4A/NS4B, NS4B/NS5A, and NS5A/NS5B junctions (Fig. 5). (76) The NS4A cofactor accelerates cleavage at the NS5A/NS5B junction and is essential for cleavage at the three other sites. A 14 amino acid hydrophobic region of NS4A (aa 21–34) is sufficient to act as a cofactor for protease activity.

A consensus sequence for the protease substrate has been deduced from the four cleavage sites within the polyprotein: Asp/GluXXXXCys/Thr-Ser/Ala, where X represents any amino acid (Table I). At all the sites cleaved in *trans* (NS4A/B, NS4B/NS5A, NS5A/NS5B), a cysteine residue is present at the position upstream of the cleavage site (position P1), whereas at the NS3/4A *cis* cleavage site this residue is a threonine. Mutational analysis has shown that this P1 residue is a major determinant of substrate specificity. Studies also highlight the importance of the phenylalanine residue at amino acid position 154 of NS3 in determining substrate specificity. This residue was predicted from molecular modeling to be part of the substrate-binding pocket of the enzyme, into which the P1 residue was accommodated. This prediction was confirmed subsequently

A. NS3: serine protease domain

B. NS3: helicase domain

C. NS5B: RNA-dependent RNA polymerase

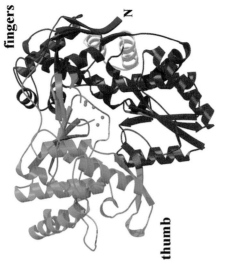

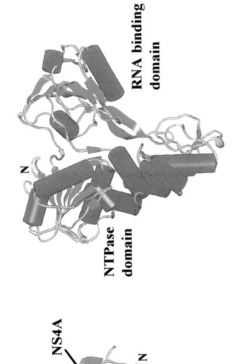

FIGURE 6 Ribbon diagrams of hepatitis C virus serine protease, helicase, and RNA-dependent RNA polymerase X-ray crystallographic structures. (A) NS3, serine protease domain–NS4A complex, viewed from above the active site, down the axis of the C-terminal β barrel. Active site residues are shown in a ball-and-stick format with the zinc-binding site indicated. The location of the NS4A peptide within the enzyme fold is shown. (B) NS3, helicase domain. NTPase- and RNA-binding domains are indicated; both face the interdomain cleft. (C) NS5B RNA-dependent RNA polymerase. This image is color coded according to the fingers (blue), palm (red), and thumb (green) subdomains with the yellow and cyan regions highlighted to indicate intersubdomain structural linkages. The small cyan balls indicate unobserved residues. The diagrams were generated and kindly provided by Dr. Nanhua Yao (NS3) and Dr. Charles Lesburg (NS5B), Schering-Plough Research Institute (Kenilworth, NJ).

TABLE I **Amino Acid Sequence at Cleavage Sites of NS3 Serine Protease**

Cleavage site	P1 residue position in HCV polyprotein	Amino acid sequence[a]
NS3/NS4A	1657	DLEVVT/STWVL
NS4A/NS4B	1711	DEMEEC/SQHLP
NS4B/NS5A	1972	ECTTPC/SGSWL
NS5A/NS5B	2420	EDVVCC/SMSYS
Consensus		DXXXXC/S
		E T

[a] Based on the sequence of the HCV genotype 1a infectious clone (2)

by experiments showing that substitution of Phe-154 resulted in a modified cleavage pattern by the protease. (77)

The RNA helicase and NTPase activities of NS3 reside in the C-terminal 465 amino acids of NS3 and function independently of the serine protease. The helicase, which unwinds RNA duplexes in the 3′ to 5′ direction, has conserved sequences with and is structurally similar to other RNA helicases. Unique to HCV, this enzyme is also able to unwind double-stranded DNA and DNA/RNA heteroduplexes. (78) The NTPase activity is likely to be coupled with the helicase function, providing the energy necessary to disrupt nucleic acid duplexes.

Helicases, both viral and cellular, have been grouped into superfamilies on the basis of conserved sequence motifs. (79) HCV and other putative or known helicases of positive-stranded RNA viruses are classified in superfamily 2, which is characterized by six conserved sequence motifs (numbered I to VI). Motif II, containing the sequence DEXH (the DEXH box), has been proposed as the site involved in coupling NTP hydrolysis to helicase activity. Motif IV, containing the sequence SAT, and motif VI, containing the sequence QRXGRXGR, are implicated in the helicase function; the latter motif is specifically required for RNA binding. The importance of helicase activity in the HCV replication cycle has not been defined. It probably functions as part of the viral replication complex to separate positive and negative strands following RNA synthesis.

NS4

NS4A and NS4B are 6- and 27-kDa proteins, respectively, and are cleaved from the HCV polyprotein by the serine protease of NS3. As described in the preceding section, NS4A is a cofactor for NS3 serine protease. Additionally, NS4A has been shown to facilitate phosphorylation of NS5A. (80) To date it is not known what function NS4B serves in HCV replication.

X-ray crystallography studies have shown that the NS4A peptide intercalates within a β sheet of the NS3 protease core. All of the contact points predicted in this model of NS3–NS4A interaction occur in the region spanning residues 21 to 32 of NS4A. (72) Although the contact surface is relatively extensive, an overall weak association between NS3 and NS4A seems to be sufficient for protease activation *in vitro*. (81)

There are a number of hypotheses on how NS4A functions as a cofactor for NS3 protease. It may act as a molecular chaperone to facilitate correct folding of the protease and/or to stabilize the conformation of the enzyme once it is folded. It has been shown to form a nonionic, detergent-stable complex with the NS4B–NS5A polyprotein substrate, explaining in part its requirement for cleavage at this junction. (82) Hydrophobicity plots predict that the N-terminal portion of NS4A forms a transmembrane helix, which probably anchors the NS4A/NS3 complex to the cellular membrane. (83)

NS5A

The NS5A protein of HCV is a phosphoprotein, generated by cleavage from the polyprotein at the junctions with NS4B and NS5B by the NS3 protease. The function of NS5A in the viral replication cycle has not yet been determined, but it is thought to be important for viral replication. The C-terminal portion of NS5A has been shown to function as a transcriptional activator in yeast and in human hepatoma cells. (84) This function may be important in viral replication and in hepatocarcinogenesis. Expression studies in mammalian cells have demonstrated two forms of NS5A (56 and 58 kDa), varying only in their degree of phosphorylation. (85) The level of phosphorylation can vary between HCV genotypes. (86) Phosphorylation occurs in the region between amino acids 2200 and 2250 and in the C-terminal region, predominantly on serine residues and, to a lesser extent, on threonine residues. A HeLa cell protein kinase has been identified that phosphorylated NS5A serine residues *in vitro*. (87) Hyperphosphorylation of NS5A to the p58 form occurs if the protein is expressed from the polyprotein, but not if expressed on its own or with other viral proteins provided in *trans*. Mutations in NS3, NS4A, or NS4B can alter the degree of phosphorylation, indicating that these nonstructural proteins interact to form a complex with NS5A. (88)

Several studies have provided evidence that NS5A is involved in mediating the resistance of HCV to interferon-α therapy. (89) Comparison of viral isolates from patients with varying sensitivity to interferon therapy showed a cluster of amino acid variations within NS5A. These differences occurred predominantly in the central region of the protein (amino acids 2209 to 2248), termed the interferon sensitivity determining region (ISDR). However, subsequent studies did not demonstrate such an association. (90) At present it is not clear why these reports are contradictory. Regarding a possible mechanism for determining interferon resistance by this region, evidence shows that NS5A interacts structurally and functionally with PKR, an interferon-induced protein kinase. (91) On induction, PKR phosphorylates eIF-2α, leading to the inhibition of protein synthesis and hence viral replication. Binding of NS5A to PKR results in repression of the kinase function and a block in eIF-2a phosphorylation. Mutational analysis of NS5A has shown that the PKR-binding domain is located within the ISDR, suggesting that interferon sensitivity may be determined in part by the sequence of the PKR-binding region.

NS5B

The NS5B protein is an RNA-dependent RNA polymerase (RdRp). This function was initially predicted by sequence comparison with other known

RdRps and has since been proven experimentally. The protein has a molecular mass of 68 kDa and is cleaved from the C terminus of the polyprotein by the NS3 protease. It is phosphorylated and has been shown to localize predominantly to the perinuclear region of mammalian and insect cells. (92)

NS5B has been overexpressed in insect cells and bacteria and requires high salt and detergent concentrations for solubilization. A cellular terminal transferase activity typically copurifies with NS5B derived from insect cells. (93) Truncation of the hydrophobic C-terminal region has been shown to facilitate solubilization without impairing the polymerase activity. This 21 amino acid region contains a putative membrane-anchoring domain important for localizing the protein to the perinuclear region. (94) Partially purified NS5B has been shown to bind specifically with the 3′ terminus of HCV RNA. Interestingly, this interaction occurred between the 3′ coding region and not the 3′-untranslated region, including the X region. (95) The crystal structure of C-terminally truncated NS5B has been determined (Fig. 6C). (96) Unlike other RNA-dependent RNA polymerases, the finger and thumb subdomains of this molecule were found to interact extensively, completely encircling the active site. The palm and fingers subdomains were also linked, thus rendering the overall structure of NS5B relatively inflexible.

The polymerase function of NS5B has been well characterized with respect to its kinetics and biochemical requirements. (97, 98) Four motifs within NS5B conserved among viral RdRps have been confirmed by mutational analyses as essential for polymerase activity. (93) NS5B requires a nucleic acid primer for polymerization and has been shown to copy the complete HCV genome. (99) However, similar to the RdRps of other RNA viruses, NS5B on its own is not sufficient to confer template specificity. (100) It is likely that template specificity is determined through interaction of the polymerase with other viral proteins or cellular factors. (101) NS5B has been shown to bind to homopolymeric templates. (93) The degree of binding was inversely related to polymerase activity, suggesting that high-binding affinity interferes with the polymerization reaction. In these studies it was necessary to use RNA or DNA oligonucleotide primers for the RdRp to function. For other RNA templates, NS5B is able to use the 3′OH group as primer. It is thought that the 3′ terminus of HCV RNA contains a hairpin secondary structure, thereby providing the primer for the initiation of RNA synthesis.

It is not known what factors are involved in the regulation of HCV replication. However, evidence from studies of other RNA viruses suggests that the RNA template itself is partly responsible. More specifically, the 5′ and 3′ termini of the genome may interact through complementary sequences, influencing the polymerization reaction as well as translation. Following synthesis of negative-strand RNA, it is not known how new positive strands are synthesized, how the genomic ends are processed, and how the newly synthesized HCV genomes are assembled into virions. Presumably the original positive strand template is removed from the negative strand by the actions of the viral helicase and/or cellular RNAse(s). Daughter-positive strand RNAs are then synthesized from the negative-strand RNA template and interact with the structural proteins to assemble into virions.

HCV REPLICATION CYCLE

Cell Entry and Uncoating

Figure 7 delineates a proposed model of the HCV replication cycle, based on current understanding of the function of the HCV proteins and on information drawn from other positive strand viruses. In order to enter the host cell, the virus must first bind to a cell surface receptor. This is a specific interaction mediated through the viral envelope proteins and determines in part the host range and tissue tropism of the virus. A few receptors have been identified for flaviviruses and pestiviruses. For example, a 65-kDa protein found on a neuroblastoma cell line but not on a nonsusceptible cell line was proposed to be the receptor for dengue-2 virus (102); a 50-kDa protein as the putative receptor for bovine viral diarrhea virus was identified on bovine kidney cells using an anti-idiotypic antibody. (103) Receptor identification for HCV is problematic partly because it has not been possible to purify sufficient viral particles to perform receptor-binding experiments. Studies demonstrated that binding of purified envelope proteins to human cells is mediated through the E2 protein. (58) In addition, the C-terminally truncated E2 was shown to bind CD81, a cell surface protein expressed on various cell lines, including hepatocytes and B lymphocytes. The major extracellular loop of CD81 bound HCV E2 protein and this binding was inhibited by HCV neutralizing antibodies. Another hypothesis proposes that HCV uptake is mediated by an LDL receptor and is supported by evidence that HCV persistence in cell culture is assisted by LDL receptor stimulation. (104)

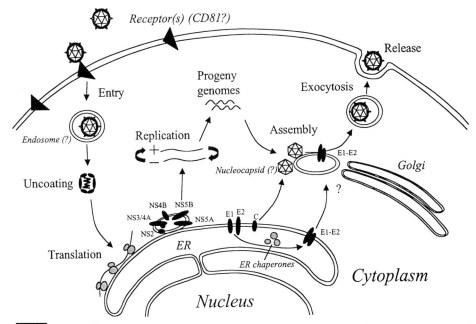

FIGURE 7 Schematic diagram of the postulated HCV replication cycle, derived from research on HCV and other positive-strand viruses. Each step of the cycle is described in detail in the text.

Following uptake, the virus must uncoat and release the genome to begin the replication cycle. Flaviviruses are thought to uncoat within acidic compartments such as endosomes following receptor-mediated endocytosis. (105) Mild acidity results in an irreversible change in the conformation of the envelope proteins and subsequent fusion to the endosomal membrane. (106) Evidence from studies with alphaviruses suggests that the nucleocapsid is released into the cytoplasm following endosomal fusion. Here it becomes associated with ribosomes, an interaction that is sufficient to release the capsid protein from the nucleocapsid. (107) The genomic RNA then serves as a template for protein translation.

Replication

As described in the preceding sections, translation of the HCV genome yields a polyprotein that is cleaved to form structural and nonstructural viral proteins. Nonstructural proteins, along with the HCV RNA template and host cell factors, are thought to form a replication ribonucleoprotein complex, such as has been described for poliovirus. (108) Cellular proteins that bind to the RNA template may function by bringing particular regions of the RNA together, thus presenting the initiation sites to the viral polymerase. These factors may also determine the specificity of the complex for the viral RNA and consequently contribute to viral tropism.

Electron microscopic studies with flavivirus-infected cells have demonstrated the localization of some nonstructural proteins and double-stranded RNA to virus-induced membrane structures or vesicles in the perinuclear region of the host cell. (109) It is thought that these membranous structures are the sites of RNA replication and are thus part of the viral replication complex. The replication complex of HCV has not been isolated, but accumulating evidence shows that NS5B associates with other HCV nonstructural proteins, in particular NS3 and NS4A. (110) Within such a complex the strategy for replication would be to produce a negative-strand copy of the RNA genome, which would in turn serve as the template for the production of progeny positive-strand RNA.

Virion Assembly

The mature HCV virion is thought to possess a nucleocapsid and an outer envelope composed of a lipid membrane and envelope proteins. Virion assembly presumably begins with the interaction of capsid proteins and genomic RNA to form a nucleocapsid. The nucleocapsid then acquires an envelope and the mature virion is released from the infected cell.

The mechanism of HCV RNA packaging has not been determined, but research with other RNA viruses suggests that the packaging reaction specifically incorporates viral RNA into the capsid with the total exclusion of cellular RNAs and negative-strand viral RNA. To achieve this specificity the positive-strand RNA is thought to possess an encapsidation signal, which exhibits a specific binding affinity for the capsid protein. Evidence from flavivirus and alphavirus research has shown that such a signal resides in the nonstructural coding region of the genome. (111, 112) Another explanation for packaging specificity, described for poliovirus, is that viral RNA replication is directly coupled to RNA packaging and only genomes being actively replicated are packaged. (113)

Enveloped viruses acquire their envelope by the process of budding, either through intracellular membranes or through the plasma membrane. Electron microscopy studies with flaviviruses have shown that nucleocapsids form in the cytoplasm and bud into intracellular vesicles derived from the ER, acquiring envelopes in the process. (114) The assembled virions are then released from cells via the exocytosis pathway. (115) Because HCV glycoprotein complexes are mostly retained in the ER, it is thought that HCV budding may occur in the ER or ER-like structures. (57) It is not known how the envelope is added to the nucleocapsid, but presumably the envelope proteins have a binding affinity for the assembled capsid proteins as has been described for alphaviruses. (116) The budding process may be driven by interactions between the virion envelope proteins and the nucleocapsid. Alternatively, the process may involve a lateral interaction of the envelope proteins, as has been suggested for alphavirus budding. Such a mechanism would explain how viral and cellular membrane proteins are distinguished so that only viral envelope proteins are incorporated into the mature virion. (117) It remains to be determined whether such a mechanism exists for HCV.

CONCLUSION

Since the identification of HCV in 1989 as the causative agent of non-A, non-B hepatitis, many advances have been made in the molecular biology of this virus, including the characterization of the genome, the role of *cis*-acting genomic structure elements, and the structure and function of virally encoded proteins. These advances were made despite a lack of a cell culture system for efficiently propagating the virus. Clearly there are several areas of the virus replication cycle that require elucidation, including the mechanism of cell entry, the precise roles of the nonstructural proteins for replication, and the means by which the virus is assembled and released from the infected cell. Determination of these aspects may prove invaluable in developing therapeutic and prophylactic modalities for HCV infection.

REFERENCES

1. Choo Q L, Kuo G, Weiner A J, Overby L R, Bradley D W, Houghton M. Isolation of a cDNA clone derived from a blood-borne non-A, non-B viral hepatitis genome. Science 1989;244: 359–62.
2. Kolykhalov A A, Agapov E V, Blight K J, Mihalik K, Feinstone S M, Rice C M. Transmission of hepatitis C by intrahepatic inoculation with transcribed RNA. Science 1997;277:570–4.
3. Yanagi M, Purcell R H, Emerson S U, Bukh J. Transcripts from a single full-length cDNA clone of hepatitis C virus are infectious when directly transfected into the liver of a chimpanzee. Proc Natl Acad Sci U S A 1997;94:8738–43.
4. Beard M R, Abell G, Honda M, et al. An infectious molecular clone of a Japanese genotype 1b hepatitis C virus. Hepatology 1999;30:316–24.
5. Yanagi M, St. Claire M, Shapiro M, Emerson S U, Purcell R H, Bukh J. Transcripts of a chimeric cDNA clone of hepatitis C virus genotype 1b are infectious in vivo. Virology 1998;244:161–72.

6. Hong Z, Beaudet-Miller M, Lanford R E, et al. Generation of transmissible hepatitis C virions from a molecular clone in chimpanzees. Virology 1999;256:36–44.
7. He L F, Alling D, Popkin T, Shapiro M, Alter H J, Purcell R H. Determining the size of non-A, non-B hepatitis virus by filtration. J Infect Dis 1987;156:636–40.
8. Shimizu Y K, Feinstone S M, Kohara M, Purcell R H, Yoshikura H. Hepatitis C virus: detection of intracellular virus particles by electron microscopy. Hepatology 1996;23:205–9.
9. Shimizu Y K, Igarashi H, Kiyohara T, et al. Infection of a chimpanzee with hepatitis C virus grown in cell culture. J Gen Virol 1998;79:1383–6.
10. Baumert T F, Ito S, Wong D T, Liang T J. Hepatitis C virus structural proteins assemble into viruslike particles in insect cells. J Virol 1998;72:3827–36.
11. Xiang J, Klinzman D, McLinden J, et al. Characterization of hepatitis G virus (GB-C virus) particles: evidence for a nucleocapsid and expression of sequences upstream of the E1 protein. J Virol 1998;72:2738–44.
12. Thomson M, Liang T J. Unpublished data. 1998.
13. Han J H, Shyamala V, Richman K H, et al. Characterization of the terminal regions of hepatitis C viral RNA: identification of conserved sequences in the 5' untranslated region and poly(A) tails at the 3' end. Proc Natl Acad Sci U S A 1991;88:1711–5.
14. Choo Q L, Richman K H, Han J H, et al. Genetic organization and diversity of the hepatitis C virus. Proc Natl Acad Sci U S A 1991;88:2451–5.
15. Lohmann V, Korner F, Koch J, Herian U, Theilmann L, Bartenschlager R. Replication of subgenomic hepatitis C virus RNAs in a hepatoma cell line. Science 1999;285:110–3.
16. Grakoui A, McCourt D W, Wychowski C, Feinstone S M, Rice C M. Characterization of the hepatitis C virus-encoded serine proteinase: determination of proteinase-dependent polyprotein cleavage sites. J Virol 1993;67:2832–43.
17. Aoki Y, Aizaki H, Shimoike T, et al. A human liver cell line exhibits efficient translation of HCV RNAs produced by a recombinant adenovirus expressing T7 RNA polymerase. Virology 1998;250:140–50.
18. Xie Z C, Riezu-Boj J I, Lasarte J J, et al. Transmission of hepatitis C virus infection to tree shrews. Virology 1998;244:513–20.
19. Moriya K, Fujie H, Shintani Y, et al. The core protein of hepatitis C virus induces hepatocellular carcinoma in transgenic mice. Nat Med 1998;4:1065–7.
20. Koike K, Moriya K, Ishibashi K, et al. Expression of hepatitis C virus envelope proteins in transgenic mice. J Gen Virol 1995;76:3031–8.
21. Kawamura T, Furusaka A, Koziel M J, et al. Transgenic expression of hepatitis C virus structural proteins in the mouse. Hepatology 1997;25:1014–21.
22. Matsuda J, Suzuki M, Nozaki C, et al. Transgenic mouse expressing a full-length hepatitis C virus cDNA. Jpn J Cancer Res 1998;89:150–8.
23. Kato T, Ahmed M, Yamamoto T, et al. Inactivation of hepatitis C virus cDNA transgene by hypermethylation in transgenic mice. Arch Virol 1996;141:951–8.
24. Wakita T, Taya C, Katsume A, et al. Efficient conditional transgene expression in hepatitis C virus cDNA transgenic mice mediated by the Cre/loxP system. J Biol Chem 1998;273:9001–6.
25. Lemon S M, Honda M. Internal ribosome entry sites within the RNA genomes of hepatitis C virus and other flaviviruses. Semin Virol 1997;8:274–88.
26. Frolov I, McBride M S, Rice C M. cis-acting RNA elements required for replication of bovine viral diarrhea virus-hepatitis C virus 5' nontranslated region chimeras. RNA 1998;4:1418–35.
27. Reynolds J E, Kaminski A, Kettinen H J, et al. Unique features of internal initiation of hepatitis C virus RNA translation. EMBO J 1995;14:6010–20.
28. Honda M, Ping L H, Rijnbrand R C, et al. Structural requirements for initiation of translation by internal ribosome entry within genome-length hepatitis C virus RNA. Virology 1996;222:31–42.
29. Honda M, Brown E A, Lemon S M. Stability of a stem-loop involving the initiator AUG controls the efficiency of internal initiation of translation on hepatitis C virus RNA. RNA 1996;2:955–68.
30. Honda M, Beard M R, Ping L H, Lemon S M. A phylogenetically conserved stem-loop structure at the 5' border of the internal ribosome entry site of hepatitis C virus is required for cap-independent viral translation. J Virol 1999;73:1165–74.
31. Honda M, Rijnbrand R, Abell G, Kim D, Lemon S M. Natural variation in translational activities of the 5' nontranslated RNAs of hepatitis C virus genotypes 1a and 1b: evidence for a long-

range RNA-RNA interaction outside of the internal ribosomal entry site. J Virol 1999;73: 4941–51.

32. Fukushi S, Kurihara C, Ishiyama N, Hoshino F B, Oya A, Katayama K. The sequence element of the internal ribosome entry site and a 25- kilodalton cellular protein contribute to efficient internal initiation of translation of hepatitis C virus RNA. J Virol 1997;71:1662–6.

33. Ali N, Siddiqui A. The La antigen binds 5′ noncoding region of the hepatitis C virus RNA in the context of the initiator AUG codon and stimulates internal ribosome entry site-mediated translation. Proc Natl Acad Sci U S A 1997;94:2249–54.

34. Hahm B, Kim Y K, Kim J H, Kim T Y, Jang S K. Heterogeneous nuclear ribonucleoprotein L interacts with the 3′ border of the internal ribosomal entry site of hepatitis C virus. J Virol 1998; 72:8782–8.

35. Kolykhalov A A, Feinstone S M, Rice C M. Identification of a highly conserved sequence element at the 3′ terminus of hepatitis C virus genome RNA. J Virol 1996;70:3363–71.

36. Tanaka T, Kato N, Cho M J, Sugiyama K, Shimotohno K. Structure of the 3′ terminus of the hepatitis C virus genome. J Virol 1996;70:3307–12.

37. Blight K J, Rice C M. Secondary structure determination of the conserved 98-base sequence at the 3′ terminus of hepatitis C virus genome RNA. J Virol 1997;71:7345–52.

38. Tsuchihara K, Tanaka T, Hijikata M, et al. Specific interaction of polypyrimidine tract-binding protein with the extreme 3′-terminal structure of the hepatitis C virus genome, the 3′X. J Virol 1997;71:6720–6.

39. Ito T, Tahara S M, Lai M M. The 3′-untranslated region of hepatitis C virus RNA enhances translation from an internal ribosomal entry site. J Virol 1998;72:8789–96.

40. Ito T, Lai M M. An internal polypyrimidine-tract-binding protein-binding site in the hepatitis C virus RNA attenuates translation, which is relieved by the 3′-untranslated sequence. Virology 1999;254:288–96.

41. Yasui K, Wakita T, Tsukiyama-Kohara K, et al. The native form and maturation process of hepatitis C virus core protein. J Virol 1998;72:6048–55.

42. Choukhi A, Ung S, Wychowski C, Dubuisson J. Involvement of endoplasmic reticulum chaperones in the folding of hepatitis C virus glycoproteins. J Virol 1998;72:3851–8.

43. Hussy P, Langen H, Mous J, Jacobsen H. Hepatitis C virus core protein: carboxy-terminal boundaries of two processed species suggest cleavage by a signal peptide peptidase. Virology 1996;224:93–104.

44. Barba G, Harper F, Harada T, et al. Hepatitis C virus core protein shows a cytoplasmic localization and associates to cellular lipid storage droplets. Proc Natl Acad Sci U S A 1997;94:1200–5.

45. Liu Q, Tackney C, Bhat R A, Prince A M, Zhang P. Regulated processing of hepatitis C virus core protein is linked to subcellular localization. J Virol 1997;71:657–62.

46. Chang S C, Yen J H, Kang H Y, Jang M H, Chang M F. Nuclear localization signals in the core protein of hepatitis C virus. Biochem Biophys Res Commun 1994;205:1284–90.

47. Santolini E, Migliaccio G, La Monica N. Biosynthesis and biochemical properties of the hepatitis C virus core protein. J Virol 1994;68:3631–41.

48. Ray R B, Lagging L M, Meyer K, Ray R. Hepatitis C virus core protein cooperates with ras and transforms primary rat embryo fibroblasts to tumorigenic phenotype. J Virol 1996;70: 4438–43.

49. Pasquinelli C, Shoenberger J M, Chung J, et al. Hepatitis C virus core and E2 protein expression in transgenic mice. Hepatology 1997;25:719–27.

50. Zhu N, Khoshnan A, Schneider R, et al. Hepatitis C virus core protein binds to the cytoplasmic domain of tumor necrosis factor (TNF) receptor 1 and enhances TNF-induced apoptosis. J Virol 1998;72:3691–7.

51. Hsieh T Y, Matsumoto M, Chou H C, et al. Hepatitis C virus core protein interacts with heterogeneous nuclear ribonucleoprotein K. J Biol Chem 1998;273:17651–9.

52. You L R, Chen C M, Yeh T S, et al. Hepatitis C virus core protein interacts with cellular putative RNA helicase. J Virol 1999;73:2841–53.

53. You L R, Chen C M, Lee Y H W. Hepatitis C virus core protein enhances NF-kappaB signal pathway triggering by lymphotoxin-beta receptor ligand and tumor necrosis factor alpha. J Virol 1999;73:1672–81.

54. Cocquerel L, Duvet S, Meunier J C, et al. The transmembrane domain of hepatitis C virus glycoprotein E1 is a signal for static retention in the endoplasmic reticulum. J Virol 1999;73:2641–9.

55. Miyamura T, Matsuura Y. Structural proteins of hepatitis C virus. Trends Microbiol 1993;1: 229–31.

56. Deleersnyder V, Pillez A, Wychowski C, et al. Formation of native hepatitis C virus glycoprotein complexes. J Virol 1997;71:697–704.

57. Duvet S, Cocquerel L, Pillez A, et al. Hepatitis C virus glycoprotein complex localization in the endoplasmic reticulum involves a determinant for retention and not retrieval. J Biol Chem 1998; 273:32088–95.

58. Pileri P, Uematsu Y, Campagnoli S, et al. Binding of hepatitis C virus to CD81. Science 1998; 282:938–41.

59. Flint M, Maidens C, Loomis-Price L D, et al. Characterization of hepatitis C virus E2 glycoprotein interaction with a putative cellular receptor, CD81. J Virol 1999;73:6235–44.

60. Kato N, Ootsuyama Y, Ohkoshi S, et al. Characterization of hypervariable regions in the putative envelope protein of hepatitis C virus. Biochem Biophys Res Commun 1992;189:119–27.

61. Kato N, Sekiya H, Ootsuyama Y, et al. Humoral immune response to hypervariable region 1 of the putative envelope glycoprotein (gp70) of hepatitis C virus. J Virol 1993;67:3923–30.

62. Manzin A, Solforosi L, Petrelli E, et al. Evolution of hypervariable region 1 of hepatitis C virus in primary infection. J Virol 1998;72:6271–6.

63. McAllister J, Casino C, Davidson F, et al. Long-term evolution of the hypervariable region of hepatitis C virus in a common-source-infected cohort. J Virol 1998;72:4893–905.

64. Rosa D, Campagnoli S, Moretto C, et al. A quantitative test to estimate neutralizing antibodies to the hepatitis C virus: cytofluorimetric assessment of envelope glycoprotein 2 binding to target cells. Proc Natl Acad Sci U S A 1996;93:1759–63.

65. Habersetzer F, Fournillier A, Dubuisson J, et al. Characterization of human monoclonal antibodies specific to the hepatitis C virus glycoprotein E2 with in vitro binding neutralization properties. Virology 1998;249:32–41.

66. Elbers K, Tautz N, Becher P, Stoll D, Rumenapf T, Thiel H J. Processing in the pestivirus E2-NS2 region: identification of proteins p7 and E2p7. J Virol 1996;70:4131–5.

67. Santolini E, Pacini L, Fipaldini C, Migliaccio G, Monica N. The NS2 protein of hepatitis C virus is a transmembrane polypeptide. J Virol 1995;69:7461–71.

68. Reed K E, Grakoui A, Rice C M. Hepatitis C virus-encoded NS2-3 protease: cleavage-site mutagenesis and requirements for bimolecular cleavage. J Virol 1995;69:4127–36.

69. Wu Z, Yao N, Le H V, Weber P C. Mechanism of autoproteolysis at the NS2-NS3 junction of the hepatitis C virus polyprotein. Trends Biochem Sci 1998;23:92–4.

70. Hijikata M, Mizushima H, Akagi T, et al. Two distinct proteinase activities required for the processing of a putative nonstructural precursor protein of hepatitis C virus. J Virol 1993;67: 4665–75.

71. Gallinari P, Brennan D, Nardi C, et al. Multiple enzymatic activities associated with recombinant NS3 protein of hepatitis C virus. J Virol 1998;72:6758–69.

72. Kim J L, Morgenstern K A, Lin C, et al. Crystal structure of the hepatitis C virus NS3 protease domain complexed with a synthetic NS4A cofactor peptide. Cell 1996;87:343–55.

73. Love R A, Parge H E, Wickersham J A, et al. The crystal structure of hepatitis C virus NS3 proteinase reveals a trypsin-like fold and a structural zinc binding site. Cell 1996;87:331–42.

74. Cho H S, Ha N C, Kang L W, et al. Crystal structure of RNA helicase from genotype 1b hepatitis C virus. A feasible mechanism of unwinding duplex RNA. J Biol Chem 1998;273: 15045–52.

75. Shoji I, Suzuki T, Sato M, et al. Internal processing of hepatitis C virus NS3 protein. Virology 1999;254:315–23.

76. Lin C, Pragai B M, Grakoui A, Xu J, Rice C M. Hepatitis C virus NS3 serine proteinase: trans-cleavage requirements and processing kinetics. J Virol 1994;68:8147–57.

77. Koch J O, Bartenschlager R. Determinants of substrate specificity in the NS3 serine proteinase of the hepatitis C virus. Virology 1997;237:78–88.

78. Tai C L, Chi W K, Chen D S, Hwang L H. The helicase activity associated with hepatitis C virus nonstructural protein 3 (NS3). J Virol 1996;70:8477–84.

79. Buck K W. Comparison of the replication of positive-stranded RNA viruses of plants and animals. Adv Virus Res 1996;47:159–251.

80. Tanji Y, Kaneko T, Satoh S, Shimotohno K. Phosphorylation of hepatitis C virus-encoded nonstructural protein NS5A. J Virol 1995;69:3980–6.

81. Koch J O, Lohmann V, Herian U, Bartenschlager R. In vitro studies on the activation of the hepatitis C virus NS3 proteinase by the NS4A cofactor. Virology 1996;221:54–66.
82. Lin C, Wu J W, Hsiao K, Su M S. The hepatitis C virus NS4A protein: interactions with the NS4B and NS5A proteins. J Virol 1997;71:6465–71.
83. Tanji Y, Hijikata M, Satoh S, Kaneko T, Shimotohno K. Hepatitis C virus-encoded nonstructural protein NS4A has versatile functions in viral protein processing. J Virol 1995;69:1575–81.
84. Kato N, Lan K H, Ono-Nita S K, Shiratori Y, Omata M. Hepatitis C virus nonstructural region 5A protein is a potent transcriptional activator. J Virol 1997;71:8856–9.
85. Reed K E, Xu J, Rice C M. Phosphorylation of the hepatitis C virus NS5A protein in vitro and in vivo: properties of the NS5A-associated kinase. J Virol 1997;71:7187–97.
86. Hirota M, Satoh S, Asabe S, et al. Phosphorylation of nonstructural 5A protein of hepatitis C virus: HCV group-specific hyperphosphorylation. Virology 1999;257:130–7.
87. Ide Y, Tanimoto A, Sasaguri Y, Padmanabhan R. Hepatitis C virus NS5A protein is phosphorylated in vitro by a stably bound protein kinase from HeLa cells and by cAMP-dependent protein kinase A-alpha catalytic subunit. Gene 1997;201:151–8.
88. Oliver Koch J, Bartenschlager R. Modulation of hepatitis C virus NS5A hyperphosphorylation by nonstructural proteins NS3, NS4A, and NS4B. J Virol 1999;73:7138–46.
89. Enomoto N, Sakuma I, Asahina Y, et al. Mutations in the nonstructural protein 5A gene and response to interferon in patients with chronic hepatitis C virus 1b infection. N Engl J Med 1996;334:77–81.
90. Herion D, Hoofnagle J H. The interferon sensitivity determining region: all hepatitis C virus isolates are not the same. Hepatology 1997;25:769–71.
91. Gale M, Jr, Kwieciszewski B, Dossett M, Nakao H, Katze M G. Antiapoptotic and oncogenic potentials of hepatitis C virus are linked to interferon resistance by viral repression of the PKR protein kinase. J Virol 1999;73:6506–16.
92. Hwang S B, Park K J, Kim Y S, Sung Y C, Lai M M. Hepatitis C virus NS5B protein is a membrane-associated phosphoprotein with a predominantly perinuclear localization. Virology 1997;227:439–46.
93. Lohmann V, Korner F, Herian U, Bartenschlager R. Biochemical properties of hepatitis C virus NS5B RNA-dependent RNA polymerase and identification of amino acid sequence motifs essential for enzymatic activity. J Virol 1997;71:8416–28.
94. Yamashita T, Kaneko S, Shirota Y, et al. RNA-dependent RNA polymerase activity of the soluble recombinant hepatitis C virus NS5B protein truncated at the C-terminal region. J Biol Chem 1998;273:15479–86.
95. Cheng J C, Chang M F, Chang S C. Specific interaction between the hepatitis C virus NS5B RNA polymerase and the 3′ end of the viral RNA. J Virol 1999;73:7044–9.
96. Lesburg C A, Cable M B, Ferrari E, Hong Z, Mannarino A F, Weber P C. Crystal structure of the RNA-dependent RNA polymerase from hepatitis C virus reveals a fully encircled active site. Nat Struct Biol 1999;6:937–43.
97. Lohmann V, Roos A, Korner F, Koch J O, Bartenschlager R. Biochemical and kinetic analyses of NS5B RNA-dependent RNA polymerase of the hepatitis C virus. Virology 1998;249:108–18.
98. Ferrari E, Wright-Minogue J, Fang J W S, Baroudy B M, Lau J Y N, Hong Z. Characterization of soluble hepatitis C virus RNA-dependent RNA polymerase expressed in Escherichia coli. J Virol 1999;73:1649–54.
99. Oh J W, Ito T, Lai M M. A recombinant hepatitis C virus RNA-dependent RNA polymerase capable of copying the full-length viral RNA. J Virol 1999;73:7694–702.
100. Behrens S E, Tomei L, De Francesco R. Identification and properties of the RNA-dependent RNA polymerase of hepatitis C virus. EMBO J 1996;15:12–22.
101. Lai M M. Cellular factors in the transcription and replication of viral RNA genomes: a parallel to DNA-dependent RNA transcription. Virology 1998;244:1–12.
102. Ramos-Castaneda J, Imbert J L, Barron B L, Ramos C. A 65-kDa trypsin-sensible membrane cell protein as a possible receptor for dengue virus in cultured neuroblastoma cells. J Neurovirol 1997;3:435–40.
103. Minocha H C, Xue W, Reddy J R. A 50 kDa membrane protein from bovine kidney cells is a putative receptor for bovine viral diarrhea virus (BVDV). Adv Exp Med Biol 1997;412:145–8.

104. Seipp S, Mueller H M, Pfaff E, Stremmel W, Theilmann L, Goeser T. Establishment of persistent hepatitis C virus infection and replication in vitro. J Gen Virol 1997;78:2467–76.

105. Nawa M. Effects of bafilomycin A1 on Japanese encephalitis virus in C6/36 mosquito cells. Arch Virol 1998;143:1555–68.

106. Allison S L, Schalich J, Stiasny K, Mandl C W, Kunz C, Heinz F X. Oligomeric rearrangement of tick-borne encephalitis virus envelope proteins induced by an acidic pH. J Virol 1995;69:695–700.

107. Singh I, Helenius A. Role of ribosomes in Semliki Forest virus nucleocapsid uncoating. J Virol 1992;66:7049–58.

108. Egger D, Pasamontes L, Bolten R, Boyko V, Bienz K. Reversible dissociation of the poliovirus replication complex: functions and interactions of its components in viral RNA synthesis. J Virol 1996;70:8675–83.

109. Mackenzie J M, Khromykh A A, Jones M K, Westaway E G. Subcellular localization and some biochemical properties of the flavivirus Kunjin nonstructural proteins NS2A and NS4A. Virology 1998;245:203–15.

110. Ishido S, Fujita T, Hotta H. Complex formation of NS5B with NS3 and NS4A proteins of hepatitis C virus. Biochem Biophys Res Commun 1998;244:35–40.

111. Khromykh A A, Varnavski A N, Westaway E G. Encapsidation of the flavivirus kunjin replicon RNA by using a complementation system providing Kunjin virus structural proteins in trans. J Virol 1998;72:5967–77.

112. White C L, Thomson M, Dimmock N J. Deletion analysis of a defective interfering Semliki Forest virus RNA genome defines a region in the nsP2 sequence that is required for efficient packaging of the genome into virus particles. J Virol 1998;72:4320–6.

113. Nugent C I, Johnson K L, Sarnow P, Kirkegaard K. Functional coupling between replication and packaging of poliovirus replicon RNA. J Virol 1999;73:427–35.

114. Hase T, Summers P L, Eckels K H, Baze W B. An electron and immunoelectron microscopic study of dengue-2 virus infection of cultured mosquito cells: maturation events. Arch Virol 1987;92:273–91.

115. Pettersson R F. Protein localization and virus assembly at intracellular membranes. Curr Top Microbiol Immunol 1991;170:67–106.

116. Cheng R H, Kuhn R J, Olson N H, et al. Nucleocapsid and glycoprotein organization in an enveloped virus. Cell 1995;80:621–30.

117. Garoff H, Hewson R, Opstelten D J E. Virus maturation by budding. Microbiol Mol Biol Rev 1998;62:1171–90.

2

HEPATITIS C: VIRAL MARKERS AND QUASISPECIES

JEAN-MICHEL PAWLOTSKY

Department of Bacteriology and Virology and INSERM U99
Hôpital Henri Mondor, Université Paris XII
Créteil, France

INTRODUCTION

Infection of a human host by hepatitis C virus (HCV) leads to active viral replication, mainly in the liver. Nonspecific antiviral defenses are triggered in the very early stages of infection, and various cytokines appear to play an important role. Later, specific humoral and cellular responses participate in the control of viral replication. When the infection becomes chronic, an unstable equilibrium is reached between HCV replication and host defenses. The state of this "cold war" can be assessed at any time of the infection by measuring several virological parameters.

HEPATITIS C VIRAL MARKERS

HCV Genotypes

HCV strains can be classified into several genotypes, including types and subtypes. On the basis of phylogenetic analysis, HCV types, subtypes and isolates can be distinguished on the basis of average sequence divergence rates of approximately 30, 20, and 10%, respectively. (1–3) Six main HCV types (numbered 1 to 6) have been recognized, which are themselves divided into more than 80 subtypes identified by lower-case letters (1a, 1b, 1c, etc.). The genotype is an intrinsic characteristic of the transmitted HCV strain(s) and does not change during the course of the infection. However, it is not known whether different genotypes (or different strains of the same genotype) can recombine in a single host.

Some viral genotypes initially restricted to geographically isolated human populations are thought to have spread through population mixing and the emergence of efficient routes of infection. For instance, blood transfusion appears to have been responsible for the worldwide spread of HCV genotype 1b, whereas intravenous drug use was clearly associated with genotype 3a transmission in most industrialized countries. (4) The HCV genotype influenced the performance of the first serological and molecular assays. (5–7) The HCV genotype

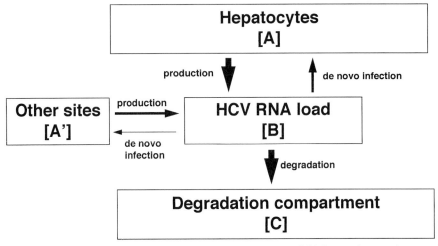

FIGURE I   Model of HCV replication kinetics [from Zeuzem et al. (12)]. During chronic infection and in the absence of antiviral treatment, the system is at steady state.

is also strongly associated with sensitivity to therapy with interferon (IFN)-α and the interferon plus ribavirin combination. (8–11)

Seropositivity

Seropositivity is defined as the presence, in peripheral blood, of antibodies specifically directed to HCV antigens as a result of past or ongoing infection. Antibodies directed to both structural (core or envelope) and nonstructural HCV antigens are present at various levels. HCV genetic variability, together with genetic differences among infected individuals, may explain the apparent heterogeneity of anti-HCV humoral responses. This phenomenon can be used for diagnostic purposes because genotype-specific antibodies can be diagnostic of the infecting genotype.

Viremia and Viral Load

HCV viremia is defined as the presence of HCV RNA in serum or plasma. It is a reliable marker of active HCV replication. As shown in Fig. 1, (12) HCV is produced mainly in the liver and, to a lesser extent, in extrahepatic replication sites. (13,14) A minority of virions produced *de novo* infect new cells, whereas the remainder are released continuously into the general circulation. The circulating HCV particles are catabolized continuously into a virtual degradation compartment, in which the immune response appears to play a major role. The minimum daily HCV production-clearance rate has been estimated at about 10^{12} virions a day, with a maximum virion half-life in serum of less than 3 hr. (15) A steady state is reached during chronic infection. Viral load, i.e., the amount of circulating genomes per volume of serum or plasma, does not vary to a significant degree over periods of months to years in most patients. (16) Quantitative assays can be used to measure HCV viral load. Data based on mathematical modeling of HCV replication kinetics during treatment has shown that viral load provides an accurate estimate of the rate of virion production in the liver, i.e., the level of HCV replication. (12,15)

Quasispecies

HCV, like many other RNA viruses, does not circulate in infected individuals as a homogeneous population of identical viral particles, but as a pool of genetically distinct but closely related variants referred to collectively as a "quasispecies." (17,18) The quasispecies nature of HCV confers a significant survival advantage, as the simultaneous presence of multiple variant genomes and the high rate at which new variants are generated allow rapid selection of mutants better suited to new environmental conditions. (19–21) It should be kept in mind that the quasispecies nature of HCV plays an important role in all aspects of the infection.

QUASISPECIES DISTRIBUTION OF HCV GENOMES: CLINICAL IMPLICATIONS

Quasispecies Distribution of HCV Genomes

Viral heterogeneity results primarily from a high error rate of RNA-dependent RNA polymerase, an enzyme encoded by the NS5B gene (Fig. 2) (22): misincorporation frequencies average about 10^{-4} to 10^{-5} per base site, and no proofreading mechanism has been identified. (20) Thus, in a given individual, the rate at which mutations accumulate during replication depends on the fidelity level of the viral RNA polymerase (which may itself vary from one genotype, strain, or quasispecies variant to the next, due to a variety of mutations in the relevant gene) and on viral replication kinetics. Most mutant viral particles are replication deficient, but some propagate efficiently. The "fittest" infectious particles are selected continuously on the basis of their replication capacities and by the selective pressure resulting from immune responses. (23–28) Figure 3 summarizes the mechanisms by which quasispecies emerge during acute HCV infection (from Ref. 29). During the chronic stage of infection, viral quasispecies are in a state of equilibrium at any given time. Their composition may, however, be altered slightly or markedly by a change in the environment. These changes can be spontaneous, related to complex metabolic interactions in the host, or triggered by external factors such as intercurrent infections, drug intake, or antiviral treatments.

The characteristics of HCV quasispecies can be studied by means of molecular biology. The quasispecies nature of HCV genomes has major implications for viral persistence, compartmentalization, and cell tropism; the severity and outcome of HCV disease; and HCV resistance to interferon therapy.

Tools for Studying HCV Quasispecies

The reference method for HCV quasispecies analysis is to generate a series of molecular clones from a given specimen after polymerase chain reaction (PCR)

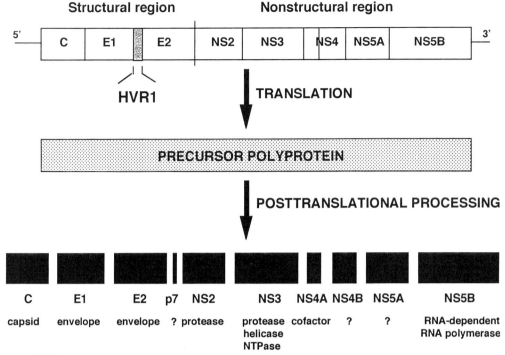

FIGURE 2 Hepatitis C virus genome, open reading frame translation, and posttranslational processing of viral proteins [from Grakoui et al. (22)]. HVR1, hypervariable region 1; NS, nonstructural.

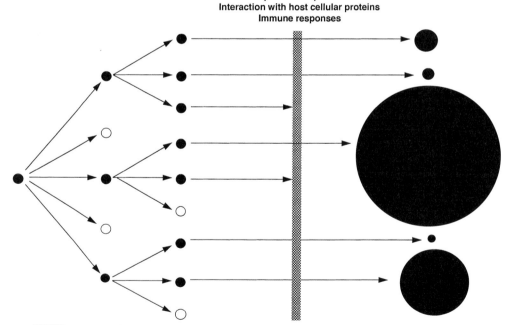

FIGURE 3 Schematic representation of the emergence of an HCV quasispecies [from Pawlotsky (29), with permission from Blackwell Science Ltd.]. Replication leads to the production of mutant viral particles, including defective and infectious particles. Infectious particles are selected by the "genetic bottleneck" composed of their own replication capacities, complex interactions with host cell proteins, and humoral and cellular immune responses. This leads to a complex mixture of genetically distinct but closely related variants in various proportions, referred to collectively as a quasispecies.

amplification and to conduct nucleotide sequence analysis. A minimum of 20 clones should be analyzed to obtain a 95% level of confidence that all major variants within a quasispecies population have been sampled. (20,30) Various parameters can be derived from sequence data. (i) Genetic complexity is defined as the total number of genetic variants within a quasispecies population. (ii) Quasispecies entropy is defined as the probability that different nucleotide or amino acid sequences or clusters of sequences will appear at a given time. Entropy provides information on the quasispecies repertoire, including the number of variants and their relative abundance. (iii) Genetic diversity is defined as the average genetic distance between the variants in a quasispecies population. (iv) "Synonymous" nucleotide substitutions are not associated with amino acid changes, contrary to "nonsynonymous" substitutions. The ratio of synonymous mutations per synonymous site to nonsynonymous mutations per nonsynonymous site provides information on whether the observed variations are related to random genetic drift or are driven by positive selection pressure. (v) Phylogenetic analysis assesses evolutionary relationships between specific variants of a quasispecies population.

Rapid methods developed to study HCV quasispecies include direct sequencing and polymorphism analysis, (31) heteroduplex analysis by temperature gradient gel electrophoresis (TGGE), (32) heteroduplex gel shift technology, (33) single-strand conformation polymorphism (SSCP) analysis, (34,35) and a combination of heteroduplex analysis and SSCP in a single gel. (36) Heteroduplex gel shift technology proved to be useful for estimating quasispecies genetic complexity, for studying the evolution of a given patient's quasispecies over time, and for clonal frequency analysis aimed at selecting clones for sequencing. (33,37) SSCP proved to be useful for estimating quasispecies genetic complexity, for studying the evolution of HCV quasispecies over time, and for clonal frequency analysis (examples: Fig. 4). (35,38,39)

Implications of Quasispecies Distribution of HCV Genomes

Viral Persistence

After the acute stage of infection, HCV replication persists in up to 85% of cases, leading to chronic disease. (40) The quasispecies nature of HCV genomes appears to play a role. Indeed, patients with persistent viremia have higher early quasispecies genetic complexity than those with spontaneous clearance. (41) In addition, new variants capable of escaping host defenses are generated continuously during replication. Hypervariable region 1 (HVR1) is located at the 5' end of the second envelope gene (Fig. 2) and is one of the main targets of neutralizing antibodies. (23,27) During acute infection, a high replication rate, together with the fact that this hypervariable region probably tolerates most, but not all amino acid substitutions, leads to a continuous generation of new HVR1 variants. The major variants are eliminated continuously by the neutralizing antibodies they elicit and are replaced by selected minor variants, which subsequently become major variants. In response to the new neutralizing response, the latter are themselves replaced by selected minor variants, and so the cycle continues. It is now accepted that viral persistence is associated with the continuous generation of new HVR1 mutants and the continuous selection of

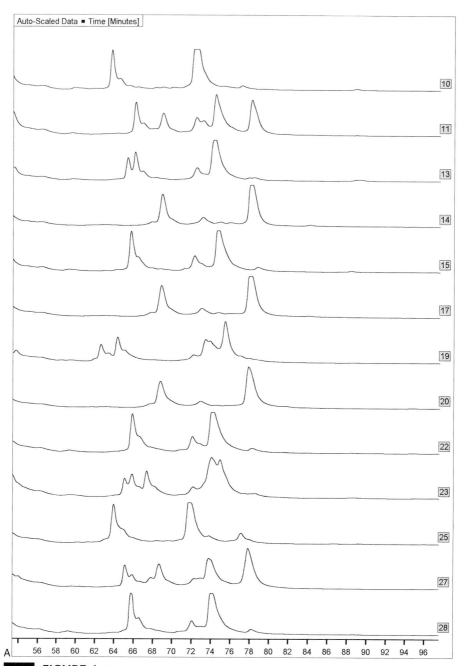

FIGURE 4 Examples of HCV quasispecies analysis with polymerase chain reaction (PCR)–fluorescence single-strand conformation polymorphism (F-SSCP). The technique includes (i) extraction of viral RNA; (ii) reverse transcription of genomic RNA; (iii) PCR amplification of the target regions, generating double-strand DNAs; (iv) heat denaturation and rapid cooling of PCR products generating single-strand DNA molecules; (v) renaturation in conditions allowing single-strand DNA molecules to assume secondary structures strictly dependent on their nucleotide sequence; (vi) nondenaturing polyacrylamide gel

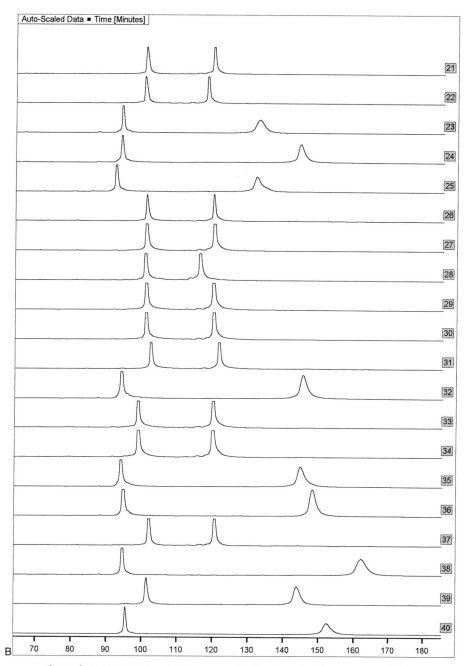

electrophoresis separating variant genomes with different nucleotide sequences; and (vii) computer analysis of the fluorescence of single DNA strand peaks. Each line corresponds to a different sample and each peak corresponds to a different quasispecies major variant present in the initial mixture. (A) Study of the evolution of the composition of a NS5A central region quasispecies over time in a patient treated with IFN-α. (B) Clonal frequency analysis of NS5A quasispecies in a sample from an HCV-infected patient before IFN therapy.

HOST DEFENSES

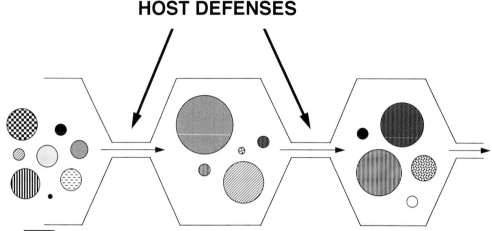

FIGURE 5 Schematic representation of the mechanisms of HCV persistence. Patients are infected with a viral quasispecies composed of a complex mixture of viral populations of different sizes (represented by circles of different diameters) composed of genetically distinct but closely related viral variants. New variants are generated continuously. Minor variants escape the host's defenses continuously (mainly the immune response), acting on the quasispecies as a bottleneck, and propagate as major variants that later undergo a similar selection process.

mutants escaping recognition by neutralizing antibodies. (23,25,42–45) Other neutralizing epitopes encoded by the HCV genome may similarly escape specific antibody responses. Cytotoxic T lymphocyte (CTL) selection of epitope variants corresponding to various genomic regions also appears to play an important role in viral persistence. (46–48) Specific interactions between viral and host proteins seem to attenuate immune responses, thus favoring the propagation of escape variants. Figure 5 summarizes this mechanism of HCV persistence.

During the course of chronic infection, random genetic drift gradually induces qualitative HVR1 quasispecies changes. (49–54) Shifts in the populations of viruses may also be observed in response to major environmental changes, such as those induced by antiviral drugs. (38,39) Similar changes in genomic regions other than HVR1 are likely but remain to be documented.

Compartmentalization and Cell Tropism

As shown in Fig. 1, HCV replication takes place mostly in the liver. However, experiments based on the specific detection of negative-stranded HCV RNA point to extrahepatic sites of replication. HCV appears to replicate in at least certain subsets of peripheral blood mononuclear cells (PBMCs), although at a much lower level than in the liver. (13,14) It has been shown that quasispecies variants isolated from various body compartments, such as the liver, general circulation, and PBMC, have different sequences, although they are closely related, being derived from the same inoculum. (13,55–58)

Compartmentalization of quasispecies variants may be due to differences in variant turnover kinetics in the various compartments and/or different tissue tropism. Indeed, the rates of production, release into the general circulation, and degradation in peripheral blood may vary from one variant population to another. Nakajima et al. (59) observed that only one variant found to be "lymphotropic" in a chimpanzee infected with the prototype HCV strain H77 was able to persist in human lymphocytic cell lines infected *in vitro* with strain H77. Infection of another chimpanzee with the culture supernatant resulted in predominant replication of the major variant of the H77 inoculum (likely "hepatotropic" and replicating at undetectable levels in the culture), whereas only the sequence recovered from PBMC was the same as the major variant found in the cell culture. (60) These findings, which need to be confirmed, might have important implications for the pathogenesis of hepatic and extrahepatic HCV disease. It is therefore necessary to consider the compartmentalization and tissue tropism of quasispecies variants in experiments aimed at establishing stable cell culture models.

Severity and Outcome of HCV Disease

Discordant results have been reported regarding the possible relationship among HCV quasispecies genetic complexity or diversity and serum alanine aminotransferase (ALT) level, the severity of liver disease, the development of cirrhosis and hepatocellular carcinoma, and the occurrence and severity of HCV-related extrahepatic immunological disorders. (61–67) These discrepancies appear to be due mainly to technical limitations and difficulties in establishing causal links between observed phenomena. Because viral replication is associated with accumulation of mutations and genetic diversification of the quasispecies over time, one would expect to find a significant relationship between the duration of infection (itself associated with HCV-related liver disease) and the genetic complexity and diversity of HCV quasispecies. However, successive shifts in the viral populations may gradually eliminate a large number of the variants. In addition, only a minority of variants would replicate at sufficiently high levels to circulate in adequate amounts to be isolated from peripheral blood with current techniques, including those based on the generation of numerous molecular clones. More sensitive techniques, as well as methods studying intrahepatic HCV quasispecies, might help resolve this intriguing issue. The observation that the quasispecies variants that associate with immunoglobulins to form immune complexes in the general circulation are different from those not associated with immunoglobulins (likely due to differences in envelope protein sequences) (44,68) suggests that the quasispecies distribution of HCV could play a role in HCV-related mixed cryoglobulinemias.

The capacity of certain quasispecies variants to induce more severe liver damage than others has been suggested in the model of HCV recurrence after orthotopic liver transplantation for HCV-related cirrhosis. (37) These findings raise the controversial issue of a direct cytopathogenic effect of HCV in the liver. It is generally accepted that liver lesions in chronic hepatitis C are principally induced by the immune response, including the specific action of CTLs on infected hepatocytes and local production of large amounts of cytokines by both CD4 positive T cells and CTLs. (29) Nevertheless, the possible relationship between certain viral sequences and the severity of HCV-related liver disease cannot be ruled out. It remains to be determined whether such a relationship might be related to differences in variant pathogenicity or the intensity of the immune responses the variants induce.

Resistance to Antiviral Therapy

A sustained virological response of chronic hepatitis C to antiviral therapy is defined by normal ALT and negative HCV RNA by PCR in serum 6 months after treatment is stopped. It is achieved in about 25% of naive patients receiving IFN-α, 3 mega units three times a week for 12 months, (69) and in about 40% of naive patients receiving the combination of IFN-α, 3 mega units three times a week, and ribavirin 1000 to 1200 mg/day for 6 to 12 months. (9,10) Like other viral parameters, such as pretreatment viral load and the HCV genotype, the genetic complexity of HCV quasispecies at the outset of therapy is an independent predictor of sustained virological responses to IFN monotherapy in multivariate analysis. (35,70) Only patients with low HCV complexity, i.e., a small quasispecies sequence repertoire, appear to have sustained HCV clearance. In contrast, patients with a large quasispecies sequence repertoire are less likely to have a sustained virological response, probably because of a much higher chance that one or several pretreatment variants could be selected. (38)

Whatever the biochemical and virological features (transient response with relapse, transient response with breakthrough, partial response, or nonresponse), failure of antiviral therapy to clear HCV RNA is almost always associated with significant changes in the composition of the HCV quasispecies in various genomic regions, such as HVR1 or NS5A (Fig. 4). (34,38,39,71–74) These evolving changes are characterized by successive shifts in the virus populations. (38,39) They appear to be related to selection pressure induced by interferon. (39) It remains to be shown whether hepatic or extrahepatic sanctuary sites serve as sources for reinfection of the liver by selected variants after transiently successful antiviral treatment. It is noteworthy that the qualitative quasispecies shifts observed after unsuccessful therapy are possibly associated with changes in the natural history of HCV disease. (39)

The existence of an "interferon sensitivity determining region" in the NS5A gene of HCV genotype 1b is highly controversial, (75) but raises the more general issue of whether specific HCV sequences confer sensitivity or resistance to interferon. The NS5A gene has a quasispecies distribution, meaning that several NS5A sequences may coexist at a given time in a given individual. (38,74, 76,77) No particular NS5A sequence appears to be intrinsically sensitive or resistant to interferon. (38) Nevertheless, some NS5A amino acid sequences appear to be more associated with nonresponders than sustained virological responders. (38) It is conceivable that variants bearing these sequences have functional properties partly or fully protecting the quasispecies mixture against the actions of interferon. This is currently under investigation in several laboratories. The principal NS5A features possibly involved in HCV resistance to IFN are the transcription-activating properties of the C-terminal half of NS5A, (78,79) the inhibitory action of NS5A on IFN-induced double-strand RNA-dependent protein kinase (PKR), (80,81) and its hypothetical capacity to inhibit the IFN-induced Jak–Stat pathway upstream of PKR. (82)

Posttransplantation Recurrence

HCV recurrence is inevitable after liver transplantation for HCV-related end-stage liver disease. The source of graft reinfection is unknown, but may be free virions, and/or extrahepatic sites of replication such as PBMC. HCV recurrence is characterized either by the propagation of major pretransplantation quasispecies variants or by the selection and propagation of minor pretransplantation populations. (37,83) The diversity of the posttransplantation quasispecies has been tentatively linked to the severity of recurrent hepatitis on the graft. (84)

VIROLOGICAL TOOLS

Performance of Assays: Definitions

Sensitivity

The analytical sensitivity of an assay is reflected by its cutoff, i.e., the smallest amount of virions, antigens, antibodies, or genomes detected and, if relevant, reliably quantified. In contrast, the clinical sensitivity of an assay is defined as its capacity to detect and, where relevant, reliably quantify clinical thresholds in given diseases. The clinical sensitivity of an assay depends on its analytical sensitivity, which should exceed its expected clinical sensitivity.

Specificity

The specificity of an assay is defined as its capacity to give a negative result for a sample that does not contain the relevant marker. The specificity of virological assays is often tested in low-risk seronegative populations such as blood donors. Any increase in the sensitivity of an assay often results in a loss of specificity. The optimal balance between these two parameters must be found in the specific context of the disease and the indications of the assay.

Predictive Value

The predictive value of an assay can be defined as its capacity to give results in keeping with the observed biological situation. The positive and negative predictive values are the probability that a positive or negative result is correct, respectively. With quantitative assays, the predictive value partly depends on the accurate determination of values corresponding to clinically important thresholds.

Precision and Reproducibility

The reproducibility of an assay can be tested in various ways, such as by determining the within-assay reproducibility (precision) and between-assay reproducibility (including between-run, between-performer, and between-lab reproducibility). The variability of an assay can be expressed as a coefficient of variation (CV) or a standard deviation (SD) after repeated testing of the same specimens. The intrinsic variability of an assay, especially semiquantitative and quantitative assays, must be known in order to avoid overinterpretation of minor changes in a virological parameter over time. Assay reproducibility may be improved by standardizing reagents and procedures and by automation.

Linearity of Quantitative Assays

The linear or dynamic range of a quantitative assay is the range of titers within which quantitation remains linear. Any concentration outside the linear range will be assigned a wrong (over- or underestimated) titer. It is particularly important that end users know the lower and upper cut offs of linear quantification, especially when clinical decisions are based on precise thresholds.

Accuracy

Viral characteristics, the intrinsic properties of the assays, and the conditions of sampling and storage can affect accuracy. Serological assays can be applied to any kind of blood sample, although old samples or samples kept at high temperatures may yield falsely positive or negative results. In molecular biology-based assays both serum and plasma can be used, excepting heparinized plasma for PCR. (85,86) They must be decanted quickly and frozen after sampling, ideally within less than 3 hr. (86,87) Storage at $-20°C$ is acceptable when the sample is processed within a few days, but for longer periods storage at -70 or $-80°C$ is mandatory. Freeze–thaw cycles must be avoided, and thawed samples should never be kept at a temperature higher than 4°C before processing. (86–90)

The accuracy of the assays may also be influenced by genotype-dependent variations in the viral genomic or protein sequences used for antigen, antibody, primer, or probe design. This may lead to lower sensitivity and underestimation of quantitative values for certain genotypes relative to others in both serological and molecular biology-based assays. (5–7) The limits of the dynamic range of quantification are also crucial, as quantification outside this range is inaccurate.

Standardization

In-house assays are developed regularly for research or diagnostic purposes and are generally evaluated only by their inventors. Quality control studies suggest that nonstandard "home-made" assays should only be used for research purposes. Conversely, in the routine settings of population screening, virological diagnosis, and patient management, only well-standardized commercial assays should be used.

A commercial assay should be used routinely in clinical laboratories and blood banks only if it meets the following conditions: (i) careful assessment of intrinsic performance and reported results by the manufacturer; (ii) careful evaluation of performance by outside laboratories, especially in routine indications; (iii) well-chosen internal and external controls; and (iv) repeated quality controls and proficiency panel testing. Universal standardization of quantitative units is also necessary.

Serological Assays

Enzyme Immunoassays

The detection of anti-HCV antibodies in plasma or serum is based on the use of enzyme immunoassays (EIAs). These tests use recombinant or synthetic viral antigens to capture circulating anti-HCV antibodies on the wells of microtiter plates or on the surface of microbeads. The presence of anti-HCV antibodies is revealed by anti-IgG antibodies labeled with an enzyme that catalyzes the transformation of a substrate into a colored compound. The optical density (OD) ratio of the reaction (sample OD/internal control OD) is roughly proportional to the amount of antibodies in the sample. Second-generation EIAs detect antibodies directed to structural (core) and nonstructural (NS3 and NS4) proteins.

Third-generation EIAs detect the same antibodies with better sensitivity, plus antibodies directed to the NS5 protein. It is noteworthy that the addition of an NS5 antigen yielded frequent false-positive results in low-prevalence populations such as healthy blood donors. (91) The sensitivity of HCV EIAs could be improved further in the future by the inclusion of envelope antigens.

EIAs are easy to use and inexpensive. They are partly or fully automated and well adapted to large runs. In the absence of a "gold standard" for HCV seropositivity, the sensitivity of anti-HCV screening assays cannot be determined precisely. In high-prevalence immunocompetent populations it has been estimated to range from 98.8 to 100%, (92,93) indicating that the vast majority of immunocompetent patients with active HCV infection can be identified by EIAs. In hemodialyzed and immunocompromized patients, such as solid organ or bone marrow transplant recipients and human immunodeficiency virus (HIV)-infected patients, the sensitivity of EIAs for the detection of anti-HCV antibodies is lower, ranging from 50 to 95% according to the degree of immunodeficiency. (94–98) False-negative results in HCV EIAs have also been reported with samples from patients with HCV-associated mixed cryoglobulinemia and are probably explained by the sequestration of anti-HCV antibodies within cryoglobulin complexes.

In acute HCV infection, anti-HCV antibodies can be detected in 50 to 70% of patients at the onset of symptoms. (99) In the remaining patients, anti-HCV antibodies usually emerge after 3 to 6 weeks. Overall, the "serologic window" between HCV infection and the detection of specific antibodies varies from one patient to the next; on average, it appears to be 7 to 8 weeks on the basis of current third-generation assays. As a result, the residual risk of HCV transmission by anti-HCV-negative blood products is low. It was estimated at 1/280,000 donations in France for the period 1995–1997, with a 95% confidence interval ranging from 1/830,000 to 1/140,000 (Anne-Marie Couroucé, personal communication).

The specificity of third-generation EIAs in the low-prevalence population represented by healthy blood donors has been estimated at 99.3 to 100%. (92,93,100) Falsely positive results can, however, be observed due to cross-reactivity with other viral antigens or immunological disorders. Some patients have detectable anti-HCV antibodies without detectable HCV RNA. Existing assays cannot distinguish among false-positive EIA results, patients having recovered from acute infection, and patients with chronic HCV infection but replication below the HCV RNA detection limit.

Immunoblot Assays

First-generation anti-HCV EIAs lacked both sensitivity and specificity. First-generation confirmatory assays based on immunoblot testing were developed to resolve false-positive EIA results and were applied systematically to samples positive in EIA, both in routine diagnosis of HCV infection and in blood screening. Second- and third-generation immunoblot tests are based on the detection of anti-HCV antibodies with structural and nonstructural viral antigens coated as parallel bands on nitrocellulose strips. Immunoblot tests are useless as confirmatory assays in routine diagnosis of HCV infection in clinical laboratories, (101) but can resolve false-positive results in the blood donor screening context.

IgM Assays

The significance of present anti-HCV IgM antibodies is not clear. Anti-HCV IgM is found in 50 to 93% of patients with acute hepatitis C and in 50 to 70% of patients with chronic hepatitis C. (102–104) Anti-HCV IgM cannot thus be used as a reliable marker of acute HCV infection. The presence and the titer of anti-HCV core IgM antibodies prior to therapy appear to be related to the HCV genotype and have been identified as independent predictors of sustained virological responses of chronic hepatitis C to IFN monotherapy, (105) although the clinical relevance of these observations is unclear. Overall, anti-HCV IgM assays have not been useful in clinical practice.

HCV Core Antigen Assay

An enzyme immunoassay for HCV core antigen in blood samples is currently available. It has been shown to be useful in reducing the "serological window" in blood donor screening. Quantitative HCV core antigen assays have also been developed to measure viral replication, but they lack sensitivity compared to molecular biology-based assays.

Serological Determination of the HCV Genotype

Serotyping techniques are based on the detection of antibodies directed to genotype-specific HCV epitopes generally located in the NS4 and/or core proteins. Two assays have been developed, based on competitive EIA (Abbott HC1–6 Serotyping Assay, Abbott Diagnostics, Chicago, IL) (106) or immunoblotting (RIBA HCV Serotyping Assay, Chiron Diagnostics, Emeryville, CA). (107) In immunocompetent HCV-infected patients, i.e., patients who may need routine HCV genotyping, serotyping assays have an average sensitivity of 85 to 90% relative to molecular biology-based genotyping assays. Their concordance with genotyping assays is 95% on average. (108–110) Subtyping is not possible with the existing serotyping assays, but it is not relevant to clinical practice at present. Overall, serotyping assays provide a reliable alternative to molecular biology-based genotyping assays in the routine indication for HCV genotype determination, i.e., tailoring the duration of interferon–ribavirin combination therapy. (9,10)

Detection of HCV Antigens in Tissues

Several techniques have been developed to locate HCV antigens in the liver and extrahepatic tissues based on the use of various monoclonal or polyclonal antibodies. A lack of specificity appears to be a major problem in many methods. A technique based on polyclonal human and chimpanzee antibodies has been used to detect HCV antigens in the liver and to show their disappearance during interferon treatment. (111,112)

Molecular Biology-Based Tests

Qualitative HCV RNA Detection Assays

HCV replicates at relatively low levels, meaning that HCV RNA cannot be detected in body fluids by means of classical hybridization techniques and that

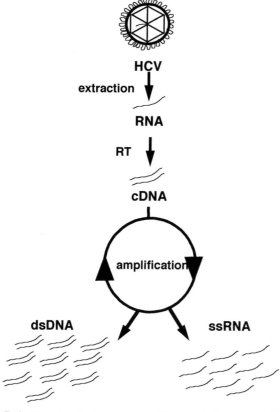

FIGURE 6 Principles of target amplification techniques for the detection of HCV RNA in body fluids.

an additional "amplification" step is necessary. In current practice HCV RNA is detected by means of target amplification techniques (Fig. 6). After extraction of viral RNA and reverse transcription into double-stranded complementary DNA (cDNA), cDNA molecules are processed in a cyclic enzymatic reaction leading to the generation of a very large number of copies, which thus become detectable. Double-stranded DNA copies of HCV cDNAs are synthesized in PCR-based methods, whereas single-stranded RNA copies are generated in transcription-mediated amplification (TMA) techniques (Fig. 6). Amplified products are usually detected by hybridization to specific probes. Real-time target amplification techniques are currently under development. In real-time PCR, each round of amplification leads to the emission of a fluorescent signal, which can be detected in the closed tube during the reaction. (113,114)

Many HCV PCR assay variants have been described in the literature, and their standardization has been difficult. (115–117) Numerous factors contribute to reverse-transcription PCR assay variability, including specimen handling and storage conditions, presence of PCR inhibitors (in 5 to 10% of samples), correct design of amplification primers, variability of biochemical reactions, DNA product contamination, and efficiency of postamplification systems. (118)

A standardized reverse-transcription PCR assay has been introduced for the qualitative detection of HCV RNA in patient's serum (Amplicor HCV, Roche Molecular Systems, Pleasanton, CA). (119) This assay was designed for use in any clinical laboratory equipped for molecular biology. The first-generation Amplicor HCV kit had a manufacturer's stated cutoff of 1000 copies/ml, but it appeared slightly less sensitive for HCV genotypes 2 and 3 than for genotype 1. The second generation of this assay has been released; the stated detection cutoff is lower (100 copies/ml), and sensitivity is claimed to be the same for all genotypes. This assay can be semiautomated, with manual extraction and automated amplification, PCR product hybridization, and interpretation in the Cobas Amplicor apparatus (Roche Molecular Systems). (120) The specificity of the second-generation Amplicor HCV kit appears to be 97 to 99%. (117)

The National Genetics Institute (NGI, Los Angeles, CA) has developed an HCV PCR assay known as Superquant, with a stated detection cutoff of 50 copies/ml. (121) The assay is not available in kit format (samples must be sent to the supplier), and a recent comparison with an assay equally quantifying HCV genotypes suggested a slightly different quantification of HCV genotypes 1, 2, and 3. (122) Finally, a TMA-based assay and real-time amplification techniques are currently in development. (113,114)

Quantitative HCV RNA Assays

Two standardized assays have been widely used: the signal amplification-based "branched DNA" assay (Quantiplex HCV RNA 2.0, Bayer Corporation, Emeryville, CA), and the competitive reverse-transcription PCR-based assay, the second generation of which is currently being released (Amplicor HCV Monitor 2.0, Roche Molecular Systems). The manufacturer's stated cutoff for the Amplicor HCV Monitor 2.0 assay is 1000 copies/ml, whereas that of bDNA version 2.0 is 200,000 genome equivalents/ml (Eq/ml). However, the Roche "copy" and the Chiron "genome equivalent" do not represent the same amount of HCV RNA in a clinical sample because they were defined independently by the two manufacturers using quantified standards (nucleic acid transcripts) of different natures, lengths, and sequences. The World Health Organization (WHO) has established international standards for the universal standardization of HCV RNA quantification units (i.e. quantification in international units (IU)/ml).

The performance of bDNA version 2.0 has been widely studied, (123) whereas less is known of the recently developed second version of the Monitor assay. The two assays appear to quantify the various HCV genotypes equally. (6,124) The dynamic range of the first-generation Monitor assay was 1000 to 5×10^5 copies/ml (i.e., 3 to 5.7 $\log_{10}$ copies/ml), and samples with a higher HCV RNA load had to be diluted for accurate quantification. (125,126) The dynamic range of the second-generation Monitor kit is 600 to 850,000 IU/ml on Cobas Amplicor. Linearity was observed within the entire range of quantification of the bDNA 2.0 kit, i.e., between 2×10^5 and 12×10^7 Eq/ml (5.3 to 8.1 $\log_{10}$ Eq/ml). (6) The specificity of bDNA assay 2.0 appears to be 97 to 100%, (124) whereas its reproducibility is slightly better than that of PCR-based assays. Variations of less than 0.5 $\log_{10}$ copies/ml or Eq/ml or IU/ml (i.e., threefold variations) must not be taken into account because they can be related to the intrin-

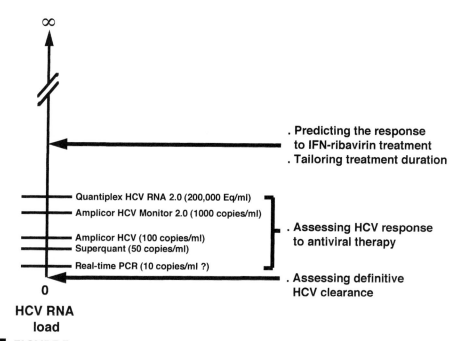

FIGURE 7 Schematic representation of the "clinical sensitivity" of HCV RNA detection and quantification assays. Horizontal bars represent the stated detection cutoffs of the various assays (in non standardized units) and arrows represent clinically relevant thresholds. All available assays appear to be able to detect and reliably quantify the threshold used to tailor the duration of IFN–ribavirin combination treatment (6 or 12 months) in patients infected by HCV genotypes 1, 4 and 5. (9,10) All can also be used to assess the virological response to antiviral therapy, but with different analytical sensitivities. Finally, none of the available assays is able to predict permanent HCV RNA clearance during therapy.

sic variability of the assays. In contrast, variations of more than $0.5 \log_{10}$ copies/ml or Eq/ml or IU/ml can reliably be considered as reflecting significant changes in HCV load.

The decisional threshold for tailoring the duration of interferon–ribavirin combination therapy in patients infected by HCV genotypes 1, 4 and 5 (2 million copies/ml or $6.3 \log_{10}$ copies/ml in the Superquant assay) (9,10) appears to be within the dynamic range of both the Monitor and the bDNA assays. The corresponding value in IU/ml is 800,000 IU/ml (Pawlotsky et al., unpublished data, February 2000). All available assays can be used to assess the HCV response to antiviral drugs during therapy, but their analytical sensitivities are different. Finally, none of the available assays can show permanent HCV clearance after therapy, which can only be established by long-term follow-up (Fig. 7).

Genotyping Assays

The reference method for HCV genotype determination is sequence analysis, followed by sequence alignment and phylogenetic analysis. Several rapid PCR-based genotyping techniques have also been developed for research and diagnostic purposes: (i) nested PCR analysis of the HCV core gene using genotype-specific primers (127); this technique is labor-intensive and yields high rates of cross-amplification; (ii) restriction fragment length polymorphism (RFLP) analysis of the highly conserved 5' noncoding region (128); this technique is inexpensive and rapid but lacks standardization; and (iii) reverse hybridization analysis using genotype-specific probes corresponding to 5′ noncoding region sequences (INNO-LiPA, Innogenetics, Gent, Belgium) (129) or 5′ noncoding and core sequences (Gen.Eti.K DEIA HCV, DiaSorin, Saluggia, Italy) (130); these techniques are standardized and available in kit format, e.g., they can be used reliably in laboratories equipped for molecular biology. A standardized assay based on direct sequencing of the 5′ noncoding region and the NS5B region has been developed (TruGene, Visible Genetics Inc., Toronto, Ontario). This technology is being evaluated in routine use.

Other Molecular Tests

Various other techniques have been developed, essentially for research purposes; they include HCV RNA negative strand-specific PCR amplification, quantitation of positive and negative HCV RNA strands in the liver and in PBMC, *in situ* hybridization, and *in situ* PCR of HCV RNA. These technologies have serious technical limitations and are not standardized. Their reliability and the interpretation of their results remain a matter of debate.

PRACTICAL USE OF VIRAL MARKERS IN THE MANAGEMENT OF HEPATITIS C PATIENTS

Screening

Systematic screening of blood donations for the presence of anti-HCV antibodies has drastically reduced the risk of posttransfusion hepatitis C. EIA testing is currently used in this indication. Although the specificity of HCV EIAs is excellent, the predictive value of a positive result in this low-risk population is relatively low. Indeed, among 1654 positive EIAs out of 444,559 new donors (0.37%) tested in 1997 at the French National Institute for Blood Transfusion, 39% were negative by immunoblotting, 21% had a isolated reactivity, and 40% had a positive immunoblot characterized by the presence of at least two reactivities (Anne-Marie Couroucé, personal communication). Therefore, confirmation of positive EIA results by immunoblot may still be of value in the specific setting of blood donor screening, at least until EIAs have been sufficiently improved to yield negligible false-positive results. HCV antigen detection by EIA and HCV RNA detection by molecular biology techniques are currently being implemented in blood donor screening to further improve blood product safety.

The consensus statement of the recent International Consensus Conference on Hepatitis C organized by the European Association for the Study of the Liver, in February 1999, recommended screening of the following patients for hepatitis C: "persons who have (or might have) received blood products prior to initiation (1991) of second-generation EIA test; hemophiliacs; hemodialyzed patients; children born to mothers who have hepatitis C; current or previous users of intravenous drugs; donors for organ or tissue transplantation." In contrast to blood donors, these groups are at risk of HCV infection, and the predictive value of a positive EIA result appears to be good. These patients are usually referred to specialists when the EIA is positive and may then undergo ALT determination, HCV RNA PCR, and liver biopsy.

Diagnosis

Acute Hepatitis C

The diagnosis of acute hepatitis C is difficult for the following reasons: (i) anti-HCV antibodies may be lacking in the acute phase of infection, emerging only months after exposure; and (ii) in the absence of a specific marker of acute infection, the presence of anti-HCV antibodies may reflect chronic HCV infection in a patient with an acute exacerbation of chronic HCV disease or acute hepatitis of another cause. In practice, anti-HCV antibodies should be tested for, together with other causes of acute hepatitis (hepatitis A, hepatitis B, autoantibodies, hepatotoxic drug or alcohol intake, metabolic disease, etc). If nothing is found, HCV RNA should be sought by PCR. In this setting, HCV RNA detection strongly suggests acute hepatitis C, which is confirmed by subsequent seroconversion. Absence of HCV RNA makes this diagnosis highly unlikely, provided that the relevant laboratory's track record with the assay is good. When anti-HCV antibodies are found at the time of acute hepatitis, liver biopsy may be useful to rule out chronic HCV infection.

Chronic Hepatitis C

The diagnosis of chronic hepatitis C is based on the detection of anti-HCV antibodies by EIA. Only one test is necessary, and immunoblot confirmation is not needed in this setting. (101) HCV RNA testing should be performed to confirm the diagnosis of HCV infection in the following cases: (i) seronegative chronic hepatitis of an unknown cause (especially in hemodialyzed and immunocompromised patients), (ii) weakly positive EIA results (i.e., an OD ratio <2), (iii) chronic hepatitis associated with HCV seropositivity and one or more other possible causes, and (iv) before initiating antiviral therapy (the presence of HCV RNA being used as a reference for the virological response). (101,131)

Special Cases

Babies born to HCV-infected mothers usually carry maternally transferred HCV antibodies for a few months to a year. (132,133) The diagnosis of HCV infection in the baby is based on HCV RNA detection by PCR. Dates at which the test should ideally be performed are not precisely known. In case of negative PCR results, the lack of transmission is confirmed by the gradual disappearance of HCV antibodies. If the baby is infected, HCV RNA detection may be positive at birth or be negative in the first weeks of life and become positive later during the first year.

In the case of accidental exposure to HCV-infected blood, HCV RNA can generally be detected in serum as early as the second week after exposure. Elevated ALT and seroconversion often occur a few weeks to months later.

Prognosis and Assessment of Severity

There are no virological parameters for the assessment of the severity of HCV-related liver disease (which is currently evaluated by means of liver biopsy). According to the most recent studies, neither the HCV genotype nor the HCV viral load at the time of liver biopsy appears to correlate with the histological activity of liver disease or the extent of fibrosis. It also remains to be determined whether the area under the viral load curve during the entire course of the infection is associated with the severity of liver disease at the time of liver biopsy. Finally, patients with end-stage liver disease have significantly lower levels of viral replication than patients with chronic hepatitis C or early-stage HCV-related cirrhosis, but this appears to be a consequence of the severity of liver disease. (134,135)

Treatment

The treatment of hepatitis C is discussed in great detail in another chapter of this book; however, some relevant issues to the practical use of HCV assays in treatment are discussed here. Qualitative HCV RNA detection assays should be used to assess the virological response of chronic hepatitis C to antiviral therapy because they are more sensitive than current quantitative assays. In patients treated with the combination of INF-α and ribavirin, HCV RNA determination at month 3 has a poor predictive value for the subsequent outcome (possibly because of the significant improvement in assay sensitivity) and should not be used. In patients with genotype 1, 4 or 5 and a high viral load, who must theoretically be treated for 12 months, HCV RNA determination must be performed at month 6 of therapy (Fig. 8): if it is positive, the treatement should be stopped because no subsequent response is observed in these patients; if it is negative, treatment should be continued for another 6 months to prevent relapse after treatment.

The end-of-treatment virological response may be evaluated at month 6 or 12 (Fig. 8). Positive HCV RNA detection at this latter time point is highly predictive of a subsequent relapse. Finally, the primary end point of treatment is a sustained virological response, characterized by normal ALT and negative HCV RNA detection 6 months after treatment cessation (Fig. 8). Long-term follow-up of sustained virological responders to the IFN–ribavirin combination is necessary to determine whether viral clearance 6 months after treatment

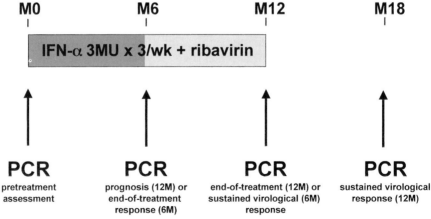

FIGURE 8 Treatment monitoring with qualitative HCV RNA detection assays (PCR) in patients receiving the combination of IFN and ribavirin for 6 months or 12 months.

withdrawal is predictive of long-term viral eradication, as shown for the sustained virological response to IFN monotherapy. (136–138)

USE OF VIRAL MARKERS IN CLINICAL RESEARCH

Epidemiology

Viral markers can be used to study the modes of HCV transmission. At the beginning of the HCV era it was observed that anti-HCV-positive blood donations were associated with transmission of the infection. (139) It was later shown that only HCV RNA-positive blood products could transmit the virus. (140) Genotype determination can be used to confirm HCV transmission from a known source. However, transmission is very unlikely when the genotypes are different, and identical genotypes do not prove transmission either. Sequence analysis of a variable region of the genome in both the source and the infected patient, followed by phylogenetic analysis, including a large number of unrelated sequences, is necessary to establish transmission. (141,142)

Both serological assays and HCV RNA detection assays have been used to determine the prevalence and incidence of HCV infection and to monitor their changes over time in various populations. These assays have also defined the pathogenetic role of HCV in several extrahepatic disorders. In addition, the HCV genotype determination has been and still is widely used to study the distribution of HCV types and subtypes in various geographic areas and epidemiologic groups.

Pathogenesis of HCV-Related Disease

Various virological techniques can be used to understand the pathogenesis of HCV-related disorders. The detection of negative-stranded HCV RNA in any tissue by a highly specific negative-strand PCR method is a strong argument for HCV replication in this tissue. Semiquantitative and quantitative techniques have been developed, but the significance of the amount of negative HCV RNA strands in a tissue is far from clear. Negative-strand RNA detection and reliable *in situ* localization of positive and negative strands and/or HCV antigens may also prove useful in the study of HCV replication and the compartmentalization of quasispecies.

Mechanisms of HCV Resistance to Antiviral Therapy

The mechanisms of resistance of HCV to interferon-α and to the interferon–ribavirin combination appear to be particularly complex. This is due to the pleiotrophic action of these drugs, which exert numerous selection pressures on various HCV genomic regions, mediated in most instances by host-specific responses. Virological tools that can be employed for this purpose include those used for analyzing HCV quasispecies and their distribution, highly sensitive quantitative assays to study the dynamics and kinetics of viral replication, and functional assays to assess the action of viral proteins on host factors possibly involved in HCV resistance.

The development of new, specific antiviral drugs requires accurate virologic assays. Functional HCV protease, helicase, polymerase, and IRES models are already available for the assessment of new inhibitory compounds. Cell culture and animal models are currently in development and could be used in the future to study the antiviral effects of these newly designed drugs. Sensitive and specific HCV RNA quantification is essential to study these drugs on HCV replication in clinical trials. The study of viral replication kinetics, quasispecies genetics, and specific mutations on target genes will be important parameters to monitor.

CONCLUSION

Clinical laboratories routinely diagnosing HCV infection will need (i) ultrasensitive HCV RNA quantitation assays with a large dynamic range, high precision, and no risk of carryover or cross-contamination. Real-time amplification techniques could meet these needs in the near future. (ii) Also needed are biologic, serological, or molecular markers for permanent HCV clearance. Recovery is currently assessed on the basis of repeatedly negative HCV RNA detection in serial samples because "seroreversion" is rare and occurs very late. (143) (iii) Reliable *in situ* hybridization and *in situ* PCR assays and (iv) Qualitative and quantitative HCV resistance assays round out the list.

REFERENCES

1. Bukh J, Miller R H, and Purcell R H. Genetic heterogeneity of hepatitis C virus: quasispecies and genotypes. Semin Liver Dis 1995;15:41–63.
2. Simmonds P. Variability of hepatitis C virus. Hepatology 1995;21:570–83.
3. Maertens G, Stuyver L. Genotypes and genetic variation of hepatitis C virus. In: Harrison T J, Zuckerman A J, eds. The molecular medicine of viral hepatitis. New York: Wiley, 1997:183–233.
4. Pawlotsky J M, Tsakiris L, Roudot-Thoraval F, et al. Relationship between hepatitis C virus genotypes and sources of infection in patients with chronic hepatitis C. J Infect Dis 1995;171:1607–10.
5. Pawlotsky J M, Roudot-Thoraval F, Pellet C, et al. Influence of hepatitis C virus (HCV) genotypes on HCV recombinant immunoblot assay patterns. J Clin Microbiol 1995;33:1357–9.
6. Detmer J, Lagier R, Flynn R, et al. Accurate quantification of hepatitis C virus (HCV) RNA from all HCV genotypes by using branched-DNA technology. J Clin Microbiol 1996;34:901–7.
7. Hawkins A, Davidson F, Simmonds P. Comparison of plasma virus loads among individuals infected with hepatitis C virus (HCV) genotypes 1, 2 and 3 by Quantiplex HCV RNA assay versions 1 and 2, Roche Monitor assay and in-house limiting dilution method. J Clin Microbiol 1997;35:187–92.
8. Martinot-Peignoux M, Marcellin P, Pouteau M, et al. Pretreatment HCV RNA levels and HCV genotype are the main and independent prognostic factors of sustained response to alpha interferon therapy in chronic hepatitis C. Hepatology 1995;22:1050–6.
9. Poynard T, Marcellin P, Lee S S, et al. Randomised trial of interferon alpha-2b plus ribavirin for 48 weeks or for 24 weeks versus interferon alpha-2b plus placebo for 48 weeks for treatment of chronic infection with hepatitis C virus. Lancet 1998;352:1426–32.
10. McHutchison J G, Gordon S C, Schiff, E R, et al. Interferon alfa-2b alone or in combination with ribavirin as initial treatment for chronic hepatitis C. N Engl J Med 1998;339:1485–92.
11. Davis G L, Esteban-Mur R, Rustgi V, et al. Interferon alfa-2b alone or in combination with ribavirin for the treatment of relapse of chronic hepatitis C. N Engl J Med 1998;339:1493–9.

12. Zeuzem S, Schmidt J M, Lee J H, Rüster B, Roth W K. Effect of interferon alfa on the dynamics of hepatitis C virus turnover in vivo. Hepatology 1996;23:366–71.
13. Shimizu Y K, Igarashi H, Kanematu T, et al. Sequence analysis of the hepatitis C virus genome recovered from serum, liver, and peripheral blood mononuclear cells of infected chimpanzees. J Virol 1997;71:5769–73.
14. Lerat H, Rumin S, Habersetzer F, et al. In vivo tropism of hepatitis C virus genomic sequences in hematopoietic cells: influence of viral load, viral genotype, and cell phenotype. Blood 1998; 91:3841–9.
15. Neumann A U, Lam N P, Dahari H, et al. Hepatitis C viral dynamics in vivo and the antiviral efficacy of interferon-α therapy. Science 1998;282:103–7.
16. N'guyen T, Sedghi-Vaziri A, Wilkes L, et al. Fluctuations in viral load (HCV RNA) are relatively insignificant in untreated patients with chronic HCV infection. J Viral Hepatitis 1996;3: 75–8.
17. Weiner A J, Brauer M J, Rosenblatt J, et al. Variable and hypervariable domains are found in the regions of HCV corresponding to the flavivirus envelope and NS1 proteins and the pestivirus envelope glycoproteins. Virology 1991;180:842–8.
18. Martell M, Esteban J I, Quer J, et al. Hepatitis C virus (HCV) circulates as a population of different but closely related genomes: quasispecies nature of HCV genome distribution. J Virol 1992;66:3225–9.
19. Duarte E A, Novella, I S, Weaver S C, et al. RNA virus quasispecies: significance for viral disease and epidemiology. Infect Agents Dis 1994;3:201–14.
20. Domingo E. Biological significance of viral quasispecies. Viral Hepatitis Rev 1996;2:247–61.
21. Domingo E, Holland J J. RNA virus mutations and fitness for survival. Annu Rev Microbiol 1997;51:151–78.
22. Grakoui A, Wychowski C, Lin C, Feinstone S M, Rice C M. Expression and identification of hepatitis C virus polyprotein cleavage products. J Virol 1993;67:1385–95.
23. Weiner A J, Geysen H M, Christopherson C, et al. Evidence for immune selection of hepatitis C virus (HCV) putative envelope glycoprotein variants: potential role in chronic HCV infections. Proc Natl Acad Sci U S A 1992;89:3468–72.
24. Higashi Y, Kakumu S, Yoshioka K, et al. Dynamics of genome change in the E2/NS1 region of hepatitis C virus in vivo. Virology 1993;197:659–68.
25. Kato N, Sekiya H, Ootsuyama Y, et al. Humoral immune response to hypervariable region 1 of the putative envelope glycoprotein (gp70) of hepatitis C virus. J Virol 1993;67:3923–30.
26. Koziel M J, Dudley D, Afdhal N, et al. Hepatitis C virus (HCV)-specific cytotoxic T-lymphocytes recognize epitopes in the core and envelope proteins of HCV. J Virol 1993;67:7522–32.
27. Farci P, Alter H J, Wong D C, et al. Prevention of hepatitis C virus infection in chimpanzees after antibody-mediated in vitro neutralization. Proc Natl Acad Sci U S A 1994;91:7792–6.
28. Ziebert A, Schreier E, Roggendorf M. Antibodies in human sera specific to hypervariable region 1 of hepatitis C virus can block viral attachment. Virology 1995;208:653–61.
29. Pawlotsky J M. Hepatitis C virus infection: virus/host interactions. J Viral Hepatitis 1998; 5(Suppl 1):3–8.
30. Gretch D R, Polyak S J. The quasispecies nature of hepatitis C virus: research methods and biological implications. In: Groupe Français d'Etudes Moléculaires des Hépatites (GEMHEP), ed. Hepatitis C virus: genetic heterogeneity and viral load. Paris: John Libbey Eurotext, 1997: 57–72.
31. Odeberg J, Yun Z, Sönnerborg A, Uhlen M, Lundeberg J. Dynamic analysis of heterogeneous hepatitis C virus populations by direct solid-phase sequencing. J Clin Microbiol 1995;33: 1870–4.
32. Lu M, Funsch B, Wiese M, Roggendorf M. Analysis of hepatitis C virus quasispecies populations by temperature gradient gel electrophoresis. J Gen Virol 1995;76:881–7.
33. Wilson J J, Polyak S J, Day T D, Gretch D R. Characterization of simple and complex hepatitis C virus quasispecies by heteroduplex gel shift analysis: correlation with nucleotide sequencing. J Gen Virol 1995;76:1763–71.
34. Enomoto N, Kurosaki M, Tanaka Y, Marumo F, Sato, C. Fluctuation of hepatitis C virus quasispecies in persistent infection and interferon treatment revealed by single-strand conformation polymorphism analysis. J Gen Virol 1994;75, 1361–9.
35. Pawlotsky J M, Pellerin M, Bouvier M, et al. Genetic complexity of the hypervariable region 1

(HVR1) of hepatitis C virus (HCV): influence on the characteristics of the infection and responses to interferon alfa therapy in patients with chronic hepatitis C. J Med Virol 1998;54: 256–64.

36. Wang Y, Ray S C, Laeyendecker O, Ticehurst J R, Thomas D L. Assessment of hepatitis C virus sequence complexity by the electrophoretic mobility of both single- and double-stranded DNA. J Clin Microbiol 1998;36:2982–9.

37. Gretch D R, Polyak S J, Wilson J J, Carithers R L, Perkins J D, Corey L. Tracking hepatitis C virus quasispecies major and minor variants in symptomatic and asymptomatic liver transplant recipients. J Virol 1996;70:7622–31.

38. Pawlotsky J M, Germanidis G, Neumann A U, Pellerin M, Frainais P O, Dhumeaux D. Interferon resistance of hepatitis C virus genotype 1b : relationship with non structural 5A (NS5A) gene quasispecies mutations. J Virol 1998;72:2795–805.

39. Pawlotsky J M, Germanidis G, Frainais P O, et al. Evolution of the hepatitis C virus second envelope hypervariable region in chronically infected patients receiving interferon-α therapy. J Virol 1999;73:6490–9.

40. Villano S A, Vlahov D, Nelson K E, Cohn S, Thomas D L. Persistence of viremia and the importance of long-term follow-up after acute hepatitis C infection. Hepatology 1999;29:908–14.

41. Ray S C, Wang Y M, Laeyendecker O, Ticehurst J R, Villano S A, Thomas D L. Acute hepatitis C virus structural gene sequences as predictors of persistent viremia: hypervariable region 1 as a decoy. J Virol 1999;73:2938–46.

42. Kojima M, Osuga T, Tsuda F, Tanaka T, Okamoto H. Influence of antibodies to the hypervariable region of E2/NS1 glycoprotein on the selective replication of hepatitis C virus in chimpanzees. Virology 1994;204:665–72.

43. Shimizu Y K, Hijikata M, Iwamoto A, Alter, H J, Purcell R H, Yoshikura H. Neutralizing antibodies against hepatitis C virus and the emergence of neutralization escape mutant viruses. J Virol 1994;65:1494–500.

44. Korenaga M, Hino K, Okazaki M, Okuda M, Okita K. Differences in hypervariable region 1 quasispecies between immune complexed and non-immune complexed hepatitis C virus particles. Biochem Biophys Res Commun 1997;240:677–82.

45. Odeberg J, Yun Z, Sönnerborg A, Björo K, Uhlen M, Lundenberg J. Variation of hepatitis C virus hypervariable region 1 in immunocompromised patients. J Infect Dis 1997;175:938–43.

46. Weiner A, Erickson A L, Kansopon J, et al. Persistent hepatitis C virus infection in a chimpanzee is associated with emergence of a cytotoxic T lymphocyte escape variant. Proc Natl Acad Sci U S A 1995;28:2755–9.

47. Chang K M, Rehermann B, McHutchison J G, et al. Immunological significance of cytotoxic T lymphocyte epitope variants in patients chronically infected by the hepatitis C virus. J Clin Invest 1997;100:2376–85.

48. Tsai S L, Chen Y M, Chen M H, et al. Hepatitis C virus variants circumventing cytotoxic T lymphocyte activity as a mechanism of chronicity. Gastroenterology 1998;115:954–65.

49. Kurosaki M, Enomoto N, Marumo F, Sato C. Rapid sequence variation of the hypervariable region of hepatitis C virus during the course of chronic infection. Hepatology 1993;18:1293–9.

50. Kao J H, Chen P J, Lai M Y, Wang T H, Chen D S. Quasispecies of hepatitis C virus and genetic drift of the hypervariable region in chronic type C hepatitis. J Infect Dis 1994;172: 261–4.

51. Kato N, Ootsuyama Y, Sekiya H, et al. Genetic drift in hypervariable region 1 of the viral genome in persistent hepatitis C virus infection. J Virol 1994;68:4776–84.

52. van Doorn L J, Quint W, Tsiquaye K, et al. Longitudinal analysis of hepatitis C virus infection and genetic drift of the hypervariable region. J Infect Dis 1994;169:1226–35.

53. van Doorn L J, Capriles I, Maertens G, et al. Sequence evolution of the hypervariable region in the putative envelope region E2/NS1 of hepatitis C virus is correlated with specific humoral immune responses. J Virol 1995;69:773–8.

54. Manzin A, Solforosi L, Petrelli E, et al. Evolution of hypervariable region 1 of hepatitis C virus in primary infection. J Virol 1998;72:6271–6.

55. Cabot B, Esteban J I, Martell M, et al. Structure of replicating hepatitis C virus (HCV) quasispecies in the liver may not be reflected by analysis of circulating HCV virions. J Virol 1997;71: 1732–34.

56. Maggi F, Fornai C, Vatteroni, M L, et al. Differences in hepatitis C virus quasispecies compo-

sition between liver, peripheral blood mononuclear cells and plasma. J Gen Virol 1997;78: 1521–5.

57. Navas S, Martin J, Quiroga, J A, Castillo I, Carreno V. Genetic diversity and tissue compartmentalization of the hepatitis C virus genome in blood mononuclear cells, liver, and serum from chronic hepatitis C patients. J Virol 1998;72:1640–6.

58. Okuda M, Hino K, Korenaga M, Yamaguchi Y, Katoh Y, Okita K. Differences in hypervariable region 1 quasispecies of hepatitis C virus in human serum, peripheral blood mononuclear cells, and liver. Hepatology 1999;29:217–22.

59. Nakajima N, Hijikata M, Yoshikura H, Shimizu Y K. Characterization of long-term cultures of hepatitis C virus. J Virol 1996;70:3325–9.

60. Shimizu, Y K, Igarashi H, Kiyohara T, et al. Infection of a chimpanzee with hepatitis C virus grown in cell culture. J Gen Virol 1998;79:1383–6.

61. Naito M, Hayashi N, Moribe T, et al. Hepatitis C viral quasispecies in hepatitis C virus carriers with normal liver enzymes and patients with type C chronic liver disease. Hepatology 1995; 22:407–12.

62. Koizumi K, Enomoto N, Kurosaki M, et al. Diversity of quasispecies in various disease stages of chronic hepatitis C virus infection and its significance in interferon treatment. Hepatology 1995;22:30–5.

63. Gonzalez-Peralta R P, Qian K, She J Y, et al. Clinical implications of viral quasispecies heterogeneity in chronic hepatitis C. J Med Virol 1996;49:242–7.

64. Yuki N, Hayashi N, Moribe T, et al. Relation of disease activity during chronic hepatitis C infection to complexity of hypervariable region 1 quasispecies. Hepatology 1997;25:439–44.

65. Hayashi J, Kishihara Y, Yamaji K, et al. Hepatitis C viral quasispecies and liver damage in patients with chronic hepatitis C virus infection. Hepatology 1997;25:697–701.

66. Leone F, Zylberberg H, Squadrito G, et al. Hepatitis C virus (HCV) hypervariable region 1 complexity does not correlate with severity of liver disease, HCV type, viral load or duration of infection. J Hepatol 1998;29:689–94.

67. Lopez-Labrador F X, Ampurdanes S, Gimenez-Barcons M, et al. Relationship of the genomic complexity of hepatitis C virus with liver disease severity and response to interferon in patients with chronic HCV genotype 1b interferon. Hepatology 1999;29:897–903.

68. Aiyama T, Yoshioka K, Okumura A, et al. Sequence analysis of hypervariable region of hepatitis C virus (HCV) associated with immune complex in patients with chronic HCV infection. J Infect Dis 1996;174:1316–20.

69. Lindsay K L. Therapy of hepatitis C: overview. Hepatology 1997;26(Suppl 1), 71S–7S.

70. Toyoda H, Kumada T, Nakano S, et al. Quasispecies nature of hepatitis C virus and response to alpha interferon: significance as a predictor of direct response to interferon. J Hepatol. 1997; 26:6–13.

71. Enomoto N, Sakuma I, Asahina Y, et al. Comparison of full-length sequences of interferon-sensitive and resistant hepatitis C virus 1b. Sensitivity to interferon is conferred by amino acid substitutions in the NS5A region. J Clin Invest 1995;96:224–30.

72. Nagasaka A, Hige S, Tsunematsu I, et al. Changes in hepatitis C virus quasispecies and density populations in patients before and after interferon therapy. J Med Virol 1996;50:214–20.

73. Shindo M, Hamada K, Koya S, Arai K, Sokawa Y, Okuno T. The clinical significance of changes in genetic heterogeneity of the hypervariable region 1 in chronic hepatitis C with interferon therapy. Hepatology 1996;24:1018–23.

74. Polyak S J, McArdle S, Liu S L, et al. Evolution of hepatitis C virus quasispecies in hypervariable region 1 and the putative interferon sensitivity-determining region during interferon therapy and natural infection. J Virol 1998;72:4288–96.

75. Pawlotsky J M, Germanidis G. The non structural (NS) 5A protein of hepatitis C virus. J Viral Hepatitis 1999;6:343–56.

76. Chayama K, Tsubota A, Kobayashi M, et al. Pretreatment virus load and multiple amino acid substitutions in the interferon sensitivity-determining region predict the outcome of interferon treatment in patients with chronic genotype 1b hepatitis C virus infection. Hepatology 1997;25: 745–9.

77. Rispeter K, Lu M, Zibert A, Wiese M, Mendes de Oliveira J, Roggendorf M. The "interferon sensitivity determining region" of hepatitis C virus is a stable sequence element. J Hepatol 1998; 29:352–61.

78. Tanimoto A, Ide Y, Arima N, Sasaguri Y, Padmanabhan R. The amino terminal deletion mutants of hepatitis C virus nonstructural protein NS5A function as transcriptional activators in yeast. Biochem Biophys Res Commun 1997;236:360–4.
79. Kato N, Lan K H, Ono-Nita, S K, Shiratori Y, Omata M. Hepatitis C virus nonstructural region 5A protein is a potent transcriptional activator. J Virol 1997;71:8856–9.
80. Gale M J Jr, Korth M J, Tang N M, et al. Evidence that hepatitis C virus resistance to interferon is mediated through repression of the PKR protein kinase by the nonstructural 5A protein. Virology 1997;230:217–27.
81. Gale M Jr, Blakely C M, Kwieciszewski B, et al. Control of PKR protein kinase by hepatitis C virus nonstructural 5A protein: molecular mechanisms of kinase regulation. Mol Cell Biol 1998;18:5208–18.
82. Heim M H, Moradpour D, Blum H E. Expression of hepatitis C virus proteins inhibits signal transduction through the Jak-Stat pathway. J Virol 1999;73:8469–75.
83. Martell M, Esteban J I, Quer J, et al. Dynamic behavior of hepatitis C virus quasispecies in patients undergoing orthotopic liver transplantation. J Virol 1994;68:3425–36.
84. Sullivan, D G, Wilson J J, Carithers R L Jr, Perkins J D, Gretch D R. Multigene tracking of hepatitis C virus quasispecies after liver transplantation: correlation of genetic diversification in the envelope region with asymptomatic or mild disease patterns. J Virol 1998;72:10036–43.
85. Wang J T, Wang T H, Sheu J C, Lin S M, Lin J T, Chen D S. Effects of anticoagulants and storage of blood samples on efficacy of the polymerase chain reaction assay for hepatitis C virus. J Clin Microbiol 1992;30:750–3.
86. Busch M P, Wilber J C, Johnson P, Tobler L, and Evans C S. Impact of specimen handling and storage on detection of hepatitis C virus RNA. Transfusion 1992;32:420–5.
87. Cuypers H T, Bresters D, Winkel I N, et al. Storage conditions of blood samples and primer selection affect the yield of cDNA polymerase chain reaction products of hepatitis C virus. J Clin Microbiol 1992;30:3220–4.
88. Davis G L, Lau J Y, Urdea M S, et al. Quantitative detection of hepatitis C virus RNA with a solid-phase signal amplification method: definition of optimal conditions for specimen collection and clinical application in interferon-treated patients. Hepatology 1994;19:1337–41.
89. Halfon P, Khiri H, Gérolami V, et al. Impact of various handling and storage conditions on quantitative detection of hepatitis C virus RNA. J Hepatol 1996;25:307–11.
90. Damen M, Sillekens P, Sjerps M, et al. Stability of hepatitis C virus RNA during specimen handling and storage prior to NASBA amplification. J Virol Methods 1998;72:175–84.
91. Pawlotsky J M, Maisonneuve P, Duval J, Dhumeaux D, Noël L. Significance of NS5 "indeterminate" third-generation anti-hepatitis C virus serological assays. Transfusion 1995;35:453–4.
92. Vrielink H, Zaaijer H L, Reesink H W, van der Poel C L, Cuypers H T, Lelie P N. Sensitivity and specificity of three third-generation anti-hepatitis C virus ELISAs. Vox Sang 1995;69:14–17.
93. Lavanchy D, Steinmann J, Moritz A, Frei P C. Evaluation of a new automated third-generation anti-HCV enzyme immunoassay. J Clin Lab Anal 1996;10:269–76.
94. Ragni M V, N'Dimbie O K, Rice E O, Bontempo F A, Nedjar S. The presence of hepatitis C virus (HCV) antibody in human immunodeficiency virus-positive hemophilic men undergoing HCV "seroreversion." Blood 1993;82:1010–5.
95. Bukh J, Wantzin P, Krogsgaard K, Knudsen F, Purcell R H, Miller R H. High prevalence of hepatitis C virus (HCV) RNA in dialysis patients: failure of commercially available antibody tests to identify a significant number of patients with HCV infection. J Infect Dis 1993;168:1343–8.
96. Quaranta J F, Delaney S R, Alleman S, Cassuto J P, Dellamonica P, Allain J P. Prevalence of antibody to hepatitis C virus (HCV) in HIV-1-infected patients (Nice SEROCO cohort). J Med Virol 1994;42:29–32.
97. Preiksaitis J K, Cockfield S M, Fenton J M, Burton N I, Chui L W. Serologic responses to hepatitis C virus in solid organ transplant recipients. Transplantation 1997;64:1775–80.
98. De Medina M, Hill M, Sullivan H O, et al. Detection of anti-hepatitis C virus antibodies in patients undergoing dialysis by utilizing a hepatitis C virus 3.0 assay: correlation with hepatitis C virus RNA. J Lab Clin Med 1998;132:73–5.
99. Consensus Development Panel. National Institutes of Health Consensus Development Conference Panel Statement: management of hepatitis C. Hepatology 1997;26 (Suppl 1):2S–10S.

100. Vrielink H, Reesink H W, van den Burg P J, et al. Performance of three generations of anti-hepatitis C virus enzyme-linked immunosorbent assays in donors and patients. Transfusion 1997;37:845–9.

101. Pawlotsky J M, Lonjon I, Hézode C, et al. What strategy should be used for diagnosis of hepatitis C virus infection in clinical laboratories? Hepatology 1998;27:1700–2.

102. Chau K H, Dawson G J, Mushahwar I K, et al. IgM antibody response to hepatitis C virus antigens in acute and chronic posttransfusion non-A, non-B hepatitis. J Virol Methods 1991;34:343–52.

103. Quiroga, J A, Campillo M, Castillo I, Bartolomé J, Porres J C, Carreno V. IgM antibody to hepatitis C virus in acute and chronic hepatitis C. Hepatology 1991;14:38–43.

104. Hellström U B, Sylvan S P E, Decker R H, Sönnerborg A. Immunoglobulin M reactivity towards the immunologically active region sp75 of the core protein of hepatitis C virus (HCV) in chronic HCV infection. J Med Virol 1993;39:325–32.

105. Pawlotsky J M, Darthuy F, Rémiré J, et al. Significance of anti-hepatitis C virus core IgM antibodies in patients with chronic hepatitis C. J Med Virol 1995;47:285–91.

106. Bhattacherjee V, Prescott L E, Pike I, et al. Use of NS-4 peptides to identify type-specific antibody to hepatitis C virus genotypes 1, 2, 3, 4, 5 and 6. J Gen Virol 1995;76:1737–48.

107. Dixit V, Quan S, Martin P, et al. Evaluation of a novel serotyping system for hepatitis C virus: strong correlation with standard genotyping methodologies. J Clin Microbiol 1995;33:2978–83.

108. Mizoguchi N, Mizokami M, Orito E, Shibata H, Shibata H. Serologically defined genotypes of hepatitis C virus among Japanese patients with chronic hepatitis C. J Virol Methods 1996;58:71–9.

109. Pawlotsky J M, Prescott L, Simmonds P, et al. Serological determination of hepatitis C virus genotype: comparison with a standardized genotyping assay. J Clin Microbiol 1997;35:1734–9.

110. Lee J H, Roth W K, Zeuzem S. Evaluation and comparison of different hepatitis C virus genotyping and serotyping assays. J Hepatol 1997;26:1001–9.

111. Krawczynski K, Beach M J, Bradley D W, et al. Hepatitis C virus antigen in hepatocytes: immunomorphologic detection and identification. Gastroenterology 1992;103:622–29.

112. Di Bisceglie A M, Hoofnagle J H, Krawczynski K. Changes in hepatitis C virus antigen in liver with antiviral therapy. Gastroenterology 1993;105:858–62.

113. Martell M, Gomez J, Esteban J I, et al. High-throughput real-time reverse transcription-PCR quantitation of hepatitis C virus RNA. J Clin Microbiol 1999;37:327–32.

114. Takeuchi T, Katsume A, Tanaka T, et al. Real-Time detection system for quantification of hepatitis C virus genome. Gastroenterology 1999;116:636–42.

115. Zaaijer H L, Cuypers H T, Reesink H W, Winkel I N, Gerken G, Lelie P N. Reliability of polymerase chain reaction for detection of hepatitis C virus. Lancet 1993;341:722–4.

116. French Study Group for the Standardization of Hepatitis C Virus PCR. Improvement of hepatitis C virus RNA polymerase chain reaction through a multicentre quality control study. J Virol Methods 1994;49:79–88.

117. Damen M, Cuypers H T, Zaaijer H L, et al. International collaborative study on the second EUROHEP HCV-RNA reference panel. J Virol Methods 1996;58:175–85.

118. Gretch D R. Diagnostic tests for hepatitis C. Hepatology 1997;26(Suppl 1):43S–7S.

119. Wolfe L, Tamatsukuri S, Sayada C, Ryff J C. Detection of HCV RNA in serum using a single-tube, single-enzyme PCR in combination with a colorimetric microwell assay. In: Groupe Français d'Etudes Moléculaires des Hépatites (GEMHEP), ed. Hepatitis C virus: new diagnostic tools. Paris: John Libbey Eurotext, 1994:83–94.

120. Albadalejo J, Alonso R, Antinozzi R, et al. Multicenter evaluation of the COBAS AMPLICOR HCV assay, an integrated PCR system for rapid detection of hepatitis C virus RNA in the diagnostic laboratory. J Clin Microbiol 1998;36:862–5.

121. Tong M J, Blatt L M, Conrad A, et al. The changes in quantitative HCV RNA titers during interferon alpha-2b therapy in patients with chronic hepatitis C infection. Am J Gastroenterol 1998;93:601–5.

122. Fang J W S, Albrecht J K, Jacobs S, Lau J Y N. Quantification of serum hepatitis C virus RNA. Hepatology 1999;29:997–8.

123. Pawlotsky J M. Measuring hepatitis C viremia in clinical samples: can we trust the assays? Hepatology 1997;26:1–4.

124. Pawlotsky J M, Martinot-Peignoux M, Poveda J D, et al. Quantification of hepatitis C virus RNA in serum by branched DNA-based signal amplification assays. J Virol Methods 1999;79:227–35.

125. Roth W K, Lee J H, Rüster B, Zeuzem S. Comparison of two quantitative hepatitis C virus reverse transcriptase PCR assays. J Clin Microbiol 1996;34:261–4.

126. Hadziyannis E, Fried M W, and Nolte F S. Evaluation of two methods for quantitation of hepatitis C virus RNA. Mol Diagn 1997;2:39–46.

127. Okamoto H, Kobata S, Tokita H, et al. A second-generation method of genotyping hepatitis C virus by the polymerase chain reaction with sense and antisense primers deduced from the core gene. J Virol Methods 1996;57:31–45.

128. Davidson F, Simmonds P, Ferguson J C, et al. Survey of major genotypes and subtypes of hepatitis C virus using RFLP of sequences amplified from the 5′ non coding region. J Gen Virol 1995;76:1197–204.

129. Stuyver L, Rossau R, Wyseur A, et al. Typing of hepatitis C virus isolates and characterization of new subtypes using a line probe assay. J Gen Virol 1993;74:1093–102.

130. Biasin M R, Fiordalisi G, Zanella I, Cavicchini A, Marchelle G, Infantolino D. A DNA hybridization method for typing hepatitis C virus genotype 2c. J Virol Methods 1997;65:307–15.

131. Dhumeaux D, Doffoël M, Galmiche J P. French consensus conference on hepatitis C: screening and treatment. J Hepatol 1997;27:941–4.

132. Roudot-Thoraval F, Pawlotsky J M, Thiers V, et al. Lack of mother-to-infant transmission of hepatitis C virus in HIV-negative women. A prospective study using HCV-RNA testing. Hepatology 1993;17:772–7.

133. Thomas D L, Villano S A, Riester K A, et al. Perinatal transmission of hepatitis C virus from human immunodeficiency virus type 1-infected mothers. Women and Infants Transmission Study. J Infect Dis 1998;177:1480–8.

134. Chazouillères O, Kim M, Combs C, et al. Quantitation of hepatitis C virus RNA in liver transplant recipients. Gastroenterology 1994;106:994–9.

135. Duvoux C, Pawlotsky J M, Bastie A, Cherqui D, Soussy C J, Dhumeaux D. Low HCV replication levels in end-stage hepatitis C virus-related liver disease. J Hepatol 1999;31:593–7.

136. Chemello L, Cavalletto L, Casarin C, et al. Persistent hepatitis C viremia predicts late relapse after sustained response to interferon-α in chronic hepatitis C. Ann Intern Med 1996;124:1058–60.

137. Marcellin P, Boyer N, Gervais A, et al. Long-term histologic improvement and loss of detectable intrahepatic HCV RNA in patients with chronic hepatitis C and sustained response to interferon-α therapy. Ann Intern Med 1997;127:875–81.

138. Lau D T Y, Kleiner D E, Ghany M G, Park Y, Schmid P, Hoofnagle J H. 10-year follow-up after interferon-α therapy for chronic hepatitis C. Hepatology 1998;28:1121–7.

139. van der Poel C L, Reesink H W, Schaasberg W, et al. Infectivity of blood seropositive for hepatitis C virus antibodies. Lancet 1990;335:558–60.

140. Garson J A, Tedder R S, Briggs M, et al. Detection of hepatitis C viral sequences in blood donations by "nested" polymerase chain reaction and prediction of infectivity. Lancet 1990;335:1419–22.

141. Power J P, Davidson F, O'Riordan J, Simmonds P, Yap P L, and Lawlor E. Hepatitis C infection from anti-D immunoglobulin. Lancet 1995;346:372–3.

142. Allander T, Gruber A, Naghavi M, et al. Frequent patient-to-patient transmission of hepatitis C virus in a haematology ward. Lancet 1995;345:603–7.

143. Lefrère J J, Guiramand S, Lefrère F, et al. Full or partial seroreversion in patients infected by hepatitis C virus. J Infect Dis 1997;175:316–22

3

HEPATITIS C VIRUS GENOTYPES

PETER SIMMONDS

Laboratory for Clinical and Molecular Virology
University of Edinburgh
Edinburgh, United Kingdom

INTRODUCTION

The hepatitis C virus (HCV) genome displays considerable heterogeneity. No fewer than six genotypes and more than 50 subtypes of HCV have been identified. Tests for HCV genotypes include both genotyping and serotyping methods. Genotyping is valuable both in epidemiological studies, whereas the biological and clinical differences between genotypes make genotyping important for decisions regarding antiviral therapy. This chapter describes the classification and nomenclature of HCV genotypes and reviews methods currently available to identify HCV genotypes and the impact that HCV sequence heterogeneity has on diagnosis, on the development of vaccines, and on the treatment of infection.

NUCLEOTIDE SEQUENCE VARIATION

HCV shows considerable genetic heterogeneity, a fact that was immediately apparent when variants that were detected and sequenced in Japan were compared with the prototype HCV variant (HCV-PT) isolated in the United States. (1) The current classification of HCV has evolved since the initial terminology, which used "type I" HCV for United States strains (HCV-PT and H strain) and "type II" for Japanese variants. With more extensive sampling, nucleotide sequencing and analysis of variants from many parts of the world, it has become clear that there are many divergent variants of HCV. (2–5) Subsequent discussions and a series of consensus meeting led to the proposal of and adoption of an extended classification of HCV into types and subtypes.

HCV Genotype Classification

In the currently widely used classification system, variants of HCV collected from different parts of the world are divided into six main "genotypes," many of which contain more closely related variants (Fig. 1). (6–8) For ease of nomenclature, HCV is classified into types, corresponding to the main branches in the phylogenetic tree, and into subtypes corresponding to the more closely related sequences within some of the major groups. (8,9) The types have been numbered 1 to 6 and the subtypes a, b, and c, in both cases in order of discovery.

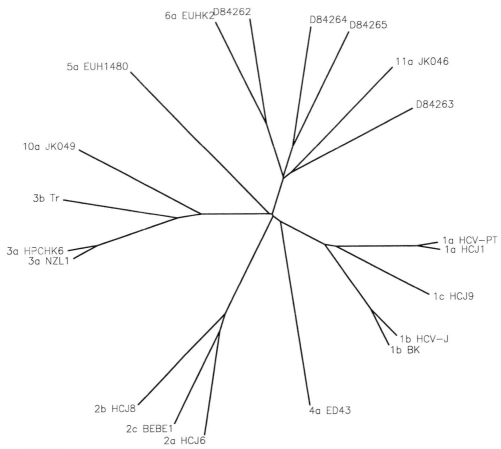

FIGURE I Sequence relationships among genotypes I and 6 using comparisons of currently available complete genomic sequences (6) (tree generated using the programs DNADIST and NEIGHBOR in the PHYLIP package). (7) Nomenclature of HCV variants follows the consensus proposal for the classification of HCV, (8) i.e., the prototype sequence cloned by Houghton and co-workers is referred to as type Ia; HCV-J and BK sequences as type Ib; HCJ6 as type 2a; and HCJ8 as type 2b.

Therefore, the original prototype sequence cloned by Houghton and co-workers was assigned type 1a, whereas the Japanese types HCV-J and -BK were assigned type 1b, HC-J6 as type 2a and HC-J8 as type 2b.

The sequence relationships depicted in Fig. 1 were derived from comparisons over the length of the genome, but it is now clear that short subgenomic regions, such as the E1 (10) or NS5B (11) regions, can be used reliably for classification. (12,13) Use of subgenomic regions makes the survey and identification of genotypes more practical. Indeed, comparisons of HCV isolates from a much wider range of geographical locations has now provided evidence for the existence of an extremely large number of subtypes recognized within five of the six main genotypes (Fig. 2). (14–17)

Each of the six main genotypes of HCV are equally divergent from each other, differing at 31 to 34% of nucleotide positions on pairwise comparisons of complete genomic sequences, and leading to approximately 30% amino acid sequence divergence between the encoded polyproteins. Different regions of the

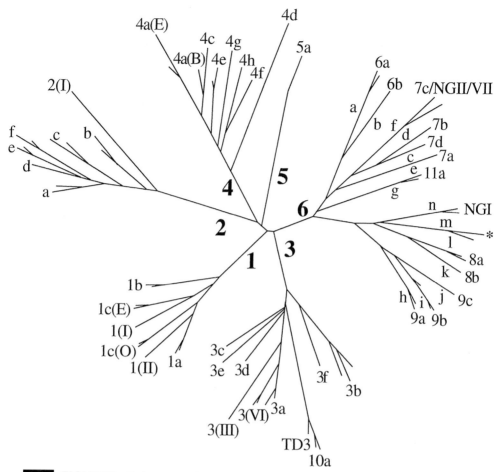

FIGURE 2 Phylogenetic analysis of nucleotide sequences from part of the HCV NS5B region amplified from samples of HCV-infected blood donors and patients with hepatitis C from several countries. Six main groups of sequence variants are found corresponding to types 1–6; each group contains a number of more closely related subtypes. Recently discovered variants from southeast Asia cluster with type 6a but are labeled according to the original publications. (14–17) See Mellor et al., (14) for a more detailed discussion of current issues in HCV classification.

genome show varying levels of sequence diversity. The ends of the genome that contain elements involved in virus replication and in guiding protein translation are highly conserved between genotypes, as is the initial structural coding region (the core gene). Other regions, such as the E1 and E2 genes coding from the envelope glycoproteins, are highly variable, typically differing at over 50% of sites between genotypes.

Within genotypes, the further clustering of HCV variants into subtypes is remarkably uniform, with subtypes within a genotype typically differing from each other by 20 to 23%, a range of values not overlapping with those between genotypes. However, there is a problem with the classification of variants from SE Asia (Thailand, Vietnam, and Burma), as they do not fit neatly into the type/subtype scheme used for nomenclature. These variants group with type 6 by phylogenetic analysis (Fig. 2), but are more divergent from each other than subtypes of other genotypes. A similarly divergent variant from Indonesia, described originally as type 10a, groups among type 3 sequences.

To resolve these problems with HCV classification, a representative group of investigators involved in the description of HCV heterogeneity reached agreement that the primary method for classifying HCV genotypes should be phylogenetic analysis. (18) Using this method, the division of currently described HCV variants into only six clades supports previous suggestions that genotypes 7, 8, 9, 10, and 11 should not be considered as separate genotypes, but rather as subtypes within types 3 and 6. (19–21)

Genotypic classification remains an essentially man-made labeling system, which attempts to categorize or compartmentalize what is, by definition, a continuous variable. In the final analysis, such classifications are only of value if they can usefully divide HCV into variants with useful differences in biological, antigenic, and/or epidemiological properties. The remainder of this chapter explores the differences that exist between and within the six currently described genetic groups of HCV.

GEOGRAPHICAL DISTRIBUTION AND EPIDEMIOLOGY

Some genotypes of HCV (types 1a, 2a, and 2b) have a broad worldwide distribution, whereas others such as type 5a and 6a are found only in specific geographical regions. HCV-infected blood donors and patients with chronic hepatitis from countries in western Europe and the North America most frequently have genotypes 1a, 1b, 2a, 2b, and 3a, although the relative frequencies of each may vary within the region. Type 1b tends to be more frequent in southern and eastern Europe than in northern Europe or the United States. In many European countries, genotype distributions vary with age of patients, reflecting rapid changes in genotype distribution with time within a single geographic area.

A striking geographical shift in genotype distribution is apparent between southeastern Europe and Turkey (where type 1b predominates) and countries in the Middle East and northern and central Africa (where type 4 predominates). (22,23) For example, a high frequency of HCV infection is found in Egypt (20–30%), which is predominantly due to type 4a HCV. (24,25) HCV genotype 5a is found frequently among patients with chronic hepatitis C and HCV-infected blood donors in south Africa but is found only rarely in other parts of Africa or elsewhere. In west Africa, genotypes 1 and 2 are predominant but show an extraordinary diversity of subtypes; by combining results from three relatively small-scale surveys, more than 10–20 distinct subtypes within the genotype 1 and 2 clades have been found. (14,26,27)

In Japan and Taiwan and probably parts of China, genotypes 1b, 2a, and 2b are found most frequently. A genotype with a highly restricted geographical range is type 6a, which was originally found in Hong Kong, where approximately one-third of anti-HCV positive blood donors were infected with this genotype, as were an equivalent proportion in neighboring Macau and Vietnam. Other genotypes have been found in Vietnam, (15) Thailand, (15–17) and Indonesia, (28) which group within the genotype 3 and 6 clades (Fig. 2), although their divergence from other variants led to the original proposal that they be described as types 7 to 11. (15,16,28) The genetic diversity of genotypes 3 and 6 in southeast Asia rivals that of genotypes 1, 2, and 4 in sub-Saharan Africa. For example, sequence comparisons of variants recovered from 14 individuals infected in Nepal or Bangladesh revealed a total of eight different subtypes of genotype 3, six of which had not been identified in other geographical areas.

ORIGINS OF HCV GENOTYPES

Attempts to identify the origins and spread of HCV in historical and prehistorical times can only be based on indirect evidence. Archived clinical material is extremely restricted, and it is unlikely that there are any plasma or liver samples available from more than 50 years from which HCV could be recovered by polymerase chain reaction (PCR). Furthermore, as primary HCV infection is generally asymptomatic and its long-term disease associations are nonspecific, it is unlikely that any historical written account could provide evidence for its presence in previous eras.

Nevertheless, indirect evidence for the origins of HCV is provided by its current epidemiological distribution, particularly the pattern of sequence diversity of HCV in different populations and risk groups. For example, separate origins for the different HCV genotypes are suggested by the current preponderance of types 3 and 6 in India and southeast Asia and of types 1, 2, and 4 in central and west Africa. Furthermore, their presence is associated with a diversity of subtypes not observed in Europe, North America, or the Far East. This high degree of population complexity is likely the result of their long-term presence within these human populations, even though there is little insight into the mechanisms of HCV transmission in such communities.

To estimate the time scale of the spread of HCV in different populations, it is necessary to combine information on the genetic diversity of HCV in different risk groups and populations with estimates of the rate of change of HCV sequences over time. The latter has been estimated previously by sequence comparisons of variants recovered from chronically infected humans or chimpanzees over periods of several years. (29,30) More recently, an opportunity to measure this rate more accurately arose from the analysis of HCV variants infecting several individuals infected through treatment with a batch of anti-D immunoglobulin that had been comtaminated inadvertently with HCV. (31) Phylogenetic clustering was apparent from NS5 sequences amplified from samples collected 17 years after this common source exposure when compared with sequences of epidemiologically unlinked type 1b-infected individuals (Fig. 3). (32–34) Comparison of sequences derived from HCV variants obtained from immunoglobulin recipients 17 years after exposure to sequences from HCV recovered from archived vials of the implicated batch of anti-D immunoglobulin demonstrated a mean rate of nucleotide sequence change of 0.14 to 0.19% per neutral (i.e, synonymous) site per year. (35)

Using nucleotide sequence data currently available from NS5 and E1 genes, one can predict the time of origin of different HCV genotypes, although the accuracy of this approach may be compromised by the availability of only short DNA sequences. (36,37) Sequence diversity among type 1b HCV variants infecting epidemiologically unlinked patients with hepatitis patients in the United States, Japan, and Europe predicts a time of divergence approximately 60–70

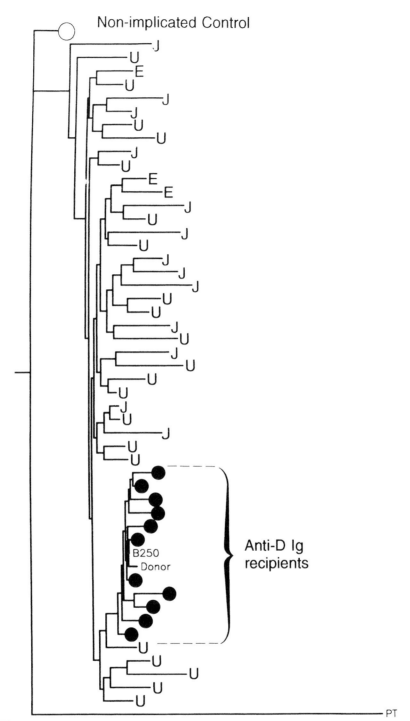

FIGURE 3 Phylogenetic relationships between sequences from the NS5B region from those exposed to HCV-contaminated batch of anti-D immunoglobulin in 1977 (●) with well-characterized but epidemiologically unrelated type 1b variants from Japan (J), the United States (U), and Europe (E). B250: NS-5 sequence of HCV recovered from batch B250 of anti-D immunoglobulin (Ig). Donor: sequence of variant infecting suspected donor to plasma pool used to manufacture batch B250. Phylogenetic analysis was carried out on a segment (222 bp; positions 7975–8196) of the NS-5 gene amplified, sequenced, and analyzed as described previously. (32) Sequence distances were calculated using the program DNAML in a data set containing HCV-PT (type 1a) as an out-group. Sequences were obtained from published sources. (32,33) [Figure reproduced from Power et al. (34)]

years ago. The lack of any observable country-specific groupings among type 1b sequences further suggests that the original outbreak was disseminated widely over a short period. The transmission events that allowed this to occur at that time remain formally undetermined, although nosocomial routes (immunization, early blood transfusion) were probably relevant. There is some evidence for less diversity among the two genotypes found most frequently in populations of injection drug users of western Europe, types 1a and 3a. The increase in drug abuse and the practice of needle sharing since the 1960s have produced a large and growing risk group for HCV infection in the United States and Europe. This is reflected in the genetic evidence for a more recent common origin for the genotypes found in current members of this group. (38)

Further extending these investigations to attempt to date the origins of different subtypes and the six genotypes of HCV is fraught with hazard. At present, evolutionary reconstructions are dominated by neutral theory, which postulates that the genetic distance between organisms should remain proportional to the time of divergence over a wide range of genetic distances. Although fossil-based studies of vertebrate evolution have provided a dramatic confirmation of the predictions from neutral theory, virus evolution may be subject to additional constraints that severely limit the ability to reconstruct their history. (39) For example, secondary structure formation in the GB virus C (GBV-C) or hepatitis G virus (HGV) genome limits the accumulation of nucleotide substitutions at sites involved in internal base pairing. Although the short rate of sequence change of HGV/GBV-C (which is actually similar to that of HCV and other positive-stranded RNA viruses) predicts that the currently described variants originated only 100 years ago, it is more likely that the virus coevolved with modern humans as they migrated out of Africa over the last 100,000 to 150,000 years. (39,40) It is also likely that the homologous viruses of HGV/GBV-C, which are found in Old and New World primates, originated with their hosts during primate speciation, beginning 35 million years ago. (41)

The considerable similarities in the genetic organization, structure, and method of replication of HCV and HGV/GBV-C suggest that the evolution of HCV may be subject to similar constraints, although direct evidence for this is lacking. The assumption of no constraints and constancy in the rate of sequence change over time predicts that different subtypes of HCV originated approximately 200 years ago, whereas the six genotypes of HCV diverged from a common ancestor approximately 400 years ago. However, it is difficult to accept that this virus originated over such a short period of human history, particularly because HCV is transmitted principally by the parenteral route and the virus has such a global distribution, being found even in the most remote communities in all areas of the world. Clearly, a more detailed understanding of the factors that govern RNA virus sequence evolution is required before this issue can be resolved.

HCV GENOTYPING ASSAYS

Although nucleotide sequence analysis is the most reliable method for identifying different genotypes of HCV, this technique is not practical for routine use or for large-scale clinical studies. A number of methods have been developed that allow the rapid identification of a limited range of HCV genotypes, typically genotypes 1a, 1b, types 2, 3, and 4, that are found in patients and study populations in Western countries. Most assays for HCV genotypes are based on the amplification of virus sequences in clinical specimens by PCR. One commonly used method is a modified PCR that uses several sets of primers, each of which selectively amplifies sequences from different HCV genotypes. For example, DNA amplified by primers specific for the core region of type 1a are a different size from those produced from the amplification of types 1b, 2a, 2b and 3a and can therefore be differentiated by agarose gel electrophoresis of the PCR product. (42–44) Other assays are based on the analysis of amplified DNA sequences. For example, the genotype of an amplified sequence can be determined by hybridization to genotype-specific probes (45–47) or through restriction fragment length polymorphisms (RFLP) in sequences amplified from the 5′ NCR. (48)

Serological typing methods are based on the detection of a type-specific antibody to epitopes of HCV that differ among genotypes. (49,50) Serotyping has advantages over PCR-based methods in terms of speed and simplicity of sample preparation and in the use of standard equipment that is found in most diagnostic virology laboratories. By careful optimization of reagents, serological typing assays can attain a high degree of sensitivity and reproducibility. For example, the type-specific antibody to NS4 peptides of genotypes 1 to 6 can be detected in 85 to 90% of patients with chronic hepatitis C. (9) Serological typing assays are generally unable to distinquish subtypes, such as 1a from 1b, because of their antigenic similarity. Nevertheless, a method that is claimed to achieve this separation has been described. (51)

A crucial assumption of all genotyping assays is that the region analyzed (5′ UTR, core, NS4, NS5B) is representative of the genome as a whole. This assumption would not hold if recombination occurred between HCV genotypes during virus replication. In patients infected with two genotypes, recombination would produce hybrid viruses containing contributions from different genotypes in different parts of the genome. (52) So far, remarkably consistent results have been obtained by comparing results of genotyping assays based on the sequence analysis of different regions of the genome and between PCR-based and serological typing assays. (33,53,54) These findings suggest that genotyping is a valid procedure, despite the theoretical possibility of recombination. Many assays can reliably identify infection with those HCV genotypes likely to be encountered in clinical practice in the Western world (1a, 1b, 2a, 2b, and 3a).

ANTIGENIC AND BIOLOGICAL DIFFERENCES BETWEEN GENOTYPES

Despite the sequence diversity found among variants of HCV, there are no differences in overall genome organization between genotypes, each encoding the same range of proteins of similar amino acid compositions and which are likely to undergo the same posttranslational modifications. However, the extensive amino acid sequence variability found in both structural and nonstructural proteins leads to antigenic and potentially biological differences between genotypes that carry implications for diagnostics, vaccine design, and clinical management of HCV-infected patients. These aspects are each reviewed briefly.

Diagnostic Assays for HCV

The discovery of HCV was followed rapidly by the development of serological screening assays for anti-HCV, as well as highly sensitive methods for the detection of HCV RNA sequences in plasma and for the quantitation of circulating virus load. Each of these assays may be affected adversely by the genetic heterogeneity of HCV.

Antigenic variability of HCV and the resulting partial type specificity of antibody responses to HCV infection could cause significant problems in serological screening for infection. Most currently available enzyme immunoassays (EIAs) for anti-HCV employ recombinant proteins produced by type 1 HCV strains. Thus, significant antigenic variation among genotypes might render the assays for anti-HCV suboptimal for screening individuals infected with genotypes other than type 1. Among the components used in second- and third-generation EIAs, antigenic variation is greatest in nonstructural proteins, such as c33c (NS3), c100 (NS4), and NS5 (NS5a). (55–58) In contrast, the core protein is highly conserved in the amino acid sequence, and it is likely that this component is the most effective at detecting cross-reactivity with antibody produced to other genotypes. (55) Overall, individuals infected with HCV type 2 or 3 have a fivefold less median reactivity in the currently available third-generation EIA compared to patients with type 1 HCV infection. (59) Although most HCV-infected individuals show a polyclonal serological response to a range of different type-common and -specific epitopes, antigenic differences may influence the detection of anti-HCV in situations where antibody production is low or modest. Of particular importance is the initial serological response in acutely infected individuals, which can be delayed and low titered as if often directed at the antigenically variable NS3 protein. (60) Thus, patients with type 2 and 3 HCV infections may seroconvert to anti-HCV reactivity later during the course of acute hepatitis C than patients with type 1 infection, and rarely such patients may test negative using type 1-based serological assays.

Standardization and genotype independence of methods used to quantify HCV RNA is necessary if they are used as clinical markers for disease progression and for predicting the likelihood of a beneficial outcome to treatment. Commercially available methods to measure HCV virus load include PCR-based (Roche Monitor) and hybridization-based (Quantiplex bDNA-2) methods. The currently used version 1 of the Roche Monitor substantially underestimates concentrations of RNA transcripts of types 2b, 3a, 4a, 5a, and 6a and virus loads in individuals infected with genotypes 2–6 relative to reference tests. (61–64) However, version 2.0 achieved equivalent quantitation of each genotype over a narrow quantitative range (10^3–5×10^5 copies of RNA/ml), but significantly underestimated RNA concentrations above this value. (64) The currently available Chiron bDNA assay (version 2) showed equivalent sensitivity for genotypes 1 to 5; however, type 6a RNA transcripts and virus loads in clinical specimens were underestimated by a factor of 2 to 4. (64)

Vaccine Development

Currently, a vaccine for HCV remains a distant prospect. Generally weak and only transient serological responses are elicited by the immunization of chimpanzees with recombinant envelope proteins. However, even these low-level responses may provide some protection against infection or at least modulate the severity of disease arising from challenge with low doses of the homologous virus strain. (65)

There is currently controversy on the relative importance of humoral and cell-mediated immunity in vaccine protection, (65–68) which influences the potential effect that HCV genotype variation may have on vaccine development (see Chapter 25). If the effectiveness of an HCV vaccine depends on eliciting neutralizing antibodies, the degree of sequence variation between genotypes is likely to be problematic. HCV sequence variation is similar to that observed between serotypes of other viruses, such as those of dengue virus types 1–4, or between poliovirus types 1–3. Fully protective vaccines for dengue and polio are multivalent and contain antigens or attenuated virus strains of each of the serotypes. Despite the current unavailability of neutralization assays for HCV, it would be reasonable to assume that antigenic variation, particularly in the envelope proteins, E1 and E2, would have a significant effect on vaccine protection, and an effective HCV vaccine may have to multivalent in a manner similar to that of the poliovirus or dengue vaccines.

However, the T-cell-mediated component to the immune response elicited by an HCV vaccine may also be important in determining the outcome of exposure. The HCV core and NS3 regions, in particular, contain a number of highly conserved T-cell epitopes whose incorporation in a vaccine may provide protection against a range of HCV genotypes and circumvent the need to produce a multicomponent vaccine. In any case, assessment of efficacy of HCV vaccines will have to incorporate analysis of genotype differences.

Disease Progression

For most RNA viruses, the existence of extensive sequence differences between serotypes has remarkably little effect on the phenotype of a virus, other than in its antigenic properties. For example, poliovirus types 1, 2, and 3 appear equally infectious and equally likely to cause paralytic disease by spread into the nervous system. Similarly, different serotypes of dengue virus show similar propensities to cause viral hemorrhagic fever. On the basis of these and observations of other RNA viruses, there would be no *a priori* reason to suspect the existence of major differences between genotypes of HCV in their clinical course or disease associations.

The issue of clinical differences associated with HCV genotype has been investigated extensively, largely in cross-sectional studies where the frequencies of infection with different genotypes are compared in patients with different disease outcomes, such as in the development of cirrhosis, hepatocellular carcinoma (HCC), and extrahepatic manifestations such as cryoglobulinemia. These studies have frequently produced conflicting results. For instance, at least 11 studies published since 1994 concluded that HCV type 1b infection was no more likely to cause cirrhosis than other genotypes, (37, 69–78) whereas 10 similarly conducted investigations found a significantly greater proportion of type 1b infections among patients with cirrhosis. (79–88) Many studies have reported an increased frequency of alanine aminotransferase (ALT) elevations in patients infected with type 1b compared with type 2 HCV, although the ALT elevations were not necessarily associated with more severe disease as assessed by liver biopsy. (89–91) Importantly, these investigations may have been affected by different epidemiological characteristics of infection with different genotypes that cannot be corrected adequately using multivariate analysis. For example, it could be argued that the higher frequency of cirrhosis in HCV type 1-infected individuals was due to the longer mean duration of infection with genotype 1 than with other genotypes. For this reason, disease associations of genotype 3 HCV infections are particularly difficult to assess because of the association of this genotype with injection drug use and infection at a younger age. However, HCV type 1b- and type 2-infected individuals generally have similar age distributions and risk factors, yet often differ in the frequency of disease complications.

Most studies provide evidence that infection with HCV genotype 1b is more likely to lead to hepatocellular carcinoma than infection with other genotypes, (82,88,92–96) with few negative or contrary reports where significant numbers have been analyzed. (97,98) There are also several reports that after liver transplantation patients with HCV type 1b infection have a higher rate of progressive disease and graft loss. (99–104) Overall, it remains difficult to conclude with absolute certainty that type 1b (or type 1 generally) has a greater pathogenic potential than other genotypes, although the weight of evidence from numerous cross-sectional studies, particularly the more recent ones, supports this hypothesis. One can conclude that severe outcomes are possible with any genotype HCV infection. A controlled prospective investigation of disease progression among individuals with known durations of infection with different HCV genotypes is hampered by the variable, unpredictable, and slow course of disease.

Treatment

Interferon (IFN)-α has been investigated extensively as a treatment for HCV infection. In initial studies, the response to treatment was assessed biochemically by whether ALT levels fell to normal and histologically by whether there were improvements in liver histology after treatment. More recently, monitoring of HCV RNA by PCR has been used and responses defined on the basis of disappearance of viremia. Sustained responses to treatment are usually marked by improvements in all three factors. A sustained loss of HCV RNA appears to be the most reliable marker of long-term benefit.

While the association of HCV genotypes with different outcomes of infection is still debated, there is a clear association between HCV genotypes and the likelihood of a response to antiviral therapy in hepatitis C. A significant difference in response rates to interferon by genotype was found in 42 of 45 published studies, representing the collective experience of treating at least 4745 patients. In most trials, a sustained response was achieved in patients with genotypes 2 and 3 at a rate threefold higher than in patients with genotype 1. (105)

Higher rates of response, particularly patients infected with HCV type 1, have been achieved using higher doses of interferon (106,107) and, most strikingly, by a combination of INF-α with ribavirin. (108–111) The importance of genotyping was firmly documented in the recent controlled trials comparing IFN-α with combination therapy of interferon and ribavirin: sustained virological responses occurred in 60 to 64% of patients with genotype 2 or 3, but in only 10 to 33% of those with genotype 1. Importantly, extending combination therapy from 6 to 12 months yielded higher rates of response in patients with genotype 1 (from 17 to 30%), but not in patients with genotype 2 or 3 (66 and 65%). These findings indicate that patients with genotype 2 and 3 should be treated with 6 months of combination therapy and those with genotype 1 with 12 months. Thus, genotyping is clinically important in choosing the appropriate duration of therapy. There were insufficient numbers of patients with genotypes 4, 5, and 6 to provide reliable information about the optimal duration of therapy for these genotypes.

The mechanism for the observed differences in response rate among the different genotypes is not currently known. This difficulty is compounded by our current lack of knowledge about the mechanism of action of interferon in hepatitis C. Some experimental observations suggest a direct antiviral action, whereas others suggest that interferon is principally immunomodulatory and stimulates the immune system to clear the virus, as seems to be the case for hepatitis B. Genotype 1b HCV variants may also have a greater replicative capacity than other genotypes, possibly as a consequence of genetic differences in a region of NS5A, which acts as a cofactor for RNA replication. (112,113) Genotypes of HCV have also been shown experimentally to differ in their efficiencies of translation from the internal ribosomal entry site (IRES). (114–117) However, the common finding of greater IRES activity in HCV genotype 2 strains compared with type 1 does not provide an obvious explanation for its greater susceptibility to interferon or for its apparent reduced pathogenicity compared with genotype 1.

Pretreatment assessment of the genotype is helpful in counseling patients regarding the likelihood of a response to antiviral therapy and in choosing the optimal duration of therapy to achieve a sustained clearance of virus. An appropriate use of information about the genotype is, therefore, helpful in avoiding unnecessarily prolonging therapy and in helping to reduce side effects, as well as medical costs of treatment. For this reason, genotyping can be considered clinically indicated in the diagnosis and evaluation of patients with hepatitis C. (118)

In the future, pretreatment variables such as virus genotype should be incorporated into cost–benefit analyses of HCV treatment to assist in the development of policies for the more effective management of HCV infection. (119–121) Predictions of cost-effectiveness will also be improved by better understanding of the natural history of infection and elucidation of the biological differences between genotypes and their impact on human health.

CONCLUSION

At least six genotypes and more than 50 subtypes of HCV have been identified in sequencing studies of samples collected from various parts of the world. Genotypes typically differ by 31 to 34%, whereas subtypes differ by 20 to 23%, with little overlap. Genotype 1a, the originally described, prototype strain of HCV, is found predominantly in the United States and northern Europe.

Genotype 1b, initially described from Japan, has a worldwide distribution and is the most common genotype found in most of Europe, Japan, and parts of Asia. Genotype 3 is most common in the Indian subcontinent and is also typically found in injection drug users in the United States and Europe. Genotype 4 is the predominant genotype of Africa and the Middle East. Genotype 5 is found in enclaves in South Africa and genotype 6 in southeast Asia; both are rare. Most patients circulate one genotype only; between 5 and 10% are infected with multiple genotypes.

Nucleotide sequencing of PCR-amplified HCV RNA products is the method by which most genotypes were identified, but this technique is impractical for widespread clinical use. Other methods include RFLP of sequences amplified from the 5' NCR or hybridization with genotype-specific probes. Serological testing for genotype-specific antibodies to HCV can also be used and has the advantage of being inexpensive and easily applied to large numbers of specimens. Some of the variation in the detection of anti-HCV and in quantitation of HCV RNA may be attributable to genotype variation, and differences in genotypes must be considered in the future assessment of diagnostic reagents and vaccines against hepatitis C.

The clinical significance of genotypes is somewhat controversial. Data suggesting differences in outcome and severity of illness among the different genotypes are suggestive but inconclusive. However, findings indicate that the genotype of HCV does correlate with the likelihood of a response to antiviral therapy. In most studies, patients infected with HCV type 2 or 3 are at least threefold more likely to have a sustained response to antiviral therapy than patients with type 1 HCV. Furthermore, current recommendations for an optimal regimen of therapy in hepatitis C are based on genotype. The combination of interferon-α and ribavirin should be given for 12 months to patients with genotype 1, but need only be given for 6 months to patients with genotype 2 or 3.

REFERENCES

1. Choo Q L, Richman K H, Han J H, et al. Genetic organization and diversity of the hepatitis C virus. Proc Natl Acad Sci USA 1991;88:2451–5.
2. Okamoto H, Kurai K, Okada S, et al. Full-length sequence of a hepatitis C virus genome having poor homology to reported isolates: comparative study of four distinct genotypes. Virology 1992; 188:331–41.
3. Okamoto H, Okada S, Sugiyama Y, et al. Nucleotide sequence of the genomic RNA of hepatitis C virus isolated from a human carrier: comparison with reported isolates for conserved and divergent regions. J Gen Virol 1991;72:2697–704.
4. Mori S, Kato N, Yagyu A, et al. A new type of hepatitis C virus in patients in Thailand. Biochem Biophys Res Commun 1992;183:334–42.
5. Chan S W, McOmish F, Holmes E C, et al. Analysis of a new hepatitis C virus type and its phylogenetic relationship to existing variants. J Gen Virol 1992;73:1131–41.
6. Chamberlain R W, Adams N J, Taylor L A, Simmonds P, Elliott R M. The complete coding sequence of hepatitis C virus genotype 5a, the predominant genotype in South Africa. Biochem Biophys Res Commun 1997;236:44–9.
7. Felsenstein, J. PHYLIP Inference Package version 3.5, Seattle: Department of Genetics, University of Washington, 1993.

8. Simmonds P, Alberti A, Alter H J, et al. A proposed system for the nomenclature of hepatitis C viral genotypes. Hepatology 1994;19:1321–4.

9. Enomoto N, Takada A, Nakao T, Date T. There are two major types of hepatitis C virus in Japan. Biochem Biophys Res Commun 1990;170:1021–5.

10. Bukh J, Purcell R H, Miller R H. At least 12 genotypes of hepatitis C virus predicted by sequence analysis of the putative E1 gene of isolates collected worldwide. Proc Natl Acad Sci U S A 1993; 90:8234–8.

11. Bhattacherjee V, Prescott L E, Pike I, et al. Use of NS-4 peptides to identify type-specific antibody to hepatitis C virus genotypes 1, 2, 3, 4, 5 and 6. J Gen Virol 1995;76:1737–48.

12. Stuyver L, Vanarnhem W, Wyseur A, Hernandez F, Delaporte E, Maertens G. Classification of hepatitis C viruses based on phylogenetic analysis of the envelope 1 and nonstructural 5b regions and identification of five additional subtypes. Proc Natl Acad Sci U S A 1994;91: 10134–8.

13. Simmonds P, Smith D B, McOmish F, et al. Identification of genotypes of hepatitis C virus by sequence comparisons in the core, E1 and NS-5 regions. J Gen Virol 1994;75:1053–61.

14. Mellor J, Holmes E C, Jarvis L M, Yap P L, Simmonds P, International Collaborators. Investigation of the pattern of hepatitis C virus sequence diversity in different geographical regions: implications for virus classification. J Gen Virol 1995;76:2493–507.

15. Tokita H, Okamoto H, Tsuda F, et al. Hepatitis C virus variants from Vietnam are classifiable into the seventh, eighth, and ninth major genetic groups. Proc Natl Acad Sci U S A 1994;91: 11022–6.

16. Tokita H, Okamoto H, Luengrojanakul P, et al. Hepatitis C virus variants from Thailand classifiable into five novel genotypes in the sixth (6b), seventh (7c, 7d) and ninth (9b, 9c) major genetic groups. J Gen Virol 1995;76:2329–35.

17. Sugiyama K, Kato N, Nakazawa T, et al. Novel genotypes of hepatitis C virus in Thailand. J Gen Virol 1995;76:2323–7.

18. Robertson B, Myers G, Howard C, et al. Classification, nomenclature, and database development for hepatitis C virus (HCV) and related viruses: proposals for standardization. Arch Virol 1998;143:2493–503.

19. Simmonds P, Mellor J, Sakuldamrongpanich T, et al. Evolutionary analysis of variants of hepatitis C virus found in South-East Asia: Comparison with classifications based upon sequence similarity. J Gen Virol 1996;77:3013–24.

20. Mizokami M, Gojobori T, Ohba K I, et al. Hepatitis C virus types 7, 8 and 9 should be classified as type 6 subtypes. J Hepatol 1996;24:622–4.

21. Delamballerie X, Charrel R N, Attoui H, Demicco P. Classification of hepatitis C virus variants in six major types based on analysis of the envelope 1 and nonstructural 5B genome regions and complete polyprotein sequences. J Gen Virol 1997;78:45–51.

22. Fretz C, Jeannel D, Stuyver L, et al. HCV infection in a rural population of the Central African Republic (CAR): Evidence for three additional subtypes of genotype 4. J Med Virol 1995;47: 435–7.

23. Rapicetta M, Argentini C, Dettori S, Spada E, Pellizzer G, Gandin C. Molecular heterogeneity and new subtypes of HCV genotype 4. Res Virol 1998;149:293–7.

24. Simmonds P, McOmish F, Yap P L, et al. Sequence variability in the 5′ non coding region of hepatitis C virus: identification of a new virus type and restrictions on sequence diversity. J Gen Virol 1993;74:661–8.

25. McOmish F, Yap P L, Dow B C, et al. Geographical distribution of hepatitis C virus genotypes in blood donors—an international collaborative survey. J Clin Microbiol 1994;32:884–92.

26. Ruggieri A, Argentini C, Kouruma F, et al. Heterogeneity of hepatitis C virus genotype 2 variants in West Central Africa (Guinea Conakry). J Gen Virol 1996;77:2073–6.

27. Jeannel D, Fretz C, Traore Y, et al. Evidence for high genetic diversity and long-term endemicity of hepatitis C virus genotypes 1 and 2 in West Africa. J Med Virol 1998;55:92–7.

28. Tokita H, et al. Hepatitis C virus variants from Jakarta, Indonesia can be classified into the tenth and eleventh genetic groups. J Gen Virol 1996.

29. Okamoto H, Kojima M, Okada S-I, et al. Genetic drift of hepatitis C virus during an 8.2 year infection in a chimpanzee: variability and stability. Virology 1992;190:894–9.

30. Ogata N, Alter H J, Miller R H, Purcell RH. Nucleotide sequence and mutation rate of the H strain of hepatitis C virus. Proc Natl Acad Sci U S A 1991;88:3392–6.

31. Power J P, Lawlor E, Davidson F, et al. Hepatitis C viraemia in recipients of Irish intravenous anti-D immunoglobulin. Lancet 1994;344:1166–7.

32. Simmonds P, Holmes E C, Cha T A, et al. Classification of hepatitis C virus into six major genotypes and a series of subtypes by phylogenetic analysis of the NS-5 region. J Gen Virol 1993; 74:2391–9.

33. Lau J Y N, Mizokami M, Kolberg J A, et al. Application of six hepatitis C virus genotyping systems to sera from chronic hepatitis C patients in the United States. J Infect Dis 1995;171:281–9.

34. Power J P, Lawlor E, Davidson F, Holmes E C, Yap P L, Simmonds P. Molecular epidemiology of an outbreak of infection with hepatitis C virus in recipients of anti-D immunoglobulin. Lancet 1995;345:1211–3.

35. Smith D B, Pathirana S, Davidson F, et al. The origin of hepatitis C virus genotypes. J Gen Virol 1997;78:321–8.

36. Simmonds P, Smith D B. Investigation of the pattern of diversity of hepatitis C virus in relation to times of transmission. In: Anonymous. Hepatitis C virus: genetic heterogeneity and viral load. Paris: John Libbey Eurotext, 1997, 37–43.

37. Simmonds P, Mellor J, Craxi A, et al. Epidemiological, clinical and therapeutic associations of hepatitis C types in western European patients. J Hepatol 1996;24:517–24.

38. Simmonds P. Evolution of hepatitis C virus. In: Roberts D M, Sharp P, Alderson G, Collins M A, eds. Evolution of microbial life. Cambridge, UK: Cambridge University Press, 1996, 145–66.

39. Simmonds P, Smith D B. Structural constraints on RNA virus evolution. J Virol 1999;73: 5787–94.

40. Tanaka Y, Mizokami M, Orito E, et al. African origin of GB virus C hepatitis G virus. FEBS Lett 1998;423:143–8.

41. Charrel R N, de Micco P, de Lamballerie X. Phylogenetic analysis of GB viruses A and C: evidence for cospeciation between virus isolates and their primate hosts. J Gen Virol 1999;80: 2329–35.

42. Okamoto H, Sugiyama Y, Okada S, et al. Typing hepatitis C virus by polymerase chain reaction with type-specific primers: application to clinical surveys and tracing infectious sources. J Gen Virol 1992;73:673–9.

43. Okamoto H, Tokita H, Sakamoto M, et al. Characterization of the genomic sequence of type V (or 3a) hepatitis C virus isolates and PCR primers for specific detection. J Gen Virol 1993;74: 2385–90.

44. Ohno T, Mizokami M, Wu R R, et al. New hepatitis C virus (HCV) genotyping system that allows for identification of HCV genotypes 1a, 1b, 2a, 2b, 3a, 3b, 4, 5a, and 6a. J Clin Microbiol 1997;35:201–7.

45. Stuyver L, Rossau R, Wyseur A, et al. Typing of hepatitis C virus isolates and characterization of new subtypes using a line probe assay. J Gen Virol 1993;74:1093–102.

46. Tisminetzky S G, Gerotto M, Pontisso P, et al. Genotypes of hepatitis C virus in Italian patients with chronic hepatitis C. Int Hepatol Commun 1994;2:105–12.

47. Viazov S, Zibert A, Ramakrishnan K, et al. Typing of hepatitis C virus isolates by DNA enzyme immunoassay. J Virol Methods 1994;48:81–91.

48. Davidson F, Simmonds P, Ferguson J C, et al. Survey of major genotypes and subtypes of hepatitis C virus using RFLP of sequences amplified from the 5' non-coding region. J Gen Virol 1995; 76:1197–204.

49. Machida A, Ohnuma H, Tsuda F, et al. Two distinct subtypes of hepatitis C virus defined by antibodies directed to the putative core protein. Hepatology 1992;16:886–91.

50. Dixit V, Quan S, Martin P, et al. Evaluation of a novel serotyping system for hepatitis C virus: strong correlation with standard genotyping methodologies. J Clin Microbiol 1995;33:2978–83.

51. Schroter M, Feucht H H, Schafer P, Zollner B, Laufs R. Serological determination of hepatitis C virus subtypes 1a, 1b, 2a, 2b, 3a and 4a by a recombinant immunoblot assay. J Clin Microbiol 1999;37:2576–80.

52. Prescott L E, Berger A, Pawlotsky J M, Conjeevaram P, Pike I, Simmonds P. Sequence analysis of hepatitis C virus variants producing discrepant results with two different genotyping assays. J Med Virol 1997;53:237–44.

53. Simmonds P, Rose K A, Graham S, et al. Mapping of serotype-specific, immunodominant epitopes in the NS-4 region of hepatitis C virus (HCV)—use of type-specific peptides to serologi-

cally differentiate infections with HCV type 1, type 2, and type 3. J Clin Microbiol 1993;31: 1493–503.

54. Tanaka T, Tsukiyamakohara K, Yamaguchi K, et al. Significance of specific antibody assay for genotyping of hepatitis C virus. Hepatology 1994;19:1347–53.

55. McOmish F, Chan S-W, Dow B C, et al. Detection of three types of hepatitis C virus in blood donors: investigation of type-specific differences in serological reactivity and rate of alanine aminotransferase abnormalities. Transfusion 1993;33:7–13.

56. Pawlotsky J M, Roudotthoraval F, Pellet C, et al. Influence of hepatitis C virus (HCV) geno-types on HCV recombinant immunoblot assay patterns. J Clin Microbiol 1995;33:1357–9.

57. Neville J A, Prescott L E, Bhattacherjee V, et al. Antigenic variation of core, NS3, and NS5 pro-teins among genotypes of hepatitis C virus. J Clin Microbiol 1997;35:3062–70.

58. Beld M, Penning M, VanPutten M, et al. Quantitative antibody responses to structural (Core) and nonstructural (NS3, NS4, and NS5) hepatitis C virus proteins among seroconverting in-jecting drug users: Impact of epitope variation and relationship to detection of HCV RNA in blood. Hepatology 1999;29:1288–98.

59. Dhaliwal S K, Prescott L E, Dow B C, et al. Influence of viraemia and genotype upon serologi-cal reactivity in screening assays for antibody to hepatitis C virus. J Med Virol 1996;48:184–90.

60. Lelie P N, Cuypers H T M, Reesink H W, et al. Patterns of serological markers in transfusion-transmitted hepatitis-c virus infection using 2nd-generation HCV assays. J Med Virol 1992;37: 203–9.

61. Hawkins A, Davidson F, Simmonds P. Comparison of plasma virus loads among individuals in-fected with hepatitis C virus (HCV) genotypes 1, 2, and 3 by Quantiplex HCV RNA assay ver-sions 1 and 2, Roche monitor assay, and an in-house limiting dilution method. J Clin Microbiol 1997;35:187–92.

62. Olmedo E, Costa J, Lopez Labrador F X, et al. Comparative study of a modified competitive RT-PCR and Amplicor HCV monitor assays for quantitation of hepatitis C virus RNA in serum. J Med Virol 1999;58:35–43.

63. Tong C Y W, Hollingsworth R C, Williams H, Irving W L, Gilmore I T. Effect of genotypes on the quantification of hepatitis C virus (HCV) RNA in clinical samples using the amplicor HCV monitor test and the quantiplex HCV RNA 2.0 assay (BDNA). J Med Virol 1998;55:191–6.

64. Mellor J, Hawkins A, Simmonds P. Genotype dependence of hepatitis C virus load measure-ment in commercially available quantitative assays. J Clin Microbiol 1999;37:2525–32.

65. Choo Q L, Kuo G, Ralston R, et al. Vaccination of chimpanzees against infection by the hepa-titis C virus. Proc Natl Acad Sci U S A 1994;91:1294–8.

66. Encke J, Putlitz J Z, Geissler M, Wands J R. Genetic immunization generates cellular and hu-moral immune responses against the nonstructural proteins of the hepatitis C virus in a murine model. J Immunol 1998;161:4917–23.

67. Lee S W, Cho J H, Lee K J, Sung Y C. Hepatitis C virus envelope DNA-based immunization elicits humoral and cellular immune responses. Mol Cells 1998;8:444–51.

68. Cooper S, Erickson A L, Adams E J, et al. Analysis of a successful immune response against hepatitis C virus. Immunity 1999;10:439–49.

69. Mita E, Hayashi N, Kanazawa Y, et al. Hepatitis C virus genotype and RNA titer in the pro-gression of type c chronic liver disease. J Hepatol 1994;21:468–73.

70. Yamada M, Kakumu S, Yoshioka K, et al. Hepatitis C virus genotypes are not responsible for development of serious liver disease. Dig Dis Sci 1994;39:234–9.

71. Dusheiko G, Schmilovitzweiss H, Brown D, et al. Hepatitis C virus genotypes—an investiga-tion of type- specific differences in geographic origin and disease. Hepatology 1994;19:13–8.

72. Lau J Y N, Davis G L, Prescott L E, et al. Distribution of hepatitis C virus genotypes determined by line probe assay in patients with chronic hepatitis C seen at tertiary referral centers in the United States. Ann Intern Med 1996;124:868.

73. Kleter B, Brouwer J T, Nevens F, et al. Hepatitis C virus genotypes: Epidemiological and clini-cal associations. Liver 1998;18:32–8.

74. Benvegnu L B, Pontisso P, Cavalletto D, Noventa F, Chemello L, Alberti A. Lack of correlation between hepatitis C virus genotypes and clinical course of hepatitis C virus-related cirrhosis. Hepatology 1997;25:211–5.

75. Cicciarello S, Borgia G, Crowell J, et al. Prevalence of hepatitis C virus genotypes in southern Italy. Eur J Epidemiol 1997;13:49–54.

76. Mangia A, Cascavilla I, Lezzi G, et al. HCV genotypes in patients with liver disease of different stages and severity. J Hepatol 1997;26:1173–8.

77. Poynard T, Bedossa P, Opolon P. Natural history of liver fibrosis progression in patients with chronic hepatitis C. Lancet 1997;349:825–32.

78. Puoti C, Magrini A, Stati T, et al. Clinical, histological, and virological features of hepatitis C virus carriers with persistently normal or abnormal alanine transaminase levels. Hepatology 1997;26:1393–8.

79. Booth J C L, Foster G R, Kumar U, et al. Chronic hepatitis C virus infections: predictive value of genotype and level of viraemia on disease progression and response to interferon alpha. Gut 1995;36:427–32.

80. Kasahara A, Hayashi N, Hiramatsu N, et al. Ability of prolonged interferon treatment to suppress relapse after cessation of therapy in patients with chronic hepatitis C: a multicenter randomized controlled trial. Hepatology 1995;21:291–7.

81. Kobayashi M, Tanaka E, Sodeyama T, Urushihara A, Matsumoto A, Kiyosawa K. The natural course of chronic hepatitis C: A comparison between patients with genotypes 1 and 2 hepatitis C viruses. Hepatology 1996;23:695–9.

82. Takada A, Tsutsumi M, Zhang S C, et al. Relationship between hepatocellular carcinoma and subtypes of hepatitis C virus: A nationwide analysis. J Gastroenterol Hepatol 1996;1:166–9.

83. Watson J P, Brind A M, Chapman C E, et al. Hepatitis C virus: Epidemiology and genotypes in the north east of England. Gut 1996;38:269–76.

84. Goeser T, Tox U, Muller H M, Arnold J C, Theilmann L. Genotypes in chronic hepatitis C virus (HCV) infection and in liver cirrhosis caused by HCV in Germany. Dtsch Med Wochenschr 1995;120:1070–3.

85. Tassopoulos N C, Papatheodoridis G V, Katsoulidou A, et al. Factors associated with severity and disease progression in chronic hepatitis C. Hepatogastroenterology 1998;45:1678–83.

86. Booth J C L, Foster G R, Levine T, Thomas H C, Goldin R D. The relationship of histology to genotype in chronic HCV infection. Liver 1997;17:144–51.

87. Fernandez I, Castellano G, Domingo M J, et al. Influence of viral genotype and level of viremia on the severity of liver injury and the response to interferon therapy in Spanish patients with chronic C infection. Scand J Gastroenterol 1997;32:70–6.

88. LopezLabrador F X, Ampurdanes S, Forns X, et al. Hepatitis C virus (HCV) genotypes in Spanish patients with HCV infection: relationship between HCV genotype 1b, cirrhosis and hepatocellular carcinoma. J Hepatol 1997;27:959–65.

89. Prati D, Capelli C, Zanella A, et al. Influence of different hepatitis C virus genotypes on the course of asymptomatic hepatitis C virus infection. Gastroenterology 1996;110:178–83.

90. Zignego A L, Ferri C, Giannini C, et al. Hepatitis C virus genotype analysis in patients with type II mixed cryoglobulinemia. Ann Intern Med 1996;124:31–4.

91. Tsuji H, Shimomura H, Wato M, Kondo J, Tsuji T. Virological and serological characterization of asymptomatic blood donors positive for anti-hepatitis C virus antibody. Acta Med Okayama 1995;49:137–44.

92. Yamauchi M, Nakahara M, Nakajima H, Sakamoto K, Hirakawa J, Toda G. Different prevalence of hepatocellular carcinoma between patients with liver cirrhosis due to genotype II and III of hepatitis C virus. Int Hepatol Commun 1994;2:328–32.

93. Chen C H, Sheu J C, Wang J T, et al. Genotypes of hepatitis C virus in chronic liver disease in Taiwan. J Med Virol 1994;44:234–6.

94. Haydon G H, Jarvis L M, Simmonds P, Hayes P C. Association between chronic hepatitis C infection and hepatocellular carcinoma. Lancet 1995;345:928–9.

95. Tanaka K, Ikematsu H, Hirohata T, Kashiwagi S. Hepatitis C virus infection and risk of hepatocellular carcinoma among Japanese: Possible role of type 1b (II) infection. J Natl Cancer Inst 1996;88:742–6.

96. Bruno S, Silini E, Crosignani A, et al. Hepatitis C virus genotypes and risk of hepatocellular carcinoma in cirrhosis: A prospective study. Hepatology 1997;25:754–8.

97. Yotsuyanagi H, Koike K, Yasuda K, et al. Hepatitis C virus genotypes and development of hepatocellular carcinoma. Cancer 1995;76:1352–5.

98. Lee D S, Sung Y C, Whang Y S. Distribution of HCV genotypes among blood donors, patients with chronic liver disease, hepatocellular carcinoma, and patients on maintenance hemodialysis in Korea. J Med Virol 1996;49:55–60.

99. Feray C, Gigou M, Samuel D, et al. Influence of the genotypes of hepatitis C virus on the severity of recurrent liver disease after liver transplantation. Gastroenterology 1995;108:1088–96.

100. Gane E J, Naoumov N V, Qian K P, et al. A longitudinal analysis of hepatitis C virus replication following liver transplantation. Gastroenterology 1996;110:167–77.

101. Cane E J, Portmann B C, Naoumov N V, et al. Long-term outcome of hepatitis C infection after liver transplantation. N Engl J Med 1996;334:815–20.

102. Casino C, Lilli D, Rivanera D, et al. Recurrence of hepatitis c virus infection after orthotopic liver transplantation: Role of genotypes. Microbiologica 1999;22:11–8.

103. Costes V, Durand L, Pageaux G P, et al. Hepatitis C virus genotypes and quantification of serum hepatitis C RNA in liver transplant recipients—relationship with histologic outcome of recurrent hepatitis C. Am J Clin Pathol 1999;111:252–8.

104. Berg T, Hopf U, Bechstein W O, et al. Pretransplant virological markers hepatitis C virus genotype and viremia level are not helpful in predicting individual outcome after orthotopic liver transplantation. Transplantation 1998;66:225–8.

105. Bell H, Hellum K, Harthug S, et al. Genotype, viral load and age as independent predictors of treatment outcome of interferon-alpha 2a treatment in patients with chronic hepatitis C. Scand J Infect Dis 1997;29:17–22.

106. Ideo G, Bellobuono A, Mondazzi L, et al. Alpha interferon treatment in chronic hepatitis C. Clin Exp Rheumatol 1995;13:S167-73.

107. Chemello L, Bonetti P, Cavalletto L, et al. Randomized trial comparing three different regimens of alpha-2a-interferon in chronic hepatitis C. Hepatology 1995;22:700–6.

108. Braconier J H, Paulsen O, Engman K, Widell A. Combined alpha-interferon and ribavirin treatment in chronic hepatitis C: a pilot study. Scand J Infect Dis 1995;27:325–9.

109. Chemello L, Cavalletto L, Bernardinello E, Guido M, Pontisso P, Alberti A. The effect of interferon alfa and ribavirin combination therapy in naive patients with chronic hepatitis C. J Hepatol 1995;23:8–12.

110. McHutchison J G, Gordon S C, Schiff E R, et al. Interferon alfa-2b alone or in combination with ribavirin as initial treatment for chronic hepatitis C. N Engl J Med 1998;339:1485–92.

111. Davis G L, EstebanMur R, Rustgi V, et al. Interferon alfa-2b alone or in combination with ribavirin for the treatment of relapse of chronic hepatitis C. N Engl J Med 1998;339:1493–9.

112. Enomoto N, Sakuma I, Asahina Y, et al. Mutations in the nonstructural protein 5A gene and response to interferon in patients with chronic hepatitis C virus 1b infection. N Engl J Med 1996;334:77–81.

113. Enomoto N, Sakuma I, Asahina Y, et al. Comparison of full-length sequences of interferon-sensitive and resistant hepatitis C virus 1b—sensitivity to interferon is conferred by amino acid substitutions in the NS5a region. J Clin Invest 1995;96:224–30.

114. Honda M, Rijnbrand R, Abell G, Kim D S, Lemon S M. Natural variation in translational activities of the 5′ nontranslated RNAs of hepatitis C virus genotypes 1a and 1b: Evidence for a long-range RNA-RNA interaction outside of the internal ribosomal entry site. J Virol 1999;73:4941–51.

115. Collier A J, Tang S X, Elliott R M. Translation efficiencies of the 5′ untranslated region from representatives of the six major genotypes of hepatitis C virus using a novel bicistronic reporter assay system. J Gen Virol 1998;79:2359–66.

116. Buratti E, Gerotto M, Pontisso P, Alberti A, Tisminetzky S G, Baralle F E. In vivo translational efficiency of different hepatitis C virus 5′-UTRs. FEBS Lett 1997;411:275–80.

117. Tsukiyama Kohara K, Iizuka N, Kohara M, Nomoto A. Internal ribosome entry site within hepatitis C virus RNA. J Virol 1992;66:1476–83.

118. Anonymous. EASL International Consensus Conference on Hepatitis C—Consensus Statement. J Hepatol 1999;30:956–61.

119. Bennett W G, Inoue Y, Beck J R, Wong J B, Pauker S G, Davis G L. Estimates of the cost-effectiveness of a single course of interferon- alpha 2b in patients with histologically mild chronic hepatitis C. Ann Intern Med 1997;127:855.

120. Koff R S. Therapy of hepatitis C: Cost-effectiveness analysis. Hepatology 1997;26:S152–5.

121. Dusheiko G M, Roberts J A. Treatment of chronic type B and C hepatitis with interferon alpha: an economic appraisal. Hepatology 1995;22:1880–2.

4
ACUTE HEPATITIS C

JAY H. HOOFNAGLE
Liver Diseases Section, Digestive Diseases Branch
National Institute of Diabetes and Digestive and Kidney Diseases
National Institutes of Health
Bethesda, Maryland

INTRODUCTION

Acute hepatitis C accounts for 15 to 16% of cases of acute, icteric hepatitis in the United States, ranking below acute hepatitis A (47 to 49%) and B (33 to 35%). (1) The incidence of acute hepatitis C appears to be falling. The Centers for Disease Control and Prevention (CDC) estimate that in 1996 there were 36,000 new cases of hepatitis C, which was down from 230,000 cases per year in the 1980s and probably a greater number in the 1960s and 1970s. (2) Reasons for the decrease in incidence of hepatitis C are multiple and include the disappearance of posttransfusion hepatitis C with the introduction of screening for anti-HCV (3), more rigorous use of universal precautions in medical settings, and a decrease either in injection drug use or in transmission of hepatitis C during drug use. Whatever the cause, acute hepatitis C is now becoming an uncommon disease in the United States.

At present, the majority of cases of acute hepatitis C can be attributed to parenteral exposures, most commonly injection drug use and accidental needlestick. (4) In an analysis of 170 cases of acute hepatitis C identified in a population-based surveillance system in the United States, (5) 43% of cases were associated with injection drug use, 17% were attributed to sexual exposure to an infected individual or high-risk sexual behavior, and less than 10% to other known risk factors (medical care occupation, blood transfusion, household exposures). The source of infection was unknown in 31% of cases. Whether the source of infection in these patients was unacknowledged injection drug use, sexual exposure, or other inapparent parenteral exposures remains unclear.

CLINICAL COURSE: ACUTE, SELF-LIMITED HEPATITIS C

Clinical symptoms and signs, biochemical laboratory tests results, and liver histology in acute hepatitis C resemble those of other forms of acute viral hepatitis. The disease can be distinguished as HCV related only by serological or virological testing. (2,6) The clinical hallmarks of acute hepatitis C are the frequency of progression to chronicity (6–8) and the infrequency of fulminant disease. (9)

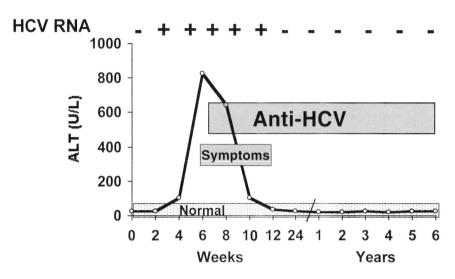

FIGURE I Self-limited acute hepatitis C. ALT, alanine aminotransferase; HCV RNA, hepatitis C viral RNA.

The clinical, biochemical, and serological course of a typical case of acute hepatitis C with recovery is shown in Fig. 1.

Incubation Period

The *incubation period* of acute hepatitis C, defined as the time from exposure to onset of symptoms, ranges from 2 to 12 weeks and averages 7 weeks. (6–8, 10–16) The wide range of incubation periods between that of hepatitis A (averaging 3 to 4 weeks) and hepatitis B (averaging 9 to 12 weeks) and the difficulty of defining the time of exposure make the incubation period an unreliable indicator of serological diagnosis. In addition, virological testing shows that HCV RNA becomes detectable well before the onset of symptoms and that most patients become HCV RNA positive within 1 to 2 weeks of exposure. (17) Subsequently, levels of HCV RNA rise and reach titers of 10^5 to 10^7 copies per milliliter by the onset of dark urine or jaundice. (18)

Preicteric Phase

The preicteric phase of hepatitis C is defined as the period between the onset of nonspecific symptoms and the onset of jaundice or dark urine. This period usually lasts for 2 to 10 days. Symptoms include fatigue, poor appetite, feverishness, nausea, and right upper quadrant discomfort. Because symptoms are nonspecific, the diagnosis of acute hepatitis C is rarely made at this time, unless patients are being monitored after a parenteral or other exposure. Some patients develop a serum sickness-like syndrome during the preicteric phase of hepatitis C, marked clinically by rash, hives, arthalgias, and low-grade fever. This syndrome probably represents the effects of circulating immune complexes: serum complement levels are generally low. The symptoms are generally short-lived and resolve quickly with the onset of jaundice. This syndrome occurs most frequently with acute hepatitis B, but can also occur with HCV infection.

Icteric Phase

The icteric phase of hepatitis C is initiated with the onset of dark urine or jaundice. Rarely, jaundice is the first clinical symptom, and there is no preicteric phase of nonspecific constitutional symptoms. Symptoms and jaundice typically worsen for 1 to 2 weeks and then begin to abate. The most common symptoms are fatigue, lethargy, weakness, muscle and headaches, low-grade fever, nausea, and right upper quadrant pain. The duration of jaundice and symptoms in acute hepatitis C is variable. Prolonged symptoms and fatigue are not uncommon. Most patients are reactive for HCV RNA during the preicteric and icteric phases of disease, but titers of viral genome fluctuate greatly and some patients test intermittently negative for HCV RNA, even by sensitive assays. (16–18) Anti-HCV generally first becomes detected during the icteric phase (or occasionally the late preicteric phase) of illness. (6–8,11–16) Immunoblot assays demonstrate that the earliest reactivities are to the core and NS3 regions of the viral genome (anti-22c and c33 by recombinant immunoblot assay; RIBA). Antibodies to NS4 and the envelope regions (anti-E1 and anti-E2) arise somewhat later. Using second-generation assays, approximately 70% of patients have detectable anti-HCV by enzyme immunoassays (EIA) by the time of onset of symptoms or jaundice, and almost all patients are reactive within 2 months of onset. (16)

Convalescence

The convalescent phase of hepatitis C is usually demarcated by the disappearance of jaundice. Mild constitutional symptoms may persist for several months. The return of appetite and weight gain are the most reliable symptoms of beginning convalescence. Of course, clinical convalescence and disappearance of symptoms and signs of hepatitis do not always indicate resolution of the infection or disease. In hepatitis C, between 55 and 90% of patients develop chronic HCV infection, averaging 75% among adults and 55% in children. (6–8,15–21) Titers of anti-HCV tend to be low during the acute phase of hepatitis C, gradually rising thereafter, particularly in patients who develop chronic infection. Few studies have addressed the issue of whether anti-HCV titers or profiles during the acute illness can distinguish patients who ultimately recover from those who develop chronic infection. A proportion of patients with self-limited hepatitis C either do not produce anti-HCV or produce anti-HCV for a short time only. (16–21) In long-term follow-up studies, at least 10% of patients ultimately lose anti-HCV reactivity and are left without serological evidence of previous hepatitis C. In these patients without anti-HCV, T-cell responses to HCV can be detected. (22) The immunological features that accompany recovery and determine the outcome of acute hepatitis C are discussed in more detail in Chapters 7 and 8.

Patients who have acute self-limited hepatitis C in follow-up appear to have truly recovered from the infection: serum aminotransferase (ALT) levels are normal and there appears to be no symptoms of liver disease and no long-term consequences. Interestingly, patients with anti-HCV without HCV RNA may have minor abnormalities on liver biopsy, spotty inflammation, and occasional areas of focal necrosis. (23) Reasons for these abnormalities are not clear, whether they represent residual viral replication, presence of low levels of viral antigens, an autoimmune phenomenon induced by the previous hepatitis, or an incidental and nonspecific finding unrelated to hepatitis C. The persistence of low levels of virus or integrated genomic material that occur in many viral infections, including hepatitis B, does not appear to occur with hepatitis C.

CLINICAL COURSE: DEVELOPMENT OF CHRONIC HEPATITIS C

The course of a patient developing chronic hepatitis C is shown in Fig. 2. The initial clinical, biochemical, and virological features are similar to what occurs with acute, self-limited disease. Approximately one-third of patients who develop chronic hepatitis C have clinical symptoms or signs that are compatible with the diagnosis of acute hepatitis C at the time of onset of infection. (10–13, 15,16) During this phase, there are no clinical or biochemical features that distinguish whether the patient is developing chronic infection. In general, titers

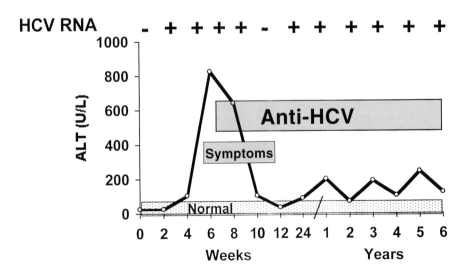

FIGURE 2 Acute hepatitis C with progression to chronic infection. See legend to Fig. 1.

of HCV RNA reach higher and more sustained levels during the acute phase of infection in patients who develop chronic viremia, but the amount of variability in the quantitative assays for HCV RNA and the spontaneous fluctuations in levels of viremia make this clinically unhelpful. (11) Indeed, in several instances patients can become transiently HCV RNA negative, despite having chronic viremia during follow-up. (17,24) This typically occurs during the acute phase of infection. Once the infection is chronic, levels of HCV RNA tend to be stable and spontaneous clearance of virus is uncommon.

The diagnosis of chronic hepatitis C is generally dependent on the persistence of ALT elevations and HCV RNA in serum for 6 months or longer. Follow-up of humans at a high risk of developing HCV infection and experimental animals inoculated with infectious material demonstrates that self-limited infection may be associated with a delayed clearance of HCV RNA. (24) However, loss of HCV RNA more than 6 months after the onset of hepatitis C is relatively uncommon and may be best described as early spontaneous recovery from chronic hepatitis C rather than late recovery from acute (self-limited) disease.

Not all patients who develop chronic hepatitis C persist in having elevations in serum aminotransferase levels. In prospective and retrospective–prospective studies, between 25 and 50% of patients who develop chronic HCV infection have persistently normal ALT values. (6,7,10–16,19,20,24,25,26) These patients are sometimes referred to as "healthy HCV carriers," but the term is inappropriate and almost all have chronic hepatitis with an active inflammatory component on liver biopsy. (23,25) Indeed, in some patients the disease appears to be progressive and severe despite normal ALT levels. In most patients with moderate or severe hepatitis by liver biopsy, despite normal ALT levels, there are other features that indicate significant disease, such as elevations in aspartate aminotransferase (AST) or γ-glutamyl transpeptidase (GGTP) levels or abnormalities of serum albumin, bilirubin, prothrombin time, or platelet counts. Further discussion of chronic hepatitis C is given in Chapter 13.

DIAGNOSIS

Anti-HCV Testing

The diagnosis of acute hepatitis C can be problematic. As shown in Figs. 1 and 2, anti-HCV tends to arise late during the course of disease and is not detectable in serum at the onset of symptoms or jaundice in approximately 30% of patients. (16,27) By a month after the onset of symptoms, more than 90% of patients have anti-HCV. Thus, the diagnosis of acute hepatitis C can be missed if anti-HCV testing is used alone. In addition, the presence of anti-HCV does not prove the diagnosis of acute hepatitis C; the patient may have acute hepatitis A or another form of liver injury and have preexisting anti-HCV due to previous exposures. Indeed, the high-risk patient for acquiring hepatitis C may also be at high risk for acquiring hepatitis A and B. Finally, patients may actually have chronic hepatitis C and be suffering an acute, symptomatic exacerbation of the disease. (28)

IgM Anti-HCV

In many other acute viral infections, specific IgM responses are used to distinguish between acute and chronic infections. In hepatitis C, however, IgM anti-HCV is not a reliable marker for acute disease. (29–31) IgM anti-HCV can be detected in both acute and chronic hepatitis C, and titers of IgM antibody are not particularly high during the acute phase of illness. There are no IgM anti-HCV assays available commercially as the test remains a research assay of uncertain clinical significance.

Seroconversion

More helpful in the diagnosis of acute hepatitis C than specific IgM responses is a documented seroconversion to anti-HCV positivity. (10–16) Thus, the diagnosis can confidently be made in a patient with the clinical features of acute hepatitis who initially tests nonreactive for anti-HCV but who is later positive. Similarly, immunoblot testing can provide insights; the presence of antibody to only one or two HCV antigens followed by the development of strong reactions with three or four bands in the assay is fairly reliable evidence of acute infection with HCV. (18) Furthermore, testing for antibodies to specific HCV proteins by EIA methods, such as antibodies to the envelope proteins E1 and E2, may help demonstrate an acute seroconversion. (32) However, these approaches are not particularly clinically relevant; they rely on expensive and repeat serological testing. At the present time, commercial laboratories employ immunoblot testing but usually do not report which bands are reactive and the intensity of the reaction.

HCV RNA Testing

The majority of patients with acute hepatitis C are reactive for HCV RNA during the incubation period and both icteric and anicteric phases of illness. (16–18) Testing for HCV RNA can identify the case of acute hepatitis as being due to hepatitis C. However, the presence of HCV RNA does not prove that the disease is acute as opposed to chronic. Furthermore, some patients with acute hepatitis C are only intermittently reactive for HCV RNA. (24,27) Even patients who go on to develop chronic hepatitis C may test negative for HCV RNA transiently during the icteric or early convalescent phase of illness. Thus, the presence of HCV RNA is reliable in documenting ongoing HCV infection, but does not prove that the infection is acute or chronic; furthermore, the absence of HCV RNA is evidence for but not proof of lack of ongoing hepatitis C.

Algorithm for Diagnosis of Acute Viral Hepatitis

Thus, there is no one specific serological or virological assay that proves the diagnosis of acute hepatitis C; the diagnosis relies on a combination of clinical, serological, and virological features. Table I provides a clinically useful paradigm to approach the diagnosis of a patient with clinical features of acute hepatitis.

■■■ **TABLE I** **Algorithm for Diagnosis of Acute Viral Hepatitis**

Test	Interpretation	Other tests
IgM anti-HAV	Diagnostic of acute hepatitis A	False positives occur but are rare
HBsAg	Indicates hepatitis B, but does not distinguish between acute and chronic infection	HBV DNA testing indicates active viral replication Anti-HDV should be tested to rule out delta hepatitis
IgM anti-HBc	Diagnostic of acute hepatitis B (rarely during severe exacerbation or reactivation)	False positives occur but are rare
Anti-HCV	Indicates hepatitis C, but does not distinguish between acute and chronic infection	HCV RNA suggests diagnosis of acute hepatitis C in the correct clinical setting
All markers negative	Hepatitis C can only be ruled out by retesting for anti-HCV in 4–8 weeks Consider other acute liver diseases: mononucleosis, syphilis, cholangitis, drug-induced liver disease, autoimmune hepatitis, Wilson's disease, and finally non-A-E hepatitis	Heterophile antibody Complete blood counts, VDRL, Antinuclear Antibody Ultrasound Careful history of drug intake, including vitamins and herbal preparations

THERAPY OF ACUTE HEPATITIS C

At present there are no specific therapies of proven benefit for acute hepatitis C. The mainstays of management include bed rest, adequate nutrition, and avoidance of alcohol and all but the most necessary medications. If signs and symptoms of hepatic failure supervene, patients should be referred early for consideration of emergency liver transplantation. (9) However, symptomatic acute hepatitis C usually resolves without complications and with no specific treatment. The major complication, and the rationale to attempt specific antiviral therapy during the course of acute hepatitis C, is the development of chronic infection and liver injury. Without therapy, HCV infection resolves in only 25% of cases, although this rate may be higher in children, (21) young patients, and in women. (19)

Studies of Interferon-α Therapy

The possibility that therapy during the course of acute hepatitis C might shorten the period of illness, ameliorate symptoms and hepatic injury, and prevent chronicity has led to several controlled and uncontrolled trials of therapy with interferon-α or -β. (33–42) All studies were small and limited by the infrequency of new cases of acute hepatitis C, particularly as most studies were done among recipients of blood or blood products who were being followed prospectively after transfusion. With the introduction of routine screening of blood for anti-HCV, posttransfusion hepatitis C has become rare and new cases of acute hepatitis C have all but disappeared.

■■■ **TABLE II**   Seven Randomized Controlled Trials of Type I Interferon
in Acute Hepatitis C

Authors (year/ reference) Regimen	No. patients studied	Interferon		No treatment	
		Normal ALT	HCV RNA negative	Normal ALT	HCV RNA negative
Omata et al. (1991) (33) Interferon-β (3 mu daily for 4 weeks)	25	7/11 (64%)	6/10 (60%)	1/14 (7%)	0/12 (0%)
Viladomiu et al. (1992) (34) Interferon-α2b (3 mu tiw for 12 weeks)	28	8/15 (53%)	Not reported	4/13 (31%)	Not reported
Tassopoulos et al. (1993) (35) Interferon-α2b (3 mu tiw for 6 weeks)	24	6/12 (50%)	Not reported	3/12 (25%)	Not reported
Alberti et al. (1994) (36) Interferon-α2a (6 mu tiw for 16–24 weeks)	21	8/11 (73%)	7/11 (64%)	2/10 (20%)	2/10 (20%)
Palmovic et al. (1994) (37) Interferon-α2b (3 mu tiw for 24 weeks)	30	8/16 (50%)	Not reported	4/14 (29%)	Not reported
Lampertico et al. (1994) (38) Interferon-α2b (3 mu tiw for 12 weeks)	38	3/22 (59%)	7/22 (39%)	6/16 (37%)	0/16 (0%)
Hwang et al. (1994) (39) Interferon-α2b (3 mu tiw for 3 months)	33	9/16 (56%)	7/16 (44%)	6/17 (37%)	2/17 (13%)
Total	199	59/103 (57%)	27/59 (46%)	29/96 (27%)	4/55 (7%)

There have been seven randomized controlled trials of interferon therapy of acute hepatitis C (Table II). (41) Many differed in design, dose, and regimen of interferon, type of interferon used, criteria for entry, criteria for beneficial response, and rigor of monitoring and follow-up. Nevertheless, all studies showed a decrease in the rate of chronic infection among patients treated with interferon-α or -β during the acute phase of the disease (generally 1 to 4 months after the onset of aminotransferase elevations or symptoms). The sustained response rate (loss of HCV RNA) in these studies ranged from 39 to 64% and averaged 46%. Among untreated patients in control groups, 0 to 20% (average = 7%) recovered and became negative for HCV RNA. Interestingly, patients who had a long-term response to treatment often became or remained anti-HCV negative with treatment. (34,36,38) Responding patients also had normal serum aminotransferase levels and remained HCV RNA negative during long-term follow-up.

The largest study of therapy of acute hepatitis C with interferon was a randomized, dose-ranging study from Japan that did not include an untreated control group. (40) Ninety-seven patients were enrolled, but only 90 could be analyzed, of whom only 65 were found to have HCV RNA at the start of therapy.

Patients were randomized to six regimens of interferon-β using doses of 0.3, 3, or 6 million units given intravenously for either 28 or 56 days. Thus the total dosage ranged from 8.4 to 336 million units. Of the 65 patients with HCV RNA at the start of therapy, 26 (40%) had a sustained virological response. Response rates were higher with higher total doses of interferon, being 10% (2/21) in patients given the lowest dose, 44% (11/25) given the intermediate dose, and 68% (13/19) given the highest dose. Thus, if the lowest dose regimen is considered equivalent to no treatment, higher doses were clearly associated with a significantly higher rate of virological response. Nevertheless, it is difficult to extrapolate these findings using interferon-β given daily by the intravenous route to use of interferon-α given three times weekly by subcutaneous injection. Indeed, in a more recent multicenter-randomized controlled trial of interferon-β (3 million units three times weekly intramuscularly for 4 weeks) in 40 patients with acute hepatitis C conducted in Italy, the long-term virological response rate was the same with treatment (5 of 20; 25%) as with monitoring without treatment (4 of 20; 20%). (41) The study can perhaps be faulted for the short duration of therapy (4 weeks).

There have been a large number of case series and individual case reports published describing therapy of acute hepatitis C with interferon-α. (43–46) If one assumes that the spontaneous clearance rate of virus during acute hepatitis C is 15 to 25%, many of these reports are supportive of the efficacy of interferon therapy during the acute phase of hepatitis C. In a study from Austria, (43) 22 compliant patients with acute icteric hepatitis C and HCV RNA in serum were treated with interferon in doses of 10 million units daily until serum aminotransferase levels were normal (18 to 43 days: total dose 140 to 430 million units). Patients were largely injection drug users, and initial serum bilirubin levels ranged from 5 to 12 mg/dl and ALT levels from 531 to 1940 IU/liter at the start of treatment. All 22 patients became HCV RNA negative during therapy and all except 2 remained negative during 7 to 42 months of follow-up after therapy.

Several studies have focused on the prevention of hepatitis C after needlestick accident by early treatment with interferon. In prospective studies after needlestick accidents, only 5 to 10% of subjects developed hepatitis C. (47,48) In addition, case studies have documented that early intervention with interferon treatment does not prevent infection. (49) Thus, intervention before the appearance of markers of HCV infection does not appear to be either needed or effective. However, HCV RNA is often detectable in serum within 1 to 2 weeks of exposure, and initiation of therapy immediately after the appearance of viremia might be appropriate. (50–53) Large-scale studies of early intervention have yet to be reported.

The many studies of interferon therapy in acute hepatitis C have shown that therapy can be effective. However, one cannot conclude from the results of these trials that patients should be treated during the acute phase of illness. The issue is not whether interferon therapy can lead to a sustained clearance of HCV RNA; this fact has been well documented in studies of chronic hepatitis C. The important issue is whether the initiation of treatment during the acute phase of illness is safer and more effective than the initiation of treatment once the disease has clearly become chronic. This concept is important, both from a research and biological point of view, as well as from a clinical and patient care point of view. By initiating therapy early, one treats some patients who would resolve the infection spontaneously, exposing these patients to the expense and adverse side effects of therapy. However, early therapy may be more effective than delayed therapy in eradicating the virus, leading to a more rapid resolution of symptoms. Early therapy may also allow for a shorter course of treatment and be more readily acceptable to the patient with acute disease.

The advantages of early therapy, however, have yet to be demonstrated. Studies that have suggested that a short duration of disease is associated with a higher likelihood of response to antiviral therapy have been flawed by not controlling for other important factors, such as viral genotype, titer, patient gender, and age. (54,55) Furthermore, these studies have usually considered a short duration of infection as less than 5 or 10 years, not less than a few months. Thus, the greater efficacy of early over delayed therapy has not been shown; indeed, the response rates in most studies of acute hepatitis C were similar to those reported among patients with chronic hepatitis C.

Combination Therapy with Interferon-α and Ribavirin

With the demonstration that the combination of interferon-α and ribavirin is superior to interferon monotherapy as therapy of chronic hepatitis C, (56–58) the issue of therapy of acute hepatitis C has become more difficult. This combination may be more effective than interferon-α monotherapy, but it is also more expensive and has more side effects. The side effects of ribavirin, for instance, include hemolysis, anemia, itching, and hyperbilirubinemia, adverse effects that could complicate the management of acute hepatitis and jaundice. Furthermore, the fever, muscle aches, and fatigue induced by interferon can lead to erroneous assumptions about the course of acute disease. For these reasons, early therapy of acute hepatitis C must be considered experimental and a proper topic for a controlled trial rather than routine management. For the average patient it is prudent to delay therapy until the disease has been shown to persist for more than a few months. In fact, most trials of interferon therapy in "acute" hepatitis C required that the disease was present for 2 to 4 months before initiation of therapy.

If therapy is initiated during the acute course of hepatitis C, either early or late, it is also unclear what regimen to employ. The various trials of therapy used a 1- to 3-month course of interferon, courses that are clearly suboptimal in treating chronic hepatitis C. For this reason, delayed therapy is preferable and use of standard regimens more appropriate, such as combination therapy with interferon-α (3 million units three times weekly or the equivalent) and ribavirin (1000 to 1200 mg per day) for 24 to 48 weeks, depending on viral genotype (see Chapter 16).

CONCLUSION

Acute hepatitis C accounts for 15 to 16% of acute viral hepatitis in the United States and appears to be decreasing in incidence with the introduction of screening of blood for anti-HCV, widespread recommendations for prevention of the spread of hepatitis C, and a recent decrease in injection drug use. The acute disease has an incubation period of 7 weeks, and jaundice and symptoms occur in approximately one-third of patients.

Hepatitis C virus RNA appears in the serum during the incubation period, often within 1 to 2 weeks of exposure. Viral RNA levels increase and peak at or around the time of onset of symptoms and disappear with convalescence. The antibody to HCV as detected by enzyme immunoassay and recombinant immunoblot assay appears during the course of illness, but may not be detectable at the onset of symptoms. Some patients do not produce detectable anti-HCV, whereas in other patients this antibody is short-lived, which makes serological testing for the prevalence of HCV infection somewhat inaccurate. Acute liver failure due to hepatitis C is rare, occurring in less than 0.1% of cases and rarely reported in large series from the United States and western Europe. The major complication of acute hepatitis C is a progression to chronic infection, which occurs in 75% of patients, more commonly in adults than children and in men than women. Chronic hepatitis C can be defined as the persistence of HCV RNA in serum for more than 6 months after the onset of illness, but tests for HCV RNA may occasionally be nonreactive during the early phases of chronic infection and, in some instances, HCV RNA clearance may occur later. The role and benefit of antiviral therapy for acute hepatitis C have not been defined. At present it is prudent to delay therapy until the patient has clearly developed chronic infection and to treat the infection as is recommended for chronic hepatitis C.

REFERENCES

1. Alter M J, Gallagher M, Morris T T, et al. Acute non-A-E hepatitis in the United States and the role of hepatitis G virus infection. N Engl J Med 1997;336:741–6.
2. Center for Disease Control and Prevention. Recommendations for prevention and control of hepatitis C virus (HCV) infection and HCV-related chronic disease. MMWR 1998;47(No. RR-19):1–39.
3. Donahue J G, Munoz A, Ness R M, et al. The declining risk of post-transfusion hepatitis C virus infection. N Engl J Med 1992;327:369–73.
4. Alter M J, Hadler S C, Judson F N, et al. Risk factors for acute non-A, non-B hepatitis in the United States and association with hepatitis C virus infection. JAMA 1990;264:2231–5.
5. Williams I T, Sabin K, Fleenor M, et al. Current patterns of hepatitis C virus transmission in the United States: the role of drugs and sex. Hepatology 1998l;28:497A [abstract].
6. Alter H J: Descartes before the horse: I clone, therefore I am: the hepatitis C virus in current perspective. Ann Intern Med 1991;115:644–9.
7. Alter M J, Margolis H S, Krawczynski J, et al. The natural history of community-acquired hepatitis C in the United States. N Engl J Med 1992;327:1899–905.
8. Hoofnagle J H: Hepatitis C. The clinical spectrum of disease. Hepatology 1997;26(Suppl 1): 15S-20S.
9. Lee W. Acute liver failure. N Engl J Med 1993;329:1862–72.
10. Alter H J, Purcell R H, Shih J W, et al. Detection of antibody to hepatitis C virus in prospectively followed transfusion recipients with acute and chronic non-A, non-B hepatitis. N Engl J Med 1989;321:1494–500.
11. Estaban J I, Gonzalez A, Hernandez J M, et al. Evaluation of antibodies to hepatitis C virus in a study of transfusion associated hepatitis. N Engl J Med 1990;323:1107–12.
12. Aach R D, Stevens C E, Hollinger F B, et al. Hepatitis C virus infection in post-transfusion hepatitis. An analysis with first- and second-generation assays. N Engl J Med 1991;325:1325–9.

13. Tremolada F, Casarin C, Tagger A, et al. Antibody to hepatitis C virus in post-transfusion hepatitis. Ann Intern Med 1991;114:227–81.

14. Tassopoulos N C, Hatzakis A, Delladetsima I, Koutelou M G, Todoulos A, Miriagou V. Role of hepatitis C virus in acute non-A, non-B hepatitis in Greece: a 5-year prospective study. Gastroenterology 1992;102:969–72.

15. Hino K, Sainokami S, Shimoda K, Niwa H, Iino S. Clinical course of acute hepatitis C and changes in HCV markers. Dig Dis Sci 1994;39:19–27.

16. Barrera J M, Bruguera M, Ercilla M G, et al. Persistent hepatitis C viremia after acute self-limiting posttransfusion hepatitis C. Hepatology 1995;21:639–44.

17. Farci P, Alter H J, Wong D, et al. A long-term study of hepatitis C virus replication in non-A, non-B hepatitis. N Engl J Med 1991;325:98–104.

18. Alter J H, Sanchez-Pescador R, Urdea M S, et al. Evaluation of branched DNA signal amplification for the detection of hepatitis C virus RNA. J Viral Hepatitis 1995;2:121–32.

19. Kenny-Walsh E for the Irish Hepatology Research Group. Clinical outcomes after hepatitis C infection from contaminated anti-D immune globulin. N Engl J Med 1999;340:1228–33.

20. Seeff L B, Buskell-Bales Z, Wright E C, et al. National Heart, Lung and Blood Institute Study Group: Long-term mortality after transfusion-associated non-A, non-B hepatitis. N Engl J Med 1992;327:1906–11.

21. Vogt M, Lang T, Frösner G, et al. Prevalence and clinical outcome of hepatitis C infection in children who underwent cardiac surgery before the implementation of blood-donor screening. N Engl J Med 1999;341:866–70.

22. Rehermann B, Change K M, McHutchison J, et al. Differential cytotoxic T-lymphocyte responsiveness to the hepatitis B and C viruses in chronically infected patients. J Virol 1996;70:7092–102.

23. Shakil O, Conry-Cantilena C, Alter H J, et al. Volunteer blood donors with antibodies to hepatitis C virus: clinical, biochemical, virological and histological features. Ann Intern Med 1995;123:330–7.

24. Villano S A, Vlahov D, Nelson K E, Cohn S, Thomas D L. Persistence of viremia and the importance of long-term follow-up after acute hepatitis C infection. Hepatology 1999;29:908–14.

25. Alberti A, Morsica G, Chemello L, et al. Hepatitis C viraemia and liver disease in symptom-free individuals with anti-HCV. Lancet 1992;340:697–8.

26. Lau D T Y, Kleiner D E, Ghany M G, Park Y, Schmid P, Hoofnagle J H: 10-year follow-up after interferon-alpha therapy for chronic hepatitis C. Hepatology 1998;28:1121–7.

27. Gretch D: Diagnostic tests for hepatitis C. Hepatology 1997;26(Suppl 1);43S–7S.

28. Sheen I S, Liaw T F, Lin D Y, Chu C M. Acute exacerbations in chronic hepatitis C: a clinico-pathological and prognostic study. J Hepatol 1996;24:525–31.

29. Chau K H, Dawson G J, Mushahwar I K, et al. IgM antibody response to hepatitis C virus antigens in acute and chronic post-transfusion non-A, non-B hepatitis. J Virol Methods 1991;35:343–52.

30. Yuki N, Hayashi N, Ohkawa K, et al. The significance of immunoglobulin M antibody response to hepatitis C virus core protein in patients with chronic hepatitis C. Hepatology 1995;22:402–6.

31. Quiroga J A, Binsbergen J V, Wang C Y, et al. Immunoglobulin M antibody to hepatitis C virus core antigen: correlations with viral replication, histological activity, and liver disease outcome. Hepatology 1995;22:1635–40.

32. Fournillier-Jacob A, Lunel F, Cahour A, et al. Antibody responses to hepatitis C envelope proteins in patients with acute or chronic hepatitis C. J Med Virol 1996;50:159–67.

33. Omata M, Yokosuka O, Takano S, et al. Resolution of acute hepatitis C after therapy with natural beta interferon. Lancet 1991;338:914–5.

34. Viladomiu L, Genescà J, Esteban J I, et al. Interferon-α in acute posttransfusion hepatitis C: a randomized controlled trial. Hepatology 1992;15:767–9.

35. Tassopoulos N C, Koutelou M G, Papatheodoridis G, et al. Recombinant human interferon alfa-2b treatment for acute non-A, non-B hepatitis. Gut 1993;34(Suppl):S130–2.

36. Alberti A, Chemello L, Belussi F, et al. Outcome of acute hepatitis C and role of interferon alpha therapy. In: Nishioka K, Suzuki H, Oda T, eds. Viral hepatitis and liver disease. Tokyo: Springer-Verlag, 1994:604–6.

37. Palmovic D I, Kurelac I, Crnjakovic-Palmovic J. The treatment of acute post-transfusion hepatitis C with recombinant interferon-alpha. Infection 1994;22:222–3.
38. Lampertico P, Rumi M, Romeo R, et al. A multicenter randomized controlled trial of recombinant interferon-α2b in patients with acute transfusion-associated hepatitis C. Hepatology 1994;19:19–22.
39. Hwang S-J, Lee S-D, Chang C-Y, Lu R-H, Lo K-J. A randomized controlled trial of recombinant interferon alfa 2b in the treatment of Chinese patients with acute post-transfusion hepatitis C. J Hepatol 1994;21:831–6.
40. Takano S, Satomura Y, Omata M, Japan Acute Hepatitis Cooperative Study Group. Effects of interferon beta on non-A, non-B acute hepatitis: a prospective, randomized, controlled-dose study. Gastroenterology 1994;107:805–11.
41. Calleri G, Colombatto P, Gozzelino M, et al. Natural beta interferon in acute type-C hepatitis patients: a randomized controlled trial. Ital J Gastroenterol Hepatol 1998;30:181–4.
42. Cammá C, Almasio P, Craxí A. Interferon as treatment for acute hepatitis C: a meta-analysis. Dig Dis Sci 1996;41:1248–55.
43. Vogel W, Graziadei I, Umlauft F, et al. High dose interferon-alfa 2b treatment prevents chronicity in acute hepatitis C: a pilot study. Dig Dis Sci 1996;41:81S-5S.
44. Ohnishi K, Nomura F, Iida S. Treatment of posttransfusion non-A, non-B hepatitis acute and chronic hepatitis with human fibroblast -interferon: a preliminary report. Am J Gastroenterol 1989;84:596–600.
45. Christie J M, Healey C J, Watson J, et al. Clinical outcome of hypogammaglobulinaemic patients following outbreak of acute hepatitis C: a 2-year follow up. Clin Exp Immunol 1997;110:4–8.
46. Süleymanlar I, Sezer T, Işitan F, Yakupoğlu G, Süleymanlar G. Efficacy of interferon alpha in acute hepatitis C in patients on chronic hemodialysis. Nephron 1998;79:353–4.
47. Kiyosawa K, Sodeyama T, Tanaku E, et al. Hepatitis C in hospital employees with needlestick injuries. Ann Intern Med 1991;115:367–9.
48. Arai Y, Noda K, Enomoto V, et al. A prospective study of hepatitis C virus infection after needlestick accidents. Liver 1996;16:331–4.
49. Nakano Y, Kiyosawa K, Sodeyama T, et al. Acute hepatitis C transmitted by needlestick accident despite short duration interferon treatment. J Gastroenterol Hepatol 1995;10:609–11.
50. Poignet J-L, Dego F, Bouchardeau F, Chauveau P, Courouce A M. Complete response to interferon-alpha for acute hepatitis C after needlestick injury in a hemodialysis nurse. J Hepatol 1995;23:740–1.
51. Noguchi S, Sata M, Suzuki H, Ohba K, Mizokami M, Tanikawa K. Early therapy with interferon for acute hepatitis C acquired through a needlestick. Clin Infect Dis 1997;24:992–4.
52. Yang S S, Wu C H, Huang C S, et al. Early interferon therapy and abortion of posttransfusion hepatitis C viral infection. J Clin Gastroenterol 1995;21:38–41.
53. Sata M, Ide T, Noguchi S, et al. Timing of IFN therapy initiation for acute hepatitis C after accidental needlestick. J Hepatol 1997:27:425–6.
54. Davis GL, Lau JYN. Factors predictive of a beneficial response to therapy of hepatitis C. Hepatology 1997;26(Suppl 1):112S-27S.
55. Nousbaum J-B, Pol S, Nalpas B, et al. Hepatitis C virus type 1b infection in France and Italy. Ann Intern Med 1995;122:161–8.
56. McHutchison J G, Gordon S C, Schiff E R, et al. Interferon alfa-2b alone or in combination with ribavirin as initial treatment for chronic hepatitis C. N Engl J Med 1998;339:1485–92.
57. Poynard T, Marcellin P, Lee S S, et al. Randomised trial of interferon alpha 2b plus ribavirin for 48 weeks or for 24 weeks versus interferon alpha 2b plus placebo for 48 weeks for treatment of chronic infection with hepatitis C virus. Lancet 1998;352:1426–32.
58. Davis GL, Esteban-Mur R, Rustgi V, et al. Interferon alfa-2b alone or in combination with ribavirin for the treatment of relapse of chronic hepatitis C. N Engl J Med 1998;339:1493–9.

5
NATURAL HISTORY
OF HEPATITIS C

LEONARD B. SEEFF
Division of Digestive Diseases and Nutrition
National Institute of Diabetes and Digestive and Kidney Diseases
National Institutes of Health
Bethesda, Maryland

INTRODUCTION

Hepatitis C is the most common blood-borne infection in the United States and thus represents a major problem both in this country and abroad. (1) It is a disease characterized by onset that is largely silent because of the paucity or even total absence of clinical manifestations during the acute infection, by the fact that the majority of cases failed to resolve, and by the developing evidence that the ensuing chronic infection is responsible for the major proportion of cases of end-stage liver disease in the United States. It is therefore not surprising that hepatitis C now represents the most frequent reason for liver transplantation in adults (2) and the most frequent reason for a hepatological consultation.

In the current climate of concern, a common question posed by hepatitis C virus (HCV)-infected individuals to the consulting physician is: "What is my prognosis?" and "Will my life be shortened by my diagnosis and, if so, by how much time?" Accordingly, the major challenge to the basic scientist is to define the pathogenesis of chronic hepatitis C and to determine why the majority of infected individuals fail to clear the virus and how to predict the likelihood of progression. The challenge to the clinical investigator is to fully characterize the natural history of the chronic infection in order to provide information to patients regarding the expected long-term outcome as well as to better establish the need and place for treatment.

ISSUES THAT IMPACT ON THE STUDY OF THE NATURAL HISTORY

To accurately define the natural history of *any* medical condition—implying characterization of the consequences of the condition from its beginning to its termination (or that of the host)—it is essential to start the evaluation from onset of the disease and follow through to its *denouement*, preferably in comparison to a matched control group. In these respects, the study of the natural history of hepatitis C poses several problems. First, onset of acute hepatitis C is rarely identified. Second, the vast majority of chronically infected persons are totally asymptomatic or have minimal, nonspecific symptoms. Third, the rate of disease progression is generally leisurely, requiring decades before clinically apparent evidence of chronic liver disease emerges. Furthermore, in some persons the disease appears not to be progressive at all. Fourth, the risk of HCV infection is highest among persons whose underlying condition is itself associated with high morbidity and diminished life expectancy (e.g., transfusion recipients, particularly those undergoing cardiac surgery; injection drug users; hemodialysis patients; persons with hemophilia). Given the potential impact of the underlying condition, it is important that outcome studies include a noninfected control group for comparison.

Strategies Used to Define Long-Term Outcome

Three strategies have been used to help define the natural history of hepatitis C. (3) The prospective study is the optimal approach but has two major drawbacks: (i) outcome beginning from disease onset is not possible in the majority of cases unless the study involves at-risk groups who are monitored specifically for development of acute hepatitis or who are involved in a common source outbreak and (ii) the protracted nature of the chronic infection requires difficult to accomplish follow-up that may exceed two or even three decades. (4,5) The retrospective study, while overcoming the need for markedly prolonged follow-up, has important shortcomings: (i) tracing cases back to presumed onset is subject to the same uncertainty and vagaries and often proves to be incorrect and (ii) this approach excludes patients whose disease has resolved or who, for various reasons, did not come to clinical attention. Retrospective studies focus predominantly on patients with already established chronic disease, generally of a more severe nature. Also, retrospective analyses rarely allow comparison with an uninfected control group. A third approach is to combine the first two strategies in the form of a retrospective–prospective (or nonconcurrent prospective) study. This approach only has value if it is possible to identify a common source hepatitis outbreak or a prospective screening study that had occurred far in the past and that permits tracing of the infected individuals (and a matched, noninfected control group) many years later, thus shortening the period of long-term follow-up.

Prospective Studies of Acute Non-A, Non-B Hepatitis or Hepatitis C

Two categories of prospective studies have been performed: (i) those designed to determine long-term outcome beginning from the time of development of acute HCV infection and (ii) those designed to examine outcome among persons with already established chronic hepatitis C. Each of these strategies will be examined in turn.

Table I lists four prospective studies that describe long-term follow-up from onset of acute hepatitis C or non-A, non-B hepatitis, all focusing on transfusion-associated disease. (6–9) These studies were performed shortly after the identification of HCV, and therefore specific diagnoses of hepatitis C were based on early, less sensitive assays.

TABLE I Prospective Studies of Acute Transfusion-Associated Non-A, Non-B/C Hepatitis

Author (Ref.)	Country	No. patients	Mean follow-up (years)	Clinical symptoms (%)	Cirrhosis (%)	HCC[a] (%)	Liver death (%)
Di Bisceglie et al. (6)	USA	65	9.7	12.8	12.3	0	3.7
Koretz et al. (7)	USA	80	16.0	10.0	7.0	1.3	1.3
Mattson et al. (8)	Sweden	61	13.0	12.0	8.0	NR	1.6
Tremolada et al. (9)	Italy	135	7.6	3.7	15.6	0.7	3.7

[a] Hepatocellular carcinoma.

Di Bisceglie et al. (6) from the National Institutes of Health assessed the outcome of 65 patients 1 to 24 years (mean = 9.7 years) after onset of acute non-A, non-B transfusion-associated hepatitis. Fifty-three (82%) patients were classified as having hepatitis C based on screening with a first-generation enzyme immunoassay (EIA) supplemented by the recombinant immunoblot assay (RIBA). Forty-five of the 53 (65%) developed chronic hepatitis, of whom 33 consented to liver biopsy. The follow-up described these 33 patients as well as 6 others with transfusion-associated chronic hepatitis C who were not participating in the original follow-up study. Not discussed in the report was the outcome of the 8 patients who did not develop chronic hepatitis or the 12 patients with chronic hepatitis who did not undergo liver biopsy. Initial liver biopsies were done between 4 and 22 months after transfusion and 4 of the 39 patients already had cirrhosis. Twenty of the 39 patients underwent repeat liver biopsy 8 to 26 months later, 4 more of whom developed cirrhosis. Thus, cirrhosis was diagnosed in 20% of the 39 who were biopsied and 12.3% of the total cohort of 65 patients. Eleven had died, but only 2 from liver failure. None had developed HCC. Thus, liver-related death occurred in 2 of the 33 (6%) chronic hepatitis cohort who were biopsied or in 2 of the 53 (3.7%) who were originally identified with acute posttransfusion hepatitis C.

Koretz and co-workers (7) from Los Angeles attempted follow-up on 90 patients who had developed acute transfusion-associated hepatitis, identifying and evaluating 80 patients approximately 16 years after onset of infection. Fifty-five (69%) patients had chronic hepatitis, whereas in 4, the outcome could not be determined. Serological evidence of HCV infection was found in 64 patients using both first- and second-generation EIA. Although 40% of the original 90 patients had symptoms during the acute illness, none who developed chronic hepatitis continued to have significant symptoms. Only 8 patients underwent liver biopsy; 3 had cirrhosis and another 2 patients were reported to have cirrhosis on an earlier liver biopsy. Thus, 6.3% of the cohort had cirrhosis, but more cases may have been identified if liver biopsies were performed on all patients. Decompensated liver disease was estimated to be present in 19% of all patients and 22% of those with chronic hepatitis C. Approximately one-third of the patients who could be traced had died during the follow-up period, all but one from nonhepatic causes. The single liver-related death (1.3%) occurred in a patient with chronic hepatitis C and was the result of HCC.

Mattson et al. (8) from Scandinavia reported a 13-year follow-up of 39 of 61 patients who had developed acute transfusion-associated non-A, non-B hepatitis. Screening of archived blood samples identified acute hepatitis C in 24 patients based on second-generation EIA and RIBA as well as by testing for HCV RNA by the polymerase chain reaction (PCR) assay. Follow-up revealed that all 24 were still anti-HCV positive 13 years later and that 16 had HCV RNA (75%). Most of the patients in follow-up (79%) had abnormal aminotransferase levels with or without HCV RNA in serum. The remaining 21% of patients appeared to have recovered completely. Liver-related symptoms were present in 12% of patients. Liver biopsies showed the presence of cirrhosis in 8%. One patient (1.6%) died as a consequence of liver disease.

Tremolada et al. (9) from northern Italy reported a follow-up study (mean = 7.6 years) among 135 patients with transfusion-associated non-A, non-B hepatitis where most had undergone cardiac surgery. A little over one-half were identified in the course of a planned prospective study, with the rest representing cases diagnosed with overt transfusion-related acute hepatitis outside of the prospective study. Almost all cases of non-A, non-B hepatitis could be attributed to HCV infection based on first- and second-generation assays. Chronic hepatitis evolved in 104 patients (77%). Mild symptoms (intermittent fatigue) were found in 35%, splenomegaly in 13%, and esophageal varices in 5% of patients. Sixty-five patients were biopsied and 21 (32%) had cirrhosis, which represented a frequency of cirrhosis of 21% among patients with chronic hepatitis and 16% among all patients in the original cohort diagnosed with acute hepatitis C. Among the 104 with chronic hepatitis, 16 (16%) died, 5 (4.8%) from liver disease (3, bleeding; 1, liver failure; 1, HCC). Thus, five (3.7%) of the original 135 HCV-infected group died as a consequence of liver disease.

Two nontransfusion-related hepatitis studies involving follow-up of acute hepatitis C (10,11) focused attention on serologic and biochemical rather than clinical and histologic sequelae. Follow-up of community-acquired hepatitis C was reported by Alter et al. (10) from the Center for Disease Control and Prevention (CDC). Patients were identified with acute non-A, non-B hepatitis in four counties in the United States participating in the CDC's Hepatitis Surveillance Program. Among 130 identified cases, 106 (82%) were diagnosed as hepatitis C using sophisticated serologic markers. Of note is that the diagnosis was based on the presence of both anti-HCV and HCV RNA in 93 cases and on the presence of HCV RNA alone in 9 others. Ninety-seven of the 106 were followed for 9 to 48 months after diagnosis, 60 (62%) of whom advanced to chronic hepatitis. Liver biopsies were performed in 30 individuals with chronic hepatitis; 10 (33%) had "chronic active hepatitis," 1 of whom also had cirrhosis, 13 (43%) had "chronic persistent hepatitis," and 6 (20%) had chronic lobular hepatitis. Thus, cirrhosis was found in only 1% of the 106 hepatitis C cases followed over this relatively short time period. Follow-up of 85 anti-HCV positive patients over periods of 9 months to 6 years revealed persistence of anti-HCV in all 54 with chronic hepatitis C but loss of the antibody in 2 of the 31 patients who had had biochemical recovery. No patient with hepatitis C died over the course of the study.

In the course of a long-term natural history study of human immunodeficiency virus (HIV) infection among 142 illicit drug users, Villano et al. (11) from Baltimore, Maryland, identified 43 persons through semiannual screening who had seroconverted to anti-HCV. Seroconversion was used to signify onset of the acute HCV infection. Anti-HCV was assayed using second-generation EIA with confirmation by RIBA, and HCV RNA was assessed quantitatively by PCR assay. All but 1 patient was positive for HCV RNA. The 43 persons who seroconverted to anti-HCV positivity were reevaluated 14 to 93 (median, 74) months later for evidence of continuing viral infection and liver disease. In 5 patients, HCV RNA was no longer detected, leaving 37 (86%) with continuing viremia. No clinical, biochemical, or serological differences were found among those who cleared virus and those in whom it persisted. Serum aminotransferase levels had returned to normal in all patients who became HCV RNA negative, as well as in 43% of those with viral persistence. At last follow-up, 6 of the 43 patients had died from causes unrelated to liver disease; among those who were alive and could be interviewed, only one had evidence of continuing liver disease, and this individual also admitted to long-term heavy alcoholism.

Thus, these six prospective studies identified that progression from acute to chronic hepatitis C was common; that during the time periods of follow-up (approximately 4 to 16 years), cirrhosis, when sought, was identified in 1 to 20% of cases; that development of HCC was uncommon; and that liver-related mortality was modest in frequency, ranging from 0 to 3.7%. None of these studies included a noninfected control group for comparison. Because the transfusion studies had been performed early after identification of HCV, they failed to provide adequate information on the serologic sequelae. In contrast, serological outcome was the basis for the illicit drug use and community-acquired hepatitis studies, which, in the case of the former, identified early viral clearance in 14% of cases and, in the latter, resolution of the acute infection in 38% and even rare instances of spontaneous loss of anti-HCV. Taken together, these studies demonstrated that during the first 20 years after onset of HCV infection, liver-related morbidity and mortality certainly occur, but at a relatively low rate. These studies were unable to provide needed information on outcome in the more critical time periods of 20 and more years after acute infection.

Prospective Studies of Chronic Hepatitis C

Several studies have assessed the natural history of hepatitis C beginning with patients with already established chronic hepatitis. While these studies are prospective, they also often analyze the rate of progression of disease based on retrospective analyses dating the onset of infection as the time of possible exposure to HCV, either from blood transfusion or from injection drug use.

Poynard et al. (12) assessed the natural history of liver fibrosis progression in patients with chronic hepatitis C based on liver biopsies that were available from 2235 patients who were recruited in three large population-based studies performed in France. Fibrosis progression was determined as a ratio between the fibrosis stage (in METAVIR units) and the estimated duration of infection in years. The METAVIR scoring system incorporated fibrosis staging and activity grading using carefully defined parameters. Most data derived from single

TABLE II   **Rate of Progression of Fibrosis**[a]

Three independent risk factors associated with progression:
  Age at infection > 40 years
  Daily alcohol consumption > 50g
  Male sex

Mean rate of progression to cirrhosis:
  Men with the risk factors, 13 years
  Women without the risk factors, 42 years

[a] From Poynard et al. (12)

biopsies, although 70 patients had paired biopsy samples. Fibrosis progression was assessed in relation to nine factors: sex, age at biopsy, estimated duration of infection, age at infection, alcohol consumption, HCV genotype, hepatitis C viremia, cause of infection, and histological activity grade. The authors found a median rate of fibrosis progression of 0.133 fibrosis units per year. They identified three independent factors associated with a more rapid progression of fibrosis: age at infection older than 40 years, daily alcohol consumption of 50g or more, and male sex (Table II). They concluded that the median estimated duration of infection for progression to cirrhosis was 30 years, with a range from as little as 13 years among men infected over the age of 40 years who drank alcohol, to as long as 42 years among women infected below the age of 40 years who did not drink alcohol. Because the rate of fibrosis progression was not distributed normally, they hypothesized that the cohort comprised three separate populations: rapid fibrosers, intermediate fibrosers, and slow fibrosers. These data prompted their assumption that about one-third of HCV-infected persons will advance to cirrhosis in less than 20 years and that another one-third would either never develop cirrhosis or will do so over a span of at least 50 years.

Somewhat conflicting data were reported by Niederau et al. (13) from Germany. These investigators conducted a follow-up study on 838 patients with chronic hepatitis C as defined by the presence of both anti-HCV and HCV RNA. Most patients had been referred to this tertiary care center for therapy. The duration of follow-up ranged from 6 to 122 months (median = 50.2 months). Outcome data were compared with the general population matched for age and sex. At study entry, 141 patients (17%) had cirrhosis, mostly classified as Childs A cirrhosis, and 73% had genotype 1a or 1b. During the course of the study, 62 patients died: 18 from cirrhosis, 13 from HCC, and 31 from other causes. Overall, mortality was higher in the HCV-infected group as compared to the general population based on standardized mortality ratios (SMR) (Table III). However, as noted in Table III, mortality was strongly related to the presence of cirrhosis and estimated duration of infection. Among 696 patients without cirrhosis, mortality was no greater than that of the age- and sex-matched general population, regardless of duration of infection. In contrast, the mortality rate was significantly higher among patients with cirrhosis, regardless of the duration of infection. All patients who developed HCC either had cirrhosis at entry or developed cirrhosis during the study. Multivariate regression analyses indicated that survival was decreased by cirrhosis,

TABLE III   Standardized Mortality Rates (SMR) of Patients with and without Cirrhosis[a]

Group	No. patients	SMR	95% CI
All patients	838	1.6[b]	1.3–2.0
Cirrhosis absent	696	0.9	0.6–1.2
Cirrhosis present	141	3.9[b]	2.8–4.9
Duration ≥ 15 years	229	2.6[b]	1.9–3.3
Cirrhosis absent	150	1.2	0.6–1.9
Cirrhosis present	79	4.8[b]	3.3–6.4

[a] From Niederau et al. (13)
[b] Significant SMRs.

long disease duration, chronic alcoholism, injection drug use, and older age, whereas survival was improved among patients treated with interferon, although treatment did not reduce the risk of HCC.

The effect of cirrhosis on long-term outcome of hepatitis C was carefully assessed by Fattovich et al. (14) in a follow-up study of 384 European patients with compensated HCV-related cirrhosis. The period of follow-up ranged from 6 to 153 months (mean = 61 months). During follow-up, 59% of the patients were treated, the vast majority with interferon-α. HCC developed in 29 (8%) of patients over periods of 7 to 134 months (mean = 48 months). The cumulative probability of occurrence of HCC was 4% at 3 years after recognition of cirrhosis, 7% at 5 years, and 14% at 10 years. The calculated yearly incidence of HCC development was 1.4%. Among the remaining 355 patients, 65 (18%) developed evidence of decompensation at a mean interval of 3 to 137 months (mean = 37 months). Fifty-one patients died during follow-up: 17 from HCC, 16 from liver failure, 3 from bleeding, and 15 from causes unrelated to cirrhosis. Thus, 9% died from liver-related causes 9 to 124 months (mean = 50 months) after study entry. Survival probability was 96% at 3 years, 91% at 5 years, and 79% at 10 years unless decompensation ensued, in which case survival fell to 50% at year 5. The annual mortality rate was 1.9% during the first 5 years. Multivariate analysis identified bilirubin, manifestations of liver disease on physical examination, age, and platelet counts as independent risk factors for survival. Treatment with interferon was not identified to be an independent prognostic factor for survival.

A similar analysis was undertaken by Serfaty et al. (15) from France (Table IV). Among 668 patient with HCV infection referred to a tertiary care

TABLE IV   Outcome among HCV-Positive Patients with Compensated Cirrhosis

Author (Ref.)	No. patients	Mean follow-up (months)	Hepatic decompensation (%)	HCC[a] (%)	Annual HCC rate (%)	Death (%)	Annual mortality rate (%)
Fattovich et al. (14)	384	61	18.0	8.0	1.4	9.0	1.9
Serfaty et al. (15)	103	40	14.5	10.6	3.3	16.0	5.5

[a] Hepatocellular carcinoma.

institution in Paris, 103 (15%) had cirrhosis. These patients were followed for a median period of 40 months (range = 6 to 72 months). Fifty-nine of the 103 were treated with interferon-α, only 3 of whom had a sustained virological response. Twenty-six patients (25%) developed hepatic complications, consisting of HCC in 11 and hepatic decompensation in 15. The calculated annual incidence of HCC was 3.3%, based on the calculated cumulative probability of its development in 3% of the patients at 2 years and 11.5% at 4 years. The cumulative probability of decompensation without HCC was 15% at 2 years and 20% at 4 years. Sixteen percent of patients died in follow-up, all but 1 from hepatic causes (liver failure, HCC, bleeding) and 3 patients underwent liver transplantation. The annual incidence of death or transplantation was 5.5%, and conversely, the cumulative probabilities of survival were 96% at 2 years and 84% at 4 years. Unlike the European study, multivariate analysis revealed that absence of interferon therapy was an independent predictive factor for HCC and decompensation and that low albumin and lack of treatment were independent predictive factors for death or liver transplantation.

An interesting, short-term prospective study involving chronically infected persons in the general population, namely the inhabitants of two northern Italian towns, has been reported by Bellentani et al. (16) A total of 10,151 inhabitants were invited to participate in a survey (the Dionysis study) that included an initial extensive history, physical examination, and biochemical and serological testing. A total of 6917 persons, 69% of the eligible population, agreed to participate. Individuals found to be anti-HCV positive (by third-generation EIA followed by RIBA) and those with a clinical diagnosis of cirrhosis were followed at 6-month intervals for at least 3 years with repeated biochemical, serological, and ultrasonographic evaluation. Anti-HCV was detected in 226 persons in the population (3.2%), 79% of whom were RIBA positive, 9% RIBA indeterminate, and 12% RIBA negative. HCV RNA was detected in 162 anti-HCV positive patients (2.3% of the total population), including 154 (86%) of those who were RIBA positive, 6 (30%) RIBA indeterminate, and 2 (7%) RIBA negative. Thus, the overall rate of HCV RNA positivity among individuals with anti-HCV was 72%. The authors, however, assumed that 12% of the positive anti-HCV cases were falsely positive and that, in fact, only 16% had anti-HCV without HCV RNA, indicative of recovery and clearance of virus. Risk factors for HCV transmission, based on logistic regression analysis, included a history of injection drug use, blood transfusion, sexual exposure, and animal bites. Liver biopsies were performed in the 77 of 162 HCV-positive patients who had abnormal serum aminotransferase levels or clinical evidence of cirrhosis. Twenty (26%) of the 77 persons biopsied, representing 12% of the 162 HCV RNA-positive cases, had histologically confirmed cirrhosis. Four patients with cirrhosis also had HCC, and one additional person with HCC was not reported as having cirrhosis. Almost all patients with cirrhosis, including all with HCC, also reported heavy alcohol intake. Liver biopsies in the remaining 52 HCV RNA-positive patients showed either chronic active hepatitis or minimal inflammation. Of note is that 34% of the HCV RNA-positive patients had normal serum enzymes and 18% had only minimal elevations, whereas 83% of those positive for anti-HCV but HCV RNA negative had completely normal clinical findings, with the remaining persons in this category having other reasons for liver dysfunction, predominantly chronic alcoholism. The authors concluded that disease progression that did occur among their study population was strongly associated with infection with genotype 1b and with chronic alcoholism, but that more than 50% of the HCV RNA-positive subjects had no clinical or biochemical evidence of liver damage over the 3 years of follow-up.

Thus, not surprisingly, a different pattern of outcome emerges in long-term studies that begin with already established chronic hepatitis C, particularly in studies evaluating outcome among those with existing cirrhosis. In this latter group, progression to end-stage liver disease and HCC is relatively common, as is liver-related mortality. Noteworthy is that regardless of the duration of follow-up, about 15 to 20% of HCV-infected patients seem to have cirrhosis and that HCC seems almost always to occur in the presence of cirrhosis. In general, HCV-infected patients without cirrhosis seem to suffer minimally with regard to clinical illness, although sensitive instruments do measure variable degrees of reduction of quality of life. (17,18) However, because of their relatively short durations, these studies provide insufficient information on the likelihood and frequency of progression from portal fibrosis to cirrhosis. Indeed, a critical question is whether fibrosis progresses linearly over the course of a lifetime or whether one can assume that if marked fibrosis or overt cirrhosis is not present at the end of a given period of time, such as two decades, that subsequent progression to cirrhosis is unlikely. (19) Several studies have suggested that the progression of hepatitis C is strongly enhanced by chronic alcoholism. Nevertheless, provided decompensation does not ensue, early stage cirrhosis seems compatible with considerable longevity.

Retrospective Studies

Retrospective studies involve assessment of persons with already established chronic hepatitis, attempting to define the rate of development of adverse sequelae by tracing the chronic disease back in time to the moment of acute onset. Four studies will be reviewed. (4,5,20,21)

Kiyosawa et al. (4) conducted a retrospective evaluation of 231 Japanese patients with chronic non-A, non-B hepatitis (96 with chronic hepatitis, 81 with cirrhosis, and 29 with HCC). Tests for anti-HCV, using first generation EIA, revealed that 90, 86, and 94% of these groups, respectively, were seropositive. To determine the duration of infection before evolution (or, more properly, recognition) of these serious sequelae, investigators focused attention, on the proportion within each category whose infection was believed to result from blood transfusion, hypothesizing that this event correctly established the time of onset of infection. A history of transfusion was present in 52% of patients with chronic hepatitis, 33% with cirrhosis, and 42% with HCC. Within these subsets of patients, transfusions had been give a mean of 10, 22, and 29 years earlier (Table V). Among the 21 patients with HCC, transfusions had been received as recently as 15 years and as remotely as 60 years earlier. That progression was sequential and linear was documented in several patients with HCC who had multiple liver biopsies showing progression from chronic persistent hepatitis to

TABLE V Rate of Progression of Chronic Hepatitis C
Based on Retrospective Studies[a]

Author (Ref.)	Mean interval (years) between transfusion and development of		
	Chronic hepatitis	Cirrhosis	Hepatocellular carcinoma
Kiyosawa et al. (4)	10.0	21.2	29.0
Tong et al. (5)	13.7	20.6	28.3

[a] Onset of acute hepatitis is based on the history of receipt of transfusions.

chronic active hepatitis to cirrhosis and, ultimately, to HCC. Of note was that cirrhosis was documented to precede onset of HCC in 18 of 21 patients, with the remaining 3 patients not having a liver biopsy prior to discovery of the cancer. These findings clearly show the relationship between HCV infection and the development of progressively severe liver disease, as well as the snail-like pace of the progression. Because this investigation was a retrospective evaluation of patients with chronic hepatitis, end-stage liver disease, and cirrhosis, it provided no information on the frequency of these serious outcomes.

Similar findings have been reported by Tong et al. (5) from Los Angeles on a cohort of patients with transfusion-related chronic hepatitis C. These investigators conducted a retrospective evaluation on 213 patients with chronic hepatitis C referred in consultation to their hospital and provided short-term follow-up of 131 patients in this group. The diagnosis of hepatitis C was based on second-generation EIA. Liver biopsies were performed in 101 patients. The average age of the patients at the time of transfusion was 35 years and when seen for initial evaluation at the tertiary care hospital was 57 years (range = 21 to 81 years). At initial evaluation, 67% complained of fatigue, 20% of abdominal pain, and 14% of anorexia. Physical examination revealed hepatomegaly in 68% and splenomegaly in 21%. Only 2 patients were jaundiced. Initial liver biopsies revealed chronic hepatitis in 21%, chronic active hepatitis in 23%, cirrhosis in 51%, and HCC in 5.3%. Based on the timing of the initial transfusion, the interval from onset of infection to the diagnosis of chronic hepatitis averaged 14 years, to chronic active hepatitis averaged 18 years, to cirrhosis averaged 21 years, and to HCC averaged 28 years (Table V). The patients were followed for an additional mean duration of 3.9 years (range, 1 to 15 years). During this time, a further seven cases (5.3%) developed HCC and 20 (15%) died: 8 from complications of cirrhosis, 11 from HCC, and 1 from pneumonia (Table VI). This study from the United States, like that from Japan (4), underscored the slow pace of liver disease progression and clearly demonstrated the potentially serious nature of chronic hepatitis C infection in this subset of patients. However, this study almost certainly represented the "worst-case" scenario; data were accrued at a well-known referral hospital and most patients already had severely compromised liver disease at the time of their first visit.

Yano et al. (20) from several institutions in Japan analyzed histological progression in patients with hepatitis C (Table VI). This study was based on results of repeat liver biopsies from 80 patients with HCV infection selected from

TABLE VI Long-Term Outcome of Hepatitis C Based on Evaluation of Persons with Already Established Chronic Liver Disease

Author (Ref.)	No. of patients	Follow-up (years)	Cirrhosis (%)	HCC[a] (%)	Liver deaths (%)
Tong et al. (5)	131	3.9	51.0	10.6	15.3
Yano et al. (20)	70	2–26	50.0	NR[b]	NR
Gordon et al. (21)	282[c]	NR	52.5	4.0	NR
Gordon et al. (21)	262[d]	NR	35.0	1.0	NR

[a] Hepatocellular carcinoma.
[b] Not reported.
[c] Cases of transfusion-associated hepatitis.
[d] Hepatitis cases not due to transfusions.

approximately 2000 patients with chronic liver disease seen at their institutions. Patients who underwent repeated liver biopsies generally had fluctuating serum aminotransferase levels, rising to levels at least five times the upper limit of normal. The diagnosis had been confirmed by anti-HCV testing using second-generation EIA, and the period of follow-up ranged from 5 to 26 years. Ten patients were excluded because of cirrhosis at baseline, and the remaining 70 (25 with transfusion-related, 45 with community-acquired hepatitis) underwent 2 to 10 liver biopsies (mean = 3.9) at intervals from the first to the last biopsy of 1 to 26 years. Biopsy histology was reviewed independently by four pathologists using a scoring system for necrosis and inflammation (grade or activity of liver disease) and a staging system for fibrosis. During follow-up, 50% of patients developed cirrhosis. Cirrhosis occurred in all patients with a high initial score of necroinflammatory activity, in 96% with an intermediate, and in 30% with a low grade. Furthermore, the rapidity of progression correlated directly with the histological grade. This important, frequently cited paper clearly demonstrated the potentially serious nature of this chronic infection, which was best predicted by the degree of fibrosis and histological activity. However, the patients studied were highly selected; being chosen in this retrospective study from a group of 2000 patients because they had undergone repeat liver biopsy and serious liver disease was suspected. Thus, patients with milder forms of hepatitis C and less progressive liver disease were likely to have not been chosen for repeat histological assessment and inclusion in this study.

Gordon et al. (21) from the United States assessed the possibility that the mode of HCV transmission affected the long-term outcome. They evaluated 627 consecutively admitted nonalcoholic patients with chronic hepatitis C: 282 (45%) of whom had apparently been infected through transfusions, 262 (42%) through other percutaneous exposure, and 83 (13%) through unknown sources. The duration of disease was determined on the basis of time of transfusion, time of icteric hepatitis, or first year of injection drug use. For those reporting multiple transfusions without jaundice, a midpoint between transfusions was selected. Liver biopsies were available from 463 patients; 173 (37%) had cirrhosis of whom 16 (4%) also had HCC. Cirrhosis was detected in 118 of 215 patients (55%) with a history of transfusion as compared to only 40 of 195 (21%) patients with other parenteral exposures. HCC was similarly more common among the cohort with a history of transfusion (4%) than those without (1%). The authors calculated that the cumulative risk of developing cirrhosis 25 years after exposure was 52% in the transfusion group and 35% in the other percutaneous exposure group ($p = 0.001$). Because of the potential bias of differing age ranges in the two study cohorts (younger for drug users, older for transfusion recipients), age as a predictive factor, as well as duration of infection, were each examined through univariate analysis; a significant difference was found for age but not duration of infection. Multivariate analysis, however, identified only mode of acquisition as a predictive factor for subsequent liver failure. The authors thus concluded that "the risk of liver failure is more closely related to the mode of transmission than to age at viral acquisition or to duration of infection."

As noted earlier for prospective studies of chronic hepatitis C, retrospective studies attempting to define disease onset by historical methods describe a high frequency of cirrhosis, liver failure, and HCC. The inherent bias in this approach is the omission from the analysis of individuals who have entirely recovered from an acute bout of hepatitis C or whose chronic infection was too mild to come to the attention of health care practitioners. Nevertheless, they confirm the serious sequelae that can evolve from chronic HCV infection, particularly after the development of cirrhosis. Prospective studies identify cirrhosis far less frequently than do retrospective studies, the explanation for which might simply be an issue of duration from the time of initial infection or that patients who have cirrhosis are more likely to come to clinical attention creating the potential for "referral bias."

Nonconcurrent Prospective Studies

Another approach to study the natural history of hepatitis C is the nonconcurrent prospective study in which one traces and recalls for prospective evaluation a cohort of patients who had a clearly recognized initial infection. Typically, these patients were involved in a large outbreak of hepatitis C or could be identified as having hepatitis C long in the past.

Kenny-Walsh et al. (22) have described clinical outcomes of a large group of Irish women who acquired HCV infection from the use of contaminated anti-D immune globulin given at the time of delivery for Rh incompatibility. The problem came to light when routine screening of blood donors for anti-HCV identified 15 women positive for antibody who had no identifiable risk factors for hepatitis C and who were almost all Rh negative. Twelve of the 15 had received anti-D immune globulin in 1977. Further inquiry into this finding revealed that the immune globulin product used had been contaminated by plasma from a woman with the diagnosis of "infective hepatitis" that had been added to the pool from which the globulin had been manufactured. This prompted a major inquiry that concluded with four major recommendations: that all recipients of this product from the time of its introduction until February 1994 be screened for the presence of HCV infection; that all women found to be positive should be referred to one of six hepatology centers; that a group of experts and a national tribunal of inquiry be assembled by the government to investigate the circumstances and consequences of the contamination; and that a hepatitis C compensation panel be formed to expedite the processing of related claims. The tribunal of inquiry determined that the plasma of the woman who had had icteric hepatitis was added to a pool that was used to prepare 16 batches of anti-D immune globulin, 8 of which were later found to be positive for HCV RNA. Almost 6000 doses from these lots were thought to have been administered. On the basis of the publicity, 62,667 women presented themselves for screening between 1997 and 1998, a mean of 17 years following exposure; 704 were found to be anti-HCV positive of whom 390 (55%) were also HCV RNA positive; 376 (96%) completed a thorough medical, serum biochemical, and virological evaluation. The average age of women at the time of receipt of the contaminated immune globulin was 28 years. In follow-up, 81% complained of at least one symptom (the evaluation having taken place during intense publicity, which included common reference to potential consequences), about one-third had at least one other risk factor for acquiring hepatitis C, and 5% had a history of alcoholism. Serum alanine aminotransferase (ALT) values were normal in 45% of women, mildly elevated (40 to 99 IU/ml) in 47%, and moderately elevated (exceeding 100 IU/ml) in 8%. The median ALT concentration was 42 IU/ml. Liver biopsies were performed on 363 women and examined for grade of necrosis and inflammation and stage of fibrosis. There was no evidence of necrosis and inflammation in 2%, mild (grade 1–3) necroinflammatory changes in 41%, moderate (grade 4–8) in 52%, and marked (grade 9–18) in 4%. Strikingly, 49% of liver biopsies had no fibrosis, 34% showed only portal or periportal fibrosis, 15% had bridging fibrosis, and 2% had cirrhosis (Table VII). Two of the 7 women with cirrhosis were also heavy alcohol drinkers. These investigators thus found a far more benign long-term outcome than had been reported previously. Furthermore, they indicated that their results were similar to those of another study of women who had received HCV-contaminated Rh immune globulin in Germany (23); none of 152 women evaluated approximately 15 years after exposure had chronic active hepatitis or cirrhosis. The authors hypothesized that the relatively benign outcome in these women might have been due to several factors, including the viral strain and relatively small size of the inoculum as well as the young age at the time of infection and the fact that women may have a more benign course of disease and a higher likelihood of spontaneous clearance of HCV. (24)

A large retrospective–prospective analysis of the natural history of posttransfusion hepatitis has been published by members of the National Heart, Lung, and Blood Institute Hepatitis Working Group. (25) Data were derived

TABLE VII Frequency of Development of Cirrhosis in Patients with Acute Hepatitis C: Prospective Studies

Author (Ref.)	Country	Duration of patients	Cirrhosis follow-up (years)	(%)
Kenny-Walsh et al. (22)	Ireland	376	17	2
Seeff et al. (32)	USA	146	20	15
Vogt et al. (35)	Germany	458	17	3

from five separate prospective studies of transfusion recipients conducted between 1967 and 1980, including two Veterans Administration (VA) studies, (26,27) the study conducted at the Clinical Center of the National Institutes of Health, (28) the national Transfusion-Transmitted Viruses study, (29) and a study conducted at the Walter Reed Army Hospital. (30) The diagnosis of viral hepatitis in the original five studies was based on the development of ALT elevations as detected by the bimonthly screening of transfusion recipients for periods of at least 6 months. Patients who developed hepatitis were matched, in a ratio of 1:2, with transfusion recipients from the same studies who had not developed hepatitis. The vital status of each subject was obtained from Social Security Death Tapes, the National Death Index, the Health Care Financing Administration, and the Beneficiary Identification and Records Locator System. Cause of death was determined from a review of death certificates. Also, next-of-kin proxies were interviewed by telephone if the subject was deceased or incompetent. A total of 1552 of the 6438 persons who entered the original studies were included in the follow-up study: 568 patients with non-A, non-B hepatitis and 984 matched controls (first controls, 526; second controls, 458). At the initiation of follow-up, an average of 18 years after transfusion, all-cause mortality was 51% for the group with non-A, non-B hepatitis, 52% for the first controls, and 50% for the second controls. Liver-related causes of death occurred in 3.3% (19 subjects) of the non-A, non-B cases, in 1.1% (6 subjects) of the first control group, and 2.0% (9 subjects) of the second control group ($p = 0.022$). Twenty-eight of the 34 patients with a liver-related cause of death had medical records available for examination, of whom 20 (71%) were identified as heavy drinkers following their original enrollment (78% of those with non-A, non-B hepatitis and 60% of the controls). Cirrhosis accounted for liver-related death in 1.9% of the non-A, non-B cases and 1.0% of the controls, while there was one death (0.2%) from HCC in the hepatitis group and two (0.2%) in the control group. Because most of the liver-related deaths had occurred among VA patients, the only one of the original studies that had permitted enrollment in the original transfusion study even if there had been a remote history of alcoholism, there was speculation regarding an additive role of alcoholism in mortality among both those with hepatitis C and their controls.

In a follow-up report of this study of natural history, 5 years of evaluation were added. (31) Life-table analysis showed similar increases in all-cause mortality for both non-A, non-B hepatitis cases (to 69.1%) and controls (to 69.4%) ($p = 0.67$). Liver-related death for the entire cohort was 4.0% for hepatitis cases and 1.7% for controls ($p = 0.009$); for cases identified as HCV related, liver-related death was 2.7% for the cases and 1.5% among their controls ($p = 0.31$). Thus, most deaths could be ascribed to the underlying reason for the initial transfusion rather than to liver disease, but there was clearly a trend toward increasing liver-related death among the cases with the passage of time. A third report from this same study focused on long-term morbidity over a period of approximately 20 years. (32) This analysis was accomplished by recalling all living patients for interview, physical examination, and blood testing for routine chemistries and hepatitis B and C serologies. If ALT levels were abnormal on at least two of three tests performed over a 6-month period, the patient was designated as having chronic hepatitis. The diagnosis of hepatitis C was based on second-generation EIA with supplemental testing by RIBA. Because the intention was to determine the long-term morbidity outcome according to the specific original virological diagnosis, the analysis was restricted to three of the original five transfusion studies in which original sera were archived, permitting retrospective serological testing. This approach yielded 146 patients alive at the commencement of follow-up, of whom 103 (71%) were anti-HCV positive. The remaining patients were negative for markers of active infection with hepatitis A, B, C, or G viruses. Testing of the 103 HCV-related cases approximately 18 to 20 years after transfusion identified 74% who still were positive for HCV RNA, 16% with anti-HCV without HCV RNA, and 10% with no markers whatsoever. One-half of the viremic patients had biochemical evidence of chronic hepatitis, whereas the other one-half had normal serum aminotransferase levels. Biopsies, targeted only to those with abnormal ALT values, revealed histologically defined cirrhosis in one-third and chronic hepatitis in two-thirds. Clinically apparent evidence of chronic liver disease was found almost exclusively among those with cirrhosis. Extrapolating these data to the entire group indicated that cirrhosis had developed in 15% of the original cases of acute hepatitis C.

This long-term study of the consequences of posttransfusion hepatitis C, the only one to employ a matched nonhepatitis control group, thus revealed that the majority of deaths were a consequence of the original reason for the transfusion rather than the acquisition of HCV infection (Fig. 1). Long-term mortality was no different for patient groups with or without hepatitis C, but both groups differed significantly from the normal population with respect to mortality. Deaths due to liver diseases were found to be slightly more common among patients with chronic hepatitis C than their controls, with this difference increasing slightly with time. In keeping with other reports, chronic alcoholism appeared to be a contributory factor to the morbidity and mortality of hepatitis C. Among living study patients, about one-third had lost viremia, whereas half of those who were

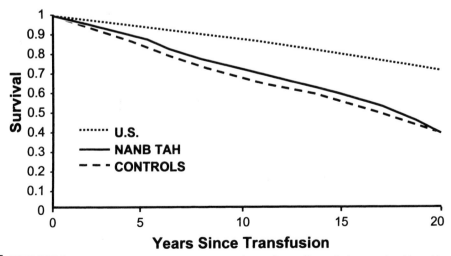

FIGURE 1 Survival curves comparing patients with non-A, non-B transfusion-associated hepatitis (NANB TAH), predominantly type C hepatitis; matched transfusion recipients without hepatitis (CONTROLS); and the general U.S. population (U.S.).

still viremic had normal ALT values. The observed and estimated frequency of cirrhosis 20 years after infection was approximately 15%, and clinically apparent disease was found almost exclusively among patients with cirrhosis (Table VII). Thus, progressive chronic liver disease appeared to be likely in about 15 to 20% of transfusion-related HCV-infected persons.

The high rate of nonhepatitis mortality, the inclusion of older patients, and the relatively restricted duration of follow-up in these transfusion studies have been viewed as confounding problems in accurately determining the true natural history of hepatitis C. More compelling data would require a study with longer follow-up, focusing on younger patients without other comorbidities. An opportunity to undertake just such a study was presented with the discovery of almost 10,000 sera that had been stored frozen since having been drawn from young Air Force recruits between 1948 and 1954 who were being studied during an analysis of an outbreak of streptococcal infection. (33) The retrieved specimens were tested for anti-HCV using third-generation EIA and RIBA methods, followed by the PCR for HCV RNA and genotyping. (34) Outcome data were available from 8568 individuals using VA and Medicare files and Social Security and National Death Index tapes. Thirty-four (0.4%) of those tested were positive for anti-HCV, but only 17 (0.2%) were RIBA positive, with the remainder being indeterminate (9 persons) or negative (8 persons). The frequency of HCV infection was significantly higher among African-Americans than Caucasian recruits. Eleven of the 17 (65%) RIBA-positive persons were HCV RNA positive; 10 could be genotyped and all were identified as 1b. All-cause morbidity comparing the anti-HCV- and RIBA-positive group with those found to be negative over the 45-year period was found to be similar (relative risk = 1.24), but liver-related events were more common in the positive group (2/17 vs 115/3566; relative risk = 8.92). Mortality in the positive group (7/17, 41%) was clearly higher than that in the negative group (26%) (relative risk for African-Americans = 9.33). Of the seven deaths, however, only one was attributed to chronic liver disease. No HCV-positive but 9 HCV-negative persons had died of HCC. Thus, only 20% of the infected cohort had continuing infection or liver disease, whereas the remainder were alive without overt liver disease or had died from nonliver-related causes. Although this study was not strictly speaking a nonconcurrent cohort study of acute hepatitis C (the actual time of onset of the infection was not known), nevertheless it provided information on the outcome of hepatitis C among a young cohort of patients (average age was 23 years) with HCV infection dating from childhood or young adulthood.

Equally interesting was a study from Germany by Vogt et al. (35) detailing the prevalence and clinical outcome of HCV infection in children who had had cardiac surgery before the implementation of blood donor screening. The study involved 458 children who had undergone cardiac surgery at a mean of 17 years (range = 12 to 27 years) earlier at a mean age at first operation of 2.8 years. None had received prior or subsequent transfusions and none had mothers with detectable HCV infection. An age- and sex-matched control group from the general population was also studied. Screening included routine chemistries and hepatitis serologies using second-generation EIA, a Western blot supplemental assay, PCR for HCV RNA, quantitation of HCV RNA levels, and genotyping. Liver biopsies were performed in 17 patients who were HCV RNA positive.

Anti-HCV was detected in 67 (14.6%) patients as compared to 3 (0.7%) controls. At follow-up evaluation, 37 patients (55%) were HCV RNA positive and all but 1 had normal ALT levels. Only 3 of the 17 liver biopsies performed showed any degree of fibrosis: 2 had portal fibrosis (and both patients had congestive heart failure) and 1 patient had cirrhosis (Table VII). Thus, these authors described a benign course for transfusion-associated hepatitis C in children over a period of 20 years. They also found that almost one-half of the patients had anti-HCV without HCV RNA in serum. They concluded that the natural history of chronic hepatitis C in childhood is either more benign or more slowly progressive than in adults.

Spontaneous Loss of HCV

In initial cross-sectional studies of patients with hepatitis C, an estimated 15% of persons with HCV infection appeared to have recovered from the viral infection and were repeatedly negative for HCV RNA during long-term follow-up evaluation. (10,36) The estimate that 15% of persons recover spontaneously from HCV infection was also reported from a prospective study done among injection drug users, in which 14% of persons with serological evidence of acute HCV infection ultimately became and remained HCV RNA negative. (11) However, more recent studies have suggested that a larger proportion of persons with HCV infection clear virus, with the spontaneous recovery rate ranging from 26 to 45% (16,17,32) (Table VIII). Similar findings were reported from the analysis of the third National Health and Nutrition Examination Survey (NHANES III). (1) Among 21,241 persons who were tested from this population-based survey, 1.8% had anti-HCV as detected by second-generation EIA and RIBA, corresponding to an estimated 3.9 million persons nationwide. Virological testing of anti-HCV-positive samples indicated that 74% were positive for HCV RNA, suggesting that 2.7 million persons in the United States are infected with HCV. Thus, serological and virological testing from this population-based, unbiased cohort suggests that 26% of persons who acquire HCV infection recover and become HCV RNA negative. This estimate may also be low because some patients have been found to lose all markers of HCV infection and thus would not be detected by anti-HCV screening. In addition, these studies could not establish when during the course of hepatitis C that HCV RNA is lost, whether spontaneous clearance of HCV RNA always occurs during the first 6 months after onset of infection, and whether patients can become HCV RNA negative

TABLE VIII "Spontaneous" Loss of Hepatitis C Virus Based on Anti-HCV Seropositivity in the Absence of HCV RNA

Author (Ref.)	Country	Percentage loss	Comments
Alter et al. (1)	USA	26	NHANES III
Kenny-Walsh et al. (22)	Ireland	45	Women receiving immune globulin
Seeff et al. (32)	USA	26	Transfusion hepatitis
Vogt et al. (35)	Germany	45	Children

after 6 months, once chronic hepatitis is believed to be established. Current information suggests that spontaneous viral loss probably occurs relatively early after infection, if not during the initial 6 months, perhaps in the first year or two, but more data are needed to confirm this suspicion.

Factors That Promote Progression of Liver Disease

An issue of great importance is whether fibrosis, the major determinant of serious sequelae in chronic hepatitis C, advances inevitably and in a linear fashion to the development of cirrhosis. If progression is not universal, then there must be reasons why some but not all HCV-infected persons progress insidiously but inexorably to cirrhosis and HCC. Factors that might determine progression may be viral related (viral levels, genotype, multiplicity of quasispecies), host related (age at infection, gender, immune defect, genetic predilection, coinfection with other viruses such as hepatitis B or HIV, comorbid conditions such as hemochromotosis or iron overload), or a consequence of external factors (chronic alcoholism, diet, smoking, concomitant medicinal or illicit drug use, undefined environmental contaminants). (37–54) Indeed, the question that lingers is whether disease progression is intrinsic to HCV infection or whether, and to what extent, inherent or external modifiers determine outcome. Clearly, this is an important area deserving further attention and exploration.

CONCLUSION

The natural history of hepatitis C continues to be a dilemma (55), but knowledge in this regard is of extreme importance both for accurate counseling of patients and for rational decisions regarding therapy. Moving from the early view that hepatitis C was an insignificant form of liver disease to the view that it is almost certainly a seriously progressive disease, engendering profound concern by anxious patients exposed to sensational newspaper, magazine, and internet reports, the pendulum seems to be slowly swinging back to a less gloomy view of the chronic illness. Evidence accruing seems to suggest that more persons than originally believed to be the case recover spontaneously from the acute infection, which most do not even realize they have suffered. Among those who develop persistent infection, progression of liver disease to cirrhosis is not inevitable and probably varies in likelihood according to certain recognized (age, gender, chronic alcoholism, viral coinfections, quasispecies characterisctics, etc.) and unrecognized factors. Among those who progress to marked fibrosis or cirrhosis, serious consequences for many can be anticipated. These facts are well characterized through retrospective studies or prospective studies of those with already well-established chronic liver disease, but that does not seem to be the complete story. Prospective studies beginning with disease onset seem to indicate that a small but given proportion of acutely infected individuals progress to serious end points over the first two to three decades after infection. If that is the case, then the number of people who will ultimately develop end-stage liver disease will be directly proportional to the total number of HCV-infected persons. It has been assumed that the number of infected patients increased in the mid-

1960s to the mid-1970s as a consequence of escalating illicit drug use and that the incidence of acute hepatitis C has declined dramatically in the last decade. Accordingly, since progression to serious end-stage liver disease requires the passage of two to three decades, it is reasonable to assume that the frequency of serious disease will increase before leveling off and declining. Models to predict the extent of the anticipated problem are being developed, but time will tell just how accurate they are. In the meantime, despite the continuing controversy about the natural history, there seems to be general internal consistency even in conflicting data. Studies describing a relatively benign course focus on acute hepatitis but few exceed three decades of follow-up. Those describing serious sequelae generally focus on persons with already well-established chronic liver disease. The seriousness of the problem in this latter category is beyond dispute.

REFERENCES

1. Alter M J, Kruszon-Moran D, Nainan O V, et al. The prevalence of hepatitis C virus infection in the United States, 1988 through 1994. N Engl J Med 1999;341:556–62.
2. Pessoa M G, Wright T L. Hepatitis C infection in transplantation. Clin Liver Dis 1997;1:663–90.
3. Seeff LB. The natural history of chronic hepatitis C virus infection. Clin Liver Dis 1997; 1:587–602.
4. Kiyosawa K, Sodeyama T, Tanaka E, et al. Interrelationship of blood transfusion, non-A non-B hepatitis and hepatocellular carcinoma: analysis by detection of antibody to hepatitis C virus. Hepatology 1990;12:671–5.
5. Tong M J, El-Farra N S, Reikes A R, Co R L. Clinical outcomes after transfusion-associated hepatitis C. N Engl J Med 1995;332:1463–6.
6. Di Bisceglie A M, Goodman Z D, Ishak K G, Hoofnagle J H, Melpolder J J, Alter H J. Long-term clinical and histopathological follow-up of chronic posttransfusion hepatitis. Hepatology 1991;14:969–74.
7. Koretz R L, Abbey H, Coleman E, Gitnick G. Non-A, non-B Post-transfusion hepatitis: looking back in the second decade. Ann Intern Med 1993;119:110–5.
8. Mattson L, Sonnerborg A, Weiland O. Outcome of acute symptomatic non-A, non-B hepatitis: a 13-year follow-up study of hepatitis C virus markers. Liver 1993;13:274–8.
9. Tremolada F, Casarin C, Alberti A, et al. Long-term follow-up of non-A, non-B (type C) post-transfusion hepatitis. J Hepatol 1992;16:273–81.
10. Alter M J, Margolis H S, Krawczynski K, et al. The natural history of community-acquired hepatitis C in the United States. N Engl J Med 1992;327:1899–905.
11. Villano S A, Vlahov D, Nelson K E, Cohn S, Thomas D L. Persistence of viremia and the importance of long-term follow-up after acute hepatitis C infection. Hepatology 1999;29:908–14.
12. Poynard T, Bedossa P, Opolon P, for the OBSVIRC, METAVIR, CLINIVIR, and DOSVIRC groups. Natural history of liver fibrosis progression in patients with chronic hepatitis C. Lancet 1997;349:825–32.
13. Niederau C, Lange S, Heintges T, et al. Prognosis of chronic hepatitis C: results of a large, prospective cohort study. Hepatology 1998;28:1687–95.
14. Fattovich G, Giustina G, Degos F, et al. Morbidity and mortality in compensated cirrhosis type C: a retrospective follow-up study of 384 patients. Gastroenterology 1997;112:463–72.
15. Serfaty L, Aumaitre H, Chazouilleres O, et al. Determinants of outcome of compensated hepatitis C virus-related cirrhosis. Hepatology 1998;27:1435–40.
16. Bellentani SW, Pozzato G, Saccoccio G, et al. Clinical course and risk factors of hepatitis C virus related liver disease in the general population: report from the Dionysos study. Gut 1999; 44:874–80.
17. Bonkovsky H l, Woolley J M. Reduction of health-related quality of life in chronic hepatitis C and improvement with interferon therapy. Hepatology 1999;29:264–70.

18. Bayliss M S, Gandek B, Bungay K M, Sugano D, Hsu M A, Ware J E Jr. A questionnaire to as-
    sess the generic and disease-specific health outcomes of patients with chronic hepatitis C. Qual
    Life Res 1998;7:39–55.
19. Chossegrossi P, Pradat P, Bailly F, et al. Natural history of chronic hepatitis C: fibrosis progres-
    sion is not linear. Hepatology 2443.
20. Yano M, Kumada H, Kage M, et al. The long-term pathological evolution of chronic hepa-
    titis C. Hepatology 1996;23:1334–40.
21. Gordon S C, Bayati N, Silverman A L. Clinical outcome of hepatitis C as a function of mode of
    transmission. Hepatology 1998;28:562–7.
22. Kenny-Walsh E, for the Irish Hepatology Research group. Clinical outcomes after hepatitis in-
    fection from contaminated anti-globulin. N Engl J Med 1999;340:1228–33.
23. Muller R. The natural history of hepatitis C: clinical experiences. J Hepatol 1996;24(Suppl):
    52–4.
24. Yamakawa Y, Sata M, Suzuki H, Noguchi S, Tanakiwa K. Higher elimination rate of hepatitis
    C virus among women. J Viral Hepatitis 1996;3:317–21.
25. Seeff L B, Buskell-Bales Z, Wright E C, et al. Long-term mortality after transfusion-associated
    non-A, non-B hepatitis. N Engl J Med 1992;327:1906–11.
26. Seeff L B, Zimmerman H J, Wright E C, et al. A randomized, double-blind, controlled trial of
    the efficacy of immune serum globulin in the prevention of post-transfusion hepatitis: a
    Veterans Administration cooperative study. Gastroenterology 1977;72:111–21.
27. Seeff L B, Wright E C, Zimmerman H J, et al. Posttransfusion hepatitis, 1973–1975: a Veterans
    Administration cooperative study. In: Vyas GN, Cohen SN, Schmid R, eds. Viral hepatitis: a
    contemporary assessment of etiology, epidemiology pathogenesis and prevention. Philadelphia:
    Franklin Institute Press, 1978:371–81.
28. Alter H J, Purcell R H, Feinstone S M, Holland P V, Morrow A G. Non-A/non-B hepatitis: a
    review and interim report of an ongoing prospective study. In: Vyas GN, Cohen SN, Schmid R.
    eds. Viral hepatitis: a contemporary assessment of etiology, epidemiology, pathogenesis and pre-
    vention. Philadelphia: Franklin Institute Press, 1978:359–69.
29. Aach R D, Szmuness W, Mosley J W, et al. Serum alanine aminotransferase of donors in relation
    to the risk of non-A, non-B hepatitis in recipients: the Transfusion-Transmitted Viruses Study.
    N Engl J Med 1981;304:989–94.
30. Knodell R G, Conrad M E, Ginsberg A L, Bell C J, Flannery E P. Efficacy of prophylactic gamma-
    globulin in preventing non-A, non-B post-transfusion hepatitis. Lancet 1976;1:557–61.
31. Wright E C, Seeff L B, Hollinger F B, et al. Updated long-term mortality of transfusion-associated
    hepatitis (TAH), non-A, non-B and C. Hepatology 1998;28:272A.
32. Seeff L B, Hollinger F B, Alter H J, Wright E C, Bales Z B, NHLBI Study Group. Long-term
    morbidity of transfusion-associated hepatitis (TAH) C. Hepatology 1998;28:407A.
33. Denny F W, Wannamaker L W, Brink W R, Rammelkamp C H. Prevention of rheumatic fever,
    treatment of preceding streptococcic infection. JAMA 1950;143:151–3.
34. Seeff L B, Miller R N, Rabkin C S, et al. Forty-five year follow-up of hepatitis C virus infection
    among healthy young adults—a retrospective cohort study. Ann Intern Med 2000;132:
    105–11.
35. Vogt M, Lang T, Frosner G, et al. Prevalence and clinical outcome of hepatitis C infection in
    children who underwent cardiac surgery before the implementation of blood-donor screening.
    N Engl J Med 1999;341:866–70.
36. Alter H J, Conry-Cantilena C, Melpolder J, et al. Hepatitis C in asymptomatic blood donors.
    Hepatology 1997;26(Suppl 1):29S–33S.
37. Mendenhall C l, Seeff L B, Diehl A M, et al. Antibodies to hepatitis B virus and hepatitis C virus
    in alcoholic hepatitis and cirrhosis: their prevalence and clinical relevance. Hepatology 1991;
    14:581–9.
38. Koff R S, Dienstag J L. Extrahepatic manifestations of hepatitis C and the association with al-
    coholic liver disease. Semin Liver Dis 1995;15:101–9.
39. Pessione F, Degos F, Marcellin P, et al. Effect of alcohol consumption on serum hepatitis C vi-
    rus RNA and histological lesions in chronic hepatitis C. Hepatology 1998;27:1717–22.
40. Ostapowicz G, Watson K J R, Locarnini A, Desmond P V. Role of alcohol in the progression
    of liver disease caused by hepatitis C virus infection. Hepatology 1998;27:1730–5.

41. Gomez M R, Nogales M C, Grande L, et al. Alcohol consumption enhances intrahepatic hepatitis C virus replication. Hepatology 1998;28:280A.

42. Wiley T E, McCarthy M, Breidi L, McCarthy M, Layden T J. Impact of alcohol on the histological and clinical progression of hepatitis C infection. Hepatology 1998;28:805–9.

43. Chiba T, Matsuzaki Y, Abei M, et al. The role of previous hepatitis B virus infection and heavy smoking in hepatitis C virus-related hepatocellular carcinoma. Am J Gastroenterol 1996;91:119–203.

44. Tzouno A, Trichopoulos D, Kaklamani E, et al. Epidemiologic assessment of interactions of hepatitis C virus with seromarkers of hepatitis-B and -D viruses, cirrhosis and tobacco smoking in hepatocellular carcinoma. Int J Cancer 1991;49:377–80.

45. Serfaty L, Costagliola D, Wendum D, et al. Does HIV infection aggravate chronic hepatitis C in IV drug users? A case-control study. Hepatology 1998;28:462A.

46. Monga H K, Breaux K, Rodriguez-Barradas M C, Yoffe B. Increased HCV-related morbidity and mortality in HIV patients. Hepatology 1998;28:565A.

47. Zhang J-Y, Dai M, Wang X, et al. A case-control study of hepatitis C and V virus infection as risk factors for hepatocellular carcinoma in Henan, China. Int J Epidemiol 1998;27:574–8.

48. Smith B C, Grove J, Guzail M A, et al. Heterozygosity for hereditary hemochromatosis is associated with more fibrosis in chronic hepatitis C. Hepatology 1998;27:1695–9.

49. Gretch D, Corey I, Wilson J, et al. Assessment of hepatitis C virus levels by quantitative competitive RNA polymerase chain reaction: high-titer viremia correlated with advanced stage of disease. J Infect Dis 1994;169:1219–25.

50. Honda M, Kaneko S, Sakai A, et al. Degree of diversity of hepatitis C quasispecies and progression of liver disease. Hepatology 1994;20:1144–51.

51. Farci P, Melpolder J C, Shimoda A, et al. Studies of HCV quasispecies in patients with acute resolving hepatitis compared to those who progress to chronic hepatitis. Hepatology 1996;24:350A.

52. Kobayashi M, Tanaka E, Sodeyama T, Urushihara A, Matsumoto A, Kiyosawa K. The natural course of chronic hepatitis C: a comparison between patients with genotypes 1 and 2 hepatitis C viruses. Hepatology 1996;23:695–9.

53. Romeo R, Tommassini M A, Rumi M G, et al. Genotypes in the progression of hepatitis C related cirrhosis and development of hepatocellular carcinoma. Hepatology 1996;24:153A.

54. Pozzatto G, Moretti M, Franzini F, et al. Severity of liver disease with different hepatitis C viral clones. Lancet 1991;338:509.

55. Seeff L B. The natural history of hepatitis C—a quandary (editorial). Hepatology 998;28:1710–2.

6
PATHOLOGY OF HEPATITIS C

DAVID E. KLEINER

Laboratory of Pathology
National Cancer Institute
National Institutes of Health
Bethesda, Maryland

INTRODUCTION

Chronic hepatitis is a pattern of liver injury characterized by immune-mediated hepatocellular destruction accompanied by progressive scarring and alteration of architecture that ends as cirrhosis. The pattern of injury is distinctive in that it may be distinguished from other forms of liver disease, particularly other patterns of chronic injury, such as chronic cholestatic liver disease and steatohepatitis. However, the pattern of injury seen with chronic hepatitis C overlaps significantly with the pattern observed in chronic hepatitis B and D, in chronic autoimmune hepatitis, and in some types of chronic drug injury. The natural history of chronic hepatitis C may take anywhere from several years to decades to progress from infection to end-stage liver disease. Therefore, it is important for the pathologist to communicate not only the pattern of injury, but also the histologic severity and stage.

The percutaneous needle biopsy is the most common method used by clinicians to obtain information about liver histology in chronic hepatitis C. It is important to obtain an adequate size sample for evaluation. For a 16-gauge trucut biopsy, a biopsy length from 1 to 1.5 cm will show sufficient numbers of portal areas to make an adequate assessment of the inflammatory activity and fibrosis. If a skinny needle is used to obtain the biopsy, about twice that length should be submitted for review. The smaller the biopsy, the greater the chance of over- or underestimating the current state of disease injury. Wedge biopsies may also be used, although there is a general tendency for fibrosis to be more prominent adjacent to the capsule. Biopsies should be fixed in formalin or another suitable fixative as soon as possible to avoid artifacts due to autolysis. Mercuric fixatives such as B5 or acid-based fixatives such as Bouin's should be avoided because they make the biopsy useless for molecular analysis. After fixation and histological processing, several levels should be cut for staining. At least one section should be stained routinely with a connective tissue stain such as Masson Trichrome. Another section may be kept in reserve for an iron stain if pigment is seen within the hepatocytes. Several levels stained with hematoxylin and eosin (or its equivalent) should be examined as the degree of inflammation or fibrosis may vary from place to place within the biopsy. If the clinical differential diagnosis is broader than chronic viral hepatitis, other special stains may also be used to characterize the pathologic changes.

Questions have been raised as to the need for a liver biopsy in patients with known chronic hepatitis C. (1) Specifically the role of the liver biopsy in making treatment decisions was questioned, in that choosing not to treat patients who had unfavorable histology (specifically cirrhosis) or to treat only patients with favorable histology would miss a proportion of responders and added a risk of biopsy-related complications. However, the National Institutes of Health (NIH) Consensus Conference on the Management of Hepatitis C concluded that a liver biopsy was very helpful in that it provides useful information on the severity of activity and stage of fibrosis as well as excluding other forms of liver injury. (2,3) Knowing the histologic stage and grade of the disease can be very useful when advising patients on the current status of their disease as well as what their short- and long-term prognosis is. Thus, for now, there are still good reasons to perform a baseline liver biopsy prior to treating patients for chronic hepatitis C. As therapies for chronic hepatitis C improve, the need for an initial liver biopsy should continue to be reassessed.

ACUTE HEPATITIS C

The histologic features of acute hepatitis C have not been studied and characterized as thoroughly as those of chronic hepatitis C because of the rarity of liver biopsies performed during the acute stage of the infection. As with chronic hepatitis C (see later) the injury pattern of acute hepatitis C is similar to acute hepatitis caused by other hepatotropic viruses, specifically hepatitis A and B. (4,5) In general, acute hepatitis is dominated by a pattern of liver cell injury, as shown histologically by ballooning degeneration, spotty necrosis, hepatocellular apoptosis, and drop out. These changes are paired with changes of regeneration, including increased mitotic activity, widened liver cell plates, and disorganization of the reticulin pattern. Hepatocellular reactive changes such as nuclear hyperchromasia and variation in cell and nuclear size and shape may be seen. In severe cases, small areas of confluent necrosis may be seen, and these zones of necrosis may span the acinus, giving rise to bridging necrosis. Zones of confluent necrosis may be easily discerned on a reticulin silver stain, where the reticulin framework will have collapsed together. The hepatocellular injury is paired with an inflammatory response characterized by a predominantly lobular infiltrate of lymphocytes and activated Kupffer cells. The lymphocytes may be seen adjacent to dying hepatocytes and in foci of spotty and confluent necrosis. Kupffer cells are present to phagocytose cellular debris and may stain positively with the periodic acid-Schiff (PAS) stain as they accumulate indigestible glycoproteins and glycolipids. Fulminant massive necrosis as a result of acute infection with hepatitis C appears to occur only rarely, if at all. (6,7)

CHRONIC HEPATITIS C

Chronic hepatitis C has a basic pattern of injury that is similar to chronic hepatitis due to hepatitis B or D and to autoimmune hepatitis (for other reviews of pathology see Refs. 4, 5, 8–11). Table I (12–14) shows the distribution of histologic findings in a population of patients referred to the NIH for protocol evalu-

■ **TABLE I** **Histologic Features of Chronic Hepatitis C: Comparison with Chronic Hepatitis B and D**[a]

	HCV		HBV		HDV	
Age Mean (STD)	43.3	11.0	40.0	12.1	35.3	7.2
Range	19–78		19–71		25–54	
	Number	%	Number	%	Number	%
Sex Male	275	60.3	226	80.4	24	92.3
Female	181	39.7	55	19.6	2	7.7
Piecemeal necrosis						
None	11	2.4	0	0	0	0
Mild	107	23.8	50	18.8	1	4
Moderate	261	58.0	125	47.0	7	27
Severe	71	15.8	91	34.2	18	69
Lobular inflammation						
None	1	0.2	1	0.4	0	0
Mild	38	8.4	23	8.6	0	0
Moderate	153	34.0	101	38.0	3	12
Severe	258	57.3	141	53.0	23	88
Bridging or multiacinar necrosis	96	21.3	100	37.6	18	69.2
Lymphoid aggregates	341	75.6	132	49.6	19	73
Germinal centers	32	7.1	17	6.4	3	11
Fibrosis						
None	99	22	25	9.4	0	0
Portal fibrotic expansion	194	43.1	104	39.1	5	19
Bridging fibrosis	118	26.2	104	39.1	12	46
Cirrhosis	39	8.7	33	12.4	9	35
Poulsen (bile duct) lesions	198	43.9	56	21.0	11	42
Steatosis						
Non/trace	256	56.2	185	69.5	14	54
Mild	142	31.5	73	27.4	11	42
Moderate/severe	55	12.2	8	3.1	1	4
Iron						
None/trace	215	60.0	99	55.0	5	28
Mild	104	29.1	61	33.9	3	17
Moderate/severe	39	10.9	20	11.1	10	55

[a]Data are based on the initial liver biopsy of patients referred for evaluation to the National Institutes of Health between 1981 and 1999. Histologic features of inflammation and fibrosis were graded according to the histology activity index, (12) as modified by Di Besceglie et al. (13) Steatosis and iron were graded on a scale from 0 to 4+, with 1+ being considered mild. (14)

ation. The histologic hallmark of chronic hepatitis is the inflammatory destruction of hepatocytes accompanied by progressive fibrosis. The inflammatory component may be conveniently divided into three compartments: the hepatocellular parenchyma, the interface zone between the hepatocytes and the portal area, and the portal area itself. The classic injury is the destruction of hepatocytes at the portal limiting plate, which is known as piecemeal necrosis or interface hepatitis. From low magnification this change is demonstrated by a loss of the smooth edge of the limiting plate, which becomes ragged and indistinct as periportal hepatocytes are destroyed and inflammatory cells infiltrate between remaining hepatocytes (Fig. 1A). Piecemeal necrosis may be very focal, involving only one or two hepatocytes and with little penetration of lymphocytes into the hepatic parenchyma (Fig. 1B), or it may be severe, involving the entire circumference of the portal area with penetration of the periportal infiltrate to a depth of several hepatocytes (Fig. 1C). Careful examination of all the portal areas of a biopsy will usually reveal at least one portal area with piecemeal necrosis. Despite the name, actual necrosis is not usually seen, although rarely one may identify apoptotic hepatocytes associated with the inflammation. This observation has led some authors to propose the alternate term "interface hepatitis" to describe this change. The inflammatory infiltrate in piecemeal necrosis is dominated by CD4-positive T cells accompanied by smaller numbers of macrophages, CD8-positive T cells, and plasma cells. (15) As the disease progresses, periportal collagen deposition replaces the destroyed hepatocytes, giving a stellate appearance to the portal areas on connective tissue stains. This is the earliest fibrotic change seen in chronic hepatitis C and is given the descriptive term of periportal fibrotic expansion. In most fibrosis scoring systems (see later), this is the first recognizable stage of fibrosis (Fig. 2E).

Although we usually speak of piecemeal necrosis as a distinct histologic feature and grade it separately, it is really just the edge of the inflammation that fills the portal area itself. Portal inflammation in hepatitis C may be one of the more striking features from low magnification, especially early in the natural history when there is little fibrosis. The pattern is dominated by dense lymphoid aggregates that fill and expand the portal areas (Fig. 2A). Lymphoid aggregates are seen more frequently in hepatitis C than in hepatitis B (Table I), and some authors have suggested this as a useful diagnostic feature favoring infection by HCV in the absence of knowledge about the patient's serological findings. (16) Lymphoid aggregates have a structure and composition similar to primary follicles of lymph nodes. They are composed mainly of a mixture of B and T cells with small numbers of macrophages and CD21-positive dendritic cells. On reticulin staining, true lymphoid aggregates push the reticulin fibers aside, resulting in a round hole in the otherwise dense reticulin network. In contrast, inflammation, which is merely dense without having a specific architecture, does not cause a discernible change in the portal reticulin pattern (Figs. 2C and 2D). Rarely is there transformation of the lymphoid aggregate into a true germinal center with a core of transformed B cells and a mantle zone of B and T cells (Fig. 2B). In portal areas without lymphoid aggregates there is often an infiltrate of T lymphocytes, macrophages, and rare plasma cells and eosinophils. Neutrophils are rarely seen unless there is bile ductular proliferation secondary to fibrosis.

A histologic feature often associated with lymphoid aggregates is the Poulsen or bile duct lesion (Fig. 1E). The injured ducts may generally be seen within or at the edges of lymphoid aggregates and are characterized by reactive epithelial changes without true destruction. The ductal epithelium may be infiltrated by lymphocytes, but bile plugs and other changes of acute cholangitis or bile duct obstruction are not seen. Epithelial cells typically show reactive changes, including nuclear enlargement with the appearance of a prominent nucleolus. The cytoplasm may become more abundant and hypereosinophilic. Poulsen lesions may be severe enough to mimic the duct damage of primary biliary cirrho-

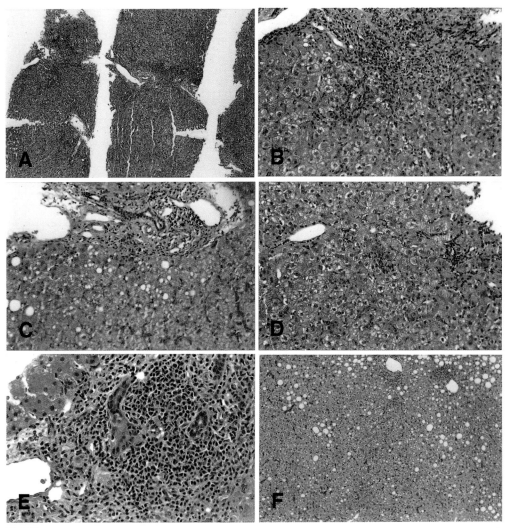

FIGURE 1 Histological changes of chronic hepatitis C. (A–C) Piecemeal necrosis (interface hepatitis). (A) From low magnification, piecemeal necrosis gives the portal area a ragged, disrupted border. Lymphocytes infiltrate between the hepatocytes of the limiting plate, separating them from their neighbors. (B) Piecemeal necrosis is severe, extending the length of the limiting plate and extending into the hepatic parenchyma to a depth of two to three hepatocytes. (C) The opposite extreme. In this portal area, the inflammation is limited and essentially involves only a single hepatocyte of the limiting plate. (D) Lobular activity. Within the hepatocellular parenchyma, small foci of lobular inflammation may be seen. These foci are composed of small collections of lymphocytes and macrophages, and the inflammation may be associated with an apoptotic hepatocyte (acidophil body, Councilman body) or an area of reticulin collapse on the reticulin stain. (E) Poulsen bile duct lesion. A bile duct lesion characteristic of those seen in hepatitis C is shown. Within a lymphoid aggregate, bile duct epithelial cells are enlarged with abundant hypereosinophilic cytoplasm and reactive nuclei. Lymphocytes are infiltrating into the bile duct. (F) Steatosis. The typical pattern of steatosis observed in chronic hepatitis C is shown. Steatosis tends to be macrovesicular (large droplet) and involves less than half of the hepatocytes. Steatosis by itself is a nonspecific finding and is not present in some biopsies of chronic hepatitis C. (A, 50×; B–D, 200×; E, 400×; F, 100×; all panels H&E stain.)

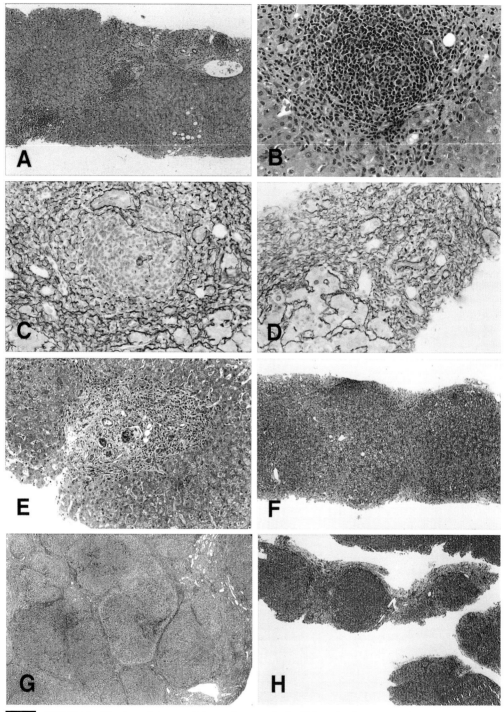

FIGURE 2 Histological changes of chronic hepatitis C. (A–D) Lymphoid aggregates. Several small lymphoid aggregates are seen in A. They appear as cohesive, round collections of small lymphocytes and may occupy all or only part of a portal area. A lymphoid aggregate may be present in a portal area without any evident piece-meal necrosis. In rare cases, the lymphoid aggregates will transform into germinal centers, as shown in B. The

(continued)

sis (PBC), but there will be no evidence of duct loss or chronic cholestasis in chronic hepatitis C, nor are Poulsen lesions associated with the granulomatous inflammation that often accompanies the early duct lesions of PBC. Finally, the ductal epithelial cells are HLA-DR negative in chronic hepatitis C, in contrast with the injured ducts of PBC, which often display this antigen. (17) Because the Poulsen lesion is seen more often in chronic hepatitis C than in chronic hepatitis B (Table I), this feature has also been recommended as a useful marker for infection with HCV. (16)

Parenchymal inflammation in chronic hepatitis C generally consists of small foci of lymphocytes and macrophages often associated with focal hepatocyte drop out or apoptosis (Fig. 1D). In some cases the number of these foci of "spotty necrosis" dominates the inflammatory pattern, and it was this type of pattern that gave rise to the obsolete term "chronic lobular hepatitis." The distinction between such cases and a pattern of resolving acute hepatitis can be difficult and it is important to correlate the pathologic pattern with the clinical information. The parenchyma may show changes in addition to the focal spots of necrosis, including areas of ballooning degeneration and focal collapse. There may also be features of regenerative activity such as hepatocellular mitotic figures and widened liver cell plates. In some cases these regenerative features will give the biopsy a vaguely nodular appearance without much fibrosis. This regenerative change can become prominent enough that a diagnosis of nodular regenerative hyperplasia may be made in addition to that of chronic hepatitis.

Steatosis, or fatty change, is another parenchymal change associated with chronic hepatitis C (Fig. 1F). At least one study has observed an increased

---

FIGURE 2 *(continued)*

germinal center shows large, transformed lymphocytes in its center. By immunophenotyping, the germinal center shows the same architecture as reactive germinal centers in lymph nodes. Lymphoid aggregates and germinal centers create a "hole" in the collagen of the portal area. The collagen fibers in C have been splayed apart by a lymphoid aggregate. The collagen fibers reorient themselves concentrically around the aggregate. This architecture recapitulates the collagen architecture of a primary follicle in a lymph node. In contrast, D shows that in a portal area with dense inflammation but without a lymphoid aggregate, there is no "hole" in the collagen. The collagen fibers remain oriented normally. (E–H) Fibrosis in chronic hepatitis C. The earliest recognizable fibrotic change in chronic hepatitis C is periportal fibrosis (E). The portal area in this panel has been enlarged by fibrosis. The collagen (stained blue) extends out from the portal area to separate and surround hepatocytes. The smooth edge of the limiting plate has been lost. As the disease of chronic hepatitis C progresses, the fibrosis gradually extends out from portal areas to form thin connections with other vascular structures, either other portal areas or central veins (F). In this biopsy, the fibrosis is seen along the top edge of the biopsy connecting three portal areas in sequence. As more and more vascular structures are connected by fibrous tissue and the architecture is further distorted by regenerative nodules, the pattern of focal bridging fibrosis gives way to cirrhosis. (G) Under low magnification, the distorted architecture of cirrhosis is readily apparent in this section from a liver removed at the time of transplantation. The normal pattern of parenchyma and vessels has been completely replaced by regenerative nodules encircled by fibrosis. Active piecemeal necrosis may continue around the edges of the nodules and foci of lobular inflammation may be seen within nodules. When a cirrhotic liver is biopsied with a needle, sometimes the nodules of liver will "pop out" of the biopsy. This results in a fragmented specimen with small round fragments of liver rimmed by fibrosis (H). This change is seen in this biopsy, in which some nodules have broken off of the main biopsy. One short fragment of the needle biopsy shows very small nodules completely encircled by fibrosis. (A, 100×; B–D, 400×; E, 200×; F, 100×; G, 25×; H, 50×; A and B, H&E; C and D, Reticulin silver stain; E–H, Masson Trichrome.)

incidence of steatosis with genotype 3A, suggesting that viral factors may be partly involved. (18) As Table I shows, about half of patients with hepatitis C will have steatosis, as opposed to less than a third of patients with hepatitis B. The steatosis tends to be mild and macrovesicular. It may be zonally distributed or random, and by itself is an entirely nonspecific change. However, in combination with lymphoid aggregates and Poulsen lesions, the presence of steatosis is more evidence in favor of a diagnosis of hepatitis C. Given that many patients will have had a hepatitis C test done prior to biopsy, this triad of findings only achieves importance when the diagnosis of HCV infection is not clear or other etiologies of liver disease are suspected clinically.

Although it is important to characterize and describe the pattern of inflammation in chronic hepatitis C, it is the progressive fibrosis with a gradual distortion of architecture that distinguishes chronic hepatitis from inflammatory disorders that resolve with little or no permanent scarring. Currently there are no clinical measures that can accurately determine the level of fibrosis in the liver before the disease has reached the level of cirrhosis. However, after the patient has progressed to cirrhosis, clinical parameters such as the Child's class become more important in determining the patient's prognosis. In all forms of chronic viral hepatitis, fibrosis follows the same natural history. At the beginning of the disease, there is no fibrosis other than the normal collagen that provides architectural support for the portal structures and a sinusoidal framework for the hepatocytes. The earliest change is an expansion of the portal area by new collagen formation. The scarring occurs between the hepatocytes of the limiting plate, splitting them apart and disrupting the smooth edge that defines the limits of the portal area. Gradually these fibrous septations extend out from portal areas until they connect to other portal areas or to central veins (Fig. 2F). Some authors distinguish between portal to portal fibrous septation and septation that bridges between portal areas and central veins. Both types of septation tend to form in conjunction with increased inflammatory activity that extends in a continuous fashion between vascular structures. This change is known as "bridging necrosis" and is used as a marker of inflammatory severity in several scoring systems. As septations form, piecemeal necrosis may extend along the length of the septa, which probably acts to gradually widen the septae. With continued inflammatory activity, the number of bridges increases, and in combination with regenerative changes and destruction of acini acts to create the distorted architectural pattern that we recognize as cirrhosis. The actual dividing line between extensive bridging fibrosis and cirrhosis can be difficult to define in a needle biopsy, as the biopsy may not be representative of the rest of the liver and biopsies of macronodular cirrhosis may show preserved portal areas and central veins.

Cirrhosis is defined as a diffuse change of the liver in which the normal architecture is replaced by regenerative nodules that are surrounded by bands of fibrosis (Fig. 2G). Within the regenerative nodules the normal relations of central veins and portal areas have been disrupted. At the extreme end, all normal vascular structures are distorted by the fibrotic changes, whereas at earlier stages there may be larger nodules in which a preserved central vein or portal area may be found. Given the sampling problems inherent in needle biopsies, it is reasonable not to make an unequivocal histologic diagnosis of cirrhosis in the presence of preserved portal areas or central veins, although elsewhere the biopsy might show micronodules completely isolated by fibrosis. If the biopsy shows only a fraction with preservation of architecture, the term "incomplete" or "incipient" cirrhosis may be used to emphasize how close the biopsy is to complete architectural disruption and to distinguish it from lesser degrees of bridging fibrosis.

Complicating the diagnosis of cirrhosis is the tendency for needle biopsies to fragment along the edge between the parenchyma and the fibrotic bands. In micronodular cirrhosis the nodules can be about the same as the width of a standard needle biopsy, leading to a biopsy composed of small spheres of liver tissue with small wisps of fibrosis clinging to the surface (Fig. 2H). This sort of fragmentation must be distinguished from mechanical fragmentation, in which the parenchyma is torn apart at random. Typically the micronodules will not show preserved portal areas or central veins and the liver cell plates will show regenerative changes on a reticulin stain. The Masson stain may show a thin layer of collagen around the edge of the nodule, but this may not completely encircle the fragment. The reticulin stain may also help by demonstrating a continuous layer of reticulin fibers on the edge of the nodules, in contrast to the broken, discontinuous pattern that is seen at a torn edge. These can be helpful clues for the pathologist when faced with a fragmented biopsy from a patient who has cirrhosis in the clinical differential.

HISTOLOGIC DIFFERENTIAL DIAGNOSIS

When a pathologist reviews a biopsy for chronic liver disease, one of two clinical situations usually prevails. In one situation, the patient has already received a thorough laboratory evaluation for liver disease, including antibody tests for hepatitis C and B, as well as autoimmune antigens, serum iron tests, platelet counts, and prothrombin times. In this scenario, the clinician is likely to be aware of an etiology for liver disease and is seeking to learn how severe or advanced the disease is. Alternatively, the liver biopsy may be done prior to significant laboratory evaluation and the clinician may be seeking guidance from the pathologist as to an etiology. It is also possible that an extensive workup has occurred and the only finding is persistently abnormal liver-associated enzymes. Again, the clinician looks to the pathologist for guidance as to possible etiologies and, even in the absence of a histologically definable etiology, is seeking an evaluation of the histologic severity. Table II lists some of the possible etiologies for chronic liver disease that have pathologic features that overlap to a greater or lesser degree with chronic hepatitis C.

The most difficult distinction histologically is that between the different viral hepatitides and between chronic viral hepatitis and autoimmune hepatitis. The distinction is usually not possible on histologic grounds alone, although some features are helpful. The finding of ground glass cells is virtually pathognomonic for hepatitis B, but it does not rule out the presence of concomitant hepatitis C. Autoimmune hepatitis is usually very severe and often has a prominent plasma cellular infiltrate. As noted earlier, the triad of steatosis, lymphoid aggregates, and Poulsen lesions is more often associated with chronic hepatitis C than other etiologies of chronic hepatitis. However, there is so much overlap

TABLE II   Histologic Differential Diagnosis for Chronic Hepatitis C

Disease entity	Useful distinguishing features
Chronic hepatitis B	Ground glass hepatocytes, immunoperoxidase staining for hepatitis B surface and core antigen
Chronic hepatitis D	Immunoperoxidase staining for hepatitis delta antigen, typically very severe inflammation
Autoimmune hepatitis	Plasma cells dominate the inflammatory infiltrate
Drug-induced chronic hepatitis	Mixed pattern of hepatocellular and cholestatic injury, zone 3 canalicular or hepatocellular cholestatis, numerous eosinophils
Primary biliary cirrhosis	Destruction of interlobular bile ducts, cholate stasis, missing bile ducts, copper accumulation in the absence of significant fibrosis
Primary sclerosing cholangitis	Bile duct loss, concentric fibrosis around ducts, cholate stasis, copper accumulation in the absence of significant fibrosis
Steatohepatitis (alcoholic or nonalcoholic)	Zone 3 ballooning degeneration, Mallory bodies, zone 3 sinusoidal fibrosis
Hemochromatosis	Hepatocellular iron accumulation most prominent in zone 1, sparse inflammatory infiltrate
Wilson's disease	Steatohepatitis-like changes, copper accumulation later in disease course, copper-associated Mallory bodies

in the histology of these lesions that a distinction between them using histology alone is not recommended. Drug-induced chronic hepatitis may also have significant histologic overlap with chronic hepatitis C, but the pathologist may be faced with a biopsy in a patient with known chronic hepatitis C in whom drug injury is suspected. In such cases the pathologist should focus on features of injury that would be atypical for chronic hepatitis C, such as cholestasis or ballooning in acinar zone 3, prominent lobular eosinophilia, and zonal necrosis. When the overall pattern of injury is not typical for hepatitis C, the pathologist should be ready to suggest other etiologies as an explanation of the injury pattern.

Outside the core of the chronic hepatitides, there are two other major patterns of chronic injury with some overlap of histologic features: chronic cholestatic liver disease and steatohepatitis. Chronic cholestatic liver diseases such as primary biliary cirrhosis and primary sclerosing cholangitis may have early patterns of injury that show little duct injury and are therefore characterized more by their inflammatory infiltrate. Both of these diseases may show disruption of the limiting plate by inflammation and focal lobular necrosis. When the etiology of liver disease is unclear, early stages of chronic cholestatic liver disease should be included in the histologic differential diagnosis. Histologic features such as loss of interlobular bile ducts, granulomatous duct injury, and cholate stasis (pseudoxanthomatous change or feathery degeneration of hepatocytes) should lead the pathologist away from the diagnosis of chronic hepatitis into the differential of chronic cholestatic liver disease.

Steatohepatitis is a pattern of injury with diverse etiologies, including chronic alchohol use, diabetes mellitus, and obesity. It may also be seen in the absence of any clear etiology or association, which puts it in the differential diagnosis of almost every case of chronic liver disease. As a further complication, it shares some features with chronic hepatitis C, including progressive fibrosis, steatosis, and spotty lobular necrosis. When these features dominate the histologic pattern, there may be confusion as to the true etiology of the changes, even with positive serology for hepatitis C. When the patient presents with positive viral markers, it is probably more accurate to ascribe the histologic changes to the virus unless there is clear histologic evidence of another chronic liver disease. In order to make the diagnosis of intercurrent steatohepatitis, there should be specific features of steatohepatitis present. These would include clear ballooning hepatocellular injury in acinar zone 3, associated with either Mallory's hyalin or sinusoidal fibrosis. The latter two features should also be present in zone 3, although as the fibrosis progresses it will become more difficult to define the location of zone 3.

A mild degree of iron overload can be observed in many patients with hepatitis C, even in the absence of a defined etiology, such as alcohol use, hemolytic anemia, transfusion therapy, or hemochromatosis. Primary genetic hemochromatosis is one of the most common genetically transmitted diseases and 2 to 3% of patients will be heterozygous for this disorder. Iron overload has been suggested to reduce the response rate to interferon-α. Because iron overload is so common in this population and because it is possible to identify individuals at risk for genetic hemochromatosis on liver biopsy, it is not unreasonable to do an iron stain on all biopsies under evaluation for medical liver disease. Small amounts of iron restricted to Kuppfer cells, endothelial cells, or other stromal cells are probably clinically insignificant. When the iron accumulation is present within hepatocytes, the pattern of deposition and the amount are worthy of comment. Iron accumulation that is strong in zone 1 and tapers off toward zone 3 is at least suggestive of hemochromatosis even in the face of chronic hepatitis C infection and the pathologist should bring this possibility to the attention of the clinician caring for the patient.

CHRONIC HEPATITIS C IN SPECIAL CLINICAL SITUATIONS

Chronic Hepatitis C in Children

Several studies have attempted to specifically address the pathology of chronic hepatitis C in children. (19–23) Children included in these studies have mostly acquired their infection via transfusion and many have other serious diseases, such as a malignancy or aplastic anemia. One study evaluated a group of children included as part of a cohort of patients who developed posttransfusion hepatitis. (19) Out of 29 children with documented posttransfusion hepatitis, 16 (55%) developed histologic evidence of chronic hepatitis C. This group included all 14 children whose serum alanine amino-transferase (ALT) remained elevated for at least 6 months and confirmed that children could acquire a chronic infection that was histologically similar to that seen in adults. Further observations in larger cohorts have shown that chronic hepatitis C in children has all of the histologic features of chronic hepatitis C in adults, including piecemeal necrosis, spotty lobular necrosis, progression of fibrosis to cirrhosis, lymphoid aggregates, Poulsen bile duct lesions, and steatosis. (21,22) When children have been compared to cohorts of adults with hepatitis C at the same institution, the findings are generally less severe. Children generally have less fibrosis and less inflammation than adults, with only eight biopsies in a total of 283 patients (3%) from five studies having cirrhosis. However, it must be remembered that there are numerous confounding factors in making comparisons with adults, including duration of infection, variation in immune response between children and adults, and intercurrent diseases. What can be concluded is that at the light microscopic level, adults and children share the same pathology and should therefore be evaluated for inflammatory activity and fibrosis by the same criteria.

Chronic Hepatitis C and Alcohol Consumption

Alcohol consumption has been identified frequently as an independent risk factor in the progress of chronic hepatitis C to cirrhosis. (24,25) That being the case, there have been several studies that have attempted to identify specific histologic features of chronic hepatitis C that could be related to alcohol use. (25–28) The major conclusion from these studies has been that the features of chronic hepatitis C are not qualitatively different between those who drink and those who do not. There is some suggestion in the literature that patients with chronic hepatitis C who drink have more severe disease (both in terms of more advanced fibrosis and more severe inflammation) than those who do not. However, it is difficult to separate out a specific effect of alcohol from other factors that covary with drinking, such as age and male sex. Specific features of alcohol-related steatohepatitis (zone 3 ballooning degeneration and Mallory bodies) are not seen in most cases and other features (steatosis, pericellular fibrosis) appear to be common to both drinkers and nondrinkers of alcohol. Subtle differences have been reported in the character of the fibrosis seen in alcoholic liver disease as opposed to chronic hepatitis C, but it would be difficult to apply these findings in routine diagnosis. (27) In general, it would appear that most of the changes in any particular biopsy should be ascribed to hepatitis C unless other patterns of injury, such as steatohepatitis, are clearly present.

Chronic Hepatitis C in HIV-Positive Individuals

Because hepatitis C and HIV have common modes of transmission, a high percentage of HIV-infected patients will also be infected with hepatitis C. Several studies have attempted to identify changes in the pathology of chronic hepatitis C when the patient is coinfected with HIV. An early study by Guido et al. (29) examined HIV$^+$ patients with HCV infection and compared their liver biopsies to patients with HCV infection alone. When the patient's immune system was still intact, as defined by CD4 counts of greater than 400 cell/mm^3, there were no discernible differences between the HIV$^+$ and HIV$^-$ groups, suggesting that in the early stages of HIV infection, the pathology of chronic hepatitis C infection was unaffected. In patients whose CD4 counts had fallen below 400 cells/mm^3, less inflammation was seen, consistent with the immunosuppression of late-stage HIV infection. Another group, examining only patients with more intact immune systems, reported higher levels of HCV viremia and more severe inflammation and fibrosis in patients with HCV/HIV coinfection than in a control group of HIV⁻ patients with chronic hepatitis C. (30) This study also reported an independent association of hepatitis severity and HCV genotype 1b, a finding that has not been confirmed in other studies. (18) Given the small amount of data available, it is probably reasonable to conclude that there is certainly no reduction in the severity of chronic hepatitis C early in the course of HIV infection. In fact, it may be worsened by a tendency toward increases in HCV viral load and from other undefined factors. Late in the course of HIV infection, as the CD4 counts fall to zero, inflammatory changes due to HCV are reduced as the body loses its ability to mount a cell-mediated immune response. At this point, opportunistic infections of the liver and involvement by lymphoma or Kaposi sarcoma may dominate the histologic picture.

Posttransplantation Evaluation of Chronic Hepatitis C

Evaluation of the liver biopsy in the posttransplant setting is complicated by the multiple potential etiologies of injury and by overlapping patterns of injury. Both acute rejection and recurrent hepatitis C infection may have significant portal lymphocytic infiltrates and both may show varied degrees of parenchymal and bile duct injury. PCR analysis of posttransplant liver biopsies has shown that essentially all patients transplanted for chronic hepatitis C will have reinfection of the graft liver. (31–34) However, not all patients will show histologic changes of chronic hepatitis C: between 20 and 40% of patients will not progress beyond mild hepatitis in the first few years following transplantation. (31,33) The histologic pattern of injury in recurrent chronic hepatitis C is very similar to that of chronic hepatitis C in the native liver, but there is a suggestion that recurrent hepatitis C may progress more rapidly to cirrhosis. Severe hepatitis may be seen as soon as a month after transplantation and cirrhosis within the first few years. Greenson et al. (33) found that serial biopsies and the time course of histologic changes are helpful in distinguishing acute rejection from recurrent hepatitis due to HCV. In their population, acute hepatitis was seen an average of 135 days posttransplantation (range 39 to 279 days) with progression to chronic hepatitis at an average of 356 days posttransplantation (range 89 to 1365 days). Acute rejection tended to occur sooner than recurrent chronic hepatitis and tended to respond to steroid therapy. Although PCR for HCV in liver biopsy tissue has been recommended as a useful test to distinguish recurrence from rejection, given the high incidence of reinfection, only a negative result would be helpful.

STAGING, GRADING, AND HISTOLOGIC SCORING OF CHRONIC HEPATITIS C

In the mid-1990s, a quiet revolution took place in the way pathologists and clinicians viewed chronic liver disease, particularly chronic hepatitis. It had become clear that the old classification of chronic hepatitis into histologic subtypes —chronic active hepatitis, chronic persistant hepatitis, and chronic lobular hepatitis—were no longer adequate descriptions in the face of what was known about the natural history and biology of chronic hepatitis. (35–38) Several editorials and reviews attempted to address this problem, and through discussion in the literature and at specific workshops, a consensus was reached that the diagnostic evaluation of a liver biopsy in a patient with chronic hepatitis should contain three elements: an etiology, a grade, and a stage. (39) Etiology is the simplest of the three and is primarily determined based on a thorough serologic evaluation. The idea of grading and staging hepatitis arose following on observations of the effects of therapy on histology. The inflammatory grade of hepatitis fluctuates over time and may be reduced by theraputic intervention. In contrast, the fibrotic stage of hepatitis is viewed as more relentlessly progressive and relatively resistant to theraputic manipulation. Grading and staging are related to histologic scoring, but may be done independantly of a specific score. Desmet et al. (39) recommended a five-level descriptive system for both grading and staging. The inflammatory activity should be graded as none, minimal, mild, moderate, and marked. Fibrosis is staged as none, mild (portal expansion), moderate (early bridging fibrosis), marked (established bridging), and cirrhosis. Grading evaluates the amount of inflammatory activity in the biopsy and should emphasize features of piecemeal and lobular necrosis rather than the absolute density of inflammation. Features such as bridging necrosis and multiacinar necrosis should push the grade to the higher levels of activity. The fibrotic stage is related more directly to scoring systems used for quantifying this feature. In fact, the METAVIR fibrosis scale shown in Table VII (40,41) is used by many pathologists to stage liver biopsies even if they choose not to use the rest of the METAVIR scoring system.

Scoring of liver biopsies for particular histologic features is still primarily a research tool. In this context, scoring is used to stratify patients according to particular histologic features, to make objective evaluations over time, to investigate the prognostic significance of histologic features, and to provide a more finely divided ruler against which overall activity is measured. Before committing to a particular scoring system in the absence of particular research protocols, the pathologist should consult with the clinical staff so that there is common understanding of the scoring tool to be used, realizing that the use of any scoring system by a particular pathologist will be subject to individual variation in how the levels of injury are interpreted. Most published studies use the METAVIR system, the HAI score, or a variation of one of these. Tables III through VII provide a comparison of the different systems and their variants without attempting to equate scores on any particular scale to each other. (12,13,40–42) The scoring systems vary as to the degree of injury deserving a particular score and the maximum score on any one scale. Although there has been some work to evaluate the interobserver reproducibility of the different systems, one should remember that these studies are generally performed using experienced hepatic pathologists who have come together and agreed on how the scoring system should be interpreted. It is more important for an individual pathologist who is asked to use a particular scoring system to assure themselves of reasonable intraobserver reproducibility. It may be necessary to restrict such scoring to one or two pathologists in a particular group in order to achieve a high level of reproducibil-

▆▆▆ **TABLE III   Comparison of Scoring Systems: Periportal Necroinflammatory Changes**

Score	Original HAI[a] (12)	Modified HAI (42)	METAVIR[b] (40)
0	None	Absent	Absent
1	Mild piecemeal necrosis	Mild (focal, few portal areas)	Focal alteration of the periportal plate in some portal tracts
2		Mild/moderate (focal, most portal areas)	Diffuse alteration of the periportal tract in some portal tracts or focal
3	Moderate piecemeal necrosis (involves less than 50% of the circumference of most portal tracts)	Moderate (continuous around <50% of tracts or septae	Diffuse alteration of the periportal plate in all portal tracts
4	Marked piecemeal necrosis (involves more than 50% of the circumference of most portal tracts)	Severe (continuous around >50% of tracts or septae)	

[a] The periportal component of the Knodell HAI has been split into a periportal piecemeal necrosis and a bridging/confluent necrosis component for better comparison to the other scoring systems. In order to recreate the original scale, the bridging/confluent necrosis component should be added to the periportal piecemeal necrosis component.

[b] The periportal component of the METAVIR score is used with the focal necrosis score to determine overall inflammatory activity.

▆▆▆ **TABLE IV   Comparison of Scoring Systems: Bridging and Confluent Necrosis**

Score	Original HAI[a] (12)	Modified HAI (42)	METAVIR[b] (40)
0	Absent	Absent	Absent
1		Focal confluent necrosis	Present
2	Bridging necrosis (more than two such bridges)	Zone 3 necrosis in some areas	
3		Zone 3 necrosis in most areas	
4		Zone 3 necrosis + occasional portal–central bridging necrosis	
5		Zone 3 necrosis + multiple portal–central bridging necrosis	
6	Multilobular necrosis	Panacinar or multiacinar necrosis	

[a] The periportal component of the Knodell HAI has been split into a periportal piecemeal necrosis and a bridging/confluent necrosis component for better comparison to the other scoring systems. In order to recreate the original scale, the bridging/confluent necrosis component should be added to the periportal piecemeal necrosis component.

[b] The METAVIR score for bridging necrosis is not used in the overall activity determination by this system and is provided only for comparison with the other scales.

■■■■ **TABLE V Comparison of Scoring Systems: Focal (Spotty) Lobular Necrosis and Hepatocellular Apoptosis**

Score	Original HAI (12)	Modified HAI (42)	METAVIR (40)
0	None	Absent	Less than one necroinflammatory focus per lobule
1	Mild (acidophilic bodies, ballooning degeneration, and/or scattered foci of hepatocellular necrosis in less than one-third of lobules/nodules)	One focus or less per 10× field	At least one necroinflammatory focus per lobule
2		Two to 4 foci per 10× field	Several necroinflammatory foci per lobule or confluent/bridging necrosis
3	Moderate (involvement of one-third to two-thirds of lobules/nodules)	Five to 10 foci per 10× field	
4	Marked (involvement of more than two-thirds of lobules/nodules)	More than 10 foci per 10× field	

ity. Scoring should be related to the stage and grade reported in the diagnostic report. Tables VIII (39) and IX (41) show how the HAI and METAVIR inflammation scores are related to the grade of histological injury. In the HAI system, the aggregate score of the various inflammation subscores is directly related to the descriptive grade of inflammation. In the METAVIR system, the grade is re-

■■■■ **TABLE VI Comparison of Scoring Systems: Portal Inflammation**

Score	Original HAI (12)	Modified HAI (13)	Modified HAI (42)	METAVIR[a] (40)
0	No portal inflammation	No portal areas with dense inflammation	None	Absent
1	Mild (sprinkling of inflammatory cells in less than one-third of portal tracts)	Mild (dense inflammation or aggregates in less than one-third of portal areas)	Mild, some or all portal areas	Presence of mononuclear aggregates in some portal tracts
2			Moderate, some or all portal areas	Mononuclear aggregates in all portal tracts
3	Moderate (increased inflammation in one-third to two-thirds of portal tracts)	Moderate (dense inflammation or aggregates in one-third to two-thirds of portal areas)	Moderate/marked, all portal areas	Large and dense mononuclear aggregates in all portal tracts
4	Marked (dense packing of inflammatory cells in more than two-thirds of portal tracts)	Marked (dense inflammation or aggregates in more than two-thirds of portal areas)	Marked, all portal areas	

[a] The METAVIR score for portal inflammation is not used in the overall activity determination by this system and is provided only for comparison with the other scales.

███ **TABLE VII** Fibrosis

Score	Original HAI (12)	Modified HAI (42)	METAVIR (40)
0	No fibrosis	No fibrosis	No fibrosis
1	Fibrous portal expansion	Fibrous expansion of some portal areas, with or without short fibrous septa	Stellate enlargement of portal tracts without septae formation
2		Fibrous expansion of most portal areas, with or without short fibrous septa	Enlargement of portal tracts with rare septae formation
3	Bridging fibrosis (portal–portal or portal–central linkage)	Fibrous expansion of most portal areas with occasional portal to portal bridging	Numerous septae without fibrosis
4	Cirrhosis	Fibrous expansion of portal areas with marked bridging (portal to portal as well as portal to central)	Cirrhosis
5		Marked bridging with occasional nodules (incomplete cirrhosis)	
6		Cirrhosis, probable or definite	

███ **TABLE VIII** Relationship of Aggregate Inflammation Scores to Grade of Activity (39)

Sum of inflammation scores in HAI or modified HAI systems	Description of activity
0	None
1–4	Minimal
5–8	Mild
9–12	Moderate
13–18	Marked

███ **TABLE IX** Relationship of Inflammation Scores to Activity in the **METAVIR** system (41).

Piecemeal necrosis score	Focal necrosis score		
	0	1	2
0	A0-None	A1-Mild	A2-Moderate
1	A1-Mild	A1-Mild	A2-Moderate
2	A2-Moderate	A2-Moderate	A3-Marked
3	A3-Marked	A3-Marked	A3-Marked

lated to two of the inflammation scores: the score for lobular inflammation and the score for piecemeal necrosis. Table IX was derived after a group of experienced pathologists were asked to grade the biopsies based on their impression of the severity of inflammation. The result was then compared to the actual scores and only the scales with high correlation to the gestalt grade were used in the final determination. It should be emphasized that grading and staging are the most important when reporting the results of a biopsy of chronic hepatitis C. Scoring of liver biopsies is a secondary activity, which should take place only if there is good understanding not only of the scoring system used but also the purpose to which the information will be helpful.

CONCLUSION

The pathology of chronic hepatitis C is characterized by a necroinflammatory/hepatocellular injury coupled with progressive fibrosis. The basic inflammatory pattern is a combination of portal, periportal, and lobular inflammation distinct from other patterns of chronic liver disease, such as chronic cholestatic liver disease and steatohepatitis. In particular, the triad of lymphoid aggregates, Poulsen bile duct lesions, and steatosis favor HCV as the etiology of hepatitis. This pattern of injury also dominates the histologic changes when chronic hepatitis C is seen in children or is complicated by alcohol use, HIV infection, or in the posttransplant setting. The diagnostic evaluation of chronic hepatitis C should include a description of the inflammatory grade and fibrotic stage, as these are most useful in guiding patient management. The utility of the liver biopsy in the clinical workup of chronic hepatitis C should continue to be assessed as our ability to treat this disease improves.

REFERENCES

1. Wong J B, Bennett W G, Koff R S, Pauker S G. Pretreatment evaluation of chronic hepatitis C—risks, benefits, and costs. JAMA 1998;280:2088–2093.
2. National Institutes of Health Consensus Development Conference Panel Statement. Management of hepatitis-C. Hepatology 1997;26:S2–S10.
3. Perrillo R P. The role of liver biopsy in hepatitis C. Hepatology 1997;26:57S–61S.
4. Gerber M A. Pathology of hepatitis C. FEMS Microbiol Rev 1994;14:205–10.
5. Goodman Z D, Ishak K G. Histopathology of hepatitis C virus infection. Semin Liver Dis 1995;15:70–81.
6. Feray C, Gigou M, Samuel D, et al. Hepatitis C virus RNA and hepatitis B virus DNA in serum and liver of patients with fulminant hepatitis [see comments]. Gastroenterology 1993;104:549–55.
7. Liang T J, Jeffers L, Reddy R K, et al. Fulminant or subfulminant non-A, non-B viral hepatitis: the role of hepatitis C and E viruses [see comments]. Gastroenterology 1993;104:556–62.
8. Dhillon A P, Dusheiko G M. Pathology of hepatitis C virus infection. Histopathology 1995;26:297–309.
9. Fischer H P, Willsch E, Bierhoff E, Pfeifer U. Histopathologic findings in chronic hepatitis C. J Hepatol 1996;24:35–42.
10. Scheuer P J, Ashrafzadeh P, Sherlock S, Brown D, Dusheiko G M. The pathology of hepatitis C. Hepatology 1992;15:567–71.

11. Scheuer P J, Krawczynski K, Dhillon A P. Histopathology and detection of hepatitis C virus in liver. Springer Semin Immunopathol 1997;19:27–45.
12. Knodell R, Ishak K, Black W, et al. Formulation and application of a numerical scoring system for assessing histological activity in asymptomatic chronic active hepatitis. Hepatology 1981; 1:431–5.
13. Di Bisceglie A M, Conjeevaram H S, Fried M W, et al. Ribavirin as therapy for chronic hepatitis C. A randomized, double- blind, placebo-controlled trial [see comments]. Ann Intern Med 1995;123:897–903.
14. Kleiner D E, Gaffey M J, Sallie R, et al. Histopathologic changes associated with fialuridine hepatotoxicity. Mod Pathol 1997;10:192–9.
15. Khakoo S I, Soni P N, Savage K, et al. Lymphocyte and macrophage phenotypes in chronic hepatitis C infection: Correlation with disease activity. Am J Pathol 1997;150:963–70.
16. Lefkowitch J H, Schiff E R, David G L, et al. Pathological diagnosis of chronis hepatitis C: a multicenter comparative study with chronic hepatitis B. The Hepatitis Interventional Therapy Group [see comments]. Gastroenterology 1993;104:595–603.
17. Danque P O V, Bach N, Schaffner F, Gerber M A, Thung S N. HLA-DR expression in bile duct damage in hepatitis C. Mod Pathol 1993;6:327–32.
18. Mihm S, Fayyazi A, Hartmann H, Ramadori G. Analysis of histopathological manifestations of chronic hepatitis C virus infection with respect to virus genotype. Hepatology 1997;25:735–9.
19. Matsouka S, Katsuyoshi T, Hayabuchi Y, et al. Serologic, virologic and histologic characteristics of chronic phase Hepatitis C virus disease in children infected by transfusion. Pediatrics 1994;94:919–22.
20. Inui A, Fujisawa T, Miyagawa Y, et al. Histologic activity of the liver in children with transfusion-associated chronic hepatitis C. J Hepatol 1994;21:748–53.
21. Kage M, Fujisawa T, Shiraki K, et al. Pathology of chronic hepatitis C in children. Child Liver Study Group of Japan. Hepatology 1997;26:771–5.
22. Badizadegan K, Jonas M M, Ott M J, Nelson S P, Perez-Atayde A R. Histopathology of the liver in children with chronic hepatitis C viral infection. Hepatology 1998;28:1416–23.
23. Guido M, Rugge M, Jara P, et al. Chronic hapatitis C in children: the pathological and clinical spectrum. Gastroenterology 1998;115:1525–9.
24. Wiley T E, McCarthy M, Breidi L, McCarthy M, Layden T J. Impact of alcohol on the histological and clinical progression of hepatitis C infection. Hepatology 1998;28:805.
25. Ostapowicz G, Watson K J R, Locarnini S A, Desmond P V. Role of alcohol in the progression of liver disease caused by hepatitis C virus infection. Hepatology 1998;27:1730.
26. Noguchi O, Yamaoka K, Ikeda T, et al. Clinicopathological analysis of alcoholic liver disease complicating chronic type C hepatitis. Liver 1991;11:225–30.
27. Nakano M, Maruyama K, Okuyama K, et al. The characteristics of alcoholics with HCV infection: histopathologic comparison with alcoholics without HCV infection and chronic type C hepatitis. Alcohol Alcohol Suppl 1993;1B:35–40.
28. Uchimura Y, Sata M, Kage M, Abe H, Tanikawa K. A histopathological study of alcoholics with chronic HCV infection: comparison with chronic hepatitis C and alcoholic liver disease. Liver 1995;15:300–6.
29. Guido M, Rugge M, Fattovich G, et al. Human immunodeficiency virus infection and hepatitis C pathology. Liver 1994;14:314–9.
30. Garcia-Samaniego J, Soriano V, Castilla J, et al. Influence of hepatitis C virus genotypes and HIV infection on histological severity of chronic hepatitis C. The Hepatitis/HIV Spanish Study Group. Am J Gastroenterol 1997;92:1130–4.
31. Ferrell L D, Wright T L, Roberts J, Ascher N, Lake J. Hepatitis C viral infection in liver transplant recipients. Hepatology 1992;16:865–76.
32. Thung S N, Shim K S, Shieh Y S, et al. Hepatitis C in liver allografts. Arch Pathol Lab Med 1993;117:145–9.
33. Greenson J K, Svoboda-Newman S M, Merion R M, Frank T S. Histologic progression of recurrent hepatitis C in liver transplant allografts. Am J Surg Pathol 1996;20:731–8.
34. Lumbreras C, Colina F, Loinaz C, et al. Clinical, virological, and histologic evolution of hepatitis C virus infection in liver transplant recipients. Clin Infect Dis 1998;26:48–55.
35. Ludwig J. The nomenclature of chronic active hepatitis: an obituary. Gastroenterology 1993; 105:274–8.

36. Czaja A. Chronic active hepatitis: the challenge for a new nomenclature. Ann Intern Med 1993; 119:510–17.

37. Ishak K. Chronic hepatitis: morphology and nomenclature. Mod Pathol 1994;7:690–713.

38. Batts K, Ludwig J. Chronic hepatitis: an update on terminology and reporting. Am J Surg Pathol 1995;19:1409–17.

39. Desmet V, Gerber M, Hoofnagle J, Manns M, Scheuer P. Classification of chronic hepatitis: Diagnosis, grading and staging. Hepatology 1994;19:1513–20.

40. The French METAVIR Cooperative Study Group. Intraobserver and interobserver variations in biopsy interpretation in patients with chronic hepatitis C. Hepatology 1994;20:15–20.

41. Bedossa P, Poynard T. An algorithm for the grading of activity in chronic hepatitis C. The METAVIR Cooperative Study Group. Hepatology 1996;24:289–93.

42. Ishak K, Baptista A, Bianchi L, et al. Histological grading and staging of chronic hepatitis. J Hepatol. 1995;22:696–9.

7
HUMORAL RESPONSE TO HEPATITIS C VIRUS

AMY J. WEINER, DAVID CHIEN, QUI-LIM CHOO, STEPHEN R. COATES, GEORGE KUO, AND MICHAEL HOUGHTON
Chiron Corporation
Emeryville, California

INTRODUCTION

The majority of individuals infected with hepatitis C virus (HCV) develop chronic infections and approximately 20–30% of those individuals experience liver disease. (1–6) Typically, the cellular and humoral arms of the immune system play critical roles in both the pathology and the clearance of viral infections. This chapter focuses on the B-cell response to natural infection as well as on approaches to stimulate a humoral response in animals by immunization with antigens produced synthetically or by recombinant DNA technologies. Understanding the humoral response to HCV and related antigens provides insight into the mechanisms and correlates of resolution of viral infection and viral persistence. Together with information on the cellular response to HCV, progress is being made toward developing vaccines and antiviral therapies for the prevention and treatment of disease resulting from HCV infection

NATURAL HUMORAL RESPONSE TO HCV INFECTION IN HUMANS AND CHIMPANZEES

Prior to the isolation of the first cDNA clone encoding part of the HCV polyprotein using λ gt11 immunoscreening (7), evidence for a humoral response to HCV was lacking. Several attempts failed to identify an antigen–antibody complex in liver tissue or sera. (8,9) Once the entire coding sequence of the HCV genome was cloned, overlapping cDNA clones expressing superoxide dismutase (SOD)-HCV fusion proteins in bacteria were screened with sera from chronic (non-A,non-B hepatitis) NANBH patients in search of immunoreactive polypeptides. (10) Results showed that all of the HCV structural and nonstructural proteins (see Fig. 1), with the exception of NS2, encoded linear B-cell epitopes. The development of three generations of immunodiagnostics for HCV antigens (1,11,12) provided clear evidence that individuals with asymptomatic and chronic HCV infections mounted a broad response to epitopes in the nonstructural proteins (NS3-NS5). The prevalence of antibodies to core (c22), NS3 helicase domain (c33c), NS4A (c100-3), and NS5 (see Fig. 1, refs. 13–15) in a cohort of patients with posttransfusion, chronic NANBH was 92, 95, 71, and

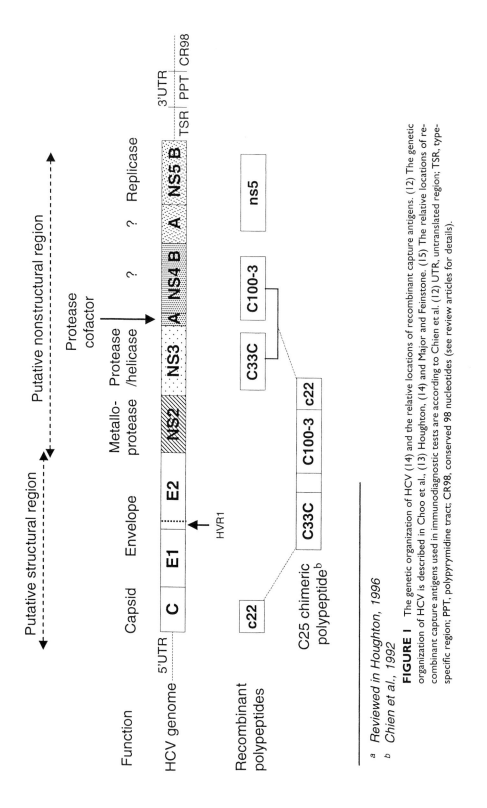

FIGURE 1 The genetic organization of HCV (14) and the relative locations of recombinant capture antigens. (12) The genetic organization of HCV is described in Choo et al., (13) Houghton, (14) and Major and Feinstone. (15) The relative locations of re-combinant capture antigens used in immunodiagnostic tests are according to Chien et al. (12) UTR, untranslated region; TSR, type-specific region; PPT, polypyrimidine tract; CR98, conserved 98 nucleotides (see review articles for details).

[a] Reviewed in Houghton, 1996
[b] Chien et al., 1992

74%, respectively. (12) Several subsequent studies have reported similar findings. (13,6–18) Chimpanzees were very poor responders to core but had a nearly equivalent humoral response to NS3-5 antigens. Reactivity of sera from 18 chimpanzees with chronic HCV infections was 56, 89, 83, and 83% for the core, NS3 helicase domain, NS4 antigen, and NS5 antigen, respectively. (19) Two separate studies found 100% seroconversion to the chimeric c25 antigen, which contained epitopes from core (c22), NS3, and NS4 (see Fig. 1) in six chimpanzees inoculated experimentally with HCV-1 (7,20,21) and eight chimpanzees inoculated with the H strain of HCV. (23) Because the reactivity of c25 was most likely due to the immunodominant c33c epitope, these findings are comparable to the 95% anti-c33c reactivity observed in humans.

Seroconversion to nonstructural antigens occurred between 2 and 8 months following transfusion in humans with a mean of 15.3 weeks with respect to c25 (12) or an average of 13.8 (range 3.6–22) weeks to any of the recombinant antigens 33c, c100, or core. (24) The mean seroconversion to c100, c33, and a combined antigen (c22, c33, and c100) was 18.4, 15.1, and 13.8 weeks, respectively, in chimpanzees (23) (see Table I). Neither the time to seroconversion nor the pattern of response to epitopes in nonstructural proteins appeared to correlate with the clinical outcome of infection. (1,25,26) Median titers of anti-NS3 (helicase domain) antibodies in genotype 1, or anti-NS3 and anti-NS4 antibodies in other genotypes, were significantly higher in individuals with persistent HCV infections than in individuals who resolved infection over the course of the follow-up period. (27) In humans, anti-C100-3 can serve as a marker for ongoing vi-

TABLE I Seroconversion[a] to Nonstructural HCV Antigens in Chronic, Transfusion-Associated NANBH and Experimentally Infected Chimpanzees

Patient ($n = 10$)[b]	Anti-C100	Anti-C33C	Anti-NS5	Anti-C25
1	14.9	11.6	11.6	11.6
2	22.4	11.4	24.0	11.6
3	53.4	12.9	49.9	10.9
4	14.9	9.0	—	9.0
5	28.3	21.3	—	21.3
6	12.6	12.6	10.4	12.6
7	7.4	15.9	44.3	7.4
8	24.1	19.9	—	16.3
9	30.7	22.4	—	22.4
10	30.6	30.6	30.6	30.6
Mean (range)	23.9 (7.4–53.4)	—	—	15.3 (7.4–53.4)

Chimpanzee ($n = 6$)[c]	Anti-C100	Anti-C33C	Anti-NS5	Combined[c,d]
Mean (range)	18.4 (13–29)	15.1 (6–36)	—	13.8 (9–29)

[a] Time in weeks.
[b] From Chien et al. (12)
[c] From Farci et al. (23)
[d] Defined as C22 + C33C + C100

remia in that anti-C100-3 titers have been observed to decline in individuals who have undetectable viral RNA. (1,28) Bassett (19) noted a similar correlation between the lower prevalence of anti-NS3 (protease domain), but not anti-NS3 (helicase domain), and the absence of viral RNA in chimpanzees. These results could be explained by differences in the antigenicity of the protease domain versus the helicase domain.

IgM responses have been described in HCV-infected individuals. (29,30) Unlike the humoral response to HBV in which an early IgM anti-Hbc had a strong association with viral replication and preceded the appearance of IgG, (31) HCV anti-capsid IgM did not necessarily precede an IgG response in acute infections nor did all patients have detectable anti-capsid IgM. (32) Therefore, IgM was not a marker for early seroconversion but was more related to viremia in HCV-infected individuals. In contrast to HBV, no correlation has been found between the frequency of IgM anticapsid antibodies in patients treated with interferon (IFN)-α and the clinical outcome of treatment. (30)

The humoral response to the structural proteins C, E1, and E2 are different in humans and chimpanzees. As indicated earlier, several groups have shown that the capsid or core antigen (c22) is highly immunogenic in humans but is weakly immunogenic in chimpanzees. (19,33–35) Similarly, although there are numerous studies showing that approximately 90–97% of humans with chronic infections develop antibodies against recombinant envelope proteins E1/E2 or E2, (25,36–43) experimentally inoculated chimpanzees had a poor humoral response to these antigens in terms of titer and prevalence of antibodies. Two studies reported that approximately 40% of chronically infected, polymerase chain reaction (PCR)-positive chimpanzees were seropositive for anti-E1/E2 (20) or anti-E2$_{715}$. (43) In a third study (44), 66% ($^2/_3$) chimpanzees seroconverted to anti-E2$_{673}$ antibodies. Despite differences in anti-E2 antibody titers between humans and chimpanzees, (20) the prevalence of anti-E2 is associated with long-term viremia (38,45,46) in both species; $^2/_6$ chimpanzees developed anti-E1E2 antibodies after 40 weeks postinfection, whereas $^4/_{10}$ long-term chronic animals had anti-E2 antibodies. (20) The underlying immunological mechanism(s) that could account for the discrepancy in the humoral response to envelope proteins in humans and chimpanzees is unknown (47) and has important implications for assessing the efficacy of vaccine antigens, as the chimpanzee is the only reliable animal model for HCV infection. (48–53)

Early work designed to detect B-cell epitopes in E1 and E2 was conducted using fusion proteins, (16) peptide-based ELISA, or pepscan (overlapping peptides attached to solid-phase pins). (54) Although these studies underestimated the number of patients and asymptomatic HCV-infected individuals with anti-E2 antibodies, (36) they were useful in identifying linear B-cell epitopes in the amino-terminal hypervariable domain (HVR 1) of E2. (35,55–67) HVR 1 is defined structurally by a highly predicted β turn at amino acids 416 to 420 based on a computer-generated secondary structure analysis (55) and contains several amino acid positions that exhibit a high degree of amino acid substitution. (68–71) Both isolate-specific and cross-reacting epitopes have been mapped to HVR 1 using synthetic peptides, *Escherichia coli* fusion proteins, (60,61,65,66,72,73) and peptide competition experiments. (65,66,74,75) Esumi (76) used mouse anti-HVR 1 peptide (amino acids 384–414) antisera to capture virus from chronic patients containing heterologous HVR 1 sequences. Because the cross-reacting antibodies in all of the studies mentioned previously have not been characterized or evaluated in virus-neutralizing assays, it is difficult to comment on their biological significance. Isolate-specific, linear B-cell epitopes have been implicated in virus neutralization.

There are many examples of viruses in which an early antibody response to envelope proteins is associated with viral clearance. The situation is unclear for HCV, as there is only limited scientific evidence on this subject. Kobayashi et al. (25) found a statistically significant correlation between seroconversion to anti-CHO E2$_{664}$ within the first month postinfection and disappearance of viremia in 26 patients with posttransfusion hepatitis. In contrast, Chen et al. (26) failed to find a similar association in 12 patients with posttransfusion hepatitis. Because both groups used the identical E2$_{664}$ antigen (38) in their assays, differences in the antigen cannot explain the conflicting results. Reevaluation of seroconversion panels using virus-like particles or recombinant E1/E2 or native antigens might clarify this issue.

NEUTRALIZING ANTIBODIES TO HCV

Studies from the early 1980s suggested that primates had a weak protective immune response at best to HCV infection. Previously infected chimpanzees and humans, who were reexposed to HCV, frequently developed characteristics of acute disease. (9) Because clinical symptoms were known to be episodic in a subset of patients, it was not clear whether nonspecific markers for disease, such as alanine aminotransferase (ALT) elevations, could be attributed to the original infection or a newly acquired infection. Reanalysis of the samples from rechallenged chimpanzees using PCR and sequencing techniques definitively showed that animals who had resolved HCV infection, as defined by a lack of detectable HCV RNA, could be reinfected with a heterologous challenge inoculum. (77–79) The lack of quantitation made it difficult to determine whether the magnitude of viremia during subsequent infection was equal to that of the primary infection. Biochemical and histological data suggested that the acute disease after rechallenge appeared less severe and suggested some functional immune response to the initial infection. (77,78)

Evidence for virus-neutralizing antibodies could be gleaned from studies in which immune globulin has been used in the passive immunization of humans and chimpanzees. (80) In one carefully performed study, a single animal was experimentally inoculated with a proven infectious dose of HCV 1 hr prior to passive immunization with hepatitis C immune globulin (HCIG) containing high titers of anti-E2 antibodies. Although the animal was infected with HCV as determined by PCR positivity, acute hepatitis was delayed significantly in this animal when compared to two control animals. The number of HCV antigen-positive hepatocytes was lower in the HCIG-treated animal than in control animals and increased as the serum titers of the anti-E2 antibody decreased over time. (80) Data strongly suggested that the natural infection of the liver was partially controlled by antibodies in the HCIG preparation. In humans, partners of heterosexual couples who received bimonthly injections of immune globulin containing high levels of anti-E2 antibodies had a statistically lower chance of becoming infected by their HCV-infected partner. (81)

The most direct evidence for virus-neutralizing antibodies came from *in vitro/in vivo* neutralization experiments in chimpanzees. One of two chimpanzees inoculated with a proven H77 inoculum, (22) which had been preincubated with plasma from the same patient 2 years after acute disease (H79), failed to contract HCV. In contrast, the H77 inoculum was infectious in chimpanzees after preincubation with either plasma from the same patient taken 11 years later (H90) or normal sera. (82,83) To define virus-neutralizing epitopes further, a similar experiment was performed with a rabbit anti-HVR 1 peptide antibody (amino acids 390–410; see Fig. 2). Again, one of two chimpanzees who received H77 preincubated with the anti-HVR 1 peptide antibody was protected from infection, whereas two control animals became PCR positive. (83) Shimizu et al. (84) obtained identical results using an *in vitro* virus-neutralizing assay in tissue culture cells. In addition, sera H91 blocked the binding of H90 virus to HPB-Ma 10.2 cells, but failed to prevent H77 from binding to cells. In contrast to results obtained with serum from patient H, rabbit antibodies raised specifically against the H77 HVR 1 peptide 390–410 did not completely block virus attachment to HPB-Ma 10.2 cells, but did prevent virus replication *in vitro*. (85) The neutralizing epitope was further mapped between amino acids 398–410 (see Fig. 2). (86) Zibert et al. (75) also reported blocking the binding of virus from in-

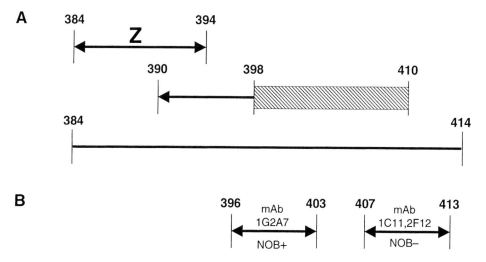

FIGURE 2 Anatomy of E2 hypervariable region 1 (HVR 1). This region describes the areas in which linear B-cell epitopes have been identified. (A) Amino-terminal epitopes associated with acute resolution of HCV infection are denoted by "Z." (66) Virus-neutralizing epitopes (83) and putative escape mutations have been mapped between amino acids (see text and Table II for references). Epitopes in the shaded area (398–410) were implicated in an *in vitro* cell culture virus-neutralizing assay. (85) (B) Monoclonal antibodies (mAb) 1G2A7, 1C11, and 2F12 react with the specific epitopes in HCV-1 E2 HVR 1 (Weiner A J, unpublished). Neutralization of binding (NOB) activity (+) or lack of activity (−) for mAb 1G2A7 (86) or 1C11 and 1F12 (Weiner A J, Rosa D: unpublished) is shown. The amino acid sequence of HCV-1 is according to Choo et al. (13)

fected individuals to human fibroblast (VH3) cells using sera obtained approximately 1 year after exposure to an HCV-contaminated anti-D immunoglobulin preparation. Sera obtained late in chronic infection from these same patients did not block virus binding to VH3 cells. The specificity of virus-neutralizing antibodies was determined by competition experiments using recombinant GST fusion–HVR 1 proteins representing the predominant HVR 1 sequences in the anti-D immunoglobulin. (65,75) In contrast to previous reports, (83,85) epitope mapping studies revealed a correlation between the resolution of acute disease with immunoreactive epitopes between amino-terminal amino acids 384–394 (see Z in Fig. 2) but not amino acids 390–410 or 398–410. (66) Van Doorn et al. (63) also found a correlation between acute resolution and high titers of anti-HVR 1 antibodies to epitopes contained between amino acids 393–416 in two chimpanzees. Taken together, data strongly suggest that E2 HVR 1 is highly immunogenic, elicits a complex humoral response, and contains isolate-specific, linear, neutralizing B-cell epitopes. These data, however, do not necessarily mean that HVR 1 contained the principle neutralizing epitope(s) of HCV. For example, dominant linear epitopes in the aminoterminus of Polio virus envelope protein VP1 (87) are neutralizing *in vitro,* (88) but they are not the principle neutralizing epitope of the Polio virus particle, which is formed by the quartinary structure of the three envelope proteins (VP1, 2, and 3). (89) In the absence of structural information on E2, the E1/E2 heterodimer, or the viral particle, it is unclear as to whether HVR 1 forms part of a conformational epitope, which might have important virus–cell membrane interactions.

Primary evidence suggesting that virus-neutralizing epitopes exist outside HVR 1 come from findings that titers of anti-HVR 1 antibodies failed to correlate with sterilizing immunity in five chimpanzees vaccinated with recombinant E1/E2 after challenge with an HCV inoculum, (90) which had been shown to be highly homogeneous with respect to the HVR 1 domain. (91) It is likely that virus-neutralizing antibodies outside HVR 1 recognize conformational rather than linear B-cell epitopes as (1) no correlation was found between the pattern of immunoreactive peptides or the magnitude of the response to particular peptides outside HVR 1 and the resolution of acute infection (54,67) and (2) sera from patients in the Zibert (67) study who had acute HCV infections reacted equally well with *in vitro*-translated $E2_{688}$ lacking the HVR 1 domain, regardless of the clinical outcome of the infection. (92)

Considering the difficulties related to using chimpanzees for *in vivo/in vitro* neutralization assays and the lack of widely available *in vitro* neutralization assays in tissue culture cells, a quantitative *in vitro* neutralization of binding (NOB) assay based on the binding of conformational, recombinant E2 to MOLT-4 cells was developed (86,93) (see Fig. 3). NOB titers of greater than $\frac{1}{600}$ correlated with sterilizing immunity in vaccinated chimpanzees. (86) Ishii et al. (94) also showed a correlation between the titer and the duration of NOB-specific antibodies with resolution of clinical disease in six of seven patients with chronic HCV infections. A mouse mAb (1G2A7), which mapped to epitopes between amino acids 396–403, but not two others (1C11 and 2F12), which mapped to epitopes between amino acids 407–413 in the HVR 1, was shown to have weak NOB titers (86; Weiner A J, Rosa D, Houghton M: unpublished). mAb data were consistent with the *in vivo* and *in vitro* identification of virus-neutralizing

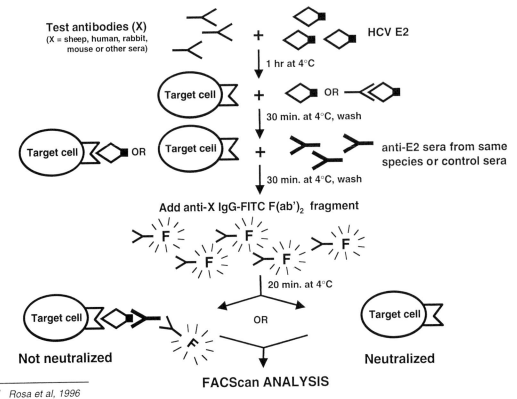

FIGURE 3 Neutralization of binding (NOB) of HCV recombinant E2. An assay to measure the NOB of recombinant E2 to target cells as described in Rosa (86) is shown. Briefly, sera from naturally infected or immunized animals such as human, rabbit, or mouse (denoted as test sera X) are incubated with the recombinant E2 protein and then incubated with target cells, e.g., MOLT-4 cells. Subsequently, antibodies raised against E2 in the same species as the test sera are added. The amount of FITC-labeled anti-X antibodies bound to the anti-E2 antibody–E2-target cell complex is quantitated by FACS analysis. The NOB titer is defined as the titer at which an antisera inhibits 50% of the E2 binding to the target cells.

epitopes between amino acids 390–410 (see Fig. 2). At least a subset of antibodies measured in the NOB assay recognized conserved and conformational epitopes. Plasma containing virus of a different genotype from the E2, type 1a antigen used in the assay exhibited NOB activity, (94) and a human mAb derived from a naturally infected patient (genotype 4) known to react specifically with a conformational epitope(s) in E2 and E1/E2 had high NOB titers. (95) Other mAbs with NOB activity, which react to conformational E2 and E1/E2 but not denatured envelope proteins of genotype 1, have also been described. (86)

IMMUNOGENICITY OF RECOMBINANT AND SYNTHETIC HCV ANTIGENS

Purification of native virus particles suitable for biochemical analysis has not been accomplished for HCV due to the relatively low levels of virus in human serum and only inefficient tissue culture systems. As a result, authentic composition and structure of the viral envelope are undescribed. The putative C, E1, and E2 polypeptides as the structural proteins of the virion are based on (1) similar genetic organization with other members of the Flaviviridae, (14) (2) direct capture of putative virus and viral core particles with anti-E2 antibodies (76,96,97) or anti-core antibodies, (97–99) respectively, and (3) the ability of a E1/E2 subunit vaccine to protect chimpanzees from a HCV challenge, as described in the previous section.

Recombinant nonstructural proteins are typically highly immunogenic in small animals and have been very useful research tools but will not be discussed. To study the humoral response to HCV structural proteins, recombinant polypeptides and synthetic peptides have been used as immunogens in small animals and nonhuman primates. C, E1, and/or E2 has been produced and characterized in a variety of systems, including recombinant vaccinia (100,101) and Sindbis (101) viral expression vectors in mammalian cells as well as in transient and stably transfected insect (102–105) and mammalian cells. (14,15,37,38, 45,104,106–108) The biogenesis of the envelope proteins has been determined from these studies. Briefly, putative structural proteins are naturally translated as a polyprotein, which is processed by host signal peptidase to generate the individual polypeptides. (100,109) E1 and E2 are directed to the endoplasmic reticulum (ER) by a signal peptide and are translocated into the ER where they undergo glycosylation (high mannose) (100,110) to form a noncovalent E1/E2 heterodimer complex, (100,101,103) in association with the molecular chaperone calnexin, (111) and remain anchored in the ER by a carboxy-terminal hydrophobic transmembrane domain. (100,101,112,113) Upon removal of the hydrophobic anchor, E1 and E2 are secreted from cells and are decorated with complex carbohydrates. (106) Although the E2 appears to fold and attain a conformation similar to that found in the E1/E2 heterodimer as assessed by reactivity with mAbs that fail to recognize denatured E2 or E1/E2 complexes, the proper folding of E1 appears to depend on the formation of the E1/E2 heterodimer. (111) As a result, the humoral response to conformational epitopes in E1, independent of E2, has been difficult to evaluate.

Antibodies to C, E1, and E2 either expressed as fusion proteins in bacterial or mammalian cells expression systems or to secreted from insect or mammalian cells have been described. Interestingly, E2$_{390-683}$ expressed in insect cells by a baculovirus vector (76) or E2$_{386-693}$ expressed as a fusion protein with human growth hormone (hGH) in CHO cells (114) both failed to induce anti-HVR 1 antibodies. However, anti-HVR 1 antibodies were generated by mice immunized with E2$_{388-664}$ (38), E2$_{384-661}$ (106) secreted from CHO cells (Coates S: unpublished), or E1/E2 HeLa cells (20; Weiner A J, Choo Q-L, Houghton M: unpublished) (see Table II). Data suggested that the HVR 1 in the context of denatured or nonnative glycosylated forms of E2 may be inefficient at inducing a humoral response to HVR 1 epitopes in mice. HVR 1 peptides are very immunogenic in mice, although the pattern of reactivity varies significantly depending on the strain (115) and possibly the method of conjugation (see Table II). In contrast to dominant linear B-cell epitopes located between amino acids 390–410 in mice, rabbits, sheep, and chimpanzees immunized with HVR 1 peptide 384–414, Esumi et al. (76) found dominant epitopes between amino acids 384–403 in three of three C57BL/6 mice. Mice immunized with KLH-conjugated peptide 384–414 reacted to immunodominant epitopes between 402 and 414,

TABLE II   **Immunogenicity of E2 HVR I**

Animal	Antigen	(conjugate)	Immunoreactivity: R/NR[a]; epitope(s) (amino acid)	Reference
Peptides				
Sheep	HCV-1	384–414 (diptheria toxoid)	P(390–410; 406–414)	Weiner A: unpublished
Rabbit	HCV-1	384–410 (diptheria toxoid)	P(390–410)	Weiner A, Chien D: unpublished
Rabbit	HCV-1	384–414 (LKH)	P(402–414)	Weiner A, Coates S: unpublished
Rabbit	H77	384–414 (LKH)	P(402–414)	Weiner A, Coates S: unpublished
Rabbit	H77	390–410 (tetanus toxoid)	P(398–410)	Farci et al. (83); Shimizu et al. (85)
Mouse	HCV-N2	384–414 (LKH)	P(384–403)[b] (394–413) (404–423)	Esumi et al. (76)
Mouse	83b	384–410 (polylysine)		Scarselli et al. (74)
Mouse	HCV-1	384–414 (diptheria toxoid)	P(399–405)	Weiner A: unpublished
			P(mAb, 396–403)	
Polypeptides			P(mAb, 407–413)	
Mouse	CHO	388–661[c]	P(384–414)	Coates S: unpublished
	CHO	384–664[d]	P(384–414)	Coates S: unpublished
Mouse	Baculovirus	390–683	**NR**	Esumi et al. (76)
Mouse	CHO hGH-E2	386–693	**NR**	Lee et al. (114)
Guinea pig	HeLa	192–906[e]	P(384–414)	Coates S: unpublished
Chimpanzee	HeLa	192–906[e]	P(384–414) (401–410)	Houghton et al. (90) Weiner A, Choo Q-L, Houghton M: unpublished

[a] R, reactive; NR, not reactive.
[b] Predominant epitope
[c] From Spaete et al. (106)
[d] From Lesniewski et al. (38,45)
[e] From Choo et al. (20)

whereas the same peptide conjugated to diptheria toxoid reacted with epitopes between 396 and 413 when immunized in the identical strain of mouse (see Table II).

Considerable effort in understanding the role and importance of HVR 1 in the development of immunity of HCV infection has focused on type-specific epitopes (see Section III). To circumvent the issue of isolate-specific anti-HVR 1 antibodies, Puntoriero et al. (116) attempted to broaden the humoral response to HVR 1 by synthesizing a library of HVR 1 sequences (amino acids 384–411), preparing a phage-display peptide library and screening the library with sera from chronic patients for sequences that were highly cross-reactive. (116) The six most reactive peptides or mimotopes, sequences that mimic sequences found in natural infections, were used to immunize mice. Antisera from the mixture of the six peptides reacted with 95% of 43 naturally occurring HVR 1 peptides in an ELISA. (116) Similarly, rabbit antisera raised against a peptide representing the consensus sequence derived from 90 type 1 HVR 1 sequences not only reacted with diverse HVR 1 peptides, but also bound to conformational type 1a and 1b E2 (Weiner A J, Chien D Y, Houghton M: unpublished). The significance of broadly cross-reacting antibodies with respect to virus neutralization is under investigation and may have value in vaccine formulations.

Data on the immunogenicity of E1/E2 complexes are limited. Using sucrose gradient-purified E1/E2 heterodimers to immunize mice, Deleersnyder et al. (112) identified a mAb (H2) that recognized conformational, high manose E1/E2 but not denatured forms of this protein. Unfortunately, H2 could not be demonstrated to capture virus. Two lines of evidence suggest that the E1/E2 heterodimer is a biologically relevant structure: (1) vaccine studies in which chimpanzees immunized with E1/E2 heterodimer were protected from challenge with a proven HCV inoculum (20) and (2) the existence of a human mAb-producing B-cell line, which bound to the conformational, intracellular E1/E2 heterodimer and not denatured E1/E2. (95) Guinea pigs immunized with the same subunit vaccine described earlier elicited significant NOB titers in assays using both E2 1a or 1b, indicating that the antigen is very immunogenic and that the immune response is directed at a conserved type 1 epitope. (90) Because immunogenicity studies in small animals or nonhuman primates do not necessarily predict the humoral response in humans, testing of HCV antigens, including E1/E2 heterodimers, await clinical trials in humans.

HUMORAL MECHANISMS OF CHRONICITY

The insidious nature of HCV is characterized by the high level of chronic infections, reportedly between 70 and 85%, and the typical slow progression to serious liver disease. (1–6) Although there are numerous strategies that host organisms utilize to clear viral infections and viruses use to evade host defenses, (117–125) this chapter only addresses aspects of virus–host interactions related to the humoral arm of the immune system.

The persistence of HCV infections has largely been attributed to viral heterogeneity and an inadequate virus-neutralizing response by the host (see Section II). With respect to viral heterogeneity, HCV is similar to other RNA viruses, (126) which lack a proofreading replicase, (127) and have been reported to have 10^{-3} to 10^{-4} nucleotide substitutions per genome site per year. (128, 129) These often quoted mutations rates for HCV were potentially flawed, as the patients used to make the calculations were not initially infected with a strictly homogeneous population of viruses. More recently, the mutation rate was calculated as approximately 1.5×10^{-3} nucleotide substitutions/site/year (130) in two chimpanzees that were inoculated with a molecular clone of HCV. (131) The mutation rate in chimpanzees may be an underestimate, as transfection with large amounts of transfected RNA was not analogous to natural infection and thus could possibly influence the kinetics of replication and the dynamics of the population. Whether as a result of mutations generated by genetic processes or by the inoculation of the host with a heterogeneous population of viral variants, HCV circulates as a quasispecies distribution in natural infections. (132,133)

According to evolutionary theory, the fittest viral species emerge from the population of variants subject to forces of positive and negative selection pressures. (134,135)

Considerable indirect evidence supports the theory that the high degree of variation observed in E2 HVR 1 results from positive immune selection in patients with chronic HCV infections and may be one mechanism by which the virus escapes clearance by neutralizing antibodies in chronic infections. Direct evidence for viral escape is limited and comes from chimpanzee experiments described previously. One of two chimpanzees was protected from challenge with the H77 inoculum, which had been preincubated with sera from patient H taken 2 years after transfusion-associated acute hepatitis (H79) or rabbit anti-HVR 1 peptide antisera. (83) The interpretation of these results with respect to the issue of escape mutations is complicated by the small number of animals used in the experiment and the complexity of the H77 inocula, which contained 19 different detectable HVR 1 sequences. (83) In both studies, the chimpanzee that was not protected was infected with a HVR 1 variant that differed from the predominant HVR 1 sequence found in the H77 inocula. One interpretation is that the animals were infected by an escape variant. A second interpretation is that either the anti-HVR 1 antibodies were of insufficient titer to neutralize the virus or that there was a weak association of virus-neutralizing antibody complexes (poor affinity or avidity) and a low titer of free virus was available to cause an infection. This free virus population would contain the same quasispecies as the H77 inoculum and a minor variant could have a selective advantage in a chimpanzee. Data in Fig. 4 suggest that the latter explanation is plausible, as one of two chimpanzees inoculated with H77 without pretreatment

		No. of clones
384**ETHVTGGNAGRTTAGLVGLLTPGAKQNIQLI**414		70/104
. . . .**S**. . . .**I**. .**FT**.		6/104
Ch561		DS[1]
Ch445 . . . .**S**. . . .**I**. .**F**$\overset{\textbf{A}}{\textbf{T}}$.		DS

---

[a] *Farci et al., 1996*
[b] *Weiner, A., Houghton, M., unpublished*

[1] *DS: direct sequencing*

FIGURE 4 Published amino acid sequences of HVR I variants in the H77 challenge innoculum (82) compared with HVR I sequences found in the plasma of chimpanzees (ch561 and ch445) infected with H77 plasma (Weiner A J, Kansopon J, Houghton M: unpublished). Dots indicate identical amino acids to those shown for the major HVR I of H77. HVR I sequences of ch561 and ch445 were determined by direct sequencing of polymerase chain reaction fragments. An alanine (A) or a threonine (T) occurred at position 401 with approximately equal frequency. DS, direct sequencing.

with anti-HCV antibodies was infected only by a minor HVR 1 variant (Weiner A J, Kansopon J, Houghton M: unpublished).

Citing a lack of sequence divergence in the HVR 1 of virus obtained from a chimpanzee (ch1536) after 46 weeks posttransfection with a molecular clone of HCV, Major et al. (130) argued that although escape mutations elsewhere in the E1 and E2 may produce virus-neutralizing escape mutants, mutations in HVR 1 could not account for persistent infection in the chimpanzee. However, shortly after the titers of anti-HVR 1 and anti-E1/E2 antibodies began to rise dramatically in ch1536 at weeks 50 and 30, respectively, the first HVR 1 variant appeared and remained the dominant HVR 1 through week 60. The second chimpanzee, which also had an early but weak anti-HVR 1 response but did not go on to have increasing titers, had no detectable HVR 1 variants by week 60. Whether the amino acid substitution generated an escape mutation was unknown. Interestingly, the mutation was at position 398, which resides in a virus-neutralizing epitope (see Fig. 2). As noted previously, the massive amounts of positive-stranded RNA with which ch1536 was inoculated may have affected the kinetics of viral quasispecies formation, the subsequent packaging of variants into virus particles, and the availability of variants subject to positive immune selective pressure. The pattern of late or no induction of anti-HVR 1 antibodies is consistent with the hypothesis that the anti-HVR 1 response is either too weak and/or late to efficiently neutralize virus and that during the progression to chronic infection, quasispecies potentially harboring escape mutants are constantly being generated.

A case can be made that HCV is capable of modifying the humoral and/or cellular immune response in order to affect the production of virus-neutralizing antibodies against the HVR 1 or unidentified principle virus-neutralizing epitope(s) on the virion envelope. HCV infection has been associated with immune dysfunction such as cryoglobulinaemia (136,137) and autoimmune disease. (138) Ray et al. (139) proposed that HVR 1 may serve as a decoy by eliciting a strong, but ineffective humoral response to HVR 1. By comparing the pattern of mutation in HVR 1 of 5 patients who resolved acute HCV infection with 10 patients who developed chronic HCV infections, a trend toward nonsynonymous HVR amino acid substitutions (those mutations that create nonconservative amino acid substitutions) and high sequence complexity in acute infection was found in patients who developed chronic HCV infections. Data strongly indicated a positive selective pressure on HVR 1, although the specific nature of the positive selection was not addressed in this study. The reduced rate of amino acid substitutions in HVR 1 of patients with common variable immunodeficiency when compared to control subjects suggested that an intact immune system seems necessary to drive the immune selection of HVR1 variants. (140) Another possible immune-modulating mechanism could involve what has been termed "original antigenic sin" (141) in which the B-cell repetoire becomes fixed such that antibodies against emerging variants would not be induced. Because seroconversion to new HVR1 variants continues to occur over the course of chronic infection, (60,79,82) this theory with respect to the HVR1 domain appears untenable. However, because many patients do not have a simple pattern of seroconversion to emerging HVR1 variants during chronic disease, it is possible that "original antigenic sin" exists but is not necessarily universal.

"Immune avoidance" has been favored as the primary mechanism by which HCV evades humoral immune surveillance. (26) HCV appears to have a low intracellular copy number, and viral antigens are difficult to detect by standard immunofluorescence techniques. Chen et al. (26) evaluated antibody profiles for structural and nonstructural proteins, including a consensus HVR1 peptide, for 12 cases of posttransfusion HCV infection in which 4 patients resolved infection and 8 patients became persistently infected. Data showed that with the exception of core, seroconversion to the structural proteins occurred late (typically after 100 weeks postinfection), the titers were low, and the antibody was predominantly of the IgG1 isotype independent of whether the patient resolved infection or developed chronic hepatitis. (26) The authors proposed that HCV might affect T-cell helper function by preventing proper IgG class switching and by decreasing IgG isotype switching. Mechanisms by which HCV manipulates the humoral and the cellular arms of the immune system and their interactions certainly are an area of intense interest and promise to expose the clever strategies by which HCV persists in a host. Further investigations into the physical characteristic of anti-HCV antibodies with respect to avidity, affinity, and specificity will be necessary in order to better understand the function of antibodies with respect to their ability to affect viral clearance.

Masking of virus-neutralizing epitopes may be yet another mechanism by which HCV eludes virus-neutralizing antibodies. Immunoprecipitation of viral particles by antiapolipoprotein B (142) and copurification of virus-associated RNA in very low density lippoproteins (VLDL) fractions of HCV containing sera (143,144) suggest that HCV can be associated with serum lipoproteins. Hijikata et al. (145) demonstrated that virus in the H77 inoculum, devoid of bound IgG, had a light density of ≤ 1.09 g/ml in sucrose, suggesting the possibility that the infectious virus was complexed with LDL. However, H77 could be neutralized by serum from the same patient or rabbit polyclonal anti-HVR1 antibodies. (82–85) Therefore, despite the association of the virus with LDL or VLDL, not all the potential neutralizing eptitopes were masked. Possibly only a subset of virion particles are associated with lipoproteins and/or a subset of B-cell epitopes that have not yet been identified are masked. Glycosylation of E1 and E2 could also have the potential to mask neutralizing epitopes.

Putative receptors for HCV have been reported, including CD81 (146), lacto ferrin (147) and the LDL receptor. (148) If in fact HCV uses multiple receptors, as do many viruses, (149) or a receptor-independent mechanism to enter hepatocytes, it is conceivable that the immune system may be incapable of mounting an efficient response to each of the epitopes involved in receptor interactions in a kinetically relevant manner, thus enabling the virus to infect hepatocytes or extrahepatic sites. As a matter of speculation, once the virus enters a hepatocyte, a possible direct cell-to-cell transmission could render the virus invisible to neutralizing antibodies.

CONCLUSION

Humans and, to a lesser extent, chimpanzees clearly mount a broad humoral response to hepatitis C and are capable of producing virus-neutralizing antibodies. However, in the face of this immune response, most individuals progress to chronic infection. Several mechanisms most likely contribute to viral persistence in the host, including the kinetics of induction of virus-neutralizing antibodies, the quantity and quality of antibodies produced, immunomodulatory consequences of viral infection, the generation of escape mutations as a result of the fluidity of the viral genome, and the ability of the virus to evade immune recognition through a variety of strategies. Although the exact composition of the virion is not known, virus-encoded proteins and peptides are typically immunogenic in animals and provide a basis for the development of vaccines.

ACKNOWLEDGMENTS

We thank Peter Anderson for the preparation of the manuscript and Nelle Cronen for the figures and tables. Thanks to Xavier Paliard for his critical reading of the manuscript and discussions related to immunology. I also appreciate the efforts of DFG in assisting me with producing this manuscript. This work was supported by Chiron Corporation.

REFERENCES

1. Alter H J. To C or Not to C: these are the questions. Blood 1995;85:1681–95.
2. Alter H J. Hepatitis C in asymptomatic blood donors. Hepatology 1997;26:29S–33S.
3. Alter M J. Epidemiology of hepatitis C. Hepatology 1997;26:62S–5S.
4. Hoofnagle J H. Hepatitis C: the clinical spectrum of disease. Hepatology 1997;26:15S–20S.
5. Seeff L B. Natural history of hepatitis C. Hepatology 1997;26:21S–8S.
6. Hu K-Q, Tong M J. The long-term outcomes of patients with compensated hepatitis C virus-related cirrhosis and history of parenteral exposure in the United States. Hepatology 1999;29:1311–6.
7. Choo Q-L, Kuo G, Weiner A J, Overby L R, Bradley D W, Houghton M. Isolation of a cDNA clone derived from a blood-borne non-A, non-B viral hepatitis genome. Science 1989;244:359–62.
8. Prince A M. Non-A, non-B hepatitis viruses. Annu Rev Microbiol 1983;37:217–32.
9. Shih W-K, Esteban J I, Alter H J. Non-A, Non-B hepatitis: Advances and unfulfilled expectations of the first decade. Liver Dis 1986;8:433–52.
10. Choo Q-L, Berger K, Kuo G, Houghton M. Detection and mapping of immunologic epitopes expressed by bacterial cDNA clones of the hepatitis C virus. In: Hollinger F B, Lemon S M, Margolis H S, eds., Viral hepatitis and liver disease. Baltimore, MD: Williams & Wilkins, 1991, 345–6.
11. Kuo G, Choo Q-L, Alter H J, et al. An assay for circulating antibodies to a major etiologic virus of human non-A, non-B hepatitis. Science 1989;244:362–4.
12. Chien D Y, Choo Q-L, Tabrizi A, et al. Diagnosis of hepatitis C virus (HCV) infection using an immunodominant chimeric polyprotein to capture circulating antibodies: reevaluation of the role of HCV in liver disease. Proc Natl Acad Sci U S A 1992;89:10011–5.
13. Choo Q-L, Richman K H, Han J H, et al. Genetic organization and diversity of the hepatitis C virus. Proc Natl Acad Sci U S A 1991;88:2451–5.
14. Houghton M. (1996a). Hepatitis C viruses. In: Fields B N, Knipe D M, Howley P M, et al., eds. Fields virology. Philadelphia: Lippincott-Raven, 1996, 1035–57.
15. Major M E, Feinstone S M. The molecular virology of hepatitis C. Hepatology 1997;25:1527–38.
16. Lok A S F, Chien D, Choo Q-L, et al. Antibody response to core, envelope and nonstructural hepatitis C virus antigens: comparison of immunocompetent and immunosuppressed patients. Hepatology 1993;18:497–502.
17. Gretch D R. Diagnostic tests for hepatitis C. Hepatology 1997;26:43S–7S.

18. Lok A S F, Gunaratnam N T. Diagnosis of hepatitis C. Hepatology 1997;26:48S–56S.
19. Bassett S E, Brasky K M, Lanford R E. Analysis of hepatitis C virus-inoculated chimpanzees reveals unexpected clinical profiles. J Virol 1998;72:2589–99.
20. Choo Q-L, Kuo G, Ralston R, et al. Vaccination of chimpanzees against infection by the hepatitis C virus. Proc Natl Acad Sci U S A 1994;91:1294–8.
21. Houghton M, Choo Q-L, Kuo G, et al. Prospects for prophylactic and therapeutic hepatitis C virus vaccines. Princess Takamatsu Symp. 1995;25:237–43.
22. Feinstone S M, Alter H J, Dienes H P, et al. Non-A, non-B hepatitis in chimpanzees and marmosets. J. Inf. Dis. 1981;144:588–598.
23. Farci P, London W T, Wong D C, et al. The natural history of infection with hepatitis C virus (HCV) in chimpanzees: comparison of serologic responses measured with first- and second-generation assays and relationship to HCV viremia. J Infect Dis 1992;165:1006–111.
24. Vallari D S, Jett B W, Alter H J, Mimms L T, Holzman R, Shih J W. Serological markers of post-transfusion hepatitis C viral infection. J Clin Microbiol 1992;30:552–6.
25. Kobayashi M, Tanaka E, Matsumoto A, Ichijo T, Kiyosawa K. Antibody response to E2/NS1 hepatitis C virus protein in patients with acute hepatitis C. J Gastroenterol Hepatol 1997;12:73–6.
26. Chen M, Sallberg M, Sonnerborg A, et al. Limited humoral immunity in hepatitis C virus infection. Gastroenterology 1999;116:135–43.
27. Beld M, Penning M, Van Putten M, et al. Quantitative antibody responses to the structural (core) and nonstructural (NS3, NS4, NS5) hepatitis C virus proteins among seroconverting injecting drug users: Impact of epitope variation and relationship to dectection of HCV RNA. Hepatology 1999;29:1288–98.
28. Lanotte P, Dubois F, Le Pogam S, et al. The kinecis of antibodies against hepatitis C virus may predict viral clearance in exposed hemophiliacs. J Infect Dis 1998;178:556–669.
29. Clemens J M, Taskar S, Chau K, et al. IgM antibody response in acute hepatitis C viral infection. Blood 1992;79:169–72.
30. Quiroga J A, van Binsbergen J, Wang C Y, et al. Immunoglobulin M antibody to hepatitis C virus core antigen: Correlations with viral replication, histological activity, and liver disease outcome. Hepatology 1995;22:1635–40.
31. Brunetto M R, Oliveri F, Rocca G, et al. Natural course and response to interferon of chronic hepatitis B accompanied by antibody to hepatitis B e antigen. Hepatology 1989;10:198–202.
32. Quinti I, Hassan N F, El Salman D, Shalaby H, El Zimatty D, Monier M K, Arthur R R. Hepatitis C virus-specific B cell activation: IgG and IgM detection in acute and chronic hepatitis C. J Hepatology 1995;23:640–7.
33. Beach M J, Meeks E L, Mimms L T, et al. Temporal relationships of hepatitis C virus RNA and antibody responses following experimental infection of chimpanzees. J Med Virol 1992;36:226–37.
34. Hilfenhaus J, Krupka U, Nowak T, Cummins L B, Fuchs K, Roggendorf M. Follow-up of hepatitis C virus infection in chimpanzees: determination of viraemia and specific humoral immune response. J Gen Virol 1992;73:1015–9.
35. Wang Y-F, Brotman B, Andrus L, Prince A M. Immune response to epitopes of hepatitis C virus (HCV) structural proteins in HCV-infected humans and chimpanzees. J Infect Dis 1996;173:808–21.
36. Chien D Y, Choo Q-L, Ralston R, Spaete R. Persistence of HCV despite antibodies to both putative envelope glycoproteins. Lancet 1993;342:933.
37. Harada S, Suzuki R, Ando A, et al. Establishment of a cell line constitutively expressing E2 glycoprotein of hepatitis C virus and humoral response of hepatitis C patients to the expressed protein. J Gen Virol 1995;76:1223–31.
38. Lesniewski R R, Watanabe S, Devare S G. Expression of HCV envelope proteins and the serological utility of the anti-E2 immune response. Princess Takamatsu Symp. 1995;25:129–37.
39. Fournillier-Jacob A, Lunel F, Cahour A, et al. Antibody responses to hepatitis C envelope proteins in patients with acute or chronic hepatitis C. J Med Virol 1996;50:159–67.
40. Lee K J, Suh Y-A, Cho Y G, et al. Hepatitis C virus E2 protein purified from mammalian cells is frequently recognized by E2-specific antibodies in patient sera. J Biol Chem 1997;272:30040–6.
41. Cerino A, Bissolati M, Cividini A, et al. Antibody responses to the hepatitis C virus E2 protein: Relationship to viraemia and prevalence in anti-HCV seronegative subjects. J Med Virol 1997;51:1–5.

42. Psichogiou M, Katsoulidou A, Vaindirli E, Francis B, Lee S R, Hatzakis A. Immunologic events during the incubation period of hepatitis C virus infection: the role of antibodies to E2 glyco-protein. Transfusion 1997;37:858–62.

43. Bassett S E, Thomas D L, Brasky K M, Lanford R E. Viral persistence, antibody to E1 and E2, and hypervariable region 1 sequence stability in hepatitis C virus-inoculated chimpanzees. J Virol 1999;73:1118–26.

44. van Doorn L-J, van Hoek K, de Martinoff G, et al. Serological and molecular analysis of hepa-titis C virus envelope regions 1 and 2 during acute and chronic infections in chimpanzees. J Med Virol 1997;52:441–50.

45. Lesniewski R, Okasinski G, Carrick R, et al. Antibody to hepatitis C virus second envelope (HCV-E2) glycoprotein: a new marker of HCV infection closely associated with viremia. J Med Virol 1995;45:415–22.

46. Yuki N, Hayashi N, Kasahara A, et al. Quantitative analysis of antibody to hepatitis C virus envelope 2 glycoprotein in patients with chronic hepatitis C virus infection. Hepatology 1996; 23:947–52.

47. Walker C M. Comparative features of hepatitis C virus infection in humans and chimpanzees. Springer Semin Immunopathol 1997;19:85–98.

48. Alter H J, Purcell R H, Holland P V, Popper H. Transmissible agent in non-A, non-B hepatitis. Lancet 1978;1:459–63.

49. Prince A M, Brotman B, van den Ende M C, Richardson L, Kellner A. Non-A, non-B hepati-tis: Identification of virus-specific antigen and antibody: a preliminary report. In: Vyas G N, Cohen S N, Schmid R, eds. Viral hepatitis. Philadelphia: Franklin Institute Press, 1978, 633–40.

50. Bradley D W, Cook E H, Maynard J E, et al. Experimental infection of chimpanzees with anti-hemophilic (factor VIII) materials: recovery of virus-like particles associated with non-A, non-B hepatitis. J Med Virol 1979;3:253–69.

51. Bradley D W. Transmission, etiology, and pathogenesis of viral hepatitis non-A, non-B in non-human primates. In: Chisari F V, ed. Advances in hepatitis research. New York: Masson, 1984; 268–80.

52. Tabor E, Gerety R J, Drucker J A, et al. Transmission of non-A, non-B hepatitis from man to chimpanzee. Lancet 1979;1:463–6.

53. Feinstone S M, Alter H J, Dienes H P, et al. Non-A, non-B hepatitis in chimpanzees and mar-mosets. J Infect Dis 1981;144:588–98.

54. Ching W M, Wychowski C, Beach M J, et al. Interaction of immune sera with synthetic pep-tides corresponding to the structural protein region of hepatitis C virus. Proc Natl Acad Sci U S A 1992;89:3190–4.

55. Weiner A J, Geysen H M, Christopherson C, et al. Evidence for immune selection of hepatitis C virus (HCV) putative envelope glycoprotein variants: potential role in chronic HCV infections. Proc Natl Acad Sci U S A 1992;89:3468–72.

56. Lesniewski R R, Boardway K M, Casey J M, et al. Hypervariable 5'-terminus of hepatitis C vi-rus E2/NS1 encodes antigenically distinct variants. J Med Virol 1993;40:150–6.

57. Taniguchi S, Okamoto H, Sakamoto M, et al. A structurally flexible and antigenically variable N-terminal domain of the hepatitis C virus (E2/NS1) protein: implication for an escape from antibody. Virology 1993;195:297.

58. Kojima M, Osuga T, Tsuda F, Tanaka T, Okamotos H. Influence of antibodies to the hyper-variable region of E2/NS1 glycoprotein on the selective replication of hepatitis C virus in chim-panzees. Virology 1994;204:665–72.

59. da Silva Cardoso M, Siemoneit K, Nemecek V, Epple S, Koerner K, Kubanek B. The serology of hepatitis C virus (HCV) infection: antibody crossreaction in the hypervariable region 1. Arch Virol 1995;140:1705–13.

60. Kato N, Sekiya H, Ootsuyama Y, et al. Humoral immune response to hypervariable region 1 of the putative envelope glycoprotein (gp70) of hepatitis C virus. J Virol 1993;67:3923.

61. Kato N, Ootsuyama Y, Sekiya H, et al. Genetic drift in the hypervariable region 1 of the viral genome in persistent hepatitis C virus infection. J Virol 1994;68:4776–84.

62. Kato N, Ootsuyama Y, Sekiya H, et al. Humoral response to linear B cell epitopes in the ter-minus of the hepatitis C virus envelope glycoprotein gp72 (E2): role in protective immunity still unknown. Hepatology 1995;22:369–71.

63. van Doorn L J, Capriles I, Maertens G, et al. Sequence evolution of the hypervariable region in the putative envelope region E2/NS1 of hepatitis C virus is correlated with specific humoral im-mune responses. J Virol 1995;69:773–8.

64. Nakamoto Y, Kaneko S, Ohno H, et al. B-cell epitopes in hypervariable region 1 of hepatitis C virus obtained from patients with chronic persistent hepatitis. J Med Virol 1996;50:35–41.

65. Zibert A, Dudziak P, Schreier E, Roggendorf M. Characterization of antibody response to hepatitis C virus protein E2 and significance of hypervariable region 1-specific antibodies in viral neutralization. Arch Virol 1997;142:523–34.

66. Zibert A, Kraas W, Meisel H, Jung G, Roggendorf M. Epitope mapping of antibodies directed against hypervariable region 1 in acute self-limiting and chronic infections due to hepatitis C virus. J Virol 1997;71:4123–7.

67. Zibert A, Kraas W, Ross S, et al. Immunodominant B-cell domains of hepatitis C virus envelope proteins E1 and E2 identified during early and late time points of infection. J Hepatol 1999;30:177–84.

68. Hijikata M, Kato N, Ootsuyama Y, Nakagawa M, Ohkoshi S, Shimotohno K. Hypervariable regions in the putative glycoprotein of hepatitis C virus. Biochem Biophys Res Commun 1991;175:220–8.

69. Weiner A J, Brauer M J, Rosenblatt J, et al. Variable and hypervariable domains are found in the regions of HCV corresponding to the flavivirus envelope and NS1 proteins and the pestivirus envelope glycoproteins. Virology 1991;180:842–8.

70. Kato N, Ootsuyama Y, Tanaka T, et al. Marked sequence diversity in the putative envelope proteins of hepatitis C viruses. Virus Res 1992;22:107–23.

71. McAllister J, Casino C, Davidson F, et al. Long-term evolution of the hypervariable region of hepatitis C virus in a common-source-infected cohort. J Virol 1998;72:4893–905.

72. Yoshioka K, Aiyama T, Okumura A, et al. Humoral immune response to the hypervariable region of hepatitis C virus differs between genotypes 1b and 2a. J Infect Dis 1996;175:505–10.

73. Hattori M, Yoshioka K, Aiyama T, et al. Broadly reactive antibodies to hypervariable region 1 in hepatitis C virus-infected patient sera: relation to viral loads and response to interferon. Hepatology 1998;27:1703–10.

74. Scarselli E, Cerino A, Esposito G, Silini E, Mondelli M U, Traboni C. Occurrence of antibodies reactive with more than one varient of the putative envelope glycoprotein (gp70) hypervariable region 1 in viremic hepatitis C virus-infected patients. J Virol 1995;69:4407–12.

75. Zibert A, Schreier E, Roggendorf M. Antibodies in human sera specific to hypervariable region 1 of hepatitis C virus can block viral attachment. Virology 1995;208:653–61.

76. Esumi M, Ahmed M, Zhou Y-H., Takahashi H, Shikata T. Murine antibodies against E2 and hypervariable region 1 cross-reactively capture hepatitis C virus. Virology 1998;251:158–64.

77. Farci P, Alter H J, Govindarajan S, et al. Lack of protective immunity against reinfection with hepatitis C virus. Science 1992;258:135–40.

78. Prince A M, Brotman B, Huima T, Pascual D, Jaffery M, Inchauspe G. Immunity in hepatitis C infection. J Infect Dis 1992;165:438–43.

79. Wyatt C A, Andrus L, Brotman B, Huang F, Lee D-H, Prince A M. Immunity in chimpanzees chronically infected with hepatitis C virus: role of minor quasispecies in reinfection. J Virol 1998;72:1725–30.

80. Krawczynski K, Alter M J, Tankersley D L, et al. Effect of immune globulin on the prevention of experimental hepatitis C virus infection. J Infect Dis 1996;173:822–8.

81. Piazza M, Sagliocca L, Tosone G, et al. Sexual transmission of the hepatitis C virus and efficacy of prophylaxis with intramuscular immune serum globulin. Arch Intern Med 1997;157:1537–44.

82. Farci P, Alter H J, Wong D C, et al. Prevention of hepatitis C virus infection in chimpanzees after antibody-mediated *in vitro* neutralization. Proc Natl Acad Sci U S A 1994;91:7792–6.

83. Farci P, Shimoda A, Wong D, et al. Prevention of hepatitis C virus infection in chimpanzees by hyperimmune serum against the hypervariable region 1 of the envelope 2 protein. Proc Natl Acad Sci U S A 1996;93:15394–9.

84. Shimizu Y K, Hijikata M, Iwamoto A, Alter H J, Purcell R H, Yoshikura H. Neutralizing antibodies against hepatitis C virus and the emergence of neutralization escape mutant viruses. J Virol 1994;68:1494–500.

85. Shimizu Y K, Igarashi H, Kiyohara T, et al. A hyperimmune serum against a synthetic peptide corresponding to the hypervariable region 1 of hepatitis C virus can prevent viral infection in cell culture. Virology 1996;223:409–12.

86. Rosa D, Campagnoli S, Moretto C, et al. A quantitative test to estimate neutralizing antibodies to the hepatitis C virus: cytofluorimetric assessment of envelope glycoprotein 2 binding to target cells. Proc Natl Acad Sci U S A 1996;93:1759–63.

87. Roivainen M, Piirainen L, Tysa T, Narvanen A, Hovi T. An immunodominant N-terminal region of VP1 protein of poliovirion that is buried in crystal structure can be exposed in solution. Virology 1993;195:762–5.

88. Li Q, Yafal A G, Lee Y M, Hogle J, Chow M. Poliovirus neutralization by antibodies to internal epitopes of VP4 and VP1 results from reversible exposure of these sequences at physiological temperature. J Virol 1994;68:3965–70.

89. Page G S, Mosser A G., Hogle J M, Filman D J, Rueckert R R, Chow M. Three-dimensional structure of poliovirus serotype 1 neutralizing determinants. J Virol 1988;62:1781–94.

90. Houghton M, Choo Q-L, Chien D, et al. Development of an HCV vaccine. In: Rizzetto M, Purcell R H, Gerin J L, Verme G, eds. Vital hepatitis and liver disease. Torino, Italy: Edizioni Minerva Medica, 1996, 656–9.

91. Weiner A J, Christopherson C, Hall J E, et al. The hypervariable amino terminus of the hepatitis C virus E2/NS1 protein appears to be under immune selection. In: Brown F, Chanock R M, Ginsberg H S, Lerner R A, eds. Vaccines 92. Modern approaches to new vaccines including prevention of AIDS. Cold Spring Harbor, NY: Cold Spring Harbor Laboratory Press, 1992, 303.

92. Lechner S, Rispeter K, Meisel H, et al. Antibodies directed to envelope proteins of hepatitis C virus outside of hypervariable region 1. Virology 1998;243:313–21.

93. Abrignani S. Immune responses throughout hepatitis C virus (HCV) infection: HCV from the immune system point of view. Springer Semin Immunopathol 1997;19:47–55.

94. Ishii K, Rosa D, Watanabe Y, et al. High titers of antibodies inhibiting the binding of envelope to human cells correlate with natural resolution of chronic hepatitis C. Hepatology 1998;28:1117–20.

95. Habersetzer F, Fournillier A, Dubuisson J, et al. Characterization of human monoclonal antibodies specific to the hepatitis C virus glycoprotein E2 with *in vitro* binding neutralization properties. Virology 1998;249:32–41.

96. Kaito M, Watanabe S, Tsukiyama-Kohara K, et al. Hepatitis C virus particle detected by immunoelectron microscopic study. J Gen Virol 1994;75:1755–60.

97. Shindo M, Di Bisceglie A M, Akatsuka T, et al. The physical state of the negative strand of hepatitis C virus RNA in serum of patients with chronic hepatitis C. Proc Natl Acad Sci U S A 1994;91:8719–23.

98. Takahashi K, Kishimoto S, Yoshizawa H, Okamoto H, Yoshikawa A, Mishiro S. p26 protein and 33-nm particle associated with nucleocapsid of hepatitis C virus recovered from the circulation of infected hosts. Virology 1992;191:431–4.

99. Takahashi K, Okamoto H, Kishimoto S, et al. Demonstration of a hepatitis C virus-specific antigen predicted from the putative core gene in the circulation of infected hosts. J Gen Virol 1992;73:667–72.

100. Ralston R, Thudium K, Berger K, et al. Characterization of hepatitis C virus envelope glycoprotein complexes expressed by recombinant vaccinia viruses. J Virol 1993;67:6753–61.

101. Dubuisson J, Hsu H H, Cheung R C, Greenberg H B, Russell D G, Rice C M. Formation and intracellular localization of hepatitis C virus envelope glycoprotein complexes expressed by recombinant vaccinia and Sindbis viruses. J Virol 1994;68:6147–60.

102. Chiba J, Ohba H, Matsuura Y, et al. Serodiagnosis of hepatitis C virus (HCV) infection with an HCV core protein molecularly expressed by a recombinant baculovirus. Proc Natl Acad Sci U S A 1991;88:4641–5.

103. Lanford R E, Notvall L, Chavez D, et al. Analysis of hepatitis C virus capsid, E1, and E2/NS1 proteins expressed in insect cells. Virology 1993;197:225–35.

104. Matsuura Y, Suzuki T, Suzuki R, et al. Processing of E1 and E2 glycoproteins of hepatitis C virus expressed in mammalian and insect cells. Virology 1994;205:141–50.

105. Baumert T F, Ito S, Wong D T, Liang T J. Hepatitis C virus structural proteins assemble into viruslike particles in insect cells. J Virol 1998;72:3827–36.

106. Spaete R R, Alexander D, Rugroden M E, et al. Characterization of the hepatitis C virus E2/NS1 gene product expressed in mammalian cells. Virology 1992;188:819–30.

107. Selby M J, Glazer E, Masiarz F, Houghton M. Complex processing and protein: Protein interactions in the E2:NS2 region of Virology 1994;204:114–22.

108. Inudoh M, Nyunoya H, Tanaka T, Hijikata M, Kato N, Shimotohno K. Antigenicity of hepatitis C virus envelope proteins expressed in Chinese hamster ovary cells. Vaccine 1996;14:1590–6.

109. Hijikata M, Kato N, Ootsuyama Y, Nakagawa M, Shimotohno K. Gene mapping of the pu-

tative structural region of the hepatitis virus genome by *in vitro* processing analysis. Proc Natl Acad Sci U S A 1991;88:5547–51.

110. Grakoui A, Wychowski C, Lin C, Feinstone S M, Rice C M. Expression and identification of hepatitis C virus polyprotein cleavage products. J Virol 1993;67:1385–95.

111. Dubuisson J, Rice C M. Hepatitis C virus glycoprotein folding: disulfide bond formation and association with calnexin. J Virol 1996;70:778–86.

112. Deleersnyder V, Pillez A, Wychowski C, et al. Formation of native hepatitis C virus glycoprotein complexes. J Virol 1997;71:697–704.

113. Cocquerel L, Duvet S, Meunier J-C, et al. The transmembrane domain of hepatitis C virus glycoprotein E1 is a signal for static retention in the endoplasmic reticulum. J Virol 1999;73:2641–94.

114. Lee J W, Kim K-M, Jung S-H, et al. Identification of a domain containing B-cell epitopes in hepatitis C virus E2 glycoprotein by using mouse monoclonal antibodies. J Virol 1999;73:11–8.

115. Ahmed M, Shikata T, Esumi M. Murine humoral immune response against recombinant structural proteins of hepatitis C virus distinct from those of patients. Microbiol Immunol 1996;40:169–76.

116. Puntoriero G, Meola A, Lahm A, et al. Towards a solution for hepatitis C virus hypervariability: mimotopes of the hypervariable region 1 can induce antibodies cross-reacting with a large number of viral variants. EMBO J 1998;17:3521–33.

117. Oldstone M B A. Molecular anatomy of viral persistence. J Virol 1991;65:6381–6.

118. Peters M, Vierling J, Gershwin M E, Milich D, Chisari F V, Hoofnagle J H. Immunology and the liver. Hepatology 1991;13:977–94.

119. Smith G L. Virus strategies for evasion of the host response to infection. Trends Microbiol 1994;2:81–8.

120. de la Torre J C, Oldstone M B. Anatomy of viral persistence: mechanisms of persistence and associated disease. Adv Virus Res 1996;46:311–43.

121. Zinkernagel R M. Immunology and immunity studied with viruses. Ciba Found Symp 1997;204:105–25.

122. Borrow P. Mechanisms of viral clearance and persistence. J Viral Hepatitis 1997;4:S216–24.

123. Ferrari C, Penna A, Bertoletti A, et al. Antiviral cell-mediated immune responses during hepatitis B and hepatitis C virus infections. Recent Results Cancer Res 1998;154:330–6.

124. Chapman M S, Rossman M G. Comparison of surface properties of picornaviruses: Strategies for hiding the receptor site from immune surveillance. Virology 1993;195:745–56.

125. Fish K N, Britt W, Nelson J A. A novel mechanism for persistence of human cytomegalovirus in macrophages. J Virol 1996;70:1855–62.

126. Domingo E, Holland J J. Mutation rates and rapid evolution of RNA viruses. In: Morse S S, ed. Evolutionary biology of viruses. New York: Raven Press, 1994, 161–84.

127. Steinhauer D A, Domingo E, Holland J J. Lack of evidence for proofreading mechanisms associated with an RNA virus polymerase. Gene 1992;122:281–8.

128. Ogata N, Alter H J, Miller R H, Purcell R H. Nucleotide sequence and mutation rate of the H strain of hepatitis C virus. Proc Natl Acad Sci U S A 1991;88:3392.

129. Okamoto H, Kojima M, Okada S-I, et al. Genetic drift of hepatitis C during an 8.2-year infection in a chimpanzee variability and stability. Virology 1992;190:894–9.

130. Major M E, Mihalik K, Fernandez J, et al. Long-term follow-up of chimpanzees inoculated with the first infectious clone for hepatitis C virus. J Virol 1999;73:3317–25.

131. Kolykahalov A A, Agapov E V, Blight K, Mihalik K, Feinstone S M, Rice C M. Transmission of hepatitis C by intrahepatic inoculation with transcribed RNA. Science 1997;277:570–4.

132. Martell M, Esteban J L, Quer J, et al. Hepatitis C virus (HCV) circulates as a population of different but closely related genomes: quasispecies nature of HCV genome distribution. J Virol 1992;66:3225.

133. Farci P, Bukh J, Purcell R H. The quasispecies of hepatitis C virus and the host immune response. Springer Semin Immunopathol 1997;19:5–26.

134. Domingo E, Martinez-Salas E, Sobrino F, et al. The quasispecies (extremely heterogeneous) nature of viral RNA genome populations: biological relevance—a review. Gene 1985;40:1–8.

135. Eigen M. On the nature of virus quasispecies. Trends Microbiol 1996;4:216–8.

136. Agnello V. The etiology and pathophysiology of mixed cryoglobulinemia secondary to hepatitis C virus infection. Springer Semin Immunopathol 1997;19:111–29.

137. Monteverde A, Ballare M, Pileri S. Hepatic lymphoid aggregates in chronic hepatitis C and mixed cryoglobulinemia. Springer Semin Immunopathol 1997;19:99–110.

138. McMurray R W. Hepatitis C-associated autoimmune disorders. Rheum Dis Clin North Am 1998;24:353–74.

139. Ray S C, Wang Y-M, Laeyendecker O, et al. Acute hepatitis C virus structural gene sequences as predictors of persistent viremia: Hypervariable region 1 as a decoy. J Virol 1999;73:2938–46.

140. Booth J C L, Kumar U, Webster D, Monjardino J, Thomas H C. Comparison of the rate of sequence variation in the hypervariable region of E2/NS1 region of hepatitis C virus in normal and hypogammaglobulinemic patients. Hepatology 1998;26:223–7.

141. Virelizier J L, Allison A C, Schild G C. Antibody responses to antigenic determinants of influenza virus hemagglutinin. II. Original antigenic sin: a bone marrow-derived lymphocyte memory phenomenon modulated by thymus-derived lymphocytes. J Exp Med 1974;140:1571–8.

142. Thomssen R, Bonk S, Propfe C, Heermann K-H, Kochel H G, Uy A. Association of hepatitis C virus in human sera with β-lipoprotein. Med Microbiol Immunol 1992;181:293–300.

143. Prince A M, Pascual D, McCarthy M, Parker T, Levine D. Apparent association of HCV RNA with very low density lipoproteins (VLDL). 4th Int. Symp. HCV, Tokyo, 1993;76.

144. Prince A M. Immunity in hepatitis C virus infection. Vox Sang 1994;67:227–8.

145. Hijikata M, Shimizu Y K, Kato H, et al. Equilibrium centrifugation studies of hepatitis C virus: evidence for circulating immune complexes. J Virol 1993;67:1953–8.

146. Pileri P, Uematsu Y, Campagnoli S, et al. Binding of hepatitis C virus to CD81. Science 1998;282:938–41.

147. Yi M, Kaneko S, Yu D Y, Murakami S. Hepatitis C virus envelope proteins bind lactoferrin. J Virol 1997;71:5997–6002.

148. Monazahian M, Bohme I, Bonk S, et al. Low density lipoprotein receptor as a candidate receptor for hepatitis C virus. J Med Virol 1999;57:223–9.

149. Haywood A M. Virus receptors: binding, adhesion strengthening and changes in viral structure. J Virol 1994;68:1–5.

8

IMMUNOPATHOGENESIS OF HEPATITIS C

BARBARA REHERMANN

Liver Diseases Section
National Institute of Diabetes and Digestive and Kidney Diseases, National Institutes of Health
Bethesda, Maryland

INTRODUCTION

More than 170 million people in the world are estimated to be infected with the hepatitis C virus (HCV) and the prevalence of HCV infection among healthy blood donors varies between 0.01 and 0.02% in northern Europe, (1,2) 6.5% in equatorial Africa, (3) and 20% in Egypt. (4,5) In the United States, infection with HCV accounts for 16–21% of all cases of acute and 45% of chronic viral hepatitis. In total, 4 million people, i.e., 1.8% of the U.S. population, are infected. (6)

The immunological correlates of viral clearance are still unknown. This is mainly due to the fact that most *de novo* HCV infections are clinically inapparent and in 40% of cases neither the time nor the routes of infection are known. Accordingly, many patients are diagnosed with hepatitis C when they present with symptoms and signs of chronic rather than acute liver disease. (7–9) For similar reasons, most studies on the HCV-specific immune response have been performed in chronically rather than in acutely infected or recovered patients. Collectively, these data imply that the immune response can mediate chronic inflammatory liver cell injury if it is not able to clear the virus early after infection.

COMPONENTS AND KINETICS OF THE CELLULAR IMMUNE RESPONSE

Induction of a Virus-Specific, Cellular Immune Response

It is generally assumed that the outcome of an acute viral infection, i.e., viral clearance or persistence, is determined in its earliest phase. Several factors, such as size, route, and genetic composition of the infecting virus as well as its rate of replication, cell tropism, and level of antigen expression, determine the kinetics with which host cells become infected and an opposing cellular immune response is induced. (10)

The cellular immune response to any infecting virus consists of an antigen nonspecific and an antigen-specific arm. The antigen nonspecific arm constitutes the first line of defense, as it is activated rapidly, and natural killer (NK) cells, neutrophils, and macrophages can be activated nonspecifically. (11) This provides time for uptake and processing of viral antigens by professional antigen presenting cells (APCs) that process and present viral antigens to T and B lymphocytes in regional lymph nodes.

The most efficient APCs are dendritic cells. These professional APCs combine the unique properties of antigen uptake in peripheral tissues and antigen transport to the regional lymph nodes as well as processing and presentation of antigen to specific T and B cells. Only 100 to 1000 antigen-pulsed dendritic cells are sufficient to induce a level of cytotoxic T lymphocyte (CTL) response that protects mice from lymphocytic chonomeningitis virus (LCMV) infection. (12) Ten thousand to 100,000 dendritic cells can induce an immune status that resembles a memory response after virus infection. Because observations show that the initial priming of the T-cell response, i.e., the original burst size, determines size and specificity of the long-term memory response, (13) the priming of the virus-specific immune response in the lymph nodes seems to be a crucial factor in the outcome of infection. In contrast, nonprofessional APCs such as hepatocytes, which are infected preferentially by hepatotropic viruses such as HCV, may induce anergy and apoptosis rather than activation of T cells as they do not convey sufficient costimulatory signals.

The acquired, virus-specific immune response, i.e., induction, activation, effector function, and interaction of virus-specific T helper (Th) cells, B cells, and cytotoxic T cells (CTL), is outlined and discussed in this chapter. Because HCV research has been hampered by the fact that neither a small, inbred animal model nor a tissue culture system is available to study virus host interaction in an infectious model, the following sections will also refer to relevant observations and results obtained in other model systems of viral infection to explain basic components and mechanisms of the immune response that may be relevant for HCV infection.

CD4-Positive T Helper Cells

CD4-positive T helper (Th) cells recognize 10 to 25 amino acid long viral peptides in the HLA class II binding groove of antigen-presenting cells. These peptides are generated intracellularly by proteolytic cleavage from larger precursors that are internalized in the form of soluble proteins (Fig. 1). Activated virus-specific CD4-positive T cells can stimulate antigen-presenting cells, antigen-nonspecific inflammatory cells, (14) antigen-specific CD8-positive T cells, and antibody-producing B cells. (15,16) Most of these interactions are mediated by distinct groups of cytokines (14,17) (Fig. 2).

T helper 1 (Th1) cytokines [interleukin (IL)-2, interferon (IFN)-γ, and tumor necrosis factor (TNF)-α] may exert antiviral effects by the stimulation of nitric oxide (NO) production in macrophages (18–21) and hepatocytes, (22) a mechanism that can induce resistance against viral infection of neighboring cells. (23) They also enhance specific immune recognition of viral antigens by the induction of HLA molecules on infected cells (23) and by activation of CD8-positive T cells and NK cells. (24) Finally, in hepatitis B virus (HBV), (25,26) as well as cytomegalovirus (CMV) (27) and rotavirus infection, (28) Th1 cytokines have been described to inhibit viral replication and gene expression.

Antigen Processing Pathways

A. Presentation by MHC I molecules

B. Presentation by MHC II molecules

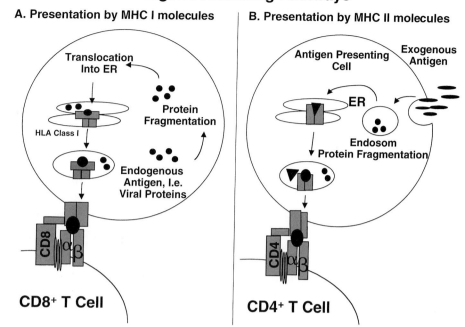

FIGURE I Antigen processing and presentation of viral peptides on MHC class I and MHC class II molecules, respectively. (A) Viral peptides are derived by cytosolic degradation of endogenously synthesized proteins and transported across the membrane of the endoplasmic reticulum (ER) by TAP 1 and 2 transporter complexes. After binding to MHC class I molecules in the endoplasmic reticulum, peptides are presented on the cell surface in the context of MHC class I molecules. (B) Exogenous, soluble viral proteins are internalized and cleaved proteolytically within endosomes. After binding to MHC class II molecules, the peptides are presented on the cell surface in the context of MHC class II molecules.

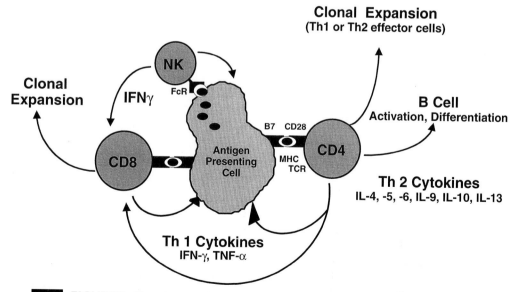

FIGURE 2 The cellular immune response to hepatitis C virus. For a description of the activation and effector function of NK cells (innate immune response) and CD4- and CD8-positive T cells (adaptive immune response), see text.

TABLE I   Factors That Influence Th1 versus Th2 Differentiation

Cytokine milieu
HLA haplotype
Costimulatory molecules
Quantity and quality of antigen
Affinity between TCR and HLA peptide complex
Density of antigenic ligand on APC

However, whether the same direct antiviral effects also apply to HCV infection is not known yet.

T helper 2 (Th2) cytokines (IL-4, IL-5, IL-6, IL-9, IL-10, and IL-13) support the humoral immune response by inducing activation and differentiation of B cells. They play an important role during infections with extracellular pathogens, (29) as they support the production of protective antibodies. This occurs at the expense of the cytotoxic T-cell response by inhibition of Th1 cytokine secretion, MHC expression, and antigen-presenting capacities of monocytes. (30–33) Efficient immune responses against intracellular viruses such as human immunodeficiency virus (HIV) (34) and intracellular pathogens such as leishmania or listeria (35) have therefore been reported to depend on Th1 rather than Th2 cytokines.

Differentiation of naïve CD4-positive T cells into either Th1 or Th2 effector cells is influenced by a large multitude of factors and conditions (Table 1). Analysis of murine T-cell responses has demonstrated that cytokines produced in the very early phase of infection, (31,36–39) as well as specific HLA alleles, (40,41) costimulatory molecules, (42) and quantity and quality of antigen, (43) determine the T-helper cell profile. In addition, Th1/2 differentiation depends on the affinity of the T-cell receptor (TCR) for a given HLA peptide complex (41,44,46): low-affinity interaction favors generation of Th1-like cells whereas high-affinity interaction induces Th2-like cells. (46) In contrast, the high density of antigenic ligands on professional antigen-presenting cells favors Th1-like responses and low ligand densities induce Th2-like responses. Although both observations seem to be contradictory at first glance, they can be reconciled by the hypothesis that Th1 differentiation requires a higher state of T-cell activation. Indeed, experimental evidence shows that low affinity between TCR and peptide–MHC complex and high density of peptide–MHC complexes on APCs allow serial engagement of many TCRs in a short time interval, thus leading to sustained signaling, subsequent TCR downmodulation, and complete T-cell activation. (47,48)

In addition to this noncognate help mediated by cytokines, T helper cells can also engage in cognate interaction with antigen-presenting cells and CD8-positive T cells and B cells. Interaction with APC is mediated via TCR-MHC and CD40L-CD40 binding and stimulates dendritic cells to upregulate costimulatory molecules, (49) to produce IL-12, and to induce CTLs. (50)

Cognate interaction between T helper cells and B cells also occurs via binding of TCR and peptide–MHC complex and of CD40L on the activated T cell and CD40 on the B cell. This cognate interaction induces B cells to produce antibodies of specific immunoglobulin classes (IgG switch). Interestingly, the antibody response does not necessarily display the same specificity as the T helper response. For example, it has been shown that Th cells specific for an internal influenza virus protein activate B cells to produce antibodies against the influenza surface antigen hemagglutinin. (51) A similar observation has been made in HBV infection: HBV core specific T helper cells provide help for HBV envelope-specific B cells. Conversely, B cells may also present viral antigens to naïve T cells. However, this interaction induces tolerance rather than stimulation of naïve T cells, (52,53) as resting B cells lack costimulatory molecules.

Finally, CD4-positive T cells have also been reported to exert antiviral as well as cytotoxic effector functions. (54–56) Specifically, HBV envelope-specific Th1 cells suppress HBV replication noncytolytically *in vivo* upon injection into HBV transgenic mice. (57) Further studies demonstrate that they also kill antigen-presenting hepatic nonparenchymal cells *in vivo* (57) as well as antigen-presenting CD8-positive T cells *in vitro* (58) and present soluble HBs antigen. CD4-positive cytotoxic T cells have even been shown to lyse infected macrophages (59) via the Fas pathway in bovine herpes virus (BHV-1) infection. Because MHC I molecules are downregulated on APCs during BHV-1 infection, this mechanism may represent a compensation for the inefficiency of the MHC I-restricted, CD8-positive T-cell response. In contrast to MHC class I-restricted, CD8-positive T cells, however, MHC class II-restricted, CD4-positive T cells exert cytotoxic effector functions only after stimulation with high concentrations of antigen that induce high TCR occupancy and IFN-γ production. (60) This observation suggests that cytotoxic activity is not the primary effector function of CD4-positive T cells, but may be an additional antiviral defense mechanism if CD8-positive cytotoxic T cells are overwhelmed and not able to reduce the concentration of viral antigen.

CD8-Positive Cytotoxic T Cells

The immune response of CD8-positive T cells is especially important during infection with noncytopathic, persistent viruses such as HCV, as these T cells recognize and lyse virus-infected cells. In virus-infected cells, viral peptides are cleaved from larger, endogenously synthesized precursors by the proteasome and other cytosolic proteases, transported across the membrane of the endoplasmatic reticulum by the heteromeric transporter complex TAP 1 and 2, and complexed with assembled MHC class I molecules (61) (Fig. 1). Importantly, each of the described steps may influence the selection of appropriate viral peptides for presentation on the cell surface. Specifically, it has been shown that intracellular peptide–MHC class I complexes are surprisingly labile, implying that a high dissociation rate of peptide–MHC class I complexes may contribute to an optimized spectrum of peptides presented on the cell surface. (62) This observation may also explain why only a fraction of all potential peptides with the appropriate HLA-binding motif are finally recognized by CTL. After recognition of a specific viral peptide in the context of the appropriate MHC molecule, CD8-positive T cells mediate antiviral effects by direct lysis of virus-infected host cells via the perforin/granzyme pathway, by induction of apoptosis via the Fas and TNF receptor-activated death pathways, or by release of cytokines that inhibit viral gene expression and replication. The latter has been shown to occur in hepatitis B virus (HBV) (25,26,63,64) and rotavirus (28) infection and is mediated by IFN-γ and TNF-α. Other cytokines, such as Rantes, MIP-1α, and MIP-1β, have been described as CD8 T-cell-derived factors that suppress HIV replication. (65)

Kinetics of the Antiviral T-cell Response

Lysis of virus-infected cells results in release of viral antigens, which are then processed and presented by local antigen-presenting cells that may prime additional T cells and amplify the antiviral immune response. (66) The abundance of each viral epitope eluted from virus-infected cells does indeed correlate with the specificity and magnitude of the CTL response: the immunodominant GP33–41 epitope, for example, that is present at 1000 copies per cell in LCMV-infected mice, primes more antigen specific CTL than two less frequently recognized epitopes that are only found at 160 and 90 copies per cell, respectively. (67) In addition, other factors, such as the avidity of CTL for a given peptide MHC complex, influence the ability of the immune response to control viral infection. The presence of high-avidity CTL capable of recognizing small amounts of antigen has been shown to correlate with protection from LCMV infection. (67) These cells may be less susceptible to induction of apoptosis by high amounts of antigen (68) and may therefore survive the downregulation of the antiviral immune response after the successful reduction of viral replication, which often leads to the death of low-affinity CTL.

A number of publications on LCMV infection report that the interaction between CD4-positive and CD8-positive T cells is crucial in maintaining the antiviral immune response in a persistent viral infection. Whereas the control of acute infection may be mediated primarily by CD8-positive T cells, the long-term control of infection is dependent on all three major components of the immune system, i.e., B cells, T helper cells, and cytotoxic T cells. (69) Obviously, sufficient and continuous production of IL-2 by T helper cells is required to sustain the CTL response. (70,71) Thus, help provided by CD4-positive T cells is critical if the virus cannot be eradicated soon after infection and CTL responses need to be maintained and protected from exhaustion. (71–74) Furthermore, CD4-positive T cells have also been shown to support the migration and effector function of CD8-positive T cells, e.g., during mouse hepatitis virus infection of the central nervous system. (75)

Interestingly, research also focuses on the interaction of CTL and virus-specific B cells, and some reports indicate that CTL memory cannot be maintained in the absence of B cells. (76) In the early acute stage of infection, however, opposite effects have been demonstrated that may potentially contribute to the late development of the humoral immune responses in acute HCV infection. Indeed, an early vigorous CTL response in LCMV-infected mice impaired or delayed the development of neutralizing antiviral antibodies. The authors hypothesize that virus-infected B cells expressing neutralizing receptors may present viral peptides on class I MHC molecules and become targets for virus-specific CTL. (76,77)

Similarly, virus-specific CD8-positive T cells have also been shown to lyse CD4-positive T cells presenting viral antigens, e.g., in HBV (58) and HIV infection. (78) They can either be targeted against specific TCR Vβ sequences of a given T-cell clone (79) or against antigenic peptides presented by CD4-positive T cells.

In summary, multiple factors have been identified that determine the strength, specificity, and especially the kinetics of the antiviral immune response. Several of these mechanisms described in other viral infections may also be relevant for HCV infection and may demonstrate that the relative inefficiency and weakness of the HCV immune response may be the result of multiple interactions between the virus and immune system as well as complex regulatory mechanisms of the immune system itself. Unfortunately, analysis of the cellular immune response and the kinetics of virus–host interaction has been hampered by the absence of a small, inbred animal model susceptible to infection by the hepatitis C virus.

CELLULAR IMMUNE RESPONSE IN HCV-INFECTED PATIENTS

Similar to the inability of the cellular immune response to control HIV, the apparent resistance of HCV to immunological control is an area of great interest and importance. Research has been hampered by the fact that the acute stage of HCV infection is usually clinically inapparent. Therefore, more human studies have concentrated on patients with chronic HCV infection than on patients with acute, self-limited hepatitis C. In particular, the intrahepatic T-cell response has only been studied in patients with chronic hepatitis C. To date, most reports suggest that the HCV-specific immune response exerts some control over virus replication but is unable to terminate persistent infection in most cases.

Acute, Self-limited Hepatitis C

Clinical observations suggest that viral and immunological events occurring during the first few weeks after infection may determine the outcome of hepatitis C. For example, patients who recover from acute HCV infection usually clear the virus within 3 months of clinical onset of acute hepatitis, and evolution into chronic infection is not a frequent outcome in patients who develop clinically evident, acute hepatitis. (80)

HCV-Specific T Helper Response

Consistent with these clinical observations, the HCV-specific proliferative Th-cell response of patients with acute, self-limited hepatitis C has been described as vigorous and multispecific. (81,82) The NS3 protein of the hepatitis C virus is an especially important antigen, as a CD4-positive T-cell response against its helicase domain is significantly stronger and is found more frequently in patients who resolve acute hepatitis C than in patients who develop persistent infection. (81) Within the NS3 protein, a short immunodominant region at amino acid 1248–1261 with a minimal epitope at amino acid 1251–1259 was identified. This epitope binds promiscuously to 10 common HLA class II alleles with high affinities (82) and is remarkably conserved within HCV 1a, 1b, 1c, 2a, and 2b genotypes. T helper cells mediating this NS3-specific immune response frequently display a Th1 or Th 0 cytokine profile, whereas a Th2 profile is associated with a chronic course of infection. (83) Tsai et al. (83) reported that peripheral blood mononuclear cells (PBMCs) of 17 patients with self-limited acute hepatitis C displayed a Th1 phenotype upon stimulation with HCV antigens, whereas PBMC of 11 patients who developed chronic hepatitis were characterized by Th2 cytokine profiles and significantly weaker proliferative T-cell responses. In another study, the levels of circulating IL-2, IL-4, IL-10, and IFN-γ were significantly higher in patients with chronic hepatitis C than in uninfected controls. (84)

After recovery from acute hepatitis C, the NS3-specific T helper cell response has been observed to persist for up to 3.5 years, i.e., the maximum time of follow-up. (85) Whether this HCV-specific memory T-cell response to HCV infection is able to protect against reinfection with the homologous or heterologous virus is not known yet and can only be analyzed in animal models of infection. Similarly, it is also a frequently discussed and controversial question whether the maintenance of a virus-specific memory response requires persisting antigen or even low levels of replicating virus for periodic *de novo* induction of virus-specific T cells. While trace amounts of persisting, replicating virus have been detected in patients with clinic and serologic evidence of recovery from hepatitis B virus, (86) varicella-zoster virus, herpes simplex virus, and measles virus infections, (87) this question has not yet been resolved for HCV.

In this respect, a recent publication seems to reconcile the previously opposing hypotheses that antigen is either required or not necessary to maintain memory responses, at least in the LCMV model. This publication by Kündig et al. (88) demonstrates that the frequency of LCMV-specific T-cell precursors remains stable in the spleen of mice independent of antigen stimulation, whereas it decreases in an antigen-dependent fashion in peripheral solid organs. Only memory T cells that are recently activated by antigen extravasate into peripheral solid organs. Therefore, protective immunity against peripheral routes of reinfection is considered to be antigen dependent and cannot be replaced by systemic immunity. Consistent with this model, it has been shown that protection against mucosal routes of vaccinia virus infection in mice correlates with CTL activity in the local mucosal sites, not with CTL activity in the spleen. (89)

How could a memory response be sustained in the absence of antigen? Interestingly, it is possible to stimulate memory cells that express IL-2 receptors and high levels of adhesion molecules by cytokines such as IL-2 and IFN-γ. These cytokines may be produced during the host's primary immune response to a second pathogen, as demonstrated for LCMV-specific memory cells in mice. (90)

HCV-Specific Cytotoxic T-cell Response

Because of the small number of patients who present with acute hepatitis C and due to technical and practical limitations inherent in CTL analysis, the CTL response to HCV during acute hepatitis is difficult to study. Only two studies have analyzed the role of the CTL response in acute hepatitis C of humans and chimpanzees. (91,92) In both cases, an early, vigorous, and multispecific CTL response was associated with a self-limited outcome of infection. Importantly, termination of infection correlated precisely with the onset of a multispecific intrahepatic CTL response. (92) Recently developed, the technique of staining peptide-specific T cells with MHC–peptide tetramers may allow a direct analysis of the frequency of HCV-specific T cells because a small number of antigen-specific cells can be stained and analyzed via FACS analysis without prior *in vitro* expansion. Applying this technique to infections other than hepatitis C, between 7 and 44% of peripheral blood CD8-positive T cells have been demonstrated to be EBV specific in acute EBV infection and 50–70% of activated CD8-positive T cells were LCMV specific during the acute phase of LCMV infection. (13) These findings suggest that, contrary to previous assumptions, the majority of cells are indeed virus specific and are not bystander cells. HCV epitope-specific T cells, however, were found at a significantly lower level in the peripheral blood of chronically infected patients. (93) Direct quantitation of HCV-specific CTL during the acute phase of infection may therefore provide a definite answer to the question of whether the HCV-specific CTL response is indeed too weak to clear the virus.

Several other studies have analyzed the CTL response of HCV-seronegative, healthy persons with frequent exposure to HCV in order to identify potentially protective CTL responses. Interestingly, individuals who were exposed repeatedly to HCV either occupationally (94) or via HCV-infected spouses (95,96) mounted peripheral blood HCV-specific helper and cytotoxic T-cell responses in the absence of either a humoral immune response or viremia. The presence of cellular immune responses in the absence of humoral responses has also been reported in HIV exposed, but uninfected persons (97) and is compatible with the hypothesis that T-cell memory may be induced by the periodic reintroduction of viral antigen via recurring, subclinical viral exposure. (98)

Chronic Hepatitis C

HCV-Specific T Helper Response

Patients with acute hepatitis C who are not able to clear the infection but proceed to develop chronic hepatitis C generally display a weaker helper and cytotoxic T-cell response in peripheral blood than patients who clear HCV. (81, 82) Th2 and Th0 rather than Th1 cytokine profiles dominate in chronic active hepatitis C. Accordingly, higher titers of nonconformational antibodies and more frequent CD30 expression and IL-10 production were seen in patients who display histological or clinical signs of disease activity. (99) These observations are consistent with the notion that Th1 cytokine responses favor cellular immune responses and Th2 responses favor humoral immune responses.

HCV-Specific Cytotoxic T-Cell Response

Studies performed in humans (100–104) and chimpanzees (105) infected chronically with the HCV as well as immunization studies in HLA-transgenic mice (106,107) identified CTL epitopes in all viral proteins. As in other viral infections, such as influenza (108–110) and HIV infection, (111,112) HCV-specific CTL have been shown to be broadly cross-reactive and able to recognize different viral subtypes. Most of these epitopes have been confirmed by several independent studies (104,106,107,113) and have been shown to be recognized in the context of several HLA haplotypes that constitute HLA supertype families. To date, four HLA class I supertypes are defined according to the A2-like, (114) B7-like, (115) B44-like, (116) and A3-like binding motif (117) that a given viral peptide needs to contain in order to bind to a given HLA allele. In total, more than 80% of the world populations displays at least one of these HLA supertypes. A vaccine that induces virus-specific immune responses restricted by these supertype motifs may therefore be beneficial for the majority of the world population.

Because repetitive *in vitro* stimulation with HCV-derived peptides is required to expand CTL from the peripheral blood, the frequency of progenitor CTL in the circulation is assumed to be rather low, ranging from one in 10^6 to one in 10^5 PBMC as determined by limiting dilution analysis. (101,118) Thus, the frequency of CTL specific for HCV is significantly lower than the frequency of CTL specific for the influenza matrix epitope as a recall antigen. (118) Although sensitive techniques employing peptide–MHC tetramers for the quantitation of CTL have demonstrated that the frequency of HCV-specific CTL is approximately 100-fold higher in the liver than in the blood, it is still much lower than the intrahepatic frequency of LCMV-specific murine CTL during self-limited LCMV infection. (119) However, the relative weakness of the HCV-specific CTL response is not due to generalized immunosuppression as the CTL response against influenza virus (118) and Epstein–Barr virus (120) is normal in HCV-infected patients.

The breadth and specificity of the intrahepatic CTL response of HCV-infected patients were assessed in a study by Wong et al. (121,122). In summary, MHC class I-restricted CTL were detected in 45% of the analyzed liver biopsies. Remarkably, each patient recognized a specific panel of HCV epitopes, only one epitope was targeted by more than one person, and immunodominant responses to a particular epitope or even protein could only be defined for a given patient and were not shared between patients.

It is important to emphasize that the repertoire of HCV-specific T cells at the site of inflammation, the HCV-infected liver, may not correspond to the T-cell population in the peripheral blood. Minutello (54) reported that the intrahepatic T helper cell response is focused on the HCV NS4 protein, mediated by T cells that are much more efficient in providing help to B cells than HCV-specific T cells in the peripheral blood and express a selective T-cell receptor that is not present in the peripheral blood compartment. The predominant use of Vβ5.1 by intrahepatic T cells (123) indicates oligoclonal expansion and intrahepatic compartmentalization of T cells and a restricted specificity for a common immunodominant HCV antigen.

Although the HCV-specific CTL response is too weak to achieve viral clearance in chronically infected subjects, it may still exert some control over viral load. Indeed, a stronger polyclonal CTL response in the peripheral blood (124) and the liver (122) is associated with lower levels of HCV viremia. This ineffective immune response leads to chronic inflammatory liver disease, which after many years to decades may result in irreversible liver cirrhosis and hepatocellular carcinoma.

PATHOGENESIS OF LIVER DISEASE

Histologic Characteristics of Hepatitis C

The liver is considered to be the primary site of HCV replication, as negative-strand RNA is only detected in the liver, not in peripheral blood mononuclear cells when highly specific techniques such as tagged polymerase chain reaction are employed. (125) HCV RNA levels are consistently greater in the liver than in the serum, (126) ranging between 10^8 and 10^{11} copies per gram of liver tissue. (126,127) HCV RNA has been detected in the cytoplasm of hepatocytes, as well as the expression of both structural and nonstructural HCV proteins. However, only 50–70% of the liver specimens from HCV-infected patients and only a small percentage of hepatocytes (5–19%) were found to be HCV RNA positive by *in situ* hybridization. (128,129) Even fewer hepatocytes (1–10%) express HCV antigens as detected by immunohistochemical analysis. Similarly, only 1–5% of mononuclear cells and a small proportion of biliary epithelial cells have detectable HCV antigen or RNA. (130) These observations may indicate a weak stimulation of the immune system due to low antigen expression. (131)

It is interesting to note that most infected hepatocytes display little or no apparent hepatocellular damage, suggesting that HCV is not a cytopathic virus. However, several histologic features characteristic of hepatitis C exist. Specifically, the presence of bile duct damage, steatosis, and lymphoid follicles is characteristic for hepatitis C. (132–134) Bile duct damage is seen in 30–90% of HCV-infected patients, but is uncommon in other form of chronic vial hepatitis. Steatosis may in part be attributed to the HCV core protein, a viral gene product with transcriptional regulatory functions. (133)

Lymphoid aggregates and even follicles with B-cell germinal centers are seen much more frequently in hepatitis C than in hepatitis B, especially in portal tracts in areas of focal or piecemeal necrosis. (135,136) T cells are the predominant liver-infiltrating cell type and represent evidence of immune-mediated liver disease. Although CD4-positive Th cells are found in portal areas, (137) CD8-positive lymphocytes infiltrate the hepatic lobules. (138) In regions of active inflammation, (139) hepatocytes express Fas antigen, and the generation of acidophil Councilman bodies is regarded as a result of CTL-induced hepatocyte apoptosis. (135,140) Presentation of HCV antigens on infected hepatocytes, recognition by CTL, and induction of liver injury are enhanced by the increased expression of HLA-A, B, C, and ICAM-1 molecules. (131) In addition, CD68-positive macrophages and monocytes are found in more aggressive forms of HCV infection. These activated cells are thought to mediate and enhance antigen presentation and hence inflammation. (141) As a result, the majority of circulating hepatitis C viruses is thought to be produced through continuous rounds of *de novo* infection and rapid turnover of cells, not through release from chronically infected cells. (142)

Mechanisms of Immune-Mediated Liver Injury

The mechanisms that regulate T-cell-induced viral clearance versus T-cell-induced liver injury are not completely understood. It is unknown whether HCV, like other viruses such as HBV, (26) CMV, (27) HIV, (65) or rotavirus, (28) is susceptible to cytokines derived from CTL or other inflammatory cells. In HBV infection, cytokines such as IFN-γ and TNF-α have been shown to inhibit viral gene expression and replication efficiently (25,26,143) and to clear hepatocytes of the infecting virus without causing liver disease. Liver-infiltrating, HCV-specific T cells are also Th1 dominant and have been shown to produce IFN-γ and TNF-α, but no or little IL-4. (144) Even antigen-nonspecific cells that form the majority of the intrahepatic inflammatory infiltrate (145) could contribute to cytokine release and amplify the antigen-specific immune response significantly. However, it is possible that the hepatitis C virus is less susceptible to these cytokines.

Inflammatory liver disease mediated by the destruction of infected hepatocytes may occur in several ways: HCV-infected hepatocytes can be killed by HCV-specific CTL clones via Fas ligand, TNF-α and/or perforin-based mechanisms. Fas ligand-induced apoptosis of hepatocytes has been implicated because expression of Fas, a mediator of apoptosis, (139) is upregulated near liver-infiltrating cells (146) and the Fas (CD95) ligand is expressed on activated, liver-infiltrating T cells. (147) TNF-α is produced predominantly by macrophages, (148) but may also be released by lymphocytes (149) and expressed on the surface of CTL. (150) Finally, the perforin-mediated mechanism may contribute to the lysis of antigen-presenting, Fas, and TNF-α resistant cells. (151)

However, CTLs do not only target antigen-presenting HCV-infected hepatocytes, but also lyse uninfected neighboring hepatocytes in which Fas expression may be upregulated in response to inflammatory cytokines. These bystander cells are killed less efficiently and usually at high effector to target cell ratios. In addition, other neighboring infected hepatocytes may be susceptible to soluble TNF-α because of altered RNA or protein synthesis (152): this mechanism does not require close cell–cell contact and may, therefore, play a more efficient role in the restriction of virus replication.

Fate of HCV-Specific, Liver-Infiltrating Lymphocytes

Finally, the origin and fate of the intrahepatic lymphocytic infiltrate are interesting areas of current research. It has been shown that intrahepatic lymphocytes do not undergo clonal expansion in the liver, but are recruited continuously from the peripheral blood. (153) This study estimates that approximately 1% of the total body lymphocytes are found in the inflamed livers of HCV-infected patients. The intrahepatic inflammatory infiltrate is significantly enriched for cells of the innate immune response, such as NK cells, TCRγ/δ-positive cells, and Vα24-positive T cells. After exerting their effector functions, the majority of these cells undergo programmed cell death themselves. Th1 cells, which are attracted preferentially into HCV-infected livers, are particularly sensitive to Fas–FasL-induced apoptosis, whereas Th2 effectors express high levels of FAP-1, a Fas-associated phophatase that presumably inhibits Fas signaling. (154) Nuti et al. (153) estimate a loss of 2×10^8 cells, i.e., 0.1% of the total body lymphocytes, per day.

POTENTIAL MECHANISMS OF HCV PERSISTENCE

The mechanisms whereby HCV circumvents the immune response, persists, and causes chronic inflammatory liver disease are currently undefined.

One hypothesis is that the HCV-specific immune response is too weak to clear HCV from all infected hepatocytes once a persistent infection is established. Hypothetically, this may be due to either an insufficient induction of the primary immune response during acute infection (see earlier discussion) or the

████ **TABLE II   Potential Mechanisms of HCV Persistence**

Quantitative or qualitative insufficiency of the virus-specific immune response
  Insufficient induction of the primary response
    Low antigenic load
    Lack of sufficient costimulatory signals on hepatocytes
    Type of antigen-presenting cell (hepatocyte versus dendritic cell)
    Cytokine profile of Th cells (Th2 versus Th1)
  Inability to maintain the primary response
    Incomplete activation and expansion of virus-specific CTL
    Insufficient T-cell help

Viral evasion of strong immune responses
  Replication in immunoprivileged sites
  Viral interference with antigen processing
  Viral suppression of host immune responses
  Viral sequence variation, selection of quasispecies
    Escape from humoral immune response
    Escape from cellular immune response
  Viral insusceptibility to cytokine-mediated inhibition of replication and gene expression

inability to maintain the T-cell response at high levels during chronic hepatitis C (Table II). As described earlier, several studies suggest that the virus-specific T helper cell response may be a crucial, early determinant for the outcome of acute HCV infection (81,82) and is also necessary for maintaining a high level of CTL reactivity during persistent viral infections. (69–71) Generally, the intensity of the initial immune response depends on antigenic load, costimulatory signals, the type of the antigen-presenting cell, and the differentiation and cytokine profile of T helper cells. Each of these factors may not be optimal in acute HCV infection, as, for example, the level of HCV antigens is relatively low in comparison to HBV antigens. Therefore, HBV is usually cleared following acute infection of immune-competent adults, whereas HCV is not. In addition, costimulatory molecules, which promote the contact between TCR and peptide–MHC complex via CD28-B7 interaction or engagement of CD4 and CD8 coreceptors, are expressed predominantly on professional antigen-presenting cells in the lymph nodes and not on hepatocytes, the preferred cell type for HCV replication. With small doses of antigen or insufficient costimulation, T-cell activation and proliferation may be suboptimal, (42) as reflected by the relatively low number of HCV-specific cytotoxic T cells in the peripheral blood of chronically infected patients.

While the number of HCV-specific CTL may therefore be too low to clear the virus from all infected cells, the HCV-specific T-cell response may still be strong enough to recognize individual, HCV-infected cells and to cause a low level of persistent intrahepatic inflammation. This may be due to the fact that the cytolytic function of HCV-specific T cells is relatively easy to elicit even by small amounts of antigen and does not require full T-cell activation. (60) In contrast, higher peptide concentrations resulting in the triggering of at least 20–50% of the T-cell receptors are necessary to elicit calcium influx, IFN-γ production, and IL-2 responsiveness of specific T cells. Finally, only the highest peptide concentration can induce the proliferation needed for the clonal expansion of virus-specific T cells.

As a second hypothetical explanation for HCV persistence, sequence variation of the quasispecies and the high mutation rate of HCV have often been discussed. Studies suggest that circulating HCV has a half-life of only about 3hr, indicating relatively efficient virus replication and release, at least in patients with high levels of viral load. (155) This dynamic process, capable of generating viral variants continuously, suggests that viral variation may be important for the establishment and maintenance of persistent infection. Due to the presence of multiple quasispecies, the main viral population can adapt quickly to a selection pressure that may be exerted by either the humoral or the cellular immune response. Depending on the heterogeneity of the infecting virus population, early escape from humoral and cellular antiviral immune responses may result. Evidence for selection pressure exerted by the humoral immune response has been obtained from several clinical studies. In immunocompromised patients the viral nucleotide sequence variability in the 27 amino acid hypervariable region 1 (HVR 1) of the hepatitis C virus was markedly lower than in immunocompetent HCV-positive patients, suggesting that immune selection, primarily by HVR 1-specific antibodies, influences sequence variation in this region. (156) However, sequence variations in HVR1 may also occur in the absence of selection pressure, as they were also found in agammaglobulinemic patients without an HCV-specific antibody response, (156) and several studies have demonstrated that persistent infection of infected chimpanzees can evolve without any HVR sequence variations. (157,158)

Viral variants that may mediate escape from the cellular immune response have been demonstrated in many viral infections, such as HBV, HTLV-I, and HIV infection. (159–163) Most recently, this phenomenon has also been described in a chimpanzee with chronically evolving hepatitis C (164) and in patients with chronic hepatitis C. (165,166) Sequence variations in CTL epitopes were found more frequently in the presence than in the absence of a CTL response and resulted in nonimmunogenic, noncross-reactive variant peptides of low binding affinity, compatible with nonrecognition by the CTL of the peptide epitope derived from the variant virus. An antagonist peptide, one that is able to inhibit recognition of both wild-type and variant virus, was detected in only one case. Because the CTL response was multispecifically targeted against several other epitopes in this patient, the clinical course did not change during the study period of 10 months during which this variant emerged. In another antigen system, simultaneous presentation of both the antagonist and the agonist peptide on the same antigen-presenting cell has been shown to block TCR internalization, thereby preventing multiple TCR engagement that is necessary to activate wild-type specific T cells. (167) Obviously, such variants would suppress the immune response against both the original and the variant epitope. Only T cells that are not cross-reactive with the variant and not susceptible to antagonism would be stimulated to proliferate. T cells that are cross-reactive with the variant, however, would not be able to reach the activation threshold for proliferation. This explains why T cells cannot expand in the presence of minute amounts of a peptide antagonist. The remaining immune response to the wild-type epitope would be weakened significantly and would focus on cells that are infected exclusively with the original virus and therefore select cells coinfected with the variant virus.

Interestingly, proliferation and expansion rather than cytotoxicity of antigen-specific T cells seem to be sensitive to inhibition by even small amounts of antagonist peptide. (166) Hence, viral antagonists may impair the expansion of HCV-specific T cells to a number that would be sufficient to clear the virus, but may still induce harmful effector functions such as a low level of cytotoxicity. This process may therefore be too weak to clear HCV, but strong enough to cause persisting chronic inflammatory liver injury, resulting in fibrosis and liver cirrhosis.

Finally, HCV could also interfere with antigen processing or presentation in APCs that prime the immune response and/or in hepatocytes that function as target cells. HCV may diminish its visibility to the immune system sufficiently to avoid clearance but not enough to prevent inflammatory liver injury. Other viruses have also been shown to interfere with antigen processing. For example, proteins encoded by the HCMV genes US11 and US12 can dislocate newly synthesized class I heavy chains from the endoplasmic reticulum to the cytosol. (168) Regarding HCV, it has been shown in an *in vivo* model that the expression of HCV core by recombinant vaccinia viruses may suppress the cytotoxic T-cell response against vaccinia virus epitopes, (169) indicating that the HCV core protein may play an important role in suppressing host immune responses.

CONCLUSION

Indirect evidence for a protective role of the cellular immune response is provided by observations that HCV-specific CTL as well as T helper cells have been shown in the blood of HCV RNA-negative persons who were exposed to HCV repeatedly and in people who resolved HCV infection spontaneously. Furthermore, both the strength and the quality of the CD4-positive T helper and the CD8-positive CTL response differ between patients who recover from acute hepatitis C and those who develop chronic infection. Despite the multispecificity of the response, a conserved, immunodominant T helper epitope with promiscuous MHC binding could be identified within the NS3 protein. A strong, Th1-dominated T helper response is also associated with a lower viral load and a more favorable course of chronic hepatitis C.

However, the high incidence of chronic hepatitis indicates that most individuals are incapable of spontaneously mounting an immune response that will clear the virus. Even after the resolution of primary infection, reinfection can occur with heterologous or homologous virus, suggesting that the immune response may be short-lived, weak, or narrowly focused to confer protection against reinfection. In addition, diverse HCV genotypes, subtypes, and quasispecies increase the potential for viral escape from immunosurveillance. Therefore, the identification of the immunologic and virologic correlates that determine resolution versus chronic evolution of HCV infection and the development of vaccines and immunotherapy for HCV will be challenging endeavors.

REFERENCES

1. Booth J C. Chronic hepatitis C: the virus, its discovery and the natural history of the disease. J Viral Hepatitis 1998;5:213–22.

2. Mutimer D J, Harrison R F, O'Donnell K B, et al. Hepatitis C virus infection in the asymptomatic British blood donor. J Viral Hepatitis 1995;2:47–53.

3. Delaporte E, Thiers V, Dazza M C, et al. High level of hepatitis C endemicity in Gabon, equatorial Africa. Trans R Soc Trop Med Hyg 1993;87:636–7.

4. Saeed A A, al-Admawi A M, al-Rasheed A, et al. Hepatitis C virus infection in Egyptian volunteer blood donors in Riyadh. Lancet 1991;338:459–60.

5. el-Ahmady O, Halim A B, Mansour O, Salman T. Incidence of hepatitis C virus in Egyptians. J Hepatol 1994;21:687.

6. Alter M J. Epidemiology of hepatitis C in the West. Semin Liver Dis 1995;15:5–14.

7. Choo Q-L, Kuo G, Weiner A J, Overby L R, Bradley D W, Houghton M. Isolation of a cDNA clone derived from a blood-borne non-A, non-B viral hepatitis genome. Science 1989;244:359–62.

8. Alter M J, Margolis H S, Krawczynski K, et al. The natural history of community-acquired hepatitis C in the United States. N Engl J Med 1992;327:1899–905.

9. Sansono D, Dammacco F. Hepatitis C virus related chronic liver disease of sporadic type: clinical, serological and histological features. Digestion 1992;51:115–20.

10. Oxenius A, Zinkernagel R M, Hengartner H. CD4+ T-cell induction and effector functions: a comparison of immunity against soluble antigens and viral infections. Adv Immunol 1998;70:313–67.

11. Moretta L, Ciccone E, Mingari M C, Biassoni R, Moretta A. Human natural killer cells: origin, clonality, specificity, receptors. Adv Immunol 1994;55:341–58.

12. Ludewig B, Ehl S, Karrer U, Odermatt B, Hengartner H, Zinkernagel R M. Dendritic cells efficiently induce protective antiviral immunity. J Virol 1998;72:3812–18.

13. Murali-Krishna K, Altman J D, Suresh M, et al. Counting antigen-specific CD8 T cells: a re-evaluation of bystander activation during viral infection. Immunity 1998;8:177–87.

14. Mosmann T R, Cherwinski H, Bond M W, Giedlin M A, Coffman R L. Two types of murine helper T cell clone. I. Definition according to profiles of lymphokine activities and secreted proteins. J Immunol 1986;136:2348–57.

15. Vitetta E S, Fernandez-Botran R, Myers C D, Sanders V M. Cellular interactions in the humoral immune response. Adv Immunol 1989;45:1–105.

16. Doherty P C, Allan W, Eichelberger M. Roles of ab and gd T cell subsets in viral immunity. Annu Rev Immunol 1992;10:123–51.

17. Kim J, Woods A, Becker-Dunn E, Bottomly K. Distinct functional phenotypes of cloned Ia-restricted helper T cells. J Exp Med 1985;162:188–201.

18. Croen K D. Evidence for an antiviral effect of nitric oxide. J Clin Invest 1993;91:2446–52.

19. Karupiah G, Xie Q-W, Buller R M L, Nathan C, Duarte C, MacMicking J D. Inhibition of viral replication by interferon gamma induced nitric oxide synthased. Science 1993;261:1445–8.

20. Harris N, Buller R M L, Karupiah G. Interferon-gamma induced, nitric oxide mediated inhibition of vaccinia viral replication. J Virol 1995;69:910–5.

21. Sharara A I, Perkins D J, Misukonis M A, Chan S U, Dominitz J A, Weinberg J B. Interferon (IFN)-alpha activation of human blood mononuclear cells in vitro and in vivo for nitric oxide synthase (NOS) type 2 mRNA and protiein expression: possible relationship of induced NOS2 to the anti-hepatitis C effects of IFN-alpha in vivo. J Exp Med 1997;186:1495–502.

22. Nussler A K, Di Silvio M, Billiar T R, et al. Stimulation f the nitric oxide synthase pathway in human hepatocytes by cytokines and endotoxin. J Exp Med 1992;176:261–4.

23. Farrar M A, Schreiber R D. The molecular cell biology of interferon gamma and its receptor. Annu Rev Immunol 1993;11:571–611.

24. Zinkernagel R M, Moskophidis D, Kundig T, Oehen S, Pircher H P, Hengartner H. Effector T-cell induction and T-cell memory versus peripheral deletion of T cells. Immunol Rev 1993;131:198–223.

25. Guidotti L G, Ando K, Hobbs M V, et al. Cytotoxic T lymphocytes inhibit hepatitis B virus gene expression by a noncytolytic mechanism in transgenic mice. Proc Natl Acad Sci U S A 1994;91:3764–3768.

26. Guidotti L G, Ishikawa T, Hobbs M V, Matzke B, Schreiber R, Chisari F V. Intracellular inactivation of the hepatitis B virus by cytotoxic T lymphocytes. Immunity 1996;4:35–6.

27. Pavic I, Polic B, Crnkovic I, Lucin P, Jonjic S, Koszinowki U H. Participation of endogenous tumor necrosis factor alpha in host resistance to cytomegalovirus infection. J Gen Virol 1993;74:2215–23.

28. Franco M A, Tin C, Rott L S, Van Cotte J L, McGhee J R, Greenberg H B. Evidence for CD8+ T-cell immunity to murine rotavirus in the absence of perforin, fas and gamma interferon. J Virol 1997;71:479–86.

29. Urban J F J, Katona I M, Paul W E, Finkelman F D. Interleukin-4 is important in protective immunity to a gastrointestinal nematode infection in mice. Proc Natl Acad Sci U S A 1991;88: 5513–7.

30. Mosmann T R, Sad S. The expanding universe of T-cell subsets: Th1, Th2 and more. Immunol Today 1996;17:138–46.

31. Abbas A K, Murphy K M, Sher A. Functional diversity of helper T lymphocytes. Nature 1996; 383:787–93.

32. Nagler A, Lanier L L, Phillips J H. The effects of IL-4 on human natural killer cells: a potent regulator of IL-2 activation and proliferation. J Immunol 1988;141:2349–51.

33. Martinez O M, Gibbons R S, Garovoy M R, Aronson F R. IL-4 inhibits IL-2 receptor expression and IL-2 dependent proliferation of human T cells. J Immunol 1990;144:2211–5.

34. Shearer G M, Clerici M. Cytokine profiles in HIV type 1 disease and protection. AIDS Res Hum Retroviruses 1998;14(Suppl 2):S149-52.

35. Dai W J, Bartens W, Kohler G, Hufnagel M, Kopf M, Brombacher F. Impaired macrophage listericidal and cytokine activities are responsible for the rapid death of Listeria monocytogenes-infected IFN- gamma receptor-deficient mice. J Immunol 1997;158:5297–304.

36. Nakajima H, Iwamoto I, Tomoe S, et al. CD4+ T-lymphocytes and interleukin-5 mediate antigen-induced eosinophil infiltration into mouse trachea. Annu Rev Respir Dis 1992;146: 374–7.

37. Scott P, Pearce E, Cheever A, Coffman R, Sher A. Role of cytokines and CD4+ T cell subsets in the regulation of parasitic immunity and disease. Innumol Rev 1989;112:161–82.

38. Gazzinelli R T, Hieny S, Wynn T A, Wolf S, Sher A. IL-12 is required for the T-lymphocyte-independent induction of interferon gamma by an intracellular parasite and induces resistance in T cell deficient hosts. Proc Natl Acad Sci U S A 1993;90:6115–9.

39. Sypek J P, Chung C L, Mayor S E H, et al. Resolution of cutaneous leishmaniasis: interleukin 12 initiates a protective T helper type 1 immune response. J Exp Med 1993;177:1797–802.

40. Tite J P, Foellmer H G, Mardi J P, Janeway, C A Jr. Inverse Ir gene control of the antibody and T cell proliferative response to human basement membrane collagen. J Immunol 1987;139: 2892–8.

41. Murray J S, Madri J, Tite J, Carding S R, Bottomly K. MHC control of CD4+ T cell subset activation. J Exp Med 1989;170:2135–40.

42. Cai Z, Sprent J. Influence of antigen dose and costimulation on the primary response of CD8+ T cells in vitro. J Exp Med 1996;183:2247–57.

43. Thompson C B. Distinct roles for the costimulatory ligands B7–1 and B7–2 in T helper cell differentiation? Cell 1995;81:979–82.

44. Pfeiffer C, Stein J, Southwood S, Ketelaar H, Sette A, Bottomly K. Altered peptide ligands can control CD4 T lymphocyte differentiation in vivo. J Exp Med 1995;181:1569–74.

45. Kawamura T, Furusaka A, Koziel M J, et al. Transgenic expression of hepatitis C virus structural proteins in the mouse. Hepatology 1997;25:1014–21.

46. Pearson CI, van Ewijk W, McDevitt HO. Induction of apoptosis and T helper 2 (Th2) responses correlates with peptide affinity for the major histocompatibility complex in self- reactive T cell receptor transgenic mice. J Exp Med 1997;185:583–99.

47. Valitutti S, Müller S, Cella M, Padovan E, Lanzavecchia A. Serial triggering of many T-cell receptors by a few peptide-MHC complexes. Nature 1995;375:148–51.

48. Gros G, Ben-Sasson S Z, Seder R, Finkelman F D, Paul W E. Generation of interleukin 4 (IL-4)-producing cells in vivo and in vitro: IL-2 and IL-4 are required for in vitro generation of IL-4 producing cells. J Exp Med 1990;172:921–9.

49. Grewal IS, Flavell RA. The role of CD40 ligand in costimulation and T-cell activation. Innumol Rev 1996;153:85–106.

50. Ridge J P, Di Rosa F, Matzinger P. A conditioned dendritic cell can be a temporal bridge between a CD4+ T-helper and a T-killer cell. Nature 1998;393:474–8.

51. Russell S M, Liew F Y. Cell cooperation in antibody responses to influenza virus. I. priming of helper t cells by internal components of virion. Eur J Immunol 1980;10:791–6.

52. Fuchs E J, Matzinger P. B cells turn off virgin but not memory T cells. Science 1992;258: 1156–9.

53. Gilbert K M, Weigle W O. Tolerogenicity of resting and activated B cells. J Exp Med 1994; 179:249–58.

54. Minutello M A, Pileri P, Unutmaz D, et al. Compartmentalization of T-lymphocyte to the site of disease: Intrahepatic CD4$^+$ T-cells specific for the protein NS4 of hepatitis C virus in patient with chronic hepatitis. J Exp Med 1993;178:17–26.

55. Jacobson S, Richert J R, Biddison W E, Satinsk A, Hartzmann R J, McFarland H F. Measles virus specific T4+ human cytotoxic T cell clones are restricted by class II HLA antigens. J Immunol 1984;133:754–7.

56. Fleischer B, Kreth H W. Clonal expansion and functional analysis of virus-specific T lymphocytes from cerebrospinal fluid in measles encephalitis. Hum Immunol 1983;7:239–48.

57. Franco A, Guidotti L G, Hobbs M V, Pasquetto V, Chisari F V. Pathogenetic effector function of CD4-positive T helper 1 cells in hepatitis B virus transgenic mice. J Immunol 1997:2001–8.

58. Franco A, Paroli M, Testa U, et al. Transferrin receptor mediates uptake and presentation of hepatitis B envelope antigen by T lymphocytes. J Exp Med 1992;175:1195–205.

59. Wang C, Splitter G A. CD4(+) cytotoxic T-lymphocyte activity against macrophages pulsed with bovine herpesvirus 1 polypeptides. J Virol 1998;72:7040–7.

60. Valitutti S, Müller S, Dessing M, Lanzavecchia A. Different responses are elicited in cytotoxic T lymphoytes by different levels of T cell receptor occupancy. J Exp Med 1996;183:1917–21.

61. Germain R N. MHC-dependent antigen processing and peptide presentation: providing ligands for T lymphocyte activation. Cell 1994;76:287–99.

62. Sijts A J, Pamer E G. Enhanced intracellular dissociation of major histocompatibility complex class I-associated peptides: a mechanism for optimizing the spectrum of cell surface-presented cytotoxic T lymphocyte epitopes. J Exp Med 1997;185:1403–11.

63. Gilles P N, Fey G, Chisari F V. Tumor necrosis factor-alpha negatively regulates hepatitis B virus gene expression in transgenic mice. J Virol 1992;66:3955–60.

64. Guidotti L G, Guilhot S, Chisari F V. Interleukin 2 and interferon alph/beta downregulate hepatitis B virus gene expression in vivo by tumor necrosis factor dependent and independent pathways. J Virol 1994;68:1265–70.

65. Cocchi F, deVico A L, Garzino-Demo A, Arya S K, Gallo R C, Lusso P. Identification of Rantes, MIP-1alpha and MIP-1beta as the major HIV-suppressive factors produced by CD8+ T cells. Science 1995;270:1811–5.

66. Battegay M, Bachmann M F, Burhkart C, et al. Antiviral immune responses of mice lacking MHC class II or its associated invariant chain. Cell Immunol 1996;167:115–21.

67. Gallimore A, Hengartner H, Zinkernagel R. Hierarchies of antigen-specific cytotoxic T-cell responses. Immunol Rev 1998;164:29–36.

68. Alexander-Miller M A, Leggatt G R, Sarin A, Berzofsky J A. Role of antigen, CD8, and cytotoxic T lymphocyte (CTL) avidity in high dose antigen induction of apoptosis of effector CTL. J Exp Med 1996;184:485–92.

69. Thomsen A R, Marker O. The complementary roles of cellular and humoral immunity in resistance to re-infection with LCM virus. Immunology 1988;65:9–15.

70. Matloubian M, Concepcion R J, Ahmed R. CD4+ T cells are required to sustain CD8+ cytotoxic T-cell responses during chronic viral infection. J Virol 1994;68:8056–63.

71. Battegay M, Moskophidis D, Rahemtulla A, Hengartner H, Mak T W, Zinkernagel R M. Enhanced establishment of a virus carrier state in adult CD4+ T-cell- deficient mice. J Virol 1994;68:4700–4.

72. von Herrath M G, Oldstone M B. Virus-induced autoimmune disease. Curr Opin Immunol 1996;8:878–85.

73. von Herrath M G, Dyrberg T, Oldstone M B. Oral insulin treatment suppresses virus-induced antigen-specific destruction of beta cells and prevents autoimmune diabetes in transgenic mice. J Clin Invest 1996;98:1324–31.

74. von Herrath M G, Evans C F, Horwitz M S, Oldstone M B. Using transgenic mouse models to dissect the pathogenesis of virus- induced autoimmune disorders of the islets of Langerhans and the central nervous system. Immunol Rev 1996;152:111–43.

75. Stohlman S A, Bergmann C C, Lin M T, Cua D J, Hinton D R. CTL effector function within the central nervous system requires CD4+ T cells. J Immunol 1998;160:2896–904.

76. Planz O, Seiler P, Hengartner H, Zinkernagel R M. Specific cytotoxic T cells eliminate B cells producing virus-neutralizing antibodies. Nature 1996;382:726–9.

77. Battegay M, Moskophidis D, Waldner H, et al. Impairment and delay of neutralizing antiviral antibody responses by virus-specific cytotoxic T cells. J Immunol 1993;151:5408–15.

78. Salemi S, Caporossi A P, Boffa L, Longobardi M G, Barnaba V. HIVgp120 activates autoreactive CD4-specific T cell responses by unveiling of hidden CD4 peptides during processing [see comments]. J Exp Med 1995;181:2253–7.

79. Ware R, Jiang H, Braunstein N, et al. Human CD8+ T lymphocyte clones specific for T cell receptor V beta families expressed on autologous CD4+ T cells. Immunity 1995;2:177–84.

80. Giuberti T, Marin M G, Ferrari C, et al. Hepatitis C virus viremia following clinical resolution of acute hepatitis C. J Hepatol 1994;20:666–71.

81. Diepolder H M, Zachoval R, Hoffmann R M, et al. Possible mechanism involving T lymphocyte response to non-structural protein 3 in viral clearance in acute hepatitis C virus infection. Lancet 1995;346:1006–7.

82. Diepolder H M, Gerlach J-T, Zachoval R, et al. Immunodominant CD4+ T-cell epitope within nonstructural protein 3 in acute hepatitis C virus infection. J Virol 1997;71:6011–9.

83. Tsai S-L, Liaw Y-L, Chen M-H, Huang C-Y, Kuo G C. Detection of type 2-like T-helper cells in hepatitis C virus infection: implications for hepatitis C virus chronicity. Hepatology 1997;25:449–58.

84. Cacciarelli T V, Martinez O M, Gish R G, Villanueva J C, Krams S M. Immunoregulatory cytokines in chronic hepatitis C virus infection: pre- and posttreatment with interferon alpha. Hepatology 1996;24:6–9.

85. Diepolder H M, Zachoval R, Hoffmann R M, Jung M C, Gerlach T, Pape G R. The role of hepatitis C virus specific CD4+ T lymphocytes in acute and chronic hepatitis C. J Mol Med 1996;74:583–8.

86. Rehermann B, Ferrari C, Pasquinelli C, Chisari F V. The hepatitis B virus persists for decades after patients' recovery from acute viral hepatitis despite active maintenance of a cytotoxic T-lymphocyte response. Nat Med 1996;2:1104–8.

87. Katayama Y, Hotta H, Nishimura A, Tatsuno Y, Homma M. Detection of measles virus nucleoprotein mRNA in autopsied brain tissues. J Gen Virol 1995;76:3201–4.

88. Kundig T M, Bachmann M F, Oehen S, et al. On the role of antigen in maintaining cytotoxic T-cell memory. Proc Natl Acad Sci U S A 1996;93:9716–23.

89. Belyakov I M, Ahlers J D, Brandwein B Y, et al. The importance of local mucosal HIV-specific CD8(+) cytotoxic T lymphocytes for resistance to mucosal viral transmission in mice and enhancement of resistance by local administration of IL-12. J Clin Invest 1998;102:2072–81.

90. Selin L K, Varga S M, Wong I C, Welsh R M. Protective heterologous antiviral immunity and enhanced immunopathogenesis mediated by memory T cell populations. J Exp Med 1998;188:1705–15.

91. Chang K M, Gruener N H, Southwood S, et al. Identification of HLA-A3 and -B7-restricted CTL response to hepatitis C virus in patients with acute and chronic hepatitis C. J Immunol 1999;162:1156–64.

92. Cooper S, Erickson AL, Adams EJ, et al. Analysis of a successful immune response against hepatitis C virus. Immunity 1999;10:439–49.

93. He X S, Rehermann B, Lopez-Labrador F X, et al. Quantitative analysis of hepatitis C virus-specific CD8(+) T cells in peripheral blood and liver using peptide-MHC tetramers. Proc Natl Acad Sci U S A 1999;96:5692–7.

94. Koziel M J, Wong D K H, Dudley D, Houghton M, Walker B D. Hepatitis C Virus-specific cytolytic T lymphocyte and T helper cell responses in seronegative persons. J Infect Dis 1997;176:859–66.

95. Scognamiglio P, Accapezzato D, Casciani A, et al. Presence of effector CD8+ T cells in hepatitis C virus-exposed healthy seronegative donors. J Immunol 1999;162:6681–9.

96. Bronowicki J-P, Vetter D, Uhl G, et al. Lymphocyte reactivity to hepatitis C virus (HCV) antigens shows evidence for exposure in HCV-seronegative spouses of HCV-infected patients. J Infect Dis 1997;176:518–22.

97. Clerici M, Giorgi J V, Chou C C, et al. Cell-mediated immune response to human immunodeficiency virus (HIV) type 1 in seronegative homosexual men with recent sexual exposure to HIV-1. J Infect Dis 1992;165:1012–9.

98. Schupper H, Hayashi P, Scheffel J, et al. Peripheral blood mononuclear cell responses to recombinant hepatitis C virus antigens in patients with chronic hepatitis C. Hepatology 1993;18:1055–60.

99. Lechmann M, Ihlenfeldt H G, Braunschweiger I, et al. T and B cell responses to different hepatitis C virus antigens in patients with chronic hepatitis C infection and in healthy anti-HCV blood donors withouth viremia. Hepatology 1996;24:790–5.

100. Battegay M, Fikes J, Di Bisceglie A M, et al. Patients with chronic hepatitis C have circulating cytotoxic T cells which recognize hepatitis C virus-encoded peptides binding to HLA-A2.1 molecules. J Virol 1995;69:2462–70.

101. Cerny A, McHutchison J G, Pasquinelli C, et al. Cytotoxic T lymphocyte response to hepatitis C virus-derived peptides containing the HLA A2.1 binding motif. J Clin Invest 1995;95: 521–30.

102. Koziel M J, Walker B D. Characteristics of the intrahepatic cytotoxic T lymphocyte response in chronic hepatitis C virus infection. Springer Semin Immunopathol 1997;19:69–83.

103. Koziel M J, Dudley D, Afdhal N, et al. Hepatitis C virus (HCV)-specific cytotoxic T lymphocytes recognize epitopes in the core and envelope proteins of HCV. J Virol 1993;67:7522–32.

104. Koziel M J, Dudley D, Wong J T, et al. Intrahepatic cytotoxic T lymphocytes specific for hepatitis C virus in persons with chronic hepatitis. J Immunol 1992;149:3339–44.

105. Erickson A L, Houghton M, Choo Q-L, et al. Hepatitis C virus-specific CTL responses in the liver of chimpanzees with acute and chronic hepatitis C. J Immunol 1993;151:4189–99.

106. Wentworth P A, Sette A, Celis E, et al. Identification of A2-restricted HCV-specific CTL epitopes from highly conserved regions of the viral genome. Int Immunol 1996;8:651–9.

107. Shirai M, Arichi T, Nishioka M, et al. CTL responses of HLA-A2.1-transgenic mice specific for hepatitis C viral peptides predict epitopes for CTL of humans carrying HLA-A2.1. J Immunol 1995;154:2733–42.

108. Ada G L, Jones P D. The immune response to influenza infection. Curr Top Microbiol Immunol 1986;128:1–54.

109. Doherty P C, Allan W, Eichelberger M, Carding S R. Roles of alpha beta and gamma delta T cell subsets in viral immunity. Annu Rev Immunol 1992;10:123–51.

110. McMichael A. Cytotoxic T lymphocytes specific for influenza virus. Curr Top Microbiol Immunol 1994;189:75–91.

111. Dorrell L, Dong T, Ogg G S, et al. Distinct recognition of non-clade B human immunodeficiency virus type 1 epitopes by cytotoxic T lymphocytes generated from donors infected in Africa. J Virol 1999;73:1708–14.

112. Rowland-Jones S L, Dong T, Fowke K R, et al. Cytotoxic T cell responses to multiple conserved HIV epitopes in HIV- resistant prostitutes in Nairobi. J Clin Invest 1998;102:1758–65.

113. Bruna-Romero O, Lasarte J J, Wilkinson G, et al. Induction of cytotoxic T-cell response against hepatitis C virus structural antigens using a defective recombinant adenovirus. Hepatology 1997;25:470–7.

114. Del Guercio M F, Sidney J, Hermanson G, et al. Binding of a peptide antigen to multiple HLA alleles allows definition of an A2-like supertype. J Immunol 1995;154:685–93.

115. Sidney J, Del Guercio M F, Southwood S, et al. Several HLA alleles share overlapping peptide specificities. J Immunol 1995;154:247–59.

116. Sidney J, Grey H M, Kubo R T, Sette A. Practical, biochemical and evolutionary implications of the discovery of HLA class I supermotifs. Immunol Today 1996;17:261–6.

117. Sidney J, Grey H M, Southwood S, et al. Definition of an HLA-A3-like supermotif demonstrates the overlapping peptide-binding repertoires of common HLA molecules. Hum Immunol 1996;45:79–93.

118. Rehermann B, Chang K M, McHutchison J G, Kokka R, Houghton M, Chisari F V. Quantitative analysis of the peripheral blood cytotoxic T lymphocyte response, disease activity and viral load in patients with chronic hepatitis C virus infection. J Clin Invest 1996;98:1432–40.

119. Byrne J A, Oldstone MBA. Biolgoy of cloned cytotoxic T lymphocytes specific for lymphocytic choriomeningitis virus: clearance of virus in vivo. J Virol 1984;51:682–6.

120. Hiroishi K, Kita H, Kojima M, et al. Cytotoxic T lymphocyte response and viral load in hepatitis C virus infection. Hepatology 1997;25:705–12.

121. Wong D K, Dudley D D, Afdhal N H, et al. Liver-derived CTL in hepatitis C virus infection: breadth and specificity of responses in a cohort of persons with chronic infection. J Immunol 1998;160:1479–88.

122. Nelson D R, Marousis C G, Davis G, et al. The role of hepatitis C virus-specific cytotoxic T lymphocytes in chronic hepatitis C. J Immunol 1997;158:1473–81.

123. Kashii Y, Shimizu Y, Nambu S, et al. Analysis of T-cell receptor V beta repertoire in liver-infiltrating lymphocytes in chronic hepatitis C. J Hepatol 1997;26:462–70.

124. Rehermann B, Chang K M, McHutchison J, et al. Differential cytotoxic T lymphocyte responsiveness to the hepatitis B and C viruses in chronically infected patients. J Virol 1996;70: 7092–102.

125. Lanford R E, Chavez D, Chisari F V, Sureau C. Lack of detection of negative-strand hepatitis C virus RNA in peripheral blood mononuclear cells and other extrahepatic tissues by the highly strand-specific rTth reverse transcriptase PCR. J Virol 1995;69:8079–83.

126. Terrault N A, Dailey P J, Ferrell L, et al. Hepatitis C virus: quantitation and distribution in liver. J Med Virol 1997;51:217–24.

127. Sugano M, Hayashi Y, Yoon S, et al. Quantitation of hepatitis C viral RNA in liver and serum samples using competitive polymerase chain reaction. J Clin Pathol 1995;48:820–5.

128. Lau G K, Davis G L, Wu S P, Gish R G, Balart L A, Lau J Y. Hepatic expression of hepatitis C virus RNA in chronic hepatitis C: a study by in situ reverse-transcription polymerase chain reaction. Hepatology 1996;23:1318–23.

129. Agnello V, Abel G, Knight G B, Muchmore E. Detection of widespread hepatocyte infection in chronic hepatitis C. Hepatology 1998;28:573–84.

130. Nouri-Aria K T, Sallie R, Mizokami M, Portmann B C, Williams R. Intrahepatic expression of hepatitis C virus antigens in chronic liver disease. J Pathol 1995;175:77–83.

131. Ballardini G, Groff P, Pontisso P, et al. Hepatitis C virus (HCV) genotype, tissue HCV antigens, hepatocellular expression of HLA-A, B, C, and intercellular adhesion-1 molecules. J Clin Invest 1995;95:2967–75.

132. Bach N, Thung S N, Schaffner F. The histological features of chronic hepatitis C and auto-immune chronic hepatitis: a comparative analysis. Hepatology 1992;15:572–7.

133. Scheuer P J, Ashrafzadeh P, Sherlock S, Brown D, Dusheiko GM. The pathology of hepatitis C. Hepatology 1992;15:567–71.

134. Lefkowitch J H, Schiff E R, Davis G L, et al. Pathological diagnosis of chronic hepatitis C: a multicenter comparative study with chronic hepatitis B. The Hepatitis Interventional Therapy Group. Gastroenterology 1993;104:595–603.

135. Onji M, Kikuchi T, Kumon I, et al. Intrahepatic lymphocyte subpopulations and HLA class I antigen expression by hepatocytes in chronic hepatitis C. Hepatogastroenterology 1992;39:340–3.

136. Gonzalez-Peralta R P, Fang J W S, Davis G L, et al. Immunopathobiology of chronic hepatitis C virus infection. Hepatology 1994;20:232A.

137. Weiner A J, Geysen H M, Christopherson C, et al. Evidence for immune selection of hepatitis C virus (HCV) putative envelope glycoprotein variants: potential role in chronic HCV infection. Proc Natl Acad Sci U S A 1992;89:3468–72.

138. Yuk K, Shimizu M, Aoyama S, et al. Analysis of lymphocyte subsets in liver biopsy specimens with lymphoid follicle like structures. Acta Hepatol Jpn 1986;27:720–5.

139. Hiramatsu N, Hayashi N, Katayama K, et al. Immunohistochemical detection of Fas antigen in liver tissue of patients with chronic hepatiits C. Hepatology 1994;19:1354–9.

140. Mosnier J F, Scoaze J Y, Marcellin P, Degott C, Benahmou J P, Feldmann G. Expression of cytokine-dependent immune adhesion molecules by hepatocytes. Gastroenterology 1994;107:1457–68.

141. Marrogi A J, Cheles M K, Gerber M A. Chronic hepatitis C. Analysis of host immune response by immunohistochemistry. Arch Pathol Lab Med 1995;119:232–7.

142. Fukumoto T, Berg T, Ku Y, et al. Viral dynamics of hepatitis C early after orthotopic liver transplantation: evidence for rapid turnover of serum virions. Hepatology 1996;24:1351–4.

143. Guidotti L G, Chisari F V. To kill or to cure: options in host defense against viral infection. Curr Opin Immunol 1996;8:478–83.

144. Lohr H F, Schlaak J F, Kollmannsperger S, Dienes H P, Meyer zum Buschenfelde K H, Gerken G. Liver-infiltrating and circulating CD4+ T cells in chronic hepatitis C: immunodominant epitopes, HLA-restriction and functional significance. Liver 1996;16:174–82.

145. Bertoletti A, D'Elios M M, Boni C, et al. Different cytokine profiles of intrahepatic T cells in chronic hepatitis B and hepatitis C virus infections. Gastroenterology 1997;112:193–9.

146. Mita E, Hayashi N, Iio S, et al. Role of Fas ligand in apoptosis induced by hepatitis C virus infection. Biochem Biophys Res Commun 1994;204:468–74.

147. Lohman B L, Razvi E S, Welsh R M. T-lymphocyte downregulation after acute viral infection is not dependent on CD95 (Fas) receptor-ligand interactions. J Virol 1996;70:8199–203.

148. Vassalli P. The pathophysiology of tumor necrosis factors. Annu Rev Immunol 1992;10:411–52.

149. Koziel M J, Dudley D, Afdhal N, et al. HLA class I-restricted cytotoxic T lymphocytes specific for hepatitis C virus. Identification of multiple epitopes and characterization of patterns of cytokine release. J Clin Invest 1995;96:2311–21.

150. Kinkhabwala M, Sehajpal P, Skolnik E, et al. A novel addition to the T cell repertory: cell surface expression of tumor necrosis factor/cachectin by activated normal human T cells. J Exp Med 1990;171:941–6.

151. Ando K, Hiroishi K, Kaneko T, et al. Perforin, fas/fas ligand, and TNF-alpha pathways as specific and bystander killing mechanisms of hepatitis C virus-specific human CTL. J Immunol 1997;158:5283–91.

152. Cuturi M C, Murphy M, Costa-Giomi M P, Weinmann R, Perussia B, Trinchieri G. Independent regulation of tumor necrosis factor and lymphotoxin production by human peripheral blood lymphocytes. J Exp Med 1987;165:1581–94.

153. Nuti S, Rosa D, Valiante N M, et al. Dynamics of intra-hepatic lymphocytes in chronic hepatitis C: enrichment for Valpha24+ T cells and rapid elimination of effector cells by apoptosis. Eur J Immunol 1998;28:3448–55.

154. Zhang X, Brunner T, Carter L, et al. Unequal death in T helper cell (Th)1 and Th2 effectors: Th1, but not Th2, effectors undergo rapid Fas/FasL-mediated apoptosis. J Exp Med 1997; 185:1837–49.

155. Neumann A U, Lam N P, Dahari H, et al. Hepatitis C viral dynamics in vivo and the antiviral efficacy of interferon-alpha therapy. Science 1998;282:103–7.

156. Odeberg J, Yun Z, Sönnerborg A, Bjoro K, Uhlen M, Lundeberg J. Variation of hepatitis C virus hypervariable region 1 in immunocompromised patients. J Infect Dis 1997;175:938–43.

157. Major M E, Mihalik K, Fernandez J, et al. Long-term follow-up of chimpanzees inoculated with the first infectious clone for hepatitis C virus. J Virol 1999;73:3317–25.

158. Bassett S E, Thomas D L, Brasky K M, Lanford R E. Viral persistence, antibody to E1 and E2, and hypervariable region 1 sequence stability in hepatitis C virus-inoculated chimpanzees. J Virol 1999;73:1118–26.

159. Bertoletti A, Sette A, Chisari F V, et al. Natural variants of cytotoxic epitopes are T-cell receptor antagonists for antiviral cytotoxic T cells. Nature 1994;369:407–10.

160. Klenerman P, Rowland-Jones S, McAdams S, et al. Cytotoxic T-cell activity antagonized by naturally occurring HIV-1 Gag variants. Nature 1994;369:403–7.

161. Niewiesk S, Daenke S, Parker C E, et al. Naturally occurring variants of human T-cell leukemia virus type I Tax protein impair its recognition by cytotoxic T lymphocytes and the transactivation function of Tax. J Virol 1995;69:2649–53.

162. Borrow P, Wei X, Horwitz M S, et al. Antiviral pressure exerted by HIV-1-specific cytotoxic T lymphocytes (CTLs) during primary infection demonstrated by rapid selection of CTL escape virus. Nat Med 1997;3:212–7.

163. Goulder P J, Phillips R E, Colbert R A, et al. Late escape from an immunodominant cytotoxic T-lymphocyte response associated with progression to AIDS. Nat Med 1997;3:212–7.

164. Weiner A, Erickson A L, Kansopon J, et al. Persistent hepatitis C virus infection in a chimpanzee is associated with emergence of a cytotoxic T lymphocyte escape variant. Proc Natl Acad Sci U S A 1995;92:2755–9.

165. Chang K M, Rehermann B, McHutchison J G, et al. Immunological significance of cytotoxic T lymphocyte epitope variants in patients chronically infected by the hepatitis C virus. J Clin Invest 1997;100:2376–85.

166. Kaneko T, Moriyama T, Udaka K, et al. Impaired induction of cytotoxic T lymphocytes by antagonism of a weak agonist borne by a variant hepatitis C virus epitope. Eur J Immunol 1997;27:1782–7.

167. Lanzavecchia A. Understanding the mechanisms of sustained signaling and T cell activation. J Exp Med 1997;185:1717–9.

168. Machold R P, Wiertz E J H J, Jones T R, Ploegh H L. The HCMV gene products US11 and US2 differ in their ability to attack allelec forms of murine major histocompatibility complex (MHC) class I heavy chains. J Exp Med 1997;185:363–6.

169. Large M K, Kittlesen D J, Hahn Y S. Suppression of host immune response by the core protein of hepatitis C virus: possible implications for hepatitis C virus persistence. J Immunol 1999;162:931–8.

9

EPIDEMIOLOGY OF HEPATITIS C

MIRIAM J. ALTER, YVAN J. F. HUTIN, * **AND**
GREGORY L. ARMSTRONG

Hepatitis Branch, National Center for Infectious Diseases
Centers for Disease Control and Prevention
Atlanta, Georgia
*Safe Injection Global Network, World Health Organization, Geneva, Switzerland

INTRODUCTION

The hepatitis C virus (HCV) is a blood-borne pathogen that appears to be endemic in most areas of the world. Differences in virus- and host-specific factors are likely responsible for the individual differences observed in the natural history of HCV-related chronic disease and in responses to antiviral therapy. Differences in the frequency and extent to which various risk factors contribute to the transmission of HCV are responsible for temporal and geographic differences that have been observed in the epidemiology of hepatitis C.

INCIDENCE OF HEPATITIS C VIRUS INFECTION

Determining the incidence of most infectious diseases relies on surveillance for clinical disease. This has been particularly problematic for hepatitis C because (1) the diagnosis of this disease prior to 1990 was based on exclusion of other etiologies (i.e., non-A, non-B hepatitis); (2) diagnostic tests available since 1990 do not distinguish among acute, chronic, or resolved infection; and (3) most persons with acute or chronic HCV infection are asymptomatic. Thus, estimates of the incidence of hepatitis C based on reported cases of acute disease have been unreliable, even in countries with well-established surveillance systems. However, estimates of the past incidence of HCV infection can be derived using the age-specific prevalence of HCV infection, as current prevalence reflects the cumulative risk for acquiring infection.

Temporal and Geographic Differences

There appear to be three distinct global patterns of age-specific HCV infection prevalence that indicate geographic differences in the time periods during which there was an increased risk for acquiring HCV infection (Fig. 1). In the United States, for example, the prevalence of HCV infection is highest among persons 30–49 years old, who account for 65% of all infections, and is lowest among persons less than 20 and greater than 60 years old. (1) This pattern indicates that

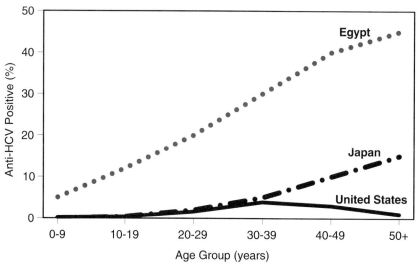

FIGURE 1   Global patterns of age-specific prevalence of hepatitis C virus infection.

most HCV transmission occurred in the recent past (i.e., 10–30 years ago), primarily among young adults, a pattern similar to that observed in Australia. (2,3) The past incidence of HCV infection in the United States has been estimated by creating catalytic models using current age-specific seroprevalence data and prior age-specific incidence data from sentinel surveillance for acute disease (CDC: unpublished data). These models showed a large increase in the incidence of newly acquired HCV infections from the late 1960s to the early 1980s. The estimated annual incidence was low (18 per 100,000) before 1965, increased steadily through 1980, and remained high (130 per 100,000) through 1989, corresponding to an average of 240,000 infections per year in the 1980s. Since 1989, the incidence of HCV infection has declined by more than 80% based on trends in reported cases of disease. (4)

Although data are not available to apply catalytic modeling techniques to estimate past incidence rates in other countries, temporal trends in incidence can be derived from their seroprevalence patterns. In Japan, the age-specific prevalence of HCV infection is low in children and younger adults and increases sharply among older persons, who account for the majority of infections (Fig. 1). (5,6) This pattern is similar to that observed in Italy, (7,8) and indicates that the risk for HCV infection was greatest in the distant past (i.e., 30–50 years ago).

The third pattern that emerges is observed in Egypt, where the prevalence of HCV infection increases steadily with age and high rates of infection are observed among persons in all age groups (Fig. 1). (9,10) This pattern indicates an increased risk in the distant past followed by an ongoing high risk for acquiring HCV infection.

Relationship to Chronic Disease Burden

Because chronic liver disease may develop many years after onset of infection, the past incidence is a major determinant of the future burden of HCV-associated complications. In the United States and other countries where the emergence of HCV infection is a more recent event, the magnitude of the burden of HCV-related chronic liver disease has yet to be realized as the duration of infection among the majority of infected persons has not reached the point at which complications from chronic liver disease typically occur. In countries where the emergence of HCV infection occurred in the distant past (such as Japan and Italy), the burden of HCV-related chronic disease already might have reached its highest magnitude, but changes in disease transmission patterns that result in younger persons acquiring infection could result in future increases in chronic disease as this cohort ages. In Egypt, where there has been an ongoing high risk for decades, the magnitude of both the current and the future burden of HCV-related chronic disease is of great concern.

DISEASE TRANSMISSION PATTERNS

The two risk factors cited most frequently as being responsible for the transmission of HCV infection are blood transfusion from unscreened donors and injecting drug use. However, the potential roles of other medical and dental procedures, cultural practices, and high-risk behaviors have not been appreciated. Furthermore, the three distinct global patterns of HCV infection indicate temporal and geographical differences in the extent to which some of these risk factors contributed to HCV transmission (Table I).

Injecting Drug Use

In the United States and Australia where the emergence of HCV infection is a more recent event that primarily affected young adults, injecting drug use has

TABLE I Global Differences in Hepatitis C Virus Transmission Patterns

Characteristic	Prevalence of HCV infection		
	Low	Moderate	High
Representative countries	United States Australia	Japan Italy	Egypt
Time period of increased incidence	Recent past (10–30 years ago)	Distant past (30–50 years ago)	Distant past/ ongoing
Age with highest prevalence	Younger adults	Older adults	All
Relative importance of exposures among prevalent infections			
Injecting drug use	++++	++	+
Transfusions	+++	+++	+++
Medical (dental) procedures	+/−	++++	++++
Unsafe injections	+/−	++++	++++
Folk medicine	−	++	No data
Occupational	+	+	+
Perinatal	+	+	+
High-risk sex	++	+	+

been the predominant mode of transmission since the 1970s, accounting for an estimated 60% of all prevalent infections in the United States and 80% in Australia. (1–3,11,12) HCV infection is acquired more rapidly after initiation of injecting drug use than other viral infections, and rates of HCV infection among young injecting drug users are four times higher than rates of human immuno-deficiency virus (HIV) infection. (13) After 5 years of injecting, 50 to 90% of users are infected with HCV. (14–16) More rapid acquisition of HCV infection compared with other viral infections among injecting drug users is likely caused by their high prevalence of chronic HCV infection, which results in a greater likelihood of exposure to an HCV-infected person.

In countries where the increased incidence of HCV infection occurred in the distant past (e.g., Japan, Italy, Egypt), injecting drug use appears to have played a minor role, although its contribution to more recent transmission in these countries may be increasing. In both Japan and Italy, the highest incidence of HCV infection is now among young adults. (17,18) In Italy, a history of inject-ing drug use has been reported by half of persons with newly acquired hepa-titis C and by 40% of persons with chronic HCV infection younger than aged 40 years. (18,19) In contrast, none of those with chronic HCV infection older than aged 40 years reported injecting drug use. (19) In one study from Egypt, a history of injecting drug use was reported by two-thirds of HCV-positive paid professional blood donors. (20)

Intranasal Cocaine Use

The role of intranasal cocaine use in transmission of HCV infection is unclear. A cross-sectional study of volunteer blood donors in the United States reported that a history of intranasal cocaine use was independently associated with HCV seropositivity. (21) Although intranasal cocaine use is a biologically plausible mode of transmission for blood-borne pathogens (i.e., mucosal exposure to in-fectious blood through sharing contaminated straws or other devices), cross-sectional studies have serious limitations for making causal inferences, particu-larly when the studies do not use random (probability) sampling. (22) The results of such studies are most useful for generating hypotheses and should be confirmed before drawing conclusions. Additional data indicate that a relatively high proportion ($\geq 10\%$) of HCV-negative volunteer blood donors report a his-tory of intranasal cocaine use, (21,23) but such a history is uncommon ($<5\%$) among patients with recently acquired hepatitis C, especially in the absence of injecting drug use. (4) Although intranasal cocaine use could be associated with HCV transmission, it may only account for a small number of infections while being practiced by a relatively high proportion of the population. Until more data are available, including data to determine if persons with a history of intra-nasal cocaine use alone are likely to be infected with HCV, it is premature to conclude that intranasal cocaine use places persons at risk for hepatitis C.

Blood and Blood Products

In developed countries, blood and organ donor screening and testing prac-tices and viral inactivation of plasma-derived products have eliminated most transfusion- and transplant-related transmission of HCV and other blood-borne pathogens. In the United States and Australia, such exposures accounted for up to 20% of infections acquired prior to 1985 and currently account for an estimated 10% of infections among persons with chronic HCV infection (i.e., prevalent infections). (2,4,11) In the latter half of the 1990s, the risk for transfusion-transmitted HCV infection has been so low that surveillance systems in these countries are unable to detect any newly acquired transfusion-associated hepatitis C.

Health-Care Related Procedures and Unsafe Injections

Transmission of HCV from other health care-related procedures has been reported rarely in most developed countries, other than in chronic hemodialysis settings. (24) In such countries, the appropriate use of disposable equipment and effective disinfection and sterilization procedures have successfully limited nosocomial transmission of HCV and other blood-borne pathogens. The few episodes of HCV transmission from patient to patient in hospitals and out-patient health care settings that have been reported were mostly associated with improper infection control practices, including unsafe phlebotomy practices, contamination of multidose vials, and inadequate cleaning and disinfection of endoscopic equipment. (25–28)

The risk for HCV transmission from an infected health care worker to patients during the performance of exposure prone invasive procedures appears to be very low. Such transmission was shown in one published report from Spain, in which a cardiothoracic surgeon transmitted HCV to five patients. (29) Although factors such as virus titer may be related to the transmission of HCV in this setting, no methods exist currently that can reliably determine infectivity, nor do data exist to determine the threshold concentration of virus required for transmission.

In countries where the increased risk for HCV infection occurred in the distant past, health care-related procedures and unsafe injections performed by both professionals and nonprofessionals appear to have been the predominant modes of HCV transmission (Table I). In Japan and Italy, studies have found geographic clustering of high HCV infection rates among older persons that appears to be associated not only with transfusions from unscreened donors, but also with unsafe injection practices (including reuse of contaminated glass syringes and administration at home by nonprofessionals in which syringes were shared with other family members, neighbors, and friends), surgical procedures, and folk medicine practices (e.g., in Japan, acupuncture performed by unlicenced therapists and traditional remedies performed by family members using nonsterile instruments). (7,19,30–32) The low HCV prevalence among children and younger adults in these countries indicates that such exposures no longer play a major role in transmission.

In Egypt, however, the increased risk for HCV infection that occurred in the past appears to be ongoing, as high prevalence rates of infection are observed among all age groups. Studies have indicated that mass campaigns to treat schistosomiasis with injection therapy during 1960 to 1987 might have been responsible for the sustained transmission of HCV during this time. (9,10,33,34) Such therapy involved a minimum of one course of 12 injections, and many were administered with reused glass syringes. (10) Although these campaigns ended in 1987, use of common syringes and a history of medical procedures involving injections or hospitalization continue to be associated with HCV infection, indicating that unsafe injection practices might be playing an ongoing role in the transmission of HCV. (10,33)

The important role of unsafe injections in the transmission of HCV and other blood-borne pathogens is being increasingly recognized. In addition to the studies mentioned earlier, therapeutic injections have been associated with the transmission of blood-borne pathogens in Romania, Moldova, and Pakistan. (35–37) Injection-associated blood-borne pathogen transmission occurs when infection control practices are inadequate, and overuse of injections to administer medications may increase opportunities for transmission. (38) In many developing countries, supplies of sterile syringes may be inadequate or nonexistent, injections are often administered outside the medical setting by nonprofessionals, and they are often given to deliver medications that could otherwise be delivered by the oral route. Reasons reported for preference for therapeutic injections include beliefs that the pain of the injection is a marker of efficacy, that medications are more effective when given by injection, and that injections represent advanced technology. (39) In addition to unsafe injection practices, lack of attention to appropriate cleaning and disinfection of equipment used in hospital and dental settings may be a major source of HCV transmission in developing countries.

Rituals and Cosmetic Services

The contribution of reused contaminated instruments and objects during rituals or cosmetic services that involve percutaneous exposures (e.g., tattooing, body piercing, commercial barbering, circumcision, scarification) to HCV transmission in developed or developing countries is unknown. The limited number of studies conducted to date either were done in highly selected groups and results cannot be extrapolated to the rest of the population or they used inappropriate control groups and valid conclusions cannot be drawn. (18,40–44) Although any percutaneous exposure has the potential for transferring infectious blood and potentially transmitting blood-borne pathogens, there are no studies demonstrating a causal link between these types of practices and HCV infection, (45,46) and there are no data showing that persons with a history of exposures such as tattooing, body piercing, or being attended by a commercial barber are at increased risk for HCV infection based on these exposures alone. Further studies are needed to determine if these types of exposures and settings in which they occur (e.g., correctional institutions, unregulated commercial establishments), are risk factors for HCV infection.

Occupational Exposures

The extent to which infections in health care workers have contributed to the overall burden of HCV infection is small, and there appears to be little variation either temporally or geographically. (1,11) Health care workers who have exposure to blood in the workplace are at risk for being infected with HCV and other blood-borne pathogens. However, the prevalence of HCV infection among health care workers, including orthopedic, general, and oral surgeons, is no greater than the general population, averaging 1–2%, and is 10 times lower than that for hepatitis B virus infection. (47–52) In a single study that evaluated risk factors for infection, a history of accidental needle stick injury was the only occupational risk factor associated independently with HCV infection. (52)

The average incidence of anti-HCV seroconversion after accidental needle sticks or sharps exposures from an HCV-positive source is 1.8% (range: 0–7%), (53–56) with one study reporting that transmission occurred only from hollow-bore needles compared with other sharps. (54) A study from Japan reported an incidence of HCV infection of 10% based on detection of HCV RNA by reverse-transcriptase polymerase chain reaction (RT-PCR). (55) Although no incidence studies have documented transmission associated with mucous membrane or nonintact skin exposures, transmission of HCV from blood splashes to the conjunctiva have been described. (57,58)

Perinatal Transmission

The contribution of perinatal infections to the overall HCV disease burden also appears to be low and varies little geographically or temporally. (11,59,60) The average rate of HCV infection among infants born to HCV-positive, HIV-negative women is 5–6% (range: 0–25%), based on detection of anti-HCV and HCV RNA, respectively. The average infection rate for infants born to women coinfected with HCV and HIV is higher; 14% (range: 5–36%) and 17%, based on detection of anti-HCV and HCV RNA, respectively. The only factor consistently found to be associated with transmission has been the presence of HCV RNA in the mother at the time of birth. Although two studies of infants born to HCV-positive, HIV-negative women reported an association with titer of HCV RNA, each study reported a different level of HCV RNA related to transmission. Studies of HCV/HIV-coinfected women have more consistently shown an association between virus titer and the transmission of HCV.

Data regarding the relationship between delivery mode and HCV transmission are limited and presently indicate no difference in infection rates between infants delivered vaginally compared with cesarean-delivered infants. The transmission of HCV infection through breast milk has not been documented. In studies that have evaluated breast feeding in infants born to HCV-infected women, the average rate of infection was 4% in both breast-fed and bottle-fed infants. (11,59) Mother-to-child transmission of HCV is discussed in further detail in Chapter 21.

Sexual Transmission

The role of sexual activity in the transmission of HCV remains controversial. Results from several types of studies indicate that sexual activity is related to HCV transmission. These included case-control studies of persons with acute hepatitis C, cross-sectional studies of highly selected groups of persons with different types of sexual behaviors [e.g., heterosexual patients attending sexually transmitted diseases (STD) clinics, men who have sex with men, and female prostitutes], and a cross-sectional study of a representative sample of the general population (in the United States). (1,11,45,46,56) These studies reported independent associations between HCV infection and exposure to an infected sex partner, increasing numbers of partners, failure to use a condom, and sexual activities involving trauma. In addition, a cross-sectional study of the partners of HCV-infected persons indicated that male-to-female transmission of HCV may be more efficient than female-to-male, (61) a pattern that is more suggestive of sexual transmission than of percutaneous transmission due to shared risk behaviors such as injecting drug use or shared contaminated personal articles such as razors.

In contrast, a low prevalence of HCV infection has been reported by studies of long-term spouses of patients with chronic HCV infection who had no other risk factors for infection. (11,56) Some of these studies demonstrated no infections among partners, but their sample sizes were small.

Only one study has found an association between HCV infection and male homosexual activity, (61) and at least in STD clinic settings, the prevalence rate of HCV infection among men who have sex with men generally has been similar to that of heterosexuals. (11,56) Because sexual transmission of blood-borne viruses is recognized to be more efficient among homosexual men compared with heterosexual men and women, it is unclear why HCV infection rates are not substantially higher among men who have sex with men compared with heterosexuals. This observation and the low prevalence of HCV infection observed among the long-term steady sex partners of persons with chronic HCV infection have raised doubts about the importance of sexual activity in the transmission of HCV. Unacknowledged percutaneous exposures (i.e., illegal injecting drug use) might contribute to the increased risk for HCV infection among persons with high-risk sexual practices. In some countries where clustering of HCV infections has been observed among sexual and other household contacts of HCV-infected persons, exposures commonly experienced in the past from contaminated equipment used in health care-related procedures or unsafe injections might have been the more likely source for their infections. (8,31,62,63)

Although considerable inconsistencies exist among studies, data indicate overall that sexual transmission of HCV can occur. The substantial contribution of sexual transmission to the disease burden in the United States relative to the inefficiency with which the virus appears to be spread in this manner can be explained by the fact that sexual activity with multiple partners is a common behavior in the population and that the large number of chronically infected persons provides multiple opportunities for exposure. (1,11) However, more data are needed to determine the risk for, and factors related to, transmission of HCV between long-term steady partners as well as among persons with high-risk sexual practices, including whether other STDs promote the transmission of HCV by influencing viral load or modifying mucosal barriers.

Persons with No Recognized Source for Their Infection

In the United States, injecting drug use currently accounts for 60% of HCV transmission and sexual activity for up to 20%. Other known exposures (occupational, hemodialysis, household, perinatal) together account for approximately 10% of infections. Thus, a potential risk factor can be identified for approximately 90% of persons with HCV infection. In the remaining 10%, no recognized source of infection can be identified. Most persons in this category are associated with a low socioeconomic level, a characteristic that consistently has been identified as independently associated with HCV infection, (1,45,46) and which might be a surrogate for high-risk behaviors.

PREVENTION AND CONTROL

Reducing the burden of HCV infection and HCV-related disease requires implementation of primary prevention activities that reduce the risks for contracting HCV infection and secondary prevention activities that reduce risks for liver and other chronic diseases in HCV-infected persons. (11,64) There is no vaccine against HCV. All countries should develop and implement programs for the primary prevention of new infections. Those countries with more developed economic, medical, and public health infrastructures should also develop programs to identify, counsel, and provide medical management for persons already infected. In many countries, the relative contribution of the various sources for HCV infection has not been defined with population-based epidemiologic studies. Wherever possible, such studies should be performed to enable countries to prioritize their preventive measures and to make the most appropriate use of available resources. (64)

Preventing New Infections

Primary prevention activities can reduce or eliminate the potential risk for HCV transmission from (a) blood, blood components, and plasma derivatives; (b) percutaneous exposures to blood in health care and other settings; and (c) such high-risk activities as injecting drug use and unprotected sex with multiple partners. In many developing countries, donor screening and testing policies for HCV and inactivation procedures for plasma-derived products have not been implemented, and transfusions and organ transplants continue to be major sources for HCV infection. In these countries, improving the safety of the blood supply should be the highest priority. (64) Programs should also be initiated to reduce the extent to which HCV is transmitted as a result of inadequate sterilization or disinfection of medical, surgical, and dental equipment, reuse of contaminated equipment, and unsafe injection practices. (38,64) Such programs should include training regarding appropriate infection control procedures and use of devices or products that prevent reuse or contamination of equipment and efforts to modify therapeutic injection practices (e.g., reducing the number of injections). Practitioners of folk medicine, rituals (e.g., circumcision and scarification), and cosmetic procedures (e.g., tattooing and body piercing) and the persons who use these services should be educated as to the risk of infection from blood-borne pathogens from nonsterile instruments or objects used in these procedures.

Primary prevention of illegal drug injecting will eliminate the greatest risk

factor for HCV infection in the United States and other countries where this behavior plays a major role in disease transmission. (11) Although consistent data
are lacking regarding the extent to which sexual activity contributes to HCV
transmission, persons having multiple sex partners are at risk for STDs (e.g.,
HIV and hepatitis B virus infections, syphilis, gonorrhea, and chlamydia).
Health care professionals in all patient care settings should routinely obtain a
history that inquires about use of illegal drugs (injecting and noninjecting) and
evidence of high-risk sexual practices (e.g., multiple sex partners or a history of
STDs). (11) Counseling and education to prevent initiation of drug injecting or
high-risk sexual practices are important, especially for adolescents. Persons
who inject drugs or who are at risk for STDs should be counseled on what they
can do to minimize their risk of becoming infected or of transmitting infectious agents to others, including a need for vaccination against hepatitis B and,
where appropriate, hepatitis A. (65–67) To reduce the risk for HCV infection
among injecting drug users, communities should consider increasing access to
sterile syringes and needles through services such as syringe and needle exchange
programs.

Identifying HCV-Infected Persons

Secondary prevention activities can reduce risks for chronic disease by identifying HCV-infected persons through diagnostic testing and by providing appropriate medical management and antiviral therapy. Identification of persons at
risk for HCV infection provides the opportunity for testing to determine their
infection status, medical evaluation to determine their disease status if infected,
and antiviral therapy, if appropriate. It also provides infected persons the opportunity to obtain information about how they can prevent further harm to
their liver and prevent transmitting the infection to others.

In countries with sufficient resources, testing should be offered routinely to
persons most likely to be infected with HCV and should be accompanied by
appropriate counseling and medical follow-up. (11,64) The determination of
which persons at risk to recommend for routine testing is based on various considerations, including a known epidemiologic relationship between a risk factor
and acquiring HCV infection, the prevalence of the risk behavior or characteristic in the population, the prevalence of infection among those with a risk behavior or characteristic, and the need for persons with a recognized exposure to be
evaluated for infection. (11)

Persons for Whom Routine HCV Testing Is Recommended

In the United States, it is recommended that testing be offered routinely to
persons who ever injected illegal drugs, including those who injected once or
a few times many years ago; persons who received plasma-derived products
known to transmit HCV infection that were not treated to inactivate viruses
(e.g., clotting factor concentrates produced before 1987); persons who were
notified that they received blood from a donor who later tested positive for HCV
infection and any person who received transfusions or solid organ transplants
before July 1992 when the more sensitive donor screening tests were widely
implemented; persons who have been on long-term hemodialysis; health care

workers after needle sticks, sharps, or mucosal exposures to HCV-positive blood; and children born to HCV-positive women. (11) Testing is not recommended routinely for health care workers or pregnant women unless an exposure or risk factor is identified. (11)

Postexposure Follow-Up

Immune globulin and antiviral agents are not recommended for postexposure prophylaxis of hepatitis C. (11) Available data indicate that immune globulin is not effective for postexposure prophylaxis of hepatitis C. (68) No assessments have been made of postexposure use of antiviral agents to prevent HCV infection. Mechanisms of the effect of interferon in treating patients with hepatitis C are poorly understood, and an established infection might need to be present for interferon to be an effective treatment. (69) Furthermore, at least in the United States, interferon (alone or combined with ribavirin) is approved only for treatment of chronic hepatitis C.

When a health care worker sustains a percutaneous or permucosal exposure to blood, the source should be tested for anti-HCV. If the source is positive, the exposed person should be tested for anti-HCV and alanine aminotransferase (ALT) at baseline and 4–6 months later. All anti-HCV results reported as positive by enzyme immunoassay should be confirmed by a supplemental assay. If earlier diagnosis of HCV infection is desired, testing for HCV RNA may be performed 4–6 weeks after the exposure.

Limited data indicate that antiviral therapy may be beneficial when started early during the course of HCV infection, (70) but no guidelines exist for the administration of therapy during the acute phase of infection. Furthermore, no data exist indicating that treatment begun during the acute phase of infection is more effective than treatment begun early during the course of chronic HCV infection. When HCV infection is identified early, the individual should be referred for medical management to a specialist knowledgeable in this area.

Because of their recognized exposure, children born to HCV-positive women also should be tested for HCV infection. (11) Testing of infants for anti-HCV should be performed no sooner than age 12–18 months, when passively transferred maternal anti-HCV declines below detectable levels. If earlier diagnosis of HCV infection is desired, RT-PCR for HCV RNA may be performed at or after the infant's first well child visit at age 1–2 months. Umbilical cord blood should not be used for the diagnosis of perinatal HCV infection because cord blood can be contaminated by maternal blood. If positive for either anti-HCV or HCV RNA, children should be evaluated for the presence or development of liver disease, and those children with persistently elevated ALT levels should be referred to a specialist for medical management.

Counseling HCV-Positive Persons

Persons who test positive should be provided with information regarding the need for reducing risks for transmitting HCV to others; preventing further harm to their liver; and medical evaluation for chronic liver disease and possible treatment. (11) To reduce the risk for transmission to others, HCV-positive persons should be advised to not donate blood, body organs, other tissue, or semen; not share toothbrushes, dental appliances, razors, or other personal care articles that might have blood on them; and cover cuts and sores on the skin to keep from spreading infectious blood or secretions.

HCV-positive persons with a long-term steady partner do not need to change their sexual practices, however, they should discuss with their partner the need for counseling and testing. If the partner chooses to be tested and tests negative, the couple should be informed of available data on risk for HCV transmission by sexual activity to assist them in making decisions about precautions, including the low, but not absent, risk for transmission. If the partner tests positive, appropriate counseling and evaluation for the presence or development of liver disease should be provided. HCV-positive persons do not need to avoid pregnancy or breast feeding, and determining the need for cesarean delivery versus vaginal delivery should not be made on the basis of HCV infection status. Persons should not be excluded from work, school, play, child care, or other settings on the basis of their HCV infection status. (11)

CONCLUSION

There is a large global reservoir of HCV-infected individuals who can serve as a source of transmission to others and who are at risk for HCV-related chronic diseases. To prevent new infections, public health programs should focus on ensuring a safe blood supply, implementing appropriate infection control practices, and preventing initiation of high-risk drug and sexual behaviors. In addition, we need to better define the risk for HCV transmission in selected settings, develop more effective therapies for treatment of persons with chronic hepatitis C, and design approaches for treating current or former injecting drug users.

REFERENCES

1. Alter M J, Kruszon-Moran D, Nainan O V, et al. Prevalence of hepatitis C virus infection in the United States. N Engl J Med 1999;341:556–62.
2. Lowe D, Cotton R. Hepatitis C: a review of Australia's response. Canberra: Publications Production Unit, Commonwealth Department of Health and Aged Care, Commonwealth of Australia, 1999.
3. Farrell G C, Weltman M, Dingley J, Lin R. Epidemiology of hepatitis C virus infection in Australia. Gastroenterol Jpn 1993;28(Suppl 5):32–6.
4. Alter M J. Epidemiology of hepatitis C. Hepatology 1997;26:62S–5S.
5. Tanaka E, Kiyosawa K, Sodeyama T, et al. Prevalence of antibody to hepatitis C virus in Japanese school children: comparison with adult blood donors. Am J Trop Med Hyg 1992;46:460–4.
6. Ishibasi M, Shinzawa H, Kuboki M, Tsuchida H, Takahashi T. Prevalence of inhabitants with anti-hepatitis C virus antibody in an area following an acute hepatitis C epidemic: age and area-related features. J Epidemiol 1996;6:1–7.
7. Guadagnino V, Stroffolini T, Rapicetta M, et al. Prevalence, risk factors, and genotype distribution of hepatitis C virus infection in the general population: a community-based survey in Southern Italy. Hepatology 1997;26:1006–11.
8. Stroffolini T, Menchinelli M, Taliani G, et al. High prevalence of hepatitis C virus infection in a small central Italian town: lack of evidence of parenteral exposure. Ital J Gastroenterol 1995;27:235–8.

9. Abdel-Wahah M F, Zakaria S, Kamel M, et al. High seroprevalence of hepatitis C infection among risk groups in Egypt. Am J Trop Med Hyg 1994;51:563–7.

10. Mohamed M K, Hussein M H, Massoud A A, et al. Study of the risk factors for viral hepatitis C infection among Egyptians applying for work abroad. J Egypt Public Health Assoc 1996; 71:113–42.

11. Centers for Disease Control and Prevention. Recommendations for prevention and control of hepatitis C virus (HCV) infection and HCV-related chronic disease. MMWR 1998;47 (No. RR-19):1–33.

12. Moaven L D, Crofts N, Locarnini S A. Hepatitis C virus infection in Victorian injecting drug users in 1971. Med J Aust 1993;158:574.

13. Garfein R S, Vlahov D, Galai N, et al. Viral infections in short-term injection drug users: the prevalence of the hepatitis C, hepatitis B, human immunodeficiency, and human T-lymphotropic viruses. Am J Public Health 1996;86:655–61.

14. Villano S A, Vlahov D, Nelson K E, Lyles C M, Cohn S, Thomas D L. Incidence and risk factors for hepatitis C among injection drug users in Baltimore, Maryland. J Clin Microbiol 1997;35:3274–7.

15. Garfein R S, Doherty M C, Monterroso E R, Thomas D L, Nelson K E, Vlahov D. Prevalence and incidence of hepatitis C virus infection among young adult injection drug users. J Acquired Immune Defic Syndr Hum Retrovirol 1998;18(Suppl 1):S11–9.

16. Crofts N, Hopper J L, Bowden D S, Breschkin A M, Milner R, Locarnini S A. Hepatitis C virus infection among a cohort of Victorian injecting drug users. Med J Aust 1993;159:237–41.

17. Tanaka H, Tsukuma H, Hori Y, et al. The risk of hepatitis C virus infection among blood donors in Osaka, Japan. J Epidemiol 1998;8:292–6.

18. Mele A, Sagliocca L, Manzillo G, et al. Risk factors for acute non-A, non-B hepatitis and their relationship to antibodies for hepatitis C virus: a case-control study. Am J Public Health 1994; 84:1640–3.

19. Chiaramonte M, Stroffolini T, Lorenzoni U, et al. Risk factors in community-acquired chronic hepatitis C virus infection: a case-control study in Italy. J Hepatol 1996;24:129–34.

20. Bassily S, Hyams K C, Fouad R A, Samaan M D, Hibbs R G. A high risk of hepatitis C infection among Egyptian blood donors: the role of parenteral drug abuse. Am J Trop Med Hyg 1995; 52:503–5.

21. Conry-Cantilena C, VanRaden M, Gibble J, et al. Routes of infection, viremia, and liver disease in blood donors found to have hepatitis C virus infection. N Engl J Med 1996;334:1691–6.

22. Lilienfeld A M, Lilienfeld D E. Foundations of epidemiology. New York: Oxford University Press, 1980.

23. Conry-Cantilena C, Melpolder J C, Alter H J. Intranasal drug use among volunteer whole-blood donors: results of Survey C. Transfusion 1998;38:512–13.

24. Moyer L A, Alter M J. Hepatitis C virus in the hemodialysis setting: a review with recommendations for control. Semin Dial 1994;7:124–7.

25. Guyer B, Bradley D W, Bryan J A, Maynard J E: Non-A, non-B hepatitis among participants in a plasmapheresis stimulation program. J Infect Dis 1979;139:634–40.

26. Schvarcz R, Johansson B, Nyström, Sönnerborg A. Nosocomial transmission of hepatitis C virus. Infection 1997;25:74–7.

27. Allander T, Gruber A, Naghavi M, et al. Frequent patient-to-patient transmission of hepatitis C virus in a haematology ward. Lancet 1995;345:603–7.

28. Bronowicki J P, Venard V, Botte C, et al. Patient to patient transmission of hepatitis C virus during colonoscopy. N Engl J Med 1997;337:237–40.

29. Esteban J I, Gomez J, Martell M, et al. Transmission of hepatitis C virus by a cardiac surgeon. N Engl J Med 1995;334:555–60.

30. Noguchi S, Sata M, Suzuki H, Mizokami M, Tanikawa K. Routes of transmission of hepatitis C virus in an epidemic rural area of Japan. Molecular epidemiologic study of hepatitis C virus infection. Scand J Infect Dis 1997;29:23–8.

31. Kiyosawa K, Tanaka E, Sodeyama T, et al. Transmission of hepatitis C in an isolated area in Japan: community-acquired infection. Gastroenterology 1994;196:1596–1602.

32. Ito S, Ito M, Cho M-J, Shimotohno K, Tajima K. Massive sero-epidemiological survey of hepatitis C virus: clustering of carriers on the Southwest coast of Tsushima, Japan. Jpn J Cancer Res 1991;82:1–3.

33. Darwish M A, Tahani R A, Perween R, Constantine N T, Rao M R, Edelman R. Risk factors associated with a high seroprevalence of hepatitis C virus infection in Egyptian blood donors. Am J Trop Med Hyg 1993;49:440–7.

34. Frank C, Mohamed M K, Lavancy D, Arthur R R, Khoby T E, Strickland G T. The role of anti-schistosomal mass injection treatment in the spread of hepatitis C virus infection in Egypt. Int Conf Emerg Infect Dis, Atlanta, GA, 1998.

35. Hutin Y J F, Harpaz R, Drobeniuc et al. Injections as a major source of hepatitis B virus infection in Moldova. Int J Epidemiol 1999;28:782–6.

36. Hersh B S, Popovici F, Jezek Z, et al. Risk factors for HIV infection among abandoned Romanian children. AIDS 1993;7:1617–24.

37. Luby S P, Qamruddin K, Shah A A, et al. The relationship between therapeutic injections and high prevalence of hepatitis C infection in Hafizabad, Pakistan. Epidemiol Infect 1997;119:349–56.

38. Centers for Disease Control and Prevention. Frequency of vaccine-related and therapeutic injections—Romania, 1998. MMWR 1999;48:271–4.

39. Reeler A V. Injections: a fatal attraction? Soc Sci Med 1990;31:1119–25.

40. Kaldor J M, Archer G T, Buring M L, et al. Risk factors for hepatitis C virus infection in blood donors: a case-control study. Med J Aust 1992;157:227–30.

41. Sun D X, Zhang F G, Geng Y Q, et al. Hepatitis C transmission by cosmetic tattooing in women. Lancet 1996;347:541.

42. Tumminelli F, Marcellin P, Rizzo S, et al. Shaving as a potential source of hepatitis C virus infection. Lancet 1995;345:658.

43. Mele A, Corona R, Tosti M E, et al. Beauty treatments and risk of parenterally transmitted hepatitis: results from the hepatitis surveillance system in Italy. Scand J Infect Dis 1995;27:441–4.

44. Balasekaran R, Bulterys M, Jamal M, et al. A case-control study of risk factors for sporadic hepatitis C virus infection in the southwestern United States. Am J Gastroenterol 1999;94:1341–6.

45. Alter M J, Gerety R J, Smallwood L, et al. Sporadic non-A, non-B hepatitis: frequency and epidemiology in an urban United States population. J Infect Dis 1982;145:886–93.

46. Alter M J, Coleman P J, Alexander W J, et al. Importance of heterosexual activity in the transmission of hepatitis B and non-A, non-B hepatitis. JAMA 1989;262:1201–5.

47. Thomas D L, Factor S H, Kelen G D, et al. Viral hepatitis in health care personnel at The Johns Hopkins Hospital. Arch Intern Med 1993;153:1705–12.

48. Cooper B W, Krusell A, Tilton R C, et al. Seroprevalence of antibodies to hepatitis C virus in high-risk hospital personnel. Infect Control Hosp Epidemiol 1992;13:82–5.

49. Panlilio A L, Shapiro C N, Schable C A, et al. Serosurvey of human immunodeficiency virus, hepatitis B virus, and hepatitis C virus infection among hospital-based surgeons. J Am Coll Surg 1995;180:16–24.

50. Shapiro C N, Tokars J I, Chamberland M E, American Academy of Orthopedic Surgeons Serosurvey Study Committee. Use of hepatitis B vaccine and infection with hepatitis B and C among orthopaedic surgeons. J Bone J Surg 1996;78-A:1791–800.

51. Thomas D L, Gruninger S E, Siew C, Joy E D, Quinn T C. Occupational risk of hepatitis C infections among general dentists and oral surgeons in North America. Am J Med 1996;100:41–5.

52. Polish L B, Tong M J, Co R L, et al. Risk factors for hepatitis C virus infection among health care personnel in a community hospital. Am J Infect Control 1993;21:196–200.

53. Lanphear B P, Linnemann C C, Cannon C G, et al. Hepatitis C virus infection in health care workers: risk of exposure and infection. Infect Control Hosp Epidemiol 1994;15:745–50.

54. Puro V, Petrosillo N, Ippolito G, Italian Study Group on Occupational Risk of HIV and Other Bloodborne Infections. Risk of hepatitis C seroconversion after occupational exposures in health care workers. Am J Infect Control 1995;23:273–7.

55. Mitsui T, Iwano K, Masuko K, et al. Hepatitis C virus infection in medical personnel after needlestick accident. Hepatology 1992;16:1109–14.

56. Alter M J. The epidemiology of acute and chronic hepatitis C. Clin Liver Dis 1997;1:559–68.

57. Sartori M, La Terra G, Aglietta M, et al. Transmission of hepatitis C via blood splash into conjunctiva. Scand J Infect Dis 1993;25:270–1.

58. Ippolito G, Puro V, Petrosillo N, De Carli G, Micheloni G, Magliano E, Coordinating Centre of the Italian Study on Occupational Risk of HIV Infection. Simultaneous infection with HIV and hepatitis C virus following occupational conjunctival blood exposure. JAMA 1998;280:28.

59. Mast E E, Alter M J. Hepatitis C. Semin Pediatr Infect Dis 1997;8:17–22.
60. Thomas D A, Villano S A, Riester K A, et al. Perinatal transmission of hepatitis C virus from human immunodeficiency virus type 1-infected mothers. Women and Infants Transmission Study. J Infect Dis 1998;177:1480–88.
61. Thomas D L, Zenilman J M, Alter H J, et al. Sexual transmission of hepatitis C virus among patients attending Baltimore sexually transmitted diseases clinics—an analysis of 309 sex partnerships. J Infect Dis 1995;171:768–75.
62. Sagnelli E, Gaeta G B, Felaco F M, et al. Hepatitis C virus infection in households of anti-HCV chronic carriers in Italy: a multicentre case-control study. Infection 1997;25:346–9.
63. Caproaso N, Ascione A, Stroffolini T, Investigators of an Italian Multicenter Group. Spread of hepatitis C virus infection within families. J Viral Hepatitis 1998;5:67–72.
64. Global surveillance and control of hepatitis C. Report of a WHO Consultation organized in collaboration with the Viral Hepatitis Prevention Board, Antwerp, Belgium. J Viral Hepatitis 1999;6:35–47.
65. Centers for Disease Control and Prevention. Hepatitis B virus: A comprehensive strategy for eliminating transmission in the United States through universal childhood vaccination: Recommendations of the immunization practices advisory committee (ACIP). MMWR 1991; 40(RR-13):1–25.
66. Centers for Disease Control and Prevention. Update: recommendations to prevent hepatitis B virus transmission—United States. MMWR 1995;44:574–5.
67. Centers for Disease Control and Prevention. Prevention of hepatitis A through active or passive immunization. Recommendations of the Advisory Committee on Immunization Practices (ACIP). MMWR 1996;45(No. RR-15):1–30.
68. Krawczynski K, Alter M J, Tankersley D L, et al. Effect of immune globulin on the prevention of experimental hepatitis C virus transmission. J Infect Dis 1996;173:822–8.
69. Peters M, Davis G L, Dooley J S, et al. The interferon system in acute and chronic viral hepatitis. Prog Liver Dis 1986;8:453–67.
70. Camma C, Almasio P, Craxi A. Interferon as treatment for acute hepatitis C. A meta-analysis. Dig Dis Sc 1996;41:1248–55.

10

WORLDWIDE PREVALENCE AND PREVENTION OF HEPATITIS C

DANIEL LAVANCHY
World Health Organization
Communicable Diseases Surveillance and Response
Geneva, Switzerland

BRIAN MCMAHON
Alaska Native Medical Center and Arctic Investigations Program
Centers for Disease Control and Prevention
Anchorage, Alaska

INTRODUCTION

The discovery of the hepatitis C virus (HCV) in 1989 and its linkage to non-A, non-B hepatitis soon led to the recognition of the global importance of this viral infection. Hepatitis C is a major global health problem that deserves widespread active interventions for prevention and control. This chapter reviews what is known about the worldwide prevalence of HCV, discusses regional factors associated with transmission, and outlines prevention strategies to reduce the spread of this infectious disease.

HEPATITIS C: A GLOBAL DISEASE

The hepatitis C virus was first identified in 1989, but already has been shown to have a worldwide distribution, occurring among persons of all ages, genders, races, and regions of the world. (1) As with most recently discovered pathogens, its prevalence, incidence, and socioeconomic burden are not yet well defined. In many countries where the epidemiology of hepatitis C has been studied, increasing rates of infection have been found. (2,3) New infections continue to occur, most likely because of the continued use of unscreened blood transfusions and failure to sterilize medical equipment adequately. Implementation of appropriate prevention measures is needed to reverse these trends. (4) Global monitoring will be necessary to evaluate results and address shortcomings.

Chronic hepatitis C has clearly been linked to the development of hepatocellular carcinoma (HCC) in many areas of the world. Of the more than 500,000 new cases of liver cancer that occur each year, 22% are attributable to HCV infection. (1) Prospective studies have shown that 75% of cases of acute hepatitis C progress to chronic infection, of which 10–20% will develop complications of chronic liver disease such as liver cirrhosis within two to three decades of onset and 1–5% will develop liver cancer. (5–8) These estimates further define hepatitis C as a health problem of global importance. (2) There is a pressing need for accurate information on the prevalence, incidence, modes of transmission, course, outcome, complications, cost, and burden of hepatitis C to the global communities.

WORLDWIDE PREVALENCE OF HEPATITIS C

Incidence and Prevalence

As most cases (60–70%) of acute hepatitis C occur without symptoms, (9–11) data on the incidence of new cases of HCV infection are scarce. Some high-risk groups clearly have a high incidence of this infection. (12–19)

Prevalence data on hepatitis C is available in some form from 134 countries (Table I). Based on a review of published data, the World Health Organization (WHO) estimated that as many as 170 million persons, or about 3% of the world's population, are infected with HCV (Table II, Fig. 1 and Fig. 2). Prevalence studies from many countries are of limited scope, usually representing only a segment of the population (i.e., pregnant women, blood donors, or hospital admissions). Only rare studies have utilized sampling techniques that would represent the entire population. Nevertheless, published data suggest that most populations in Africa, the Americas, Europe, and southeast Asia have prevalence rates of antibody to HCV (anti-HCV) under 2.5%. Anti-HCV prevalence rates for Western Pacific regions average 2.5 to 4.9%. In the Middle East, prevalence rates range from 1 to greater than 12%. In terms of absolute numbers, the majority of infected people live in southeast Asia and the Western Pacific region, a finding similar to that of hepatitis B. Representative prevalence data are still not available from many countries; prevalence studies of the general population in these countries are needed to obtain an accurate estimate of the rate of infection, the number of individuals chronically infected, and the burden of disease. As an indication of how great this burden can be, the current estimate of the annual costs of acute and chronic hepatitis C exceed $600 million for the United States alone. (20)

Global Genotype Distribution

HCV can be categorized on the basis of genomic sequence into six major genotypes (designated 1–6) and approximately 100 subtypes (designated a, b, c, etc.). (21) Information derived from the global distribution of genotypes and subtypes has been used to trace the history and spread of HCV through populations. Although there is little evidence for recombinations occurring between HCV genotypes, (22) the methodological shortcomings of molecular epidemiology of HCV make it important that the results be interpreted with caution.

Genotypes 1–3 have a worldwide distribution; subtypes 1a, 1b, 2a, 2b, and 3a represent the majority of subtypes in North and South America, Australia, western Europe, and Japan. (23–26) Genotypes 4 and 5 are found principally in Africa and genotype 6 is distributed in Asia. An extended number of subtypes

■ TABLE I Prevalence Rates for Hepatitis C[a]

Country	%HCV	Country	%HCV	Country	%HCV
Algeria	0.2	Guatemala	0.7	Portugal	0.5
Angola	1.0	Guinea	10.7	Puerto Rico	1.9
Argentina	0.6	Haiti	2.0	Qatar	2.8
Australia	0.3	Honduras	0.1	Republic of Korea	1.7
Austria	0.2	Hong Kong SAR of China	0.5	Republic of Moldova	4.9
Bangladesh	2.4	Hungary	0.9	Reunion Island	0.8
Belarus	1.4	Iceland	0.1	Romania	4.5
Belgium	0.9	India	1.8	Russian Federation	2.0
Belize	0.1	Indonesia	2.1	Rwanda	17.0
Benin	1.5	Iraq	0.5	Saudi Arabia	1.8
Bhutan	1.3	Ireland	0.1	Senegal	2.9
Bolivia	11.2	Israel	0.4	Seychelles	0.8
Botswana	0.0	Italy	0.5	Sierra Leone	2.0
Brazil	2.6	Jamaica	0.3	Singapore	0.5
Bulgaria	1.1	Japan	2.3	Slovakia	0.4
Burundi	11.1	Jordan	2.1	Solomon Islands	0.9
Cambodia	4.0	Kenya	0.9	Somalia	0.9
Cameroon	12.5	Kiribati	4.8	South Africa	1.7
Canada	0.1	Kuwait	3.3	Spain	0.7
Central African Rep.	4.5	Libyan Arab Jamahirija	7.9	Sudan	3.2
Chad	4.8	Luxembourg	0.5	Suriname	5.5
Chile	0.9	Madagascar	3.3	Swaziland	1.5
China	3.0	Malaysia	3.0	Sweden	0.003
Colombia	1.0	Mauritania	1.1	Switzerland	0.2
Costa Rica	0.3	Mauritius	2.1	Taiwan, Province of China	1.6
Croatia	1.4	Mexico	0.7	Thailand	5.6
Cuba	0.8	Micronesia, Fed. States of	1.5	Togo	3.3
Cyprus	0.1	Mongolia	10.7	Trinidad and Tobago	4.9
Czech Republic	0.2	Morocco	1.1	Tunisia	0.7
Dem. Rep. of Congo	6.4	Mozambique	2.1	Turkey	1.5
Denmark	0.2	Nepal	0.6	Uganda	1.2
Dominican Republic	2.4	Netherlands	0.1	Ukraine	1.2
Ecuador	0.7	New Zealand	0.3	United Rep. of Tanzania	0.7
Egypt	18.1	Nicaragua	0.6	United States of America	1.8
El Salvador	0.2	Niger	2.5	United Arab Emirates	0.8
Ethiopia	0.8	Nigeria	1.4	United Kingdom	0.02
Finland	0.02	Norway	0.1	Uruguay	0.5
France	1.1	Oman	0.9	Vanuatu	0.9
French Guiana	1.5	Pakistan	2.4	Venezuela	0.9
Gabon	6.5	Panama	0.1	Viet Nam	6.1
Germany	0.1	Papua New Guinea	0.6	West Bank and Gaza Strip	2.2
Ghana	2.8	Paraguay	0.3	Yemen	2.6
Greece	1.5	Peru	1.6	Zambia	0.0
Grenada	1.1	Philippines	3.6	Zimbabwe	7.7
Guadeloupe	0.8	Poland	1.4		

[a] Based on published reports by country/area. Source: WHO, June 1999.

have been reported for all but one type in distantly located regions of the world. Endemic areas for specific genotypes are found in west Africa (types 1 and 2), west central Africa (type 4), the Indian subcontinent (type 3), central Africa (type 4), and southeast Asia (type 6). An endemic area for genotype 5 has not

TABLE II Estimated HCV Prevalence per Region and Number of Infected Populations Worldwide[a]

WHO region	Total country population (in millions)	%HCV prevalence	Infected population (in millions)	Number of countries with no data available
Africa	602	5.3	31.9	12
The Americas	785	1.7	13.1	7
Eastern Mediterranean	466	4.6	21.3	5
Europe	858	1.03	8.9	19
Southeast Asia	1.5	2.15	32.3	3
Western Pacific	1.6	3.9	62.2	11
Total	5.8	3.1	170.0	57

[a] Source: WHO, June 1999.

been found. (21,27–33) The important number of subtypes reported in these areas may be attributed to a long history of endemic presence of HCV in local populations. The limited diversity of subtypes found elsewhere may be attributed to a recent introduction of HCV in the populations, as was documented for Canada, (34) Australia, (35) and Western Europe. (36)

The measure of the rate of sequence evolution in viruses introduced at a given time into a cohort provides the possibility to evaluate the history of spread of HCV through different populations. Based on the rate of development of mo-

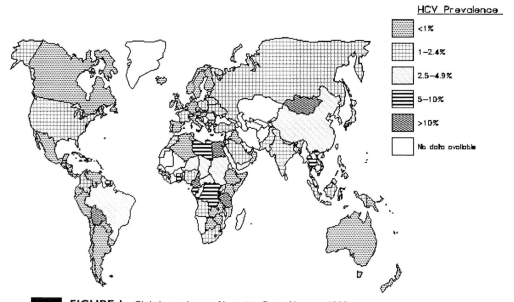

GLOBAL PREVALENCE OF HEPATITIS C
BASED ON PUBLISHED DATA, UPDATE JANUARY 1998

HCV Prevalence
<1%
1–2.4%
2.5–4.9%
5–10%
>10%
No data available

FIGURE 1 Global prevalence of hepatitis C as of January 1998.

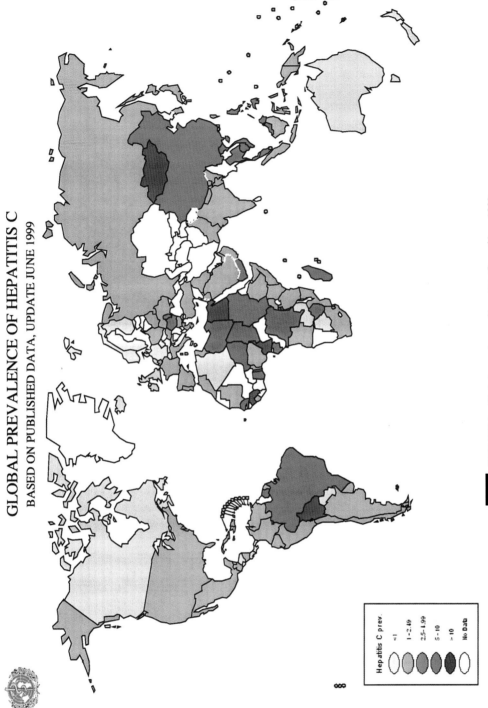

GLOBAL PREVALENCE OF HEPATITIS C
BASED ON PUBLISHED DATA, UPDATE JUNE 1999

Hepatitis C prev.
<1
1 - 2.49
2.5 - 4.99
5 - 10
> 10
No Data

FIGURE 2   Global prevalence of hepatitis C as of June 1999.

lecular diversity, the time of divergence of the HCV subtypes can be estimated to date back more than 300 years, and HCV genotypes more than 500–2000 years. (22) These figures may be an underestimate due to the saturation of substitutions anticipated to occur over time (22) and have to be interpreted with caution due to methodological limitations still inherent to molecular epidemiological techniques.

The geographic distribution of HCV genotypes and the rate of genetic variation are consistent with the global distribution of HCV and are compatible with a long history of infection in most populations of the world. Thus, HCV infection precedes the era of modern medicine by many centuries.

RISK FACTORS FOR TRANSMISSION OF HEPATITIS C

Hepatitis C is believed to be transmitted largely by the transfusion of contaminated blood or blood products and exposure to blood through the reuse of contaminated and/or inadequately sterilized syringes and needles used in medical and dental settings. (1) However, because in many countries the relative contribution of the various modes of infection has not been defined with population-based epidemiological studies, only an incomplete picture can be presented at this time. The extent to which HCV transmission is due to each of these risk factors needs to be determined or estimated in each country or region to permit the formulation and prioritization of cost-effective strategies for preventing the spread of HCV.

Blood Transfusion

Unscreened blood, blood products, and organs are a major cause of HCV infection in many populations. In the United States before 1990 and the availability of tests for hepatitis C, the risk of posttransfusion HCV infection was between 2 and 6%. (37) With the introduction of routine screening of blood and blood products for anti-HCV, this risk has been reduced substantially; the current residual risk for HCV transmission following blood transfusion with screened blood is estimated at 0.004 to 0.0004% per unit transfused. (38) Unfortunately, in many countries with developing or transitional economies, the lack of resources for anti-HCV screening and erratic or nonexistent screening policies have resulted in the continued use of blood from unscreened donors and of blood products that have not undergone viral inactivation.

Injections Used for Immunizations, Treatment, and Invasive Procedures

Parenteral exposure to blood through the reuse of contaminated and/or inadequately sterilized syringes and needles used in medical and dental procedures remains a major source of HCV infection in many countries and puts the general public in these areas at high risk of infection. The costs of disposable syringes and needles and reliable sterilizing instruments represent a major problem for many developing countries. Most countries lack programs to reduce the risk of infection from these sources, and there is a lack of education of health care providers and of the public regarding the importance of this mode of transmission of hepatitis C.

Injection Drug Users and Injection Drug Abuse

In many developed countries, injection drug use is the major source of HCV infection. (4) In many regions, injection drug users are not only represented by persons who inject drugs regularly, but also by persons who inject drugs sporadically and those who used drugs in the distant past. Thus these individuals are integrated in society to such an extent that it is often difficult to determine the prevalence of HCV infection in this high-risk population group.

Traditional Practices

Traditional practices include rituals (e.g., circumcision, scarification), traditional medicine (e.g., blood letting), and other activities that break the skin (e.g., tattooing, ear or body piercing, acupuncture). All are potential sources of infection with HCV and other blood-borne pathogens, where contaminated instruments are used, (39–46) although no association between HCV infection and such types of risk has been reported in the United States (Alter M.J. personal communication). Because most of these practices are not monitored, their importance for disease transmission is currently unknown in most parts of the world.

Other Modes of Transmission

Other modes of transmission that have been studied include a range of behaviors and practices that in theory could transmit infected blood from one individual to another. This list is not complete and an effort should be made to identify other potential modes of transmission.

HCV can be transmitted percutaneously within families and between sexual partners. Examples of potential sources of percutaneous transmission include shared use of razors or other objects that might be contaminated with blood (e.g., washcloths). The risk of sexual transmission among persons with a steady partner appears to be low. Evidence of sexual transmission among persons with multiple partners during unprotected sex or associated with sexually transmitted diseases is supported by case reports, case-control studies, and population-based surveillance data, but more research is needed to determine whether this represents sexual transmission or a failure to detect percutaneous exposures. In general, there is a considerable amount of evidence from a number of studies to conclude that the efficiency of transmission of HCV between sexual partners is limited. Higher rates of transmission may occur if there is coinfection with human immunodeficiency virus (HIV) or other sexually transmitted diseases.

Mother-to-infant transmission of HCV has been documented to occur, but the risk is probably less than 5%, unless the mother is coinfected with HIV. (47) There is no association between transmission and the type of delivery (caesarian section versus vaginal delivery) and no association with maternal breast feeding. (48–53) The long-term prognosis of HCV infection in neonates and infants is not known. From a public health perspective, there is currently no known method for preventing HCV transmission from infected mothers to infants, and more research is needed to determine the risks, outcome, and prevention of perinatal transmission.

UNIQUE REGIONAL RISK FACTORS

HCV and Schistosomiasis in Egypt

Egypt has a very high prevalence of HCV (54–56) and a high morbidity and mortality from chronic liver disease, cirrhosis, and hepatocellular carcinoma. Approximately 20% of Egyptian blood donors are anti-HCV positive. (54,57) Geographically, the desert areas of Egypt have the lowest rates of anti-HCV positivity; rural areas tend to have higher rates than cities; and rates in the Nile Delta (lower Egypt) are higher than in the Nile Valley (middle and upper Egypt). (54, 56–58)

Egypt has higher rates of HCV than neighboring countries as well as other countries in the world with comparable socioeconomic conditions and hygienic standards for invasive medical, dental, or paramedical procedures. (2) The strong homogeneity of HCV subtypes found in Egypt (mostly 4a) (24,30,59) suggests an epidemic spread of HCV. (30) A risk factor(s) originally responsible for the establishment of HCV in the general population may not be necessarily the same ones transmitting the virus today. Therefore, both traditional risk factors as well as risk factors that may be unique to Egypt need to be considered in explaining the transmission of HCV in this country.

Since a history of injection treatment has been implicated as a risk factor for HCV, a prime candidate to explain the high prevalence of HCV in Egypt is the past practice of parenteral therapy for schistosomiasis. (55,57,60–63) Initially described by J. B. Christopherson in the Sudan, the effective treatment of schistosomiasis was established in 1918 by using a series of injections with the antimony salt "tartar emetic" (potassium antimony tartrate). Because Egypt has one of the highest prevalence rates for schistosomiasis, this type of parenteral therapy was practiced extensively as mass treatment since the 1920s predominantly in rural areas. Parenteral therapy gave way to oral treatment when the latter became available in Egypt in 1982 and has been the treatment of choice there since 1988. (64)

Studies have analyzed the possibility of a causal link between the mass treatment campaigns using this drug and the presence of a large reservoir of HCV-infected individuals in rural Egypt. Data suggest that Egypt's mass campaigns indeed represent the world's largest example of iatrogenic transmission of a blood-borne pathogen. (65) The large reservoir of chronic HCV infection established in the course of these campaigns remains likely to be responsible for the high prevalence of HCV morbidity and may be largely responsible for the continued endemic transmission of HCV in Egypt today.

HCV Associated with Glass Syringes Used for Immunizations in Italy

In Italy the prevalence of anti-HCV is greater than 5% in some communities. In one region where the prevalence of anti-HCV was 12.6% overall, the rate among persons younger than 30 years of age was only 1.3% compared with 33.1% in those above 60. (66) The demographic characteristics of this community were typical of many small towns in southern Italy. The use of glass syringes for medical treatment, a common practice before 1970 in Italy, or a history of dental therapy were found to be associated with anti-HCV positivity. (66) A similar risk from immunizations in the 1950s using nondisposable syringes was reported from Japan. (67)

Other Special Associations

In addition to the factors associated with the transmission of hepatitis C cited earlier, other common practices might result in the spread of HCV. A case-control study of risk factors in volunteer blood donors in the United States who were anti-HCV positive by both enzyme immunoassay (EIA) and recombinant immunoblot assay (RIBA) compared with persons who were anti-HCV positive by EIA but negative by RIBA (false positives) showed a significant association with body piercing in men. (68) Perhaps because body piercing, especially ear piercing, is so common in women in the United States, this study did not demonstrate a difference in women. However, these findings imply that body piercing could account for some infections in persons without usual risk factors. Worldwide, body piercing is very common and cleanliness during this technique may be lacking in many areas. In Italy, a national surveillance system of acute hepatitis has been in place since 1984 in 241 local health departments. Using this data base, a study to evaluate the role of risk factors in persons who had no history of transfusion or injection drug use showed that, in addition to ear piercing, exposure to barber shop shaving in the 6 months before onset of illness was associated with acute non A, non-B hepatitis. (45)

ROLE OF HCV IN ETIOLOGY OF HCC, CIRRHOSIS, AND END-STAGE LIVER DISEASE IN DIFFERENT GEOGRAPHIC REGIONS

Hepatocellular carcinoma is a major cause of cancer and death, especially in males, in many areas of the world. (69) In several geographic regions, such as southeast Asia, the South Pacific Islands, and sub-Saharan Africa, hepatitis B virus (HBV) is the major cause of HCC. In contrast, in Japan over half of HCC is associated with HCV infection. (70,71) Similarly, in both Spain and Italy, HCV with or without alcohol abuse is the predominant risk factor associated with HCC; anti-HCV is present in over 60% of cases. (72,73)

In Japan, the prevalence of HCV is highest in persons older than 50 years and is considerably lower in children. (74) This pattern of seropositivity probably resulted from an epidemic of posttransfusion hepatitis in the 1950s and 1960s, as well as from mass immunization programs using nondisposable syringes during the same period. (67) The sequelae of this HCV epidemic, mainly

HCC and end-stage liver disease, began to appear in Japan in the 1970s. Since then, the incidence of HCC has been rising, with the number of liver cancer deaths more than tripling between 1975 and 1992. (67,75)

Although data on the prevalence of hepatitis C among patients with end-stage liver disease are not available in the countries cited earlier, HCV appears to be the major etiologic agent associated with cirrhosis in some of these regions, such as Japan and Italy. In other parts of the world, data on the prevalence of end-stage liver disease associated with HCV are limited. In the United States, a prospective study on the incidence of chronic hepatitis C in selected areas is ongoing.

STRATEGIES FOR PREVENTION OF HEPATITIS C

HCV prevention programs are needed at national, regional, and global levels if the spread of HCV and the burden of hepatitis C are to be reduced. To achieve these objectives, the implementation of measures that reduce the risk of contracting HCV infection (primary prevention) is required. Such programs need to ensure that blood supplies and related products are free of infection and that safe injection methods are practiced. The use of disposable syringes for immunizations and injections is particularly crucial in developing countries. Risk-education counseling for professionals and the public is of paramount importance.

To reduce the risk of developing HCV-related diseases (secondary prevention), and where this is affordable, persons with chronic hepatitis C should be identified and targeted for special counseling and medical management.

Surveillance of HCV is required for the monitoring and evaluation of the effectiveness of such prevention programs. In addition, prevalence studies are needed to identify populations at high risk who might be advised to undergo routine testing for HCV infection. All programs should determine/estimate the extent to which HCV is transmitted by medical and traditional health care procedures and practices, including injections, in order to sharpen the focus of their prevention and education activities.

Introduction of Global Screening of Blood, Blood Components, Organs, Tissues, and Semen

An important objective in the primary prevention of hepatitis C is the exclusion of blood, blood components, organs, tissues, and semen determined to be at risk for HCV transmission. Anti-HCV testing should be part of a comprehensive plan to improve the safety of the blood supply. Such a plan should envisage the establishment of an organized blood service that ensures standard procedures for donor selection, technologic support for serologic screening of donors for blood-borne pathogens (e.g., HIV, HBV, HCV), implementation of good laboratory practices, training of blood bank personnel, and tracking of transfusion outcomes. An important aspect is the development and implementation of inexpensive but reliable and standardized assays for screening blood products for HCV.

Implementation of Safe Injection Techniques

Education of Health Care Providers and the General Public

Health care professionals and the public should be educated about the risk of transmission of blood-borne pathogens (HCV, HBV, HIV) by contaminated injection and other medical equipment, as well as by traditional and folk medical procedures or practices. (4,76) Health care workers and the general public should receive appropriate education and training concerning the importance of controlling such infections in all medical, surgical, and dental procedures, including the use of standard precautions, safe injection practices, proper sterilization techniques, the use of high-level disinfection where appropriate, avoiding reuse and sharing of contaminated equipment and supplies, and avoiding contamination of multiuse supplies such as medication vials. The use of devices or products that prevent reuse or contamination of medical and dental equipment should be encouraged (e.g., "autodestruct" syringes).

Screening for HCV is recommended for health care workers who sustain a percutaneous or mucosal exposure to anti-HCV positive blood to determine the appropriate postexposure management. Because postexposure immunoprophylaxis has not been shown to be effective, (76,77) early detection of acute HCV infection may be important to identify persons who would be candidates for early antiviral treatment (secondary prevention). Little is known about use of antiviral agents to prevent HCV infection after exposure. (78) Health care workers found to be anti-HCV positive should not be restricted from occupational activities, but should be counseled concerning standard precautions and modes of HCV transmission.

Education Regarding Injection Drug Users and Strategies to Reduce HCV Transmission among Them

Many countries have programs to prevent the initiation of illegal drug use as part of HIV prevention strategies. Health education messages produced by these programs should include information concerning the risk of infection by other blood-borne agents, including HCV. The primary prevention of injection drug use will eliminate the greatest risk factor for HCV infection in countries where such illegal practices are present. Health care professionals working in such programs should be educated about HCV modes of transmission and disease outcomes.

Where such injection drug use-reduction programs do not exist, their establishment should be strongly considered as part of a national HCV prevention program. Harm-reduction programs should encourage injection drug users to stop using drugs and seek treatment, and those who cannot stop injecting should be counseled not to share injection or preparation equipment and be encouraged to participate in needle-syringe exchange programs. Hepatitis B and hepatitis A vaccinations should be offered to injection drug users, in the case that these infections have not already been acquired.

Education Regarding Traditional and Folk Medicine

Practitioners of traditional and folk medicine, including those who practice tattooing, body piercing, acupuncture, scarification, and circumcision, and persons who use these services should be educated as to the risk of HCV infection and infection from other blood-borne pathogens from nonsterile instruments or objects used in these procedures. Emphasis should be placed on the use of standard precautions, safe injection practices, proper sterilization techniques, the use of high-level disinfection where appropriate, and the use of devices or products that prevent reuse of equipment.

Identification and Counseling of HCV Carriers and Education to Prevent Household and Community Spread of Infection

Where programs to identify persons with HCV infection are implemented, groups at high risk of HCV infection should be tested routinely; such groups include persons with hemophilia, hemodialysis patients, persons transfused before anti-HCV testing of donors had been instituted, and persons who have ever injected drugs or who are known to have multiple sex partners or a history of sexually transmitted disease. Carriers should undergo special counseling that aims to encourage anti-infection practices and behavior. Those with multiple sex partners, for example, should be encouraged to practice safe sex.

HCV counseling programs should begin with public education of persons at highest risk who have access to sites for counseling and testing. There should be pretest counseling and counseling when testing is performed and when results are reported. Posttest counseling for persons with positive results must include an interpretation of those results and a recommendation for medical follow-up when medical care is available. These individuals also should be counseled regarding further liver injury from alcohol, and hepatitis A and B vaccinations should be considered for susceptible persons. In countries where resources are available, identification of HCV-infected persons who would benefit from antiviral treatment to prevent progression of their chronic liver disease should be a component of HCV-related public health programs. An effort should be made to identify those behaviors that might lead to transmission of HCV to others. Finally, the emotional consequences of providing information about HCV infection and its outcome must be anticipated and dealt with.

STRATEGIES FOR THE SECONDARY PREVENTION OF HCV-RELATED DISEASE BURDEN

Preventing the occurrence of complications of chronic HCV infection such as liver cirrhosis or liver cancer will substantially reduce health care costs for the community, by avoiding expensive treatments such as antiviral therapy.

Testing should only be performed in settings where an active intervention for secondary prevention is realistically envisioned and where resources are available. Consent for testing should be obtained in a way that is consistent with other medical services provided in the same setting.

Testing should be considered for persons who have ever injected illegal drugs; recipients who received blood transfusions or organ transplants before multiantigen screening was implemented (including hemophiliacs and dialysis patients) or who received blood transfusions or organ transplants from a HCV-positive donor; health care professionals after needle stick, sharps, or mucosal exposure; and children (no sooner than age 12 months) born to HCV-positive mothers.

Persons with a history of tattooing or body piercing, persons known to have multiple sex partners, or to have a history of sexually transmitted disease or long-term steady sex partners of a HCV-positive person may also be considered.

Testing of health care professionals not exposed to a blood-transmitted pathogen, pregnant women, household contacts of HCV-positive persons, and the general population is not recommended.

UNANSWERED QUESTIONS AND AREAS FOR FUTURE RESEARCH REGARDING THE GLOBAL PREVALENCE AND SPREAD OF HEPATITIS C

Prevalence and Incidence Studies

There are large gaps in our knowledge of the global epidemiology of HCV. As stated previously, the relative contribution of the various sources of infection has not been defined with population-based epidemiological studies in many countries. Wherever possible such studies should be performed to enable countries to prioritize their preventive measures and to make the most appropriate use of available resources.

In addition to limited data on the actual prevalence of HCV in the world and in most geographic areas, many unanswered questions exist concerning the role of risk factors and lifestyle conditions that are associated with HCV spread in different regions of the world. Epidemiological studies concerning the role of potential risk factors, such as medical procedures, injections for medications and immunizations, tattooing, and scarification techniques, are widely needed. Studies are also needed to determine if certain arthropods such as bed bugs, mosquitoes, and lice play a role in the transmission of HCV, especially in association with crowded living conditions.

Heavy alcohol usage may be associated with the progression of HCV liver disease, especially fibrosis. (79) Prospective longitudinal studies are needed to determine if other factors, in addition to alcohol use, are associated with disease progression. These should include certain parasitic infections, such as schistosomiasis and clonorchiasis, and the exposure to toxic solvents, a common occurrence in developing countries. As importantly, because HCV can be transmitted sexually, the role of coinfection with other sexually transmitted diseases in the spread of HCV, especially those that can result in open genital sores such as chlamydia, chancroid, and syphilis, needs to be studied.

Development of Inexpensive Oral Medications to Treat HCV

There is a great need to develop effective and inexpensive oral medications for hepatitis C that require minimal medical monitoring. The two classes of medications licensed for the treatment of HCV in the United States, interferon-α and ribavirin, are both expensive and difficult to administer. Interferon-α is licensed in several other countries, and licensing for ribavirin is under way in several other countries. The cost of combination therapy of interferon-α and ribavirin for 1 year is approximately $20,000, an estimate that does not include the costs of liver biopsy and monitoring for side effects. This regimen is clearly impractical and unaffordable for most people in the world who are chronically infected with HCV.

Potential candidates for new drugs include protease, helicase, and polymerase inhibitors. The structure of the HCV protease has been identified, (80) an important step toward the development of viral inhibitors. Experience using viral protease and nucleoside analogues in HIV has been gratifying. Unfortunately, these potent drugs have not been available to infected individuals in countries with limited resources because of their prohibitive costs. The challenge for the health care establishment will be to produce these antiviral medications inexpensively and make them widely available.

Development and Use of a Vaccine

The current and future status in the development of HCV vaccines is discussed elsewhere (Chapter 25). The spontaneous nucleotide substitution rate of HCV is very high, and isolates from around the world have shown substantial nucleotide sequence variability that is distributed throughout the viral genome. (81) Although only one species of HCV is recognized at present, reinfection with HCV has been documented both in humans and in experimentally infected chimpanzees. The lack of solid immunity after primary infection has made the development of a vaccine in the near future unlikely. Potential candidates for immunization with an HCV vaccine would include seronegative injecting drug users, patients undergoing hemodialysis, persons who receive frequent blood transfusions such as hemophiliacs, sexual partners of infected persons, and high-risk health care and public safety workers. Other possible candidates would include persons who snort cocaine, female and male sex workers, persons who have sex with multiple partners or with a history of STD, and infants of HCV-positive mothers or persons living in a household comprising a person infected with HCV. Ultimately, if an immunogenic and inexpensive vaccine can be developed, control of HCV transmission may require widespread or even universal vaccination, incorporated into routine vaccination schedules.

Models for Cost-Effective Programs to Reduce the Spread of HCV and the Need for Outcome Research on the Effect of Implementing Preventive Strategies

An initial important step in the control of HCV worldwide will be to develop model programs designed to reduce HCV transmission in a few countries and then, using outcome measurements, to test the effectiveness of these programs on the prevalence and incidence of HCV over time. These model programs could then be used for the implementation of prevention strategies in other countries. In parallel, evaluation of the cost and burden of HCV should be performed.

ACKNOWLEDGMENT

The authors thank Mr. S. Litsios for editorial comments.

REFERENCES

1. World Health Report. Geneva: World Health Organization, 1996.
2. World Health Organization. Hepatitis C: global prevalence. Wkly Epidemiol Rec 1997;72: 341–4.
3. World Health Organization. Hepatitis C. Wkly Epidemiol Rec 1997;72:65–9.
4. World Health Organization. Global surveillance and control of hepatitis C. J Med Virol 1999; 6:35–47.
5. Di Bisceglie A M, Order S E, Klein J L, et al. The role of chronic viral hepatitis in hepatocellular carcinoma in the United States. Am J Gastroenterol 1991;86(3):335–8.
6. Fattovich G, Giustina G, Degos F, et al. Morbidity and mortality in compensated cirrhosis type C: a retrospective follow-up study of 384 patients. Gastroenterology 1997;112(2): 463–72.
7. Kiyosawa K, Sodeyama T, Tanaka E, et al. Interrelationship of blood transfusion, non-A, non-B hepatitis and hepatocellular carcinoma: analysis by detection of antibody to hepatitis C virus. Hepatology 1990;12(4 Pt 1):671–5.
8. Seeff L B, Buskell-Bales Z, Wright E C, et al. Long-term mortality after transfusion-associated non-A, non-B hepatitis. N Engl J Med 1992;327(27):1906–11.
9. Alter H J, Jett B W, Polito A J, et al. Analysis of the role of hepatitis C virus in transfusion-associated hepatitis. Baltimore, MD: Williams & Wilkins, 1991.
10. Aach R D, Stevens C E, Hollinger F B, et al. Hepatitis C virus infection in post-transfusion hepatitis. An analysis with first- and second-generation assays. N Engl J Med 1991;325(19): 1325–9.
11. Koretz R L, Abbey H, Coleman E, Gitnick G. Non-A, non-B post-transfusion hepatitis. Looking back in the second decade. Ann Intern Med 1993;119(2):110–5.
12. Hagan H, McGough J P, Thiede H, Weiss N S, Hopkins S, Alexander E R. Syringe exchange and risk of infection with hepatitis B and C viruses. Am J Epidemiol 1999;149(3):203–13.
13. Tanaka H, Tsukuma H, Hori Y, et al. The risk of hepatitis C virus infection among blood donors in Osaka, Japan. J Epidemiol 1998;8(5):292–6.
14. Broers B, Junet C, Bourquin M, Deglon J J, Perrin L, Hirschel B. Prevalence and incidence rate of HIV, hepatitis B and C among drug users on methadone maintenance treatment in Geneva between 1988 and 1995. AIDS 1998;12(15):2059–66.
15. van Beek I, Dwyer R, Dore G J, Luo K, Kaldor J M. Infection with HIV and hepatitis C virus among injecting drug users in a prevention setting: retrospective cohort study. BMJ 1998;317: 433–7.
16. Dutta U, Raina V, Garg P K, et al. A prospective study on the incidence of hepatitis B & C infections amongst patients with lymphoproliferative disorders. Indian J Med Res 1998;107: 78–82.
17. Fabrizi F, Martin P, Dixit V, et al. Acquisition of hepatitis C virus in hemodialysis patients: a prospective study by branched DNA signal amplification assay. Am J Kidney Dis 1998;31(4): 647–54.
18. Crofts N, Jolley D, Kaldor J, van Beek I, Wodak A. Epidemiology of hepatitis C virus infection among injecting drug users in Australia. J Epidemiol Commun Health 1997;51(6):692–7.
19. el-Ahmady O, Halim A B, Mansour O, Salman T. Incidence of hepatitis C virus in Egyptians. J Hepatol 1994;21(4):687.
20. Moyer L A, Mast E E, Alter M J. Hepatitis C: Part I. Routine serologic testing and diagnosis. Am Fam Physician 1999;59(1):79–88, 91–2.
21. Simmonds P, Alberti A, Alter H J, et al. A proposed system for the nomenclature of hepatitis C viral genotypes. Hepatology 1994;19(5):1321–4.
22. Smith D B, Mellor J, Jarvis L M, et al. Variation of the hepatitis C virus 5′ non-coding region: implications for secondary structure, virus detection and typing. The International HCV Collaborative Study Group. J Gen Virol 1995;76(Pt 7):1749–61.
23. Bukh J, Purcell R H, Miller R H. At least 12 genotypes of hepatitis C virus predicted by sequence analysis of the putative E1 gene of isolates collected worldwide. Proc Natl Acad Sci U S A 1993;90(17):8234–8.
24. McOmish F, Yap P L, Dow B C, et al. Geographical distribution of hepatitis C virus genotypes in blood donors: an international collaborative survey. J Clin Microbiol 1994;32(4):884–92.
25. Davidson F, Simmonds P, Ferguson J C, et al. Survey of major genotypes and subtypes of hepa-

titis C virus using RFLP of sequences amplified from the 5′ non-coding region. J Gen Virol 1995; 76(Pt 5):1197–204.

26. Stuyver L, Wyseur A, van Arnhem W, Hernandez F, Maertens G. Second-generation line probe assay for hepatitis C virus genotyping. J Clin Microbiol 1996;34(9):2259–66.

27. Tokita H, Shrestha S M, Okamoto H, et al. Hepatitis C virus variants from Nepal with novel genotypes and their classification into the third major group. J Gen Virol 1994;75(Pt 4):931–6.

28. Ruggieri A, Argentini C, Kouruma F, et al. Heterogeneity of hepatitis C virus genotype 2 variants in West Central Africa (Guinea Conakry). J Gen Virol 1996;77(Pt 9):2073–6.

29. Stuyver L, van Arnhem W, Wyseur A, Hernandez F, Delaporte E, Maertens G. Classification of hepatitis C viruses based on phylogenetic analysis of the envelope 1 and nonstructural 5B regions and identification of five additional subtypes. Proc Natl Acad Sci U S A 1994;91(21): 10134–8.

30. Mellor J, Holmes E C, Jarvis L M, Yap P L, Simmonds P. Investigation of the pattern of hepatitis C virus sequence diversity in different geographical regions: implications for virus classification. The International HCV Collaborative Study Group. J Gen Virol 1995;76(Pt 10): 2493–507.

31. Tokita H, Okamoto H, Luengrojanakul P, et al. Hepatitis C virus variants from Thailand classifiable into five novel genotypes in the sixth (6b), seventh (7c, 7d) and ninth (9b, 9c) major genetic groups. J Gen Virol 1995;76(Pt 9):2329–35.

32. Mellor J, Walsh E A, Prescott L E, et al. Survey of type 6 group variants of hepatitis C virus in Southeast Asia by using a core-based genotyping assay. J Clin Microbiol 1996;34(2):417–23.

33. Tokita H, Okamoto H, Tsuda F, et al. Hepatitis C virus variants from Vietnam are classifiable into the seventh, eighth, and ninth major genetic groups. Proc Natl Acad Sci U S A 1994;91(23): 11022–6.

34. Bernier L, Willems B, Delage G, Murphy D G. Identification of numerous hepatitis C virus genotypes in Montreal, Canada. J Clin Microbiol 1996;34(11):2815–8.

35. McCaw R, Moaven L, Locarnini S A, Bowden D S. Hepatitis C virus genotypes in Australia. J Viral Hepatitis 1997;4(5):351–7.

36. van Doorn L J, Kleter G E, Stuyver L, et al. Sequence analysis of hepatitis C virus genotypes 1 to 5 reveals multiple novel subtypes in the Benelux countries. J Gen Virol 1995;76(Pt 7): 1871–6.

37. Alter M J, Hadler S C, Judson F N, et al. Risk factors for acute non-A, non-B hepatitis in the United States and association with hepatitis C virus infection. JAMA 1990;264(17):2231–5.

38. Schreiber G B, Busch M P, Kleinman S H, Korelitz J J. The risk of transfusion-transmitted viral infections. N Engl J Med 1996;334(26):1685–90.

39. Mansell C J, Locarnini S A. Epidemiology of hepatitis C in the East. Seminars Liver Dis. 1995; 15:15–32.

40. Mele A, Sagliocca L, Manzillo G, et al. Risk factors for acute non-A, non-B hepatitis and their relationship to antibodies for hepatitis C virus: a case-control study. Am J Public Health 1994; 84(10):1640–3.

41. Kiyosawa K, Tanaka E, Sodeyama T, et al. Transmission of hepatitis C in an isolated area in Japan: community-acquired infection. The South Kiso Hepatitis Study Group. Gastroenterology 1994;106(6):1596–602.

42. Kaldor J M, Archer G T, Buring M L, et al. Risk factors for hepatitis C virus infection in blood donors: a case-control study. Med J Aust 1992;157(4):227–30.

43. Tumminelli F, Marcellin P, Rizzo S, et al. Shaving as potential source of hepatitis C virus infection. Lancet 1995;345:658.

44. Stroffolini T, Menchinelli M, Taliani G, et al. High prevalence of hepatitis C virus infection in a small central Italian town: lack of evidence of parenteral exposure. Ital J Gastroenterol 1995; 27(5):235–8.

45. Mele A, Corona R, Tosti M E, et al. Beauty treatments and risk of parenterally transmitted hepatitis: results from the hepatitis surveillance system in Italy. Scand J Infect Dis 1995;27(5): 441–4.

46. Sun D X, Zhang F G, Geng Y Q, Xi D S. Hepatitis C transmission by cosmetic tattooing in women. Lancet 1996;347:541.

47. Thomas D L, Villano S A, Riester K A, et al. Perinatal transmission of hepatitis C virus from human immunodeficiency virus type 1-infected mothers. Women and Infants Transmission Study. J Infect Dis 1998;177(6):1480–8.

48. Resti M, Azzari C, Lega L, et al. Mother-to-infant transmission of hepatitis C virus. Acta Paediatr 1995;84(3):251–5.

49. Manzini P, Saracco G, Cerchier A, et al. Human immunodeficiency virus infection as risk factor for mother-to- child hepatitis C virus transmission; persistence of anti-hepatitis C virus in children is associated with the mother's anti-hepatitis C virus immunoblotting pattern. Hepatology 1995;21(2):328–32.

50. Zanetti A R, Tanzi E, Paccagnini S, et al. Mother-to-infant transmission of hepatitis C virus. Lombardy Study Group on Vertical HCV Transmission. Lancet 1995;345:289–91.

51. Paccagnini S, Principi N, Massironi E, et al. Perinatal transmission and manifestation of hepatitis C virus infection in a high risk population. Pediatr Infect Dis J 1995;14(3):195–9.

52. Lin H H, Kao J H, Hsu H Y, et al. Absence of infection in breast-fed infants born to hepatitis C virus-infected mothers. J Pediatr 1995;126(4):589–91.

53. Ohto H, Okamoto H, Mishira S. Vertical transmission of hepatitis C virus. Lancet 1994;331: 400.

54. Arthur R R, Hassan N F, Abdallah M Y, et al. Hepatitis C antibody prevalence in blood donors in different governorates in Egypt. Trans R Soc Trop Med Hyg 1997;91(3):271–4.

55. Mohamed M K, Rakhaa M, Shoeir S, Saber M. Viral hepatitis C infection among Egyptians, the magnitude of the problem: epidemiological and laboratory approach. J Egypt Public Health Assoc 1996;71(1,2):79–112.

56. el Gohary A, Hassan A, Nooman Z, et al. High prevalence of hepatitis C virus among urban and rural population groups in Egypt. Acta Trop 1995;59(2):155–61.

57. el-Sayed N M, Gomatos P J, Rodier G R, et al. Seroprevalence survey of Egyptian tourism workers for hepatitis B virus, hepatitis C virus, human immunodeficiency virus, and Treponema pallidum infections: association of hepatitis C virus infections with specific regions of Egypt. Am J Trop Med Hyg 1996;55(2):179–84.

58. Mohamed M K, Hussein M H, Massoud A A, et al. Study of the risk factors for viral hepatitis C infection among Egyptians applying for work abroad. J Egypt Public Health Assoc 1996;71(1,2):113–47.

59. Quinti I, el-Salman D, Monier M K, et al. HCV infection in Egyptian patients with acute hepatitis. Dig Dis Sci 1997;42(10):2017–23.

60. Darwish M A, Raouf T A, Rushdy P, Constantine N T, Rao M R, Edelman R. Risk factors associated with a high seroprevalence of hepatitis C virus infection in Egyptian blood donors. Am J Trop Med Hyg 1993;49(4):440–7.

61. Farghaly A G, Barakat R M. Prevalence, impact and risk factors of hepatitis C infection. J Egypt Public Health Assoc 1993;68(1–2):63–79.

62. Quinti I, Renganathan E, El Ghazzawi E, et al. Seroprevalence of HIV and HCV infections in Alexandria, Egypt. Zentralbl Bakteriol 1995;283(2):239–44.

63. el-Sayed H F, Abaza S M, Mehanna S, Winch P J. The prevalence of hepatitis B and C infections among immigrants to a newly reclaimed area endemic for Schistosoma mansoni in Sinai, Egypt. Acta Trop 1997;68(2):229–37.

64. World Health Organization. The control of schistosomiasis, 2nd report ot the WHO expert committee. W H O Tech Rep Ser 1993;930:70–1.

65. Frank C, Mohamed M, Strickland T, et al. The role of parental antischistosomal therapy in the spread of hepatitis C virus in Egypt. Submitted for publication.

66. Guadagnino V, Stroffolini T, Rapicetta M, et al. Prevalence, risk factors, and genotype distribution of hepatitis C virus infection in the general population: a community-based survey in southern Italy. Hepatology 1997;26(4):1006–11.

67. Okuda K. Hepatitis C virus and hepatocellular carcinoma. In: Okuda K, Taber E, eds. Liver cancer. New York: Churchill-Livingston, 1997:39–50.

68. Conry-Cantilena C, VanRaden M, Gibble J, et al. Routes of infection, viremia, and liver disease in blood donors found to have hepatitis C virus infection. N Engl J Med 1996;334(26):1691–6.

69. McMahon B. Hepatocellular carcinoma and viral hepatitis. In: Wilson R A, ed. Viral hepatitis. New York: Dekker, 1997:315–29.

70. Nishioka K, Watanabe J, Furuta S, et al. A high prevalence of antibody to the hepatitis C virus in patients with hepatocellular carcinoma in Japan. Cancer 1991;67(2):429–33.

71. Saito I, Miyamura T, Ohbayashi A, et al. Hepatitis C virus infection is associated with the development of hepatocellular carcinoma. Proc Natl Acad Sci U S A 1990;87(17):6547–9.

72. Simonetti R G, Camma C, Fiorello F, et al. Hepatitis C virus infection as a risk factor for hepatocellular carcinoma in patients with cirrhosis. A case-control study. Ann Intern Med 1992; 116(2):97–102.

73. Levrero M, Tagger A, Balsano C, et al. Antibodies to hepatitis C virus in patients with hepatocellular carcinoma. J Hepatol 1991;12(1):60–3.

74. Tanaka E, Kiyosawa K, Sodeyama T, et al. Prevalence of antibody to hepatitis C virus in Japanese schoolchildren: comparison with adult blood donors. Am J Trop Med Hyg 1992;46(4): 460–4.

75. Okuda K, Fujimoto I, Hanai A, Urano Y. Changing incidence of hepatocellular carcinoma in Japan. Cancer Res 1987;47(18):4967–72.

76. Recommendations for follow-up of health-care workers after occupational exposure to hepatitis C virus. Centers for Disease Control MMWR 1997;46(26):603–6.

77. Alter M J. Occupational exposure to hepatitis C virus: a dilemma. Infect Control Hosp Epidemiol 1994;15(12):742–4.

78. Camma C, Almasio P, Craxi A. Interferon as treatment for acute hepatitis C. A meta-analysis. Dig Dis Sci 1996;41(6):1248–55.

79. Poynard T, Bedossa P, Opolon P. Natural history of liver fibrosis progression in patients with chronic hepatitis C. The OBSVIRC, METAVIR, CLINIVIR, and DOSVIRC groups. Lancet 1997;349:825–32.

80. Love R A, Parge H E, Wickersham J A, et al. The crystal structure of hepatitis C virus NS3 proteinase reveals a trypsin-like fold and a structural zinc binding site. Cell 1996;87(2):331–42.

81. Fang J W S, Chow V, Lau J Y N. Virology of hepatitis C virus. Clin Liver Dis 1997;1:493–514.

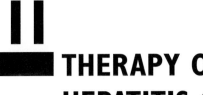

THERAPY OF CHRONIC HEPATITIS C

JOHN G. MCHUTCHISON
Division of Gastroenterology/Hepatology
Scripps Clinic and Research Foundation
La Jolla, California

JAY H. HOOFNAGLE
Division of Digestive Diseases and Nutrition
National Institute of Diabetes and Digestive and Kidney Diseases
National Institutes of Health
Bethesda, Maryland

INTRODUCTION

Chronic hepatitis C affects at least 2.7 million individuals in the United States and 170 million worldwide. (1) This disease ranks with alcoholic liver disease as the leading cause of cirrhosis and end-stage liver disease in developed countries, where it is also the single most common indication for liver transplantation. (1,2) In the United States, the number of patients with hepatitis C who suffer from complications of liver disease is estimated to double or triple over the next decade. These facts underscore the need for effective therapies for this disease.

Interferon-α was shown to have beneficial effects in hepatitis C in the late 1980s and was licensed for use in the United States and Europe in 1991. (3, 4) Subsequently, several studies demonstrated that the addition of ribavirin to interferon-α therapy increased the rate of sustained responses, (5,6) and this regimen was approved in 1998. The currently available regimens of interferon-α and ribavirin lead to eradication of hepatitis C virus (HCV) RNA from serum and a long-term remission in disease in approximately 40% of patients. The remaining patients may have a transient improvement in the liver disease but have no clear-cut long-term benefit. In addition, combination therapy must be given for 24 to 48 weeks, requires parenteral injections, has important and difficult side effects, and is quite expensive. For these reasons, the decision to use interferon or combination therapy should be made after weighing both the risks and benefits of therapy (Table I).

In view of the shortcomings of current therapies, treatment should perhaps be limited to patients in whom it is clearly needed. (7,8) Chronic hepatitis C does not always result in severe liver damage. Studies on the natural history of hepatitis C have shown that only 20 to 25% of patients develop cirrhosis during the first 20 years of infection. (9) While it would be helpful to identify which patients

**TABLE I   Benefits and Risks for Therapy
of Chronic Hepatitis C**

Benefits
    Cause of symptoms and disability in some patients
    Leads to cirrhosis in 20 to 30% of patients
    Commonest indication for liver transplantation
    Short-term benefits of therapy are clear
    Improvement in quality of life occurs in responders
    Sustained long-term benefits occur in virological responders
    In economic analyses, treatment is cost-effective

Risks
    Many patients never develop complications of hepatitis C
    Progression of disease is slow and variable
    Therapy is effective in less than half of patients
    Therapy requires parenteral administration
    Therapy has many side effects and is often poorly tolerated
    Therapy must be given for 6 to 12 months
    Therapy is costly
    Therapy is evolving and better treatments may be available soon

with chronic hepatitis C are most likely to develop cirrhosis and most warrant therapy, this is not usually possible. There are no clinical, serum biochemical, or virological features that accurately predict which patient will develop progressive disease.

Although there are published indications and contraindications for therapy of hepatitis C, the variable response rate and the evolving nature of this field make it difficult to recommend strict criteria. The aim of this chapter is to synthesize the available and most recent data regarding the treatment of chronic hepatitis C for both the clinician and the liver research investigator. Because of the many changes that have occurred in therapy of hepatitis C, the major focus will be on current recommendations rather than an exhaustive review of the many studies done since the mid-1980s.

INDICATIONS FOR THERAPY OF HEPATITIS C

The panel of 1997 National Institutes of Health Consensus Development Conference on "Management of Hepatitis C" set forth standard indications for treatment of patients with chronic hepatitis C (Table II). (7) Criteria include elevations in serum aminotransferase levels, presence of HCV RNA in serum, chronic hepatitis on liver biopsy, and no contraindications. The Consensus Conference panel stated that therapy was clearly indicated for adult patients between the ages of 18 and 60 who had histological evidence of moderate or severe disease, but was less clearly indicated for elderly patients, children, patients with cirrhosis, and patients with normal serum aminotransferase levels or with mild histological changes. These criteria are still appropriate, although there is now more enthusiasm for therapy of patients with compensated cirrhosis (see Chapter 12) and for treating elderly patients. (8)

■ **TABLE II   Minimal Criteria for Treatment of Chronic Hepatitis C** [a]

Elevations in serum aminotransferase levels for at least 6 months
Presence of HCV RNA in serum
Some degree of fibrosis or moderate inflammation on liver biopsy
Compensated liver disease
Compliance and acceptance of therapy
Abstinence from alcohol and illegal drugs
No contraindications to therapy

[a] Adapted from the National Institutes of Health and the EASL Consensus Development Conferences on hepatitis C. (7,8)

The presence of symptoms, height of serum aminotransferase elevations, viral level, and genotype may help in the decision to treat or not to treat, but these factors should not be used as strict criteria for or against treatment. Therapy should certainly not be limited to patients with symptoms. Symptoms in hepatitis C are often nonspecific (fatigue, lethargy, nonspecific gastrointestinal upset, and abdominal pain) and do not correlate with the severity or histological stage of liver disease. (10) Some patients have no symptoms of liver disease until they present with complications of advanced cirrhosis. (11) Likewise, the degree of elevation of serum aminotransferase levels (ALT and AST) should not guide decisions, as aminotransferase levels do not correlate well with histological severity of disease or prognosis. In early studies of therapy, patients were not enrolled unless ALT values were greater than 1.5 times the upper limit of normal. This criterion was arbitrary, and the fluctuating nature of ALT levels in chronic hepatitis C makes it difficult to use. In clinical practice, any abnormality of the ALT or AST that is present for 6 months or more is probably adequate to initiate evaluation for treatment. At the present time and with current therapies, patients who have persistently normal ALT and AST values should not be treated except in the context of clinical trials.

There is considerable disagreement concerning the use of histological severity of liver disease as a criterion for or against therapy. The Consensus Development panel recommended therapy only for patients with some degree of fibrosis or moderate-to-severe inflammation and necrosis on liver biopsy. (7) This recommendation was also supported by a European consensus panel. (8) The rationale for this recommendation was that the presence of fibrosis indicates that the liver disease is progressive and may ultimately lead to cirrhosis. In contrast, patients with mild disease and no fibrosis on liver biopsy are unlikely to suffer progression of disease within the ensuing 5 to 10 years (12,13) and thus can safely forego therapy and await improvements in regimens that are likely to be more effective and better tolerated.

Liver biopsy is not mandatory before starting therapy but it is recommended. (7,8) The histological information gained is important in weighing the decision for or against therapy and helps in guiding management if side effects are troublesome or therapy is ineffective in leading to clearance of virus. Liver biopsy also allows the diagnosis of cirrhosis in patients in whom this is not evident clinically and excludes other forms of liver disease and complicating factors (such as iron overload or steatosis). Presently, liver biopsy and histological assessment before therapy is prudent in all patients who have no contraindications to biopsy. If reliable and accurate noninvasive markers of fibrosis and more effective therapies become available, the role of liver biopsy will need reassessment.

CONTRAINDICATIONS TO THERAPY

The major contraindications to combination therapy with interferon and ribavirin include decompensated liver disease, a history of major depression or neurological disease, active autoimmune disease, active alcohol abuse or illicit drug use, and solid organ transplant (Table III). (7,8) Decompensated liver disease is defined by a history of variceal hemorrhage, persistent jaundice, coagulopathy, ascites, hepatic encephalopathy, and hepatorenal or hepato-pulmonary syndrome. Furthermore, patients without these clinical complications but with low albumin levels or low platelets should be assessed carefully before considering therapy. Major depression and neurological diseases are important risk factors for severe neuropsychiatric side effects of interferon. Autoimmune diseases can be exacerbated by interferon therapy, particularly systemic lupus erythematosis and rheumatoid arthritis. Patients with inactive or well-controlled thyroid disease or type I diabetes can usually be treated without complications. Patients with psoriasis and with inflammatory bowel disease should be treated with caution, as worsening of these conditions can occur on therapy. Active alcohol or drug abuse are important cofactors in promoting progressive liver disease in patients with hepatitis C and should be discontinued for at least 1 year before embarking on therapy. Other contraindications to therapy include anemia, hemolysis, or renal insufficiency if ribavirin is used. Ribavirin regularly induces a mild hemolytic anemia, which can be severe and even life-threatening in patients with preexisting hemolysis, anemia, or renal insufficiency. Because of the sudden onset of anemia with ribavirin, therapy should also be used with extreme caution

TABLE III   Contraindications to Antiviral Therapy for Chronic Hepatitis C

Interferon alone	Combination therapy with interferon and ribavirin[a]
Decompensated liver disease	Anemia (Hgb $<$ 11 g/dl)
Severe neuropsychiatric illness	Hemolysis
Severe depression or bipolar illness	Renal insufficiency
Autoimmune disease	Coronary artery disease
Active alcohol abuse	Cerebral vascular disease
Active or recent illicit drug use	Gouty arthropathy
Pregnancy	Inability to practice contraception
Significant comorbid disease	
Unstable coronary artery disease	
Uncontrolled epilepsy	
Uncontrolled diabetes	
Uncontrolled hypertension	

[a]Contraindications to interferon alone apply equally to the combination of interferon and ribavirin.

in patients with significant cardiac or cerebrovascular disease. Instances of acute myocardial infarction and death in association with the onset of anemia have been reported in patients receiving combination therapy. Ribavirin can raise uric acid levels and patients with gouty arthropathy should probably avoid use of this drug. Finally, birth control is mandatory during interferon and ribavirin therapy and for 6 months; therefore, patients unable to practice adequate contraception should not be treated.

EFFICACY OF THERAPIES OF HEPATITIS C

Definition of Responses to Antiviral Therapy

Responses to therapy in chronic hepatitis C can be categorized as *biochemical* as shown by normal alanine aminotransferase (ALT) levels, *virological* as shown by absence of detectable HCV RNA, or *histological* as shown by improvements in liver biopsy results. (14) Typically, multiple end points or a combined response is used to describe results of trials of antiviral therapy. Responses can also be categorized by timing of the measurements of success as early during treatment (*initial response*), at the end of therapy (*end-of-treatment response*), or 6 to 12 months after therapy (*sustained response*). Use of standard definitions for responses in chronic hepatitis C has been helpful in allowing for comparison of results across studies that use different regimens of therapy in different cohorts of patients.

Durability of Virological Responses to Antiviral Therapy

An important issue is whether the relatively short term (1 to 2 year) responses used in most trials of antiviral therapy are clinically meaningful and correlate with long-term benefit. The clinical validity of the short-term benefit of therapy has been confirmed in several randomized controlled trials comparing interferon-α alone to no treatment or placebo therapy using biochemical, virological, and histological criteria 6 to 12 months after stopping treatment. (4) In these studies, the majority of patients who had a sustained virological response had persistently normal serum aminotransferase levels and moderate to marked improvements in liver histology. A spontaneous loss of HCV RNA with an accompanying improvement in aminotransferase levels and liver histology was very uncommon.

A long-term benefit of interferon therapy in hepatitis C has been demonstrated by a 5- to 10-year follow-up of patients who achieved a virological or biochemical response to interferon. These studies have indicated that at least 95% of patients with a sustained virological response 6 months after completion of therapy continue to have histological improvement, normal liver tests, and no detectable HCV RNA in serum or liver. (15,16) As many as two-thirds of long-term responders will have normal hepatic histology on biopsy. In contrast, patients with a biochemical response alone (normal ALT levels but persistence of HCV RNA) usually experience a relapse in disease activity during subsequent follow-up evaluation, and with this relapse, hepatic histology usually returns to the pretreatment appearance. Thus, a sustained virological response is generally considered the best and most reliable outcome measure in studies of therapy of hepatitis C. Furthermore, a 6-month follow-up is generally adequate to document the response as relapses after 6 months are uncommon.

Whether the long-term benefits observed in patients who attain a sustained virological response ultimately translate into "cure" of the infection, prevention of cirrhosis, a decrease in complications of end-stage liver disease, and improvements in survival and need for liver transplantation are not known. In this chapter, the virological sustained response (clearance of serum HCV RNA 6 or 12 months after cessation of therapy) will be used as the standard means of defining responses to treatment.

Cost-Effectiveness of Antiviral Therapy of Hepatitis C

The documentation of both short- and long-term benefits of antiviral therapy of chronic hepatitis C has allowed for economic and cost-effectiveness analyses of this treatment. These studies have shown that antiviral therapy with interferon is cost-effective. (17,18) Future cost savings observed for treatment of hepatitis C are comparable or better than other accepted medical treatments already widely in practice (e.g., hypertension screening, renal dialysis, coronary artery bypass grafting, colorectal cancer screening). Patients who have responded to therapy (by biochemical or virological criteria) have been shown to have significant improvement in their health-related quality of life parameters. (19,20)

INITIAL THERAPY OF PATIENTS WITH CHRONIC HEPATITIS C

Interferon Monotherapy

Initial Trials of Interferon-α

Interferon-α and -β are type 1 interferons and share multiple biological effects, including antiviral, antiproliferative, and immunomodulatory actions. These characteristics led to the initial studies of interferon-α as treatment for chronic hepatitis C, which showed that treatment could lead to sustained improvements in serum aminotransferase levels and liver histology. (3) Subsequent, randomized controlled trials showed that a 6-month course of interferon-α in doses of 3 million units three times weekly led to sustained biochemical responses in 10 to 25% of patients. (4,21) The initial studies were performed before the discovery of HCV and the availability of sensitive virological testing. Application of HCV RNA assays to stored sera from these studies revealed that sustained viral eradication was achieved in only 10 to 12% of patients when this dose regimen was used, irrespective of the type of interferon (Fig. 1). (21–24) In some trials there were small but statistically significant differences in response rates between the types of interferon, which was especially observed in post hoc analysis of subgroups. The significance of these differences between subgroups are of unknown clinical significance and have not been subjected to prospective evaluation.

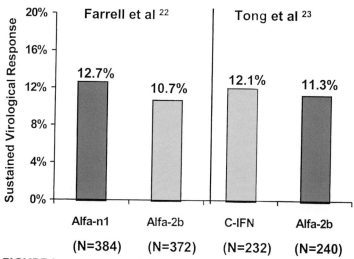

FIGURE I   Sustained virological response rates in two large trials in which there was direct comparison between different forms of type I interferon, including αn1 (Wellferon, Glaxo-Wellcome, Research Triangle Park, NC), recombinant α2b (Intron-A, Schering Plough, Kenilworth, NJ), and consensus interferon (Infergen, Amgen, Thousand Oaks, CA). (22,23)

Duration of Interferon Monotherapy

Extending the duration of interferon therapy from 6 to 12 months led to higher sustained virological response rates of approximately 15 to 20%. (25,26) Even longer courses of therapy of 18 or 24 months achieved somewhat higher rates of response. (27) These findings led to the ultimate recommendations from the NIH Consensus Development Conference panel that patients with chronic hepatitis C who meet the criteria for treatment receive a 12-month course of interferon-α in doses of 3 million units (or its equivalent) three times weekly. (7)

Higher Doses of Interferon

The efficacy of increasing the dose of interferon has been evaluated in many studies, but few have been of sufficient size and rigor to document a small increase in response rate with higher doses. Higher "fixed" dose regimens produced marginal improvements in terms of sustained virological response rates, but were associated with more severe and more frequent side effects and a high drop out rate. (4,26) Similar or higher response rates without increases in side effects were achieved by prolonging the course of therapy. At present, use of higher doses of interferon should be undertaken with caution and only in patients who tolerate interferon well.

Induction Dosing with Interferon

Various "induction" strategies have been advocated as a means of improving sustained response rates to interferon-α. Induction refers to the administration of interferon in a higher dose and/or with daily administration for the first 2 to 8 weeks of treatment. (26,27) A variety of induction regimens have been evaluated. The rationale for these regimens came from studies of the kinetics of changes in HCV RNA levels during the first days and weeks of interferon therapy. Higher doses of interferon and daily administration led to more rapid decreases in HCV RNA levels and a higher rate of initial virological response (at 2 to 8 weeks). (28,29) Whether these early changes in viral kinetics translate into enhanced long-term sustained response rates has not been shown. Preliminary findings, however, suggest that induction dosing is no more effective than routine dosing in achieving sustained response rates with interferon monotherapy. More data are needed, but at present, induction dosing with interferon-α alone cannot be recommended.

Current Recommendations for Use of Interferon Monotherapy

At present, combination therapy is recommended as the initial therapy for chronic hepatitis C. Interferon monotherapy should be reserved for patients with contraindications to or who do not qualify for use of ribavirin. For instance, the optimal dose and safety of ribavirin has not been demonstrated in children. Until there is more information on ribavirin dosing in pediatrics, children, if treated, should receive interferon alone (see Chapter 20). Similarly, ribavirin is excreted renally and patients with kidney insufficiency rapidly develop toxicity from this drug. Again, if therapy is used, patients with renal insufficiency (creatinine greater than 1.5 mg/dl or creatinine clearance of less than 60 cc/min) should receive interferon monotherapy. Interferon without ribavirin can also be used in patients with anemia and hemolysis, in patients with symptomatic coronary or cerebral vascular disease, or in patients concerned about the potential teratogenecity. The dose of interferon should be 3 million units (when using α2a or α2b interferon) and 9 μmg (when using consensus interferon) subcutaneously three times weekly for 48 weeks. (7,8) If HCV RNA remains detectable after 3 months of treatment, most investigators would recommend stopping therapy. (7)

Combination Therapy

Types of Combination Therapies Used in Hepatitis C

Because of the limited efficacy of therapy with interferon alone, combinations of antivirals, immunomodulatory, and anti-inflammatory agents have been tried, largely in small, uncontrolled, observational studies. (30) These trials of combination therapy have focused mainly on patients who did not respond to a previous course of interferon. Of course, the value of combination therapy has been shown in many infectious diseases, including chronic viral diseases such as HIV infection in which highly active antiretroviral therapy (HAART) using three or more agents has been highly effective. Among the many agents that have been tried in chronic hepatitis C, only ribavirin has been shown reproducibly to improve sustained virological response rates compared to interferon alone. (30)

Ribavirin is a synthetic nucleoside analogue with a broad spectrum of antiviral activity that was used initially in the 1970s. The putative antiviral mechanisms of action of ribavirin include inhibition of RNA-dependent RNA polymerase, depletion of intracellular GTP pools, and immunomodulatory actions, including macrophage inhibition and alteration of the Th1/Th2 cytokine balance. (31,32) Although ribavirin is well absorbed orally, it was not found to be effective or approved for use in any human viral infection, except in an aerosol form for the treatment of respiratory syncitial virus infection in children.

Because ribavirin has activity *in vitro* against several flaviviruses, it was tried as monotherapy in chronic hepatitis C shortly after HCV was characterized as a flavivirus-like agent. These studies demonstrated that ribavirin therapy led to a significant decrease in serum ALT levels in a high proportion of patients, but that treatment had little or no effect on HCV RNA levels. The effect on aminotransferase levels was transient and all patients relapsed when therapy was stopped. (33–36)

Trials of Combination Therapy

The effects of ribavirin on serum aminotransferase levels in chronic hepatitis C led to studies of the combination of ribavirin and interferon-α. To date, there have been five published, randomized controlled trials comparing the efficacy of interferon alone with the combination of interferon and ribavirin as the initial treatment of patients with chronic hepatitis C. (5,6,37–39) In all five studies, combination therapy yielded higher virological and biochemical response rates than interferon monotherapy (Table IV). Rates of histological response were also higher with the combination in the two trials that included follow-up liver biopsies.

TABLE IV Five Controlled Trials Comparing Therapy with Interferoni-α Alone to Combination Therapy with Interferon-α and Ribavirin in Chronic Hepatitis C

Author	Duration (weeks)	No.	Virological[a]	Biochemical[b]	Histological[c]
Lai et al. (37)					
Interferon alone	24	19	11%	11%	NA[d]
Combination	24	21	48%	48%	NA
Chemello et al. (38)					
Interferon alone	24	15	7%	13%	NA
Combination	24	15	4%	40%	NA
Reichard et al. (39)					
Interferon alone	24	50	18%	24%	NA
Combination	24	50	36%	44%	NA
McHutchison et al. (5)					
Interferon alone	24	23	6%	11%	44%
Interferon alone	48	225	13%	16%	41%
Combination	24	228	31%	32%	57%
Combination	48	228	38%	36%	61%
Poynard et al. (6)					
Interferon alone	48	278	19%	24%	39%
Combination	24	277	35%	39%	52%
Combination	48	277	43%	50%	63%

[a] Sustained response defined as undetectable HCV RNA at least 24 weeks after therapy
[b] Normal ALT values by end of treatment and during 24 weeks follow-up.
[c] Histological response indicates improvement in the histological activity index inflammatory score of at least two points.
[d] Not available.

Overall Response Rates to Combination Therapy

Compared to interferon-α alone, the combination of ribavirin and interferon led to higher sustained as well as end-of-treatment responses. (5,6) Thus, combination therapy increased the percentage of patients who became HCV RNA negative on therapy (both initial and end-of-treatment responses) and decreased the rate of relapse when therapy was stopped.

The two largest and most recent trials of combination therapy versus interferon monotherapy also compared 24 and 48 weeks of treatment. (5,6) In both studies, the highest rate of sustained virological response occurred with 48 weeks of combination treatment. The longer course of treatment was not associated with a higher rate of initial or end-of-therapy response, but rather with a higher sustained response. Thus, the major effect of extending the duration of therapy from 24 to 48 weeks was to decrease the relapse rate. This effect was seen both with interferon alone and with combination therapy.

Virological relapse among patients treated with interferon alone occurred in 80% of those treated for 24 weeks and in 45% of those treated for 48 weeks. Virological relapse among patients treated with the combination was seen in 45% of patients receiving 24 weeks and only 20% of those treated for 48 weeks. These results suggest that ribavirin has a synergistic effect with interferon, increasing the antiviral effect and stabilizing the response.

Predictors of a Response to Combination Therapy

Post hoc analyses of studies of combination therapy in chronic hepatitis C have identified several factors that correlated with a high likelihood of response. (5,6) The major predictive factors were viral: HCV genotype and initial serum HCV RNA level. Host factors appeared to play a lesser role in the likelihood of a sustained virological response to combination therapy, with these factors being sex, age, and degree of fibrosis on liver biopsy. Serum aminotransferase levels, inflammatory activity of the liver disease, and presence of symptoms did not correlate with a response to treatment. Several of these predictive factors may be helpful clinically in guiding therapy, in providing advice about the likelihood of a response, and in determining the duration of therapy.

Genotype and Response to Combination Therapy

Multiple studies of interferon monotherapy of hepatitis C have shown that response rates to interferon-α are lower in patients with HCV genotype 1 infection than in those with genotype 2 or 3. (21–26) This distinction was also found in trials of combination therapy. Thus, overall the sustained virological response rate to combination therapy was 30% among patients with genotype 1a or 1b as opposed to 66% in patients with genotype 2 or 3. (5,6)

Of greater clinical importance were differences in response rates by genotype and duration of treatment (Fig. 2). Results of the two trials were remarkably similar and are combined for analysis and discussion. Among patients with genotype non-1 treated with combination therapy, 62% had a sustained virological response with 24 of weeks of treatment and 63% had a response with 48 weeks of treatment. These findings indicate that patients with genotypes 2 and 3 should be treated for 24 weeks only and that continuation of ther-

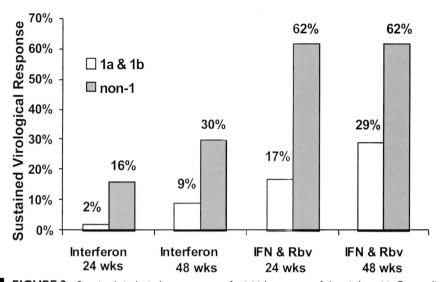

FIGURE 2 Sustained virological response rates for initial treatment of chronic hepatitis C according to HCV genotype in 1744 patients participating in the United States (5) and international trials. (6) Patients received interferon (IFN) alone for 24 or 48 weeks or combination therapy with IFN and ribavirin (Rbv) for 24 or 48 weeks. Patients with genotype 1 HCV infection had lower rates of reponse than patients with genotypes other than 1. The highest rates of response occurred with 48 weeks of combination therapy ($p < 0.008$; 48 weeks vs 24 weeks of interferon and ribavirin). Among patients with nongenotype 1 infection, response rates were identical with 24 and 48 weeks of the combination.

apy for 48 weeks does not increase the sustained response rate nor decrease the relapse rate.

In contrast, among patients with genotype 1, prolonging therapy to 48 weeks did appear to increase the sustained response rate (from 16 to 30%). This greater efficacy of 48 weeks of therapy was primarily due to a decrease in the relapse rate (from 62 to 18%). Overall, these findings indicate that determining the HCV genotype is helpful in the clinical management of patients and in determining the optimal duration of therapy. Patients with genotype 2 and 3 should be treated for 24 weeks only. Patients with genotype 1 are best treated for 48 weeks.

Most patients in the United States have infection with genotypes 1 (72%), 2 (16%), or 3 (10%). (5) In the large multicenter trials of combination therapy, there were too few patients with genotypes 4, 5, and 6 to assess response rates in these groups. Patients with mixtures of genotypes, including genotype 1, were generally grouped with patients with genotype 1 alone.

Viral Level and Response to Combination Therapy

In both large multicenter trials of combination therapy, the likelihood of response was higher among patients who had low initial levels of HCV RNA than among those with high levels. (5,6) In both trials, a serum HCV RNA level of 2 million copies/ml was determined by a quantitative polymerase chain reaction (PCR)-based assay for HCV RNA with a detection limit of 100 copies/ml. Patients were categorized as having either high ($\geq$ 2 million) or low ($<$ 2 million)

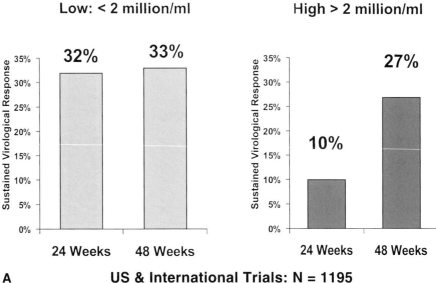

A   US & International Trials: N = 1195

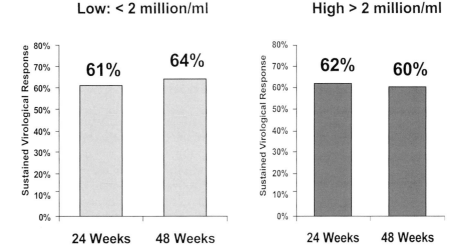

B   US & International Trials: N = 548

FIGURE 3   Sustained virological response rate to the combination of interferon-α and ribavirin given for 24 or 48 weeks in patients from two randomized controlled trials (5,6) analyzed by both HCV genotype (1 versus non-1) and pretreatment serum HCV RNA levels ($\geq$ 2 million versus < 2 million copies). (A) Among patients with genotype 1, the longer course of therapy yielded significantly higher response rates in patients with high but not with low initial levels of serum HCV RNA. (B) Among patients with genotypes other than 1, the rates of sustained virological response were the same with 24 as with 48 weeks of therapy irrespective of initial level of HCV RNA.

concentrations of virus. Sustained responses occurred in 45% of patients with low and 33% of patients with high initial HCV RNA levels. Importantly, however, the effect of viral levels was largely among patients with genotype 1 (Fig. 3 and Table V). Thus, 62% of patients with genotype 2 or 3 responded to treat-

TABLE V Response Rates to Interferon-α and Combination Therapy by Initial HCV RNA Level and Degree of Fibrosis on Liver Biopsy[a]

Pretreatment variable[b]	Interferon alone		Combination	
	24 weeks	48 weeks	24 weeks	48 weeks
HCV RNA $<2 + 10^6$	9%	30%	44%	46%
HCV RNA $>2 + 10^6$	4%	10%	27%	38%
Stage 0 or 1 fibrosis	5%	18%	36%	43%
Stage 3 or 4 fibrosis	5%	12%	23%	36%

[a] Data adapted and combined from McHutchison et al. (5) and Poynard et al. (6)
[b] The fibrosis stage was defined as absent (0), mild (1), bridging (3), or cirrhosis (4).

ment, irrespective of the initial level of HCV RNA or duration of therapy (24 or 48 weeks). Among patients with genotype 1 and low levels of HCV RNA, 33% responded to combination therapy when it was given for 24 weeks and 32% responded when treatment was given for 48 weeks. However, among patients with genotype 1 and high levels of HCV RNA, only 10% had a sustained response to a 24-week course of combination treatment, whereas 28% responded to a 48-week course of combination treatment. These findings indicate that the optimal duration of therapy among patients with genotype 1 and high levels of HCV RNA is 48 weeks, but that all other categories of patients need only receive 24 weeks of treatment. (8)

Several shortcomings of HCV RNA testing should be remembered before using HCV RNA levels as a criterion to determine the duration of therapy. First, serum levels of HCV RNA fluctuate spontaneously over time by as much as 30 to 50% (up to 0.5 log titer), and the significance of fluctuations above and below the levels chosen as "high" and "low" is not known. (40) Furthermore, different methods for determining HCV RNA levels yield quite different results. Thus, the Monitor PCR-based assay (Roche Diagnostics, Nutley, NJ) is reported to yield levels of HCV RNA that are often 1 log lower than the bDNA assay (Chiron Diagnostics, Emeryville, CA) or other PCR-based quantitative assays such as "Superquant" (National Genetics Institute, Los Angeles, CA). (41,42) Thus, using the Monitor assay, a level above 200,000 copies/ml might be best considered a "high level" of HCV RNA. For these reasons, use of the initial viral level to determine the duration of therapy should be done with caution, with full knowledge of the virological assay used and its reliability and comparability to other assays.

Other Predictive Factors

Other predictive factors of a response to interferon-α include young age (<45 years), female sex, and lesser degrees of fibrosis on liver biopsy (none or portal fibrosis only) (Table V). In a post hoc analysis of the European trial of combination therapy, a combination of these predictive factors was found helpful in guiding therapy. (6) Thus, the presence of three or more unfavorable factors (genotype 1, high HCV RNA levels, male sex, older age, and bridging fibrosis or cirrhosis) correlated well with the need to treat for 48 as opposed to 24 weeks. Such algorithms for therapy require further refinement and evaluation.

Race and Response to Antiviral Therapy

In several trials of antiviral therapy of hepatitis C, post hoc analyses identified race to be associated with differences in likelihood of a response. (42) Thus, in trials of interferon monotherapy, African-American patients were severalfold less likely to have either an end-of-treatment or a sustained virological response to a 6-month course of therapy than Hispanic or non-Hispanic whites. In analysis of the United States trial of combination therapy of previously untreated patients with chronic hepatitis C, end-of-treatment and sustained response rates among African-Americans were threefold lower than in Caucasians. (5,43) The reason for the lower response rate among African-Americans is not clear, but it may be due in part to a higher prevalence of genotype 1 and possibly other host factors such as duration of disease and degree of fibrosis. Interesting, response rates among Asian-Americans have been higher than in Caucasians, but too few such patients have been enrolled in these clinical trials for meaningful statistical analyses.

Typical Patterns of Response and Nonresponse

The course of a patient with a sustained virological response to combination therapy is shown in Fig. 4A. Serum aminotransferase levels and HCV RNA levels usually fall rapidly with treatment and typically become negative or normal within 2 months. (14) The possibility that the measurement of HCV RNA levels during the early part of therapy might demonstrate which patients will have a sustained response within 1 to 3 months of starting therapy is currently being evaluated. Most patients who have a sustained response continue to have normal serum aminotransferase levels and no detectable HCV RNA in serum for the duration of therapy. A proportion of patients with a sustained virological response, however, continue to have mild elevations in ALT levels during therapy, thus having a virological without a biochemical response (Fig. 4B). This pattern is most likely to occur in patients with cirrhosis or marked elevations before treatment. As long as these elevations are less than twice the baseline levels, therapy should be continued in patients who are HCV RNA negative, as aminotransferase levels generally fall into the normal range once therapy is stopped.

Patients who suffer a relapse have an initial pattern of response similar to patients with a sustained response, but HCV RNA reappears within 1 to 2 months of stopping treatment, usually followed by elevations in serum aminotransferase levels (Fig. 4C). Frequent testing of serum during therapy may reveal that these patients may actually have intermittent low levels of HCV RNA during treatment, but often there are no features indicating that a patient will suffer a relapse when therapy is discontinued. If such a marker were available, one could replace the rigid recommendations of 24 or 48 weeks of therapy with recommendations to continue therapy until there is reliable evidence of viral eradication and a low likelihood of relapse.

A nonresponse to combination therapy is marked by the continued presence of HCV RNA in serum despite therapy for at least 6 months. Some patients have a biochemical response to therapy despite remaining HCV RNA positive, especially when treated with combination therapy. Patients who remain HCV RNA positive usually suffer a relapse after therapy is stopped (Fig. 4D). At least half of patients who do not achieve a virological response on combination therapy

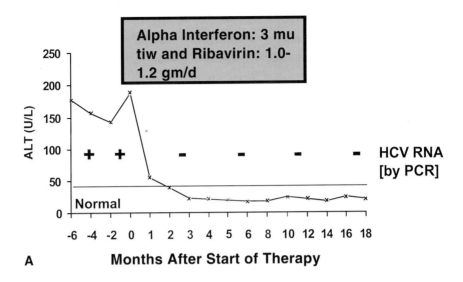

A

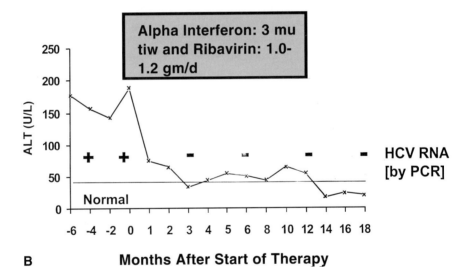

B

FIGURE 4 Six different biochemical and virological patterns of response to a 12-month course of interferon-α (3 MU three times weekly) and ribavirin (1.0–1.2 g/day) in chronic hepatitis C. (A) A typical sustained virological response with loss of HCV RNA and fall of alanine aminotransferase (ALT) levels to normal within a few months of starting therapy and absence of detectable HCV RNA during follow-up. (B) An atypical sustained virological response with loss of HCV RNA but persistence of abnormal ALT levels during therapy and fall of ALT levels to normal and persistent absence of HCV RNA during follow-up. (C) Transient virological and biochemical response with relapse after therapy. (D) Virological and biochemical nonresponse to therapy with a slight decrease in serum ALT levels but persistence of HCV RNA in serum during and after therapy. (E) Virological nonresponse to therapy with transient biochemical response but relapse after therapy. (F) Virological response to therapy intially with a breakthrough after 8 months and reappearance of HCV RNA and elevations in aminotransferase levels.

(continued)

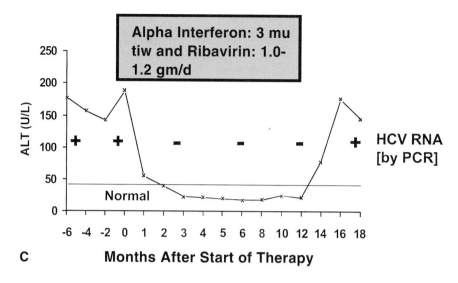

C

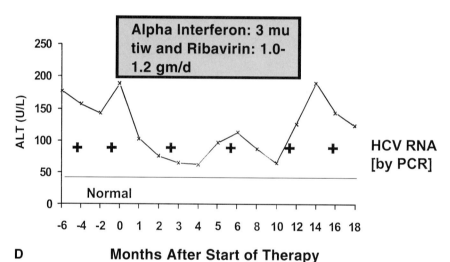

D

FIGURE 4—*Continued*

continue to have some elevation in serum aminotransferase levels during therapy, which generally rise to pretreatment levels once therapy is stopped (Fig. 4E). A final pattern is an initial response and then breakthrough with reappearance of HCV RNA in the serum, generally followed by a rise in serum aminotransferase levels (Fig. 4F).

Early Discontinuation of Therapy

Data from the large trials of combination therapy for chronic hepatitis C also provided important information about early discontinuation of therapy in patients who do not achieve a virological response. In both large trials, at least 98% of patients who had a sustained virological response became HCV RNA negative by 6 months of treatment. (8) Indeed, most patients with a sustained response became HCV RNA negative quite rapidly on therapy.

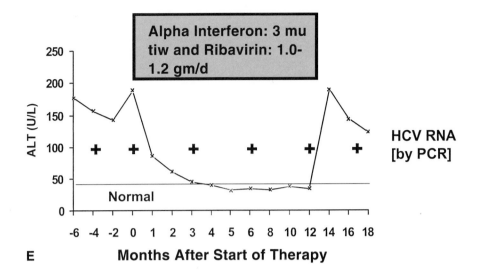

E

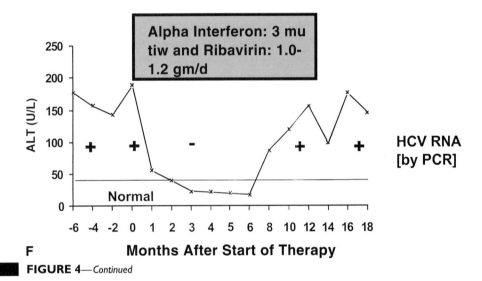

F

FIGURE 4—*Continued*

Many unresolved issues regarding the combination of interferon and riba-virin remain, including the optimal duration of therapy, the optimal dose of riba-virin, where sustained responses are maintained long term, whether predictors of response are reliable clinically, and which subsets of patients may benefit from different or "tailored" treatment regimens.

TREATMENT OF PATIENTS WHO HAVE RELAPSED

Definition of Relapse

Patients who have relapsed following interferon monotherapy represent a dis-tinct challenge for management and for further therapy. (44) As treatment mo-dalities improve and relapse becomes less frequent, this group should decrease in size. Virological relapse is defined as the loss of detectable serum HCV RNA by the end of treatment but subsequent reappearance of the viral marker after therapy is stopped. (14) In most patients, virological relapse occurs within 1 to 2 months of stopping therapy, but relapse can occur at 4 or 6 months (rarely thereafter). Biochemical relapse is defined as a fall of serum ALT levels into the normal range during and at the end of therapy, with a subsequent rise in values when therapy is stopped. Virtually all patients with a biochemical relapse also suffer virological relapse. However, some patients with a virological relapse continue to have normal serum aminotransferase levels for months to years following interferon or combination therapy. Long-term follow-up on these patients usually shows that they ultimately suffer a biochemical relapse with rises in serum ALT levels to pretreatment values. Most episodes of relapse are detected by laboratory testing and are without clinical symptoms.

Retreatment with Interferon-α

Retreatment of patients who relapsed after a previous course of interferon using the same dose or duration of interferon (such as 3 MU three times weekly for 6 months) is largely ineffective. (44–46) Increasing the dose of interferon for a 6-month period appears to be less beneficial than extending the duration of the second course to 12 or more months as defined by a sustained virological response after retreatment. (44) Several studies have compared retreatment with different regimens, doses, and forms of interferon and also indicate the beneficial effect of extending the duration of retreatment. (45)

With 12 months of retreatment with interferon-α (with or without higher doses) the reported sustained biochemical or virological response rates have ranged widely, between 20 and 58%. (44,46) A recent meta-analysis (to overcome the heterogeneity of the study populations, treatments, and response criteria) indicated that 38% of patients who relapsed after a 6-month course of treatment could achieve sustained virological remission with a 12-month course of retreatment with interferon monotherapy. (44) Sustained viral eradication in this situation occurs almost exclusively in patients who have cleared virus during the first course of therapy (irrespective of their original biochemical response). Thus, the most important predictor of a beneficial outcome to retreatment is transient viral eradication during the first course of therapy.

Retreatment with Combination Therapy

Retreatment of the patient who has relapsed using the combination of interferon and ribavirin has been evaluated in a randomized controlled trial of 350 patients. (45) The sustained virological response rate in patients who were retreated with a 24-week course of interferon and ribavirin was 49%, which was 10-fold greater than the 5% response rate to a 24-week course of retreatment with interferon alone. The combination of interferon and ribavirin for the treatment of relapsed patients with hepatitis C was approved for use in the United States in 1998 and subsequently in Europe. A hierarchal response to the com-

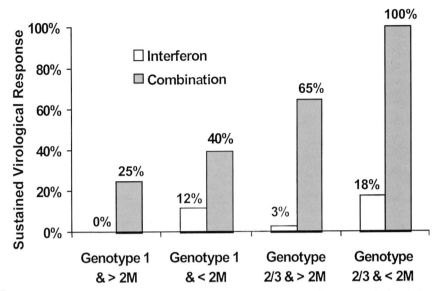

FIGURE 5 Sustained virological response rates after retreatment of patients with chronic hepatitis C who had previously responded to a course of interferon-α monotherapy and then relapsed. Patients received another course of interferon-α alone or combination therapy with interferon and ribavirin for 24 weeks. Results are according to HCV genotype and pretreatment viral level (≥ 2 million versus < 2 million copies/ml). In all categories of patients, combination therapy yielded higher response rates. The lowest rates of response to retreatment occurred in patients with genotype 1 and high levels of HCV RNA and the highest rates in patients with genotype 2 or 3 and low levels of HCV RNA.

bination of drugs was noted when the results were analyzed according to genotype and pretreatment viral RNA levels (Fig. 5).

The study of combination therapy for patients who had relapsed did not include a comparison of 24 to 48 weeks of treatment. However, the relapse rate among patients with genotype 1 with combination therapy in that study was high, averaging 40% overall. For this reason, it may be prudent to treat patients with genotype 1 and high levels of HCV RNA who have relapsed after a previous course of interferon with a full 48-week course of combination therapy—the regimen recommended for initial therapy of patients with chronic hepatitis C. A recent trial published in preliminary form has confirmed the usefulness of 48 weeks of therapy in relapsed patients with genotype 1 and high levels of HCV RNA. (47)

Thus, there are two clinically useful options for the retreatment of the patient who has relapsed following interferon monotherapy: either 24 weeks of combination therapy with interferon and ribavirin or 12 months of therapy with higher doses of interferon (e.g., 15 mcg of consensus interferon three times weekly). The response achieved with these two forms of therapy is similar (Table VI). Consideration should be given to these options for the patient who has relapsed, although these studies are different and cannot be compared directly.

Cost-effective analyses for retreatment of relapse indicate acceptable findings in terms of the cost per quality adjusted life years for both these options. The costs incurred are comparable with other acceptable medical interventions.

■ TABLE VI Comparison of Treatment Regimens for Interferon Relapse[a]

	Consensus interferon	Interferon-α2b and ribavirin
Author	Heathcote (46)	Davis (45)
Year	1998	1998
No. patients	33	173
Trial design	Retreatment	Randomized
Type of relapse	Biochemical	Virological
Therapy duration	48 weeks	24 weeks
Sustained virologic response	58%	49%
p value	0.02	<0.001
Dose reduction	33%	12–20%
Discontinuation	10%	6–8%
Cost (U.S. dollars)[b]	8–12,000	9–12,000

[a] Adapted from Davis et al. (45) and Heathcote et al. (46)
[b] Significance value compared to other treatment modalities in each trial.

TREATMENT OF PATIENTS WHO HAVE FAILED TO RESPOND

Definition of a Nonresponse to Antiviral Therapy

Patients who have failed to respond to a course of interferon-α represent a large group of patients, which is likely to expand with the addition of patients who have failed to respond to a course of combination therapy. Despite multiple studies performed in nonresponder patients, reliable and effective therapy does not exist for this heterogeneous and difficult-to-treat group. Nonresponse can be defined based on either HCV RNA or serum aminotransferase testing; differences between virological and biochemical nonresponse, however, are quite important. (14) A virological nonresponse is defined by the continued presence of HCV RNA in serum, despite an adequate dose and regimen of interferon therapy (such as 3 million units three times weekly for three months). Patients with a documented virological lack of response to interferon generally fail to respond to retreatment. (44) In contrast, a biochemical nonresponse is defined by continued abnormalities in serum aminotransferase levels during an adequate course of interferon. Some of these patients have a virological response, despite the abnormalities in serum aminotransferase levels, and thus are more similar to relapsed patients rather than nonresponders when retreated with interferon or combination therapy. Because HCV RNA testing has only recently become widely available, virological responses to therapy in patients treated in the past may not been known. Furthermore, inclusion of patients in clinical trials of retreatment who were nonresponders as defined biochemically may account for widely varying rates of response to interferon alone and combination therapy. (45,46) Thus, a nonresponse should now be defined by testing for HCV RNA and not solely by lack of changes in serum aminotransferase levels.

Retreatment of Nonresponders with Interferon-α

Many studies have approached the retreatment of nonresponder patients by attempting to optimize interferon therapy by using a higher, fixed dose regimen or

TABLE VII   Therapeutic Approaches for Interferon Nonresponse (30)

Approach	Category	ETR[a,b]	SR[c]
Fixed dose interferon		No	No
Extended duration		No	No
Induction		↑	No
IFN combined with			
NSAIDs		↑	No
Ursodeoxycholic acid		↑	No
Pentoxifylline		↑	No
Corticosteroids		No	No
Cyclosporine		↑	?
Quinolone		↑	No
Phlebotomy		↑	No

[a] End of treatment response rate.
[b] No indicates that the end of treatment or the sustained response rate was not increased compared to conventional interferon monotherapy. An arrow indicates an increase in response rate compared to published studies.
[c] Sustained response rate.

induction regimens, extending the duration of therapy, or combining interferon with ancillary agents such as ursodeoxycholic acid or corticosteroids or with iron depletion (Table VII). (30,44) These approaches have been largely unsuccessful, particularly in patients who are documented virological nonresponders.

The impact of using different forms of interferon and different regimens of treatment in patients who have previously failed to respond to interferon monotherapy is difficult to assess. Prior meta-analyses indicate that higher interferon doses may be of limited benefit. However, published results have varied; some trials of higher doses of interferon monotherapy have suggested an improvement in response rates, whereas others have not. (27,48) Theoretically, patients with genotype 1 and high viral levels might benefit from higher doses of interferon, but the documentation of such a benefit has been poor. Use of higher doses of interferon or induction regimens may lead to higher initial or end-of-treatment responses, but rarely result in sustained virological responses. Cost-effective analysis and further evaluation of the side effects, response rate, and efficacy of higher doses of interferon in previous nonresponders are needed.

Several studies have suggested that patients who do not respond to interferon may, nevertheless, have histological benefit, despite a continued presence of HCV RNA and elevations in serum aminotransferase levels. (49,50) The degree of histological improvement is less than occurs in patients with a sustained virological response and is mostly in the degree of liver inflammation and hepatocellular necrosis. These histological improvements may correlate with the magnitude of reduction in serum HCV RNA. (50) At issue is whether these improvements are clinically significant and whether they are sustained long term after interferon is stopped. However, these findings and the demonstration that interferon has antifibrotic activity in animal models of liver disease suggest that long-term, continuous or "maintenance" interferon-α therapy may be of benefit for patients who are virological nonresponders or who relapse repeatedly after courses of therapy. This hypothesis is now the focus of a large, multicenter trial of long-term interferon therapy in patients with chronic hepatitis C and significant hepatic fibrosis who have failed to have a virological response to optimal combination therapy.

Retreatment of Nonresponders with Combination Therapy

The utility of combination therapy using interferon and ribavirin for the patient who has not responded to interferon monotherapy is unknown. There are several studies in progress in this patient population, but the results to date have been sketchy and somewhat disappointing, with response rates varying between 5 to 25%. (51,52) An important shortcoming of many of these studies is the variability in the definition of nonresponse, whether biochemical, virological, or both. More complete data from these studies and possibly meta-analyses are needed before recommendations can be made regarding the effectiveness of combination therapy in the interferon nonresponder.

Because the end-of-treatment virological response rate is higher with combination therapy (approximately 50%) than with interferon monotherapy (29%), (5,6) it is probable that a proportion of patients who do not respond to interferon alone will respond to the combination at least transiently and this proportion should be between 25 and 30%, of whom approximately half should achieve a sustained response. Thus, a sustained response rate of 10 to 15% might be expected in treated patients who failed to respond to interferon alone using combination therapy. (51,52) The reliability of these calculations from studies on interferon-naïve patients and the durability of these responses need to be confirmed in prospective studies.

At least half of patients treated with the combination of interferon-α and ribavirin do not become HCV RNA negative on treatment and can be categorized as nonresponders to combination therapy. The role of retreatment and the use of other approaches in this growing group of patients has not been addressed in prospective clinical trials. Retreatment with the same regimen of interferon and ribavirin is probably inadvisable. Use of higher induction or fixed doses of interferon in combination with ribavirin is of unknown efficacy and should be avoided outside of clinical research trials. In addition, the role of continuous, long-term interferon therapy or use of long-term ribavirin in nonresponders is uncertain and is now the focus of controlled clinical studies. At present there is little to advise for such patients other than monitoring and awaiting further developments in therapy of this disease.

TREATMENT OF PATIENTS WITH NORMAL ALT VALUES

Both cross-sectional and longitudinal natural history studies indicate that at least 25% of patients with chronic hepatitis C have persistently normal aminotransferase levels, despite the presence of HCV RNA in serum. (53–56) Histological assessment in these patients has generally indicated mild liver disease with minimal inflammation, and rarely cirrhosis or fibrosis. (10) Patients with

███ **TABLE VIII** Sustained Virological Response Rates to Interferon Therapy in Patients with Normal or Near-Normal Alanine Aminotransferase Levels

Author	No.	No. with sustained virological response	No. developing abnormal ALT levels
Serfaty et al. (57)	10	0 (0%)	6 (60%)
Ideo et al. (58)	8	2 (25%)	6 (75%)
Areias et al. (59)	14	3 (21%)	Not reported
Silverman et al. (60)	15	0 (0%)	7 (47%)
Nordoy et al. (61)	23	2 (9%)	7 (30%)
Rossini et al. (62)	10	2 (20%)	5 (50%)
Orito et al. (63)	16	6 (38%)	10 (63%)
Sangiovanni et al. (64)	16	0 (0%)	6 (38%)
Total	112	15 (13%)	47 (42%)

normal ALT levels who have cirrhosis on liver biopsy often have abnormalities of other liver tests, such as elevations in aspartate aminotransferase (AST), and γ-glutamyl transpeptidase (GGT) or decreases in serum albumin or platelet counts. Thus, a careful definition should be used for patients with normal aminotransferases with documentation that both ALT and AST values are normal on multiple occasions. Using these criteria to define this group of patients, the natural history of disease is believed to be slowly, if at all, progressive and the benefits of therapy to be somewhat limited.

Patients with normal aminotransferase levels have been excluded from most large trials of antiviral therapy. Several small trials of therapy have been conducted in these patients using various formulations and regimens of interferon-α and different definitions of normal aminotransferase levels (Table VIII). (56–64) The rate of sustained virological responses in these trials ranges from 0 to 38% and averages 13%, which is similar to that rate reported with a 6-month course of interferon alone among patients with ALT elevations. Importantly, a proportion of patients with normal ALT levels who are treated with interferon-α have developed *de novo* abnormalities of aminotransferase levels during treatment, and in some cases these abnormalities have persisted during follow-up evaluation. There have been no studies reported on the combination of interferon-α and ribavirin in patients with normal serum aminotransferase levels.

Thus, at present, there is little rationale to treat patients with normal serum aminotransferase levels. (56) Further studies are warranted in these patients, particularly as safer and more effective therapies become available.

OTHER SPECIAL POPULATIONS FOR TREATMENT

Most studies of antiviral therapy of hepatitis C have been conducted in typical patients who are adults and who are highly motivated and have well-compensated liver disease without other diseases or comorbidities. The relative risks and benefits of therapy among persons who do not fit the usual profile are unclear. Many of these situations are discussed in other chapters. Such populations include children (Chapter 20); the elderly; patients with decompensated cirrhosis (Chapter 12); persons in prison, in institutions, or on public assistance; persons actively using illicit injection drugs or abusing alcohol; persons on methadone; patients with renal disease (Chapter 17) or cancer; patients receiving immunosuppressive drugs or with immune deficiencies; patients after bone marrow or solid organ transplantation (Chapters 17 and 14); and patients with HIV coinfection (Chapter 16). At present, the optimal therapy of hepatitis C is difficult to tolerate and is a major challenge to medical, personal, and financial resources. Therapeutic options for these special populations are limited and must await improvements in treatment regimens before they can be widely applicable.

NONSPECIFIC RECOMMENDATIONS IN MANAGEMENT

Both the National Institutes of Health and the European Consensus Conference panels made several nonspecific recommendations for the management of chronic hepatitis C. (7,8) Patients should be advised about the nature of the disease, its mode of spread, and natural history. Patients with chronic hepatitis C should not attempt to donate blood, cells, or tissue and should inform health care workers of their status when they undergo invasive procedures. Also, hepatitis C is rarely transmitted sexually, particularly in the situation of a monogamous relationship, and no change in monogamous sexual behavior is recommended. As for all persons, safe sex practices are recommended for patients who have multiple sexual partners and in high-risk situations. Patients with chronic hepatitis C are best advised to avoid use of alcoholic beverages for other than ceremonial purposes. Use of more than one alcoholic drink per day should be strongly discouraged. Patients found to have iron overload should undergo phlebotomy (see Chapter 22). Vaccination against hepatitis A is recommended for all patients with hepatitis C. Hepatitis B vaccination is recommended if patients belong to a high-risk group.

SIDE EFFECTS OF THERAPY

Interferon Monotherapy

Common Side Effects of Interferon

Commonly experienced side effects with interferon monotherapy are listed in Table IX. (65–68) Between 6 and 10 hr after the initial injection of interferon, most patients develop an acute, influenza-like response with fever, chills, headache, muscle aches, and fatigue. Anorexia, nausea, and diarrhea can also occur. This response is much less severe with the second and third injection, after which only a low-grade fever, chilliness, and mild body aches may occur. With continued interferon therapy, chronic side effects appear, including fatigue, muscle and headaches, diarrhea, nausea, weight loss, weakness, difficulty sleeping, difficulty concentrating, irritability, anxiety, and depression. These side effects are usually intermittent, are worse the day following interferon injection, and are somewhat unpredictable. The number and severity of side effects of in-

▆▆▆ **TABLE IX**   **Major Side Effects of Therapy for Hepatitis C**

Side effects[a]	Interferon	Ribavirin
Common	Fever and chills, fatigue, weakness, nausea, and anorexia	Hemolysis and decrease in hemoglobin/hematocrit
	Difficulty sleeping or difficulty concentrating	Pruritis or rash
	Irritability, anxiety, emotionality, depression, or difficulty concentrating	Fatigue and weakness
	Headaches, muscle aches, backache	Gastrointestinal upset
	Bone marrow suppression: anemia, thrombocytopenia, neutopenia	Nasal stuffiness, cough, or sore throat
More serious	Acute psychosis, disorientation, coma	Symptomatic anemia
	Relapse in alcohol or illicit drug abuse	Angina pectoris
	Depression and suicide	Myocardial infarction
	Induction of autoimmune disease	Cerebrovascular accident
	Thyroid dysfunction	Acute gout
	Vision or hearing loss	Gallstones
	Seizures	Fetal loss
	Acute kidney or heart failure	Fetal abnormalities
	Bacterial infections, pneumonitis	

[a] Common side effects are expected to occur in at least 5% of patients. Serious side effects occur in 1 to 2% of patients treated.

terferon vary greatly from patient to patient, and there are no clear factors that predict the severity of side effects. Side effects appear to be less in children and greater in the elderly. Healthy, physically fit and active patients tend to tolerate treatment better than those with comorbid conditions. Some patients report that side effects are less if interferon is administered in the evening. Most side effects are dose dependent and do not require discontinuation of therapy. (26,65) Eighty-five to 90% of patients can usually complete a standard 12-month course of interferon monotherapy. (5,6)

Frequency of Side Effects with Different Forms of Interferon

Different forms of interferon-α and -β appear to have similar and comparable side effect profiles. (22–24) Treatment with higher doses of interferon (daily or every other day) are usually associated with more frequent side effects and higher rates of discontinuation of therapy. (15,29,46) Whether the newer long-acting forms of interferon (see later) may have an improved side effect profile compared to equivalent doses of standard interferon monotherapy requires future evaluation, but any potential reduction in adverse events may be of benefit to patients.

Bone Marrow Suppression

Interferon-α is mildly myelosuppressive and decreases in peripheral blood counts occur in almost all patients. Typically, hemoglobin decreases minimally (less than 1 g/dl) and usually only after several months of treatment. In contrast, white blood cells decrease within 1 to 2 weeks of starting treatment and the absolute neutrophil count usually falls by 25 to 40%. The platelet count decreases

**TABLE X   Rate of Dose Reductions and Discontinuations
with Antiviral Therapy**[a]

	Interferon alone		Interferon and ribavirin	
	24 weeks	48 weeks	24 weeks	48 weeks
Discontinuation	9%	14%	8%	21%
Dose reductions				
Anemia	0%	0%	7%	9%
Other adverse events	12%	9%	13%	17%

[a] Adapted from McHutchison et al. (5)

more slowly than the white count, reaching a nadir of 25 to 40% of baseline values after 3 to 4 weeks of treatment. These decreases are usually not clinically significant and rarely require dose adjustment.

Serious Adverse Events

Serious side effects of interferon-α develop in 1 to 2% of treated patients (Table IX). The most common severe adverse events are thyroid disease and induction of autoimmune conditions. Between 10 and 25% of patients treated for 6 months with interferon-α develop autoantibodies, but only a small proportion of these develop a clinically apparent autoimmune disease. (68,69) The most common autoimmune condition induced by interferon therapy is thyroiditis. Careful monitoring shows that thyroid disturbances occur commonly before and during treatment (7 to 15%) and may be predicted by the presence of anti-TPO antibodies. (69,70) These abnormalities are usually short-lived but they can lead to need for chronic thyroid hormone replacement therapy. Frank thyrotoxicosis occurs less commonly during interferon therapy but is more likely to require discontinuation of treatment. (68,69) Other autoimmune conditions that can be induced by interferon therapy include hemolytic anemia, thrombocytopenic purpura, seronegative arthritis, a systemic-lupus-like syndrome, psoriasis, diabetes, and lichen planus. (66)

Exacerbation of Liver Disease by Interferon

A rare but clearly defined complication of interferon-α therapy of hepatitis C is a paradoxical worsening of the liver disease with therapy. (71,72) In most instances, this has been attributed to an induction of autoimmune hepatitis in a susceptible patient. Thus, most patients who have developed this complication had autoantibodies before therapy or developed high levels of antinuclear (ANA) or liver–kidney membrane (anti-LKM) antibodies during treatment. The liver disease improved with stopping therapy in most patients, but some have required corticosteroid therapy for variable periods. Patients with chronic hepatitis C who develop worsening of the liver disease on interferon (increase in ALT levels above twice the baseline values, particularly if accompanied by jaundice) should have therapy stopped and be evaluated for the possibility of an autoimmune form of hepatitis.

Psychiatric Side Effects

Psychiatric side effects are common with interferon therapy and are important to monitor and manage prospectively. Suicide has been reported during interferon therapy, seemingly the result of depression caused by the treatment. (73) Preexisting depression has been found to be common among patients with chronic hepatitis C enrolled in clinical trials of therapy and is often exacerbated by interferon therapy. (65,70) Thus, a history of depression or attempted suicide should be sought in patients being considered for therapy. Preevaluation by a psychiatrist and active management during therapy is warranted for patients who have a history of depression or significant psychiatric illness. Patients with severe psychiatric disease, neurological illness, or bipolar illness should not be treated with interferon-α without extreme caution and supervision as these patients appear to be susceptible to severe neuropsychiatric side effects of acute psychosis, confusion, encephalopathy, and coma. (65)

The most common psychiatric side effects of interferon-α therapy fall into three distinct patterns, characterized by irritability, emotionality, or depression. (65) These side effects usually appear after 1 to 2 months of treatment. Most common is gradually increasing irritability, anxiety, lack of tolerance of stress, and episodic loss of temper and self-control. Marital and job difficulties can result. In the second pattern, patients develop increased emotionality, with tearfulness and inability to tolerate emotional situations. Finally, frank sadness and depression can occur and result in loss of interest in work and daily activities and suicidal ideation. These psychological side effects usually respond to dose reduction, but are also the major reason for early discontinuation of therapy. These psychiatric problems induced by interferon are usually not predictable on the basis of pretreatment personality or psychiatric history. (65,73)

Uncommon Severe Adverse Side Effects

Other severe side effects of interferon-α include seizures, acute psychosis, confusion, coma, bacterial infections, pneumonitis, acute renal failure, acute congestive heart failure, and visual or hearing disturbances. Careful ophthalmologic evaluation of patients during interferon therapy often reveals the transient development of retinal hemorrhages and "cotton wool" spots. Instances of acute visual or hearing loss and tinnitus have been reported. These side effects appear to be more common in patients with predisposing factors, such as diabetes and hypertension.

Combination Therapy

With combination therapy, side effects are not only more common, but also more severe and more difficult to manage. Ribavirin, by itself, induces a dose-dependent red cell hemolysis and can be associated with nasal stuffiness, cough, pruritis, and skin rash. (33–36) Most of these side effects are minor and not dose limiting, but can complicate combination therapy, particularly when treatment lasts for 48 weeks.

Hemolytic Anemia

Almost all patients who receive ribavirin develop some degree of hemolysis, and 7 to 10% of treated patients develop a significant anemia. Overall, the average decrease in hemoglobin during a 24-week course of combination therapy is 2.5 to 3.0 g/dl. The fall in hemoglobin starts between weeks 2 and 3 and reaches a nadir at 6 to 8 weeks of treatment. The natural reticulocytosis of the hemolytic anemia induced by ribavirin is partially blocked by the myelosuppressive effects of interferon. (5,6) Patients have a 25% chance of a 4-g/dl or greater reduction in hemoglobulin during therapy. This degree of hemolysis dictates that patients with preexisting anemia or hemolysis, coronary artery disease, cerebrovascular disease, or those unable to tolerate anemia should not receive ribavirin in combination with interferon. The hemolysis also results in increases in iron deposition to organs of the body, particularly if therapy is prolonged. (74) Cases of biliary calculi perhaps due to the chronic hemolysis have been reported when ribavirin has been used for more than a year. (36) On completion of therapy, hemoglobin values return to baseline within 4 to 8 weeks. Dose reductions of ribavirin to 600 mg per day are recommended for patients whose hemoglobin values fall to less than 10 g/dl. This dose reduction usually leads to an increase of hemoglobin of 1.0 to 1.5 g/dl, which then stabilizes throughout therapy.

Nasal Congestion

Nasal stuffiness, cough, and shortness of breath occur in approximately 20% of patients receiving interferon and ribavirin. (34) The degree and severity of these symptoms do not correlate with the severity of anemia. The cough is usually dry, and chest X-ray is normal. Rash and pruritis occur in 10 to 20% of patients but are usually mild and rarely severe. Instances of photosensitivity have been reported in patients on ribavirin for hepatitis C.

Side Effects That Are Worse with Combination Therapy

When given in combination, ribavirin and interferon have side effect profiles that resemble addition of the side effects of both alone, suggesting that there is no actual synergism. (5,6) The exception to this is anemia, where the bone marrow suppressive activity of interferon may block the usual reticulocytosis in response to the hemolysis caused by ribavirin. The total side effects of combination therapy are greater than occurs with interferon alone, and the drop out rate and discontinuation rate of therapy with the combination are as high as 20% when the combination is given for 48 weeks (Table X).

Management of Side Effects of Interferon with or without Ribavirin

Most side effects of interferon and ribavirin are mild to moderate in severity and disappear rapidly when therapy is stopped. Because treatment is typically for 24 to 48 weeks, side effects of treatment may require intervention beyond counseling and encouragement. The major side effects that may require specific treatment or dose modification are irritability and depression, itching and rash, nasal congestion and cough, anemia, neutropenia, and thrombocytopenia. In recommending dose modification, it is important to separate side effects due to interferon from those due to ribavirin.

Psychiatric Side Effects

As many as a third of patients treated with interferon-α develop significant psychiatric symptoms, typically irritability, anxiety, emotionality or depression.

These side effects do not appear to be worse with combination therapy. Rare patients develop acute psychosis or severe anxiety or paranoia. These severe reactions are uncommon in patients without preexisting conditions, such as previous psychosis or neurological impairment. In some instances, the side effects become tolerable with a decrease in interferon dosage, such as to 2 million units three times weekly, but typically symptoms eventually recur. In some patients, specific therapy with a serotonin reuptake inhibitor (SRI) is helpful in ameliorating the depression, anxiety, and irritability associated with therapy. These drugs can be discontinued once interferon is stopped. In instances of severe irritability and difficulty concentrating, methylphenidate has been used. (65) If psychiatric symptoms are severe, interferon should be discontinued.

Sleep disturbance is also mentioned frequently as a side effect of combination therapy. In some cases, administration of the interferon in the evening causes anxiety and wakefulness and switching to giving the injections in the morning or early afternoon may be necessary. At times, the judicious use of short-acting benzodiazepines is needed.

Relapse in alcohol or drug abuse can occur during interferon therapy, perhaps as a result of the symptoms of irritability and depression. Patients with a history of recent alcohol or drug abuse should participate in active substance abuse programs during interferon therapy and receive specific counseling aimed at prevention of relapse.

With instruction, education, nursing assistance, and careful monitoring, most patients who develop the psychological side effects of interferon can complete therapy. A sympathetic, unhurried approach and use of local support groups are helpful.

Itching and Rash

Itching with or without skin rash occurs in 15 to 20% of patients receiving ribavirin. The cause may be due to a histamine-like effect of this nucleoside analogue. Accordingly, antihistamines can be helpful in managing this side effect.

Rashes are common with both interferon and ribavirin therapy. Ribavirin may also cause photosensitivity and patients should be warned against excessive sun exposure. Similarly, interferon can exacerbate psoriasis and lichen planus, which may require additional attention and therapy during the 24- or 48-week course of antiviral therapy.

Nasal Stuffiness and Cough

A myriad of upper respiratory symptoms occur commonly among patients receiving a 24- or 48-week course of interferon-α and ribavirin. Patients may believe that they are suffering from repeated "colds," ear aches, or worsening of sinus infections or asthma. Antihistamines may be helpful in these situations, but occasionally antibiotic use is needed. Rarely dose reduction or discontinuation of ribavirin is required.

Anemia

Red cell hemolysis occurs in almost all patients receiving ribavirin and is usually mild, transient, and not associated with symptoms. A fall of hemoglobin to less than 10 g/dl should trigger temporary withdrawal of ribavirin with reintroduction at a reduced dose once the hemoglobin rises above this level.

Typically, the dose reduction is by 200 mg per day. If severe anemia persists, despite reduction of dose to 600 mg per day, ribavirin should be stopped.

Neutropenia

Interferon-α has myelosuppressive actions, and neutrophils usually decrease by 25 to 40% during therapy. In contrast, ribavirin has little effect on neutrophil counts but can reduce lymphocytes by 10 to 20%. These decreases are generally mild and not clinically important. However, neutrophil counts can fall to less than 500 cells/μl in patients with preexisting neutropenia or bone marrow compromise. An important consideration is the constitutional neutropenia that occurs in at least one-third of Africans and African-Americans. In these patients, neutrophil counts of 500 to 750 cells/μl can be tolerated without apparent complications. Thus, reduction in white blood cell counts during treatment rarely necessitates a reduction in interferon dosage or early discontinuation of therapy.

Bacterial Infections

Independent of its effects on peripheral neutrophil counts, interferon-α appears to increase susceptibility to bacterial infections, particularly in patients with predisposing factors, such as ascites, chronic bronchitis and emphysema, recurrent urinary tract infections, or recurrent sinusitis. Development of fever at any time during the initial few days of a course of interferon or combination therapy should be evaluated rapidly and antibiotics started if there is any evidence of bacterial infection. In contrast, there appears to be little increased risk of viral, fungal, or mycobacterial infections during interferon therapy. Prophylactic antibiotics may be indicated in patients with a history of severe, recurrent bacterial infections who require interferon therapy.

Thrombocytopenia

Interferon-α therapy leads to a 25 to 40% decrease in platelet counts that starts within a few days and is maximal after 4 to 6 weeks of therapy. Interestingly, the decrease in platelet counts is slightly less with combination therapy (the hemolysis induced by ribavirin may stimulate platelet production). In most instances, the decrease in platelets is not clinically significant and dose reductions are rarely needed. Patients with preexisting thrombocytopenia ($< 75,000$/ml) have been treated with few adverse events, as long as platelet counts remain above 30,000/ml. If platelet counts fall by more than 50% of baseline, the possibility of autoimmune thrombocytopenic purpura should be considered and interferon-α stopped.

General Measures Helpful in Management of Side Effects

Side effects are common with combination therapy and are best managed by open and thorough discussion before therapy with both the patient and family members and monitoring and encouragement during therapy. Administration of the interferon in the evening is often helpful so that the major early side effects occur at night when the patient is at home and can rest. Attention to hydration and having adequate periods of sleep and rest are helpful. Regular physical activity should be encouraged. Patient support groups are very valuable in helping patients complete therapy.

Effect on Quality of Life

The vast majority of quality of life assessments studies indicate that some, but not all, patients with chronic hepatitis C perceive themselves to be unwell and the impairment of quality of life is not related to the degree or severity of the liver disease. (18,70) These "perceived" impairments have been shown to improve after successful antiviral therapy, but whether this is due partly to patients knowing that their tests are normal is currently unknown. Quality of life is impaired during therapy, as would be expected by the frequency of side effects, but then returns to near normal levels after a successful response to therapy. Other effects, such as the impact of time lost from work, work capacity, performance, and the effect of therapy on family dynamics, are currently unknown.

PREDICTING RESPONSE TO THERAPY

Predictors of Response to Antiviral Therapy

The cost, adverse event profile, and response rates to therapy all suggest that the ability to predict who will or will not respond to therapy may be clinically useful. Most such evaluations to date have assessed predictive variables in terms of the ability to predict a sustained virological response. Multiple pretreatment variables have been evaluated in numerous studies by both univariate and multivariate analysis (Table XI). (75) None of these pretreatment factors is sufficiently sensitive enough to predict response or lack of response in any individual patient with an acceptable degree of accuracy.

Three-Month Stop Rule with Interferon Monotherapy

Early viral clearance during therapy as a predictor of sustained virological response has been evaluated extensively. (76,77) Different interferon regimens,

TABLE XI Factors Predictive of Response to Therapy

Pretreatment variables[a] (favorable versus unfavorable)

Viral genotype (2 and 3 versus 1)
High HCV RNA levels (less than versus greater than 2 million copies/ml)
Age (younger versus older)
Sex (females versus males)
Race (Caucasians and Asians versus African-Americans)
Fibrosis on liver biopsy (lesser versus higher degrees or cirrhosis)

During treatment variables

Early loss HCV RNA (week 4 versus later)
HCV RNA at week 12 (negative versus positive)
Decrease in HCV RNA levels by 4 to 12 weeks (more than 3 logs versus less)

[a] Identified by univariate and multivariate analyses in multiple studies. Useful to predict response within a given population, but lacking accuracy to allow the prediction of response in any individual patient.

varying sensitivity of HCV RNA assays, and lack of standardization of definitions for response have hampered these studies. Despite these shortcomings, several conclusions are possible. First, the persistence of detectable HCV RNA during the first months of therapy is a better predictor of nonresponse than the early clearance of viral RNA a predictor of a sustained response. Second, the most reliable time points for prediction of a sustained response, as well as a nonresponse, appear to be 12 weeks after starting therapy. The sensitivity in terms of predicting nonresponse is 95–98% and has led to recommendations that therapy be stopped early if HCV RNA remains present after 12 weeks of therapy. Early discontinuation would result in significant cost savings and spare the patient, who is unlikely to achieve a sustained response from the side effects of continued therapy. The futility of continuing interferon monotherapy after 12 weeks in the face of persistence of detectable HCV RNA has been confirmed in studies evaluating 48-week courses of interferon therapy. (76)

Twenty-four-Week Stop Rule with Combination Therapy

The reliability of the 3-month stop rule with interferon monotherapy does not appear to apply to combination therapy. In studies of combination therapy, patients who still had detectable HCV RNA at week 12 had a 7% chance of an eventual sustained virological response. (5,6) In these same studies, late clearance of HCV RNA was not observed with interferon monotherapy. Reanalysis of results from the trials of combination therapy indicated that the persistence of serum HCV RNA at 24 weeks was predictive of a lack of sustained response in 97–98% of cases. On the basis of these results, it is recommended that therapy be discontinued in patients who remain HCV RNA positive after 24 weeks of combination therapy. This rule applies largely to patients with genotype 1 and high initial levels of HCV RNA.

These predictive factors require careful reevaluation with each new therapy and need to be refined further for different subgroups of patients. Ultimately, the use of quantitative tests for HCV RNA may provide more reliable guidance for continuing therapy in the face of persistence of detectable viral RNA or in making adjustments to dose and regimen. At present, however, decisions to discontinue therapy early should be based only on sensitive tests for HCV RNA.

FUTURE THERAPY

Despite significant advances in the therapy of chronic hepatitis C, current therapy is effective in inducing a long-term beneficial response in less than half of patients. Therapy remains costly, is associated frequently with adverse events that can be severe, and is not suitable for all patients. Further progress in antiviral therapy of hepatitis C is needed and is being actively sought.

Of greatest immediate promise as therapy of hepatitis C is the use of newer, long-acting forms of interferon-α. (78,79) The covalent attachment of polyethylene glycol to the interferon molecule produces a product that maintains the biological effects of interferon but has a longer half-life. Pegylated interferons have a slower rate of clearance, more favorable pharmacokinetics, and a longer duration of action. On a theoretical basis, these long-acting formulations might provide a more sustained level of interferon activity and avoid the peaks and troughs of interferon levels that are associated with the three-times weekly regimens and which may account for variability in response rates and frequency of side effects. Several pegylated forms of interferon-α have been developed and are now in phase 2 and 3 clinical trials with and without ribavirin in different cohorts of patients with chronic hepatitis C. Preliminary results demonstrate that a higher proportion of patients become HCV RNA negative during therapy with pegylated interferons than with standard formulations and that sustained virological response rates of 25 to 38% can be obtained. (78,79) In these preliminary trials, the relapse rates after 48 weeks of therapy with pegylated interferon have been 40 to 50%, suggesting that the combination of these formulations with ribavirin may achieve an even higher sustained response rate (by lowering the relapse rate). The safety and efficacy of combinations of pegylated interferons alone and in combination with ribavirin are currently the focus of several large-scale clinical trials in the United States and Europe.

Ultimately, better and safer antiviral agents for hepatitis C are needed (see Chapter 22). The characterization of the HCV genome and elucidation of the structural biology of the protease, helicase, and polymerase of the virus promise to provide a means of rapid development of antiviral agents that alone or in combination with interferon-α will provide effective therapy for the majority of patients with this chronic liver disease. (80–82)

Because of the rapid developments in HCV and antiviral research, recommendations for therapy of chronic hepatitis C are likely to change every 2 or 3 years. Regularly updated, simple and direct recommendations are distributed by the National Institutes of Health ("Chronic Hepatitis C: Current Disease Management") and are available through the internet. (83)

CONCLUSION

Adult patients with chronic hepatitis C who have raised serum aminotransferase levels, HCV RNA in serum, a liver biopsy with fibrosis or moderate-to-severe necroinflammatory changes, are without evidence of hepatic decompensation, and have no contraindications warrant antiviral therapy. The current recommended regimen of therapy is a 24- to 48-week course of interferon-α (3 million units three times weekly) and oral ribavirin (1000 to 1200 mg daily, depending on body weight being less than or greater than 75 kg). The duration of therapy should be 48 weeks for patients with genotype 1 and high levels of HCV RNA (greater than 2 million copies/ml), with the recommendation to stop therapy at 24 weeks if HCV RNA is still present. The duration of therapy should be 24 weeks for all other patients, such as those with genotype 2 or 3 and patients with genotype 1 and low levels of HCV RNA. Long-term sustained response rates (loss of HCV RNA on therapy which persists in follow-up) occur in approximately two-thirds of patients with genotypes 2 and 3 and one-third of patients with genotype 1. Side effects of combination therapy are common but can usually be managed conservatively. A proportion of patients may require ribavirin dose modification or early discontinuation of combination therapy.

Therapy with interferon-α alone should be reserved for patients with contra-indications to ribavirin (patients with anemia or significant renal or cardiac disease). At the present time, children should not receive ribavirin.

For patients who have relapsed following interferon monotherapy, retreatment with interferon and ribavirin for 24 to 48 weeks as described earlier is probably optimal. These patients may respond equally well to a 48-week course of higher doses of interferon monotherapy.

For patients who have not responded to interferon-α or combination therapy, the options are few and unsatisfactory. Only 10 to 15% of patients who have failed to respond to a course of interferon-α alone respond to combination therapy. Other approaches now being evaluated include the use of long-term, continuous interferon or ribavirin alone. Longer acting forms of interferon-α (pegylated interferons) may be more potent than standard interferons and may replace them in treatment regimens in the near future. New innovative therapies are still required for patients who fail to respond to the current optimal therapy, which still represents more than half the patients with chronic hepatitis C.

ACKNOWLEDGMENT

We thank E. Nunez for editing and preparing this chapter.

REFERENCES

1. Alter M J, Kruszon-Moran D, Nainan O V, et al. The prevalence of hepatitis C virus infection in the United States, 1988 through 1994. N Engl J Med 1999;341:556–62.
2. Detre K M, Belle S H, Lombardero M. Liver transplantation for chronic viral hepatitis. Viral Hepatitis Rev 1996;2:219–28.
3. Hoofnagle J H, Mullen K D, Jones D B, et al. Treatment of chronic non-A,non-B hepatitis with recombinant human alpha interferon. A preliminary report. N Engl J Med 1986;315:1575–8.
4. Carithers R L, Emerson S S. Therapy of hepatitis C: meta-analysis of interferon alfa-2b trials. Hepatology 1997;25(Suppl 1):83S–8S.
5. McHutchison J G, Gordon S C, Schiff E R, et al. Interferon alfa-2b alone or in combination with ribavirin as initial treatment for chronic hepatitis C. N Engl J Med 1998;339:1485–92.
6. Poynard T, Marcellin P, Lee S S, et al. Randomised trial of interferon alpha 2b plus ribavirin for 48 weeks or for 24 weeks versus interferon alpha 2b plus placebo for 48 weeks for treatment of chronic infection with hepatitis C virus. Lancet 1998;352:1426–32.
7. National Institutes of Health Consensus Development Conference Panel. Statement: management of hepatitis C. Hepatology 1997;26(Suppl 1):2S–10S.
8. EASL International Consensus Conference on Hepatitis C Panel. Consensus Statement. J Hepatol 1999;30:956–61.
9. Seeff L B. Natural history of hepatitis C. Hepatology 1997;26(Suppl 1):21S–8S.
10. Hoofnagle J H. Hepatitis C: the clinical spectrum of disease. Hepatology 1997;26(Suppl 1):15S–20S.
11. Fattovich G, Giustina G, Degos F, et al. Morbidity and mortality in compensated cirrhosis type C: a retrospective follow-up study of 384 patients. Gastroenterology 1997;112:463–72.
12. Poynard T, Bedossa P, Opolon P. Natural history of liver fibrosis progression in patients with chronic hepatitis C. Lancet 1997;349:825–32.
13. Mathurin P, Moussalli J, Cadranel J F, et al. Slow progression rate of fibrosis in hepatitis C virus patients with persistently normal alanine transaminase activity. Hepatology 1998;27:868–72.
14. Lindsay K L. Therapy of hepatitis C: overview. Hepatology 1997;26(Suppl 1):71S–7S.

15. Marcellin P, Boyer N, Gervais A, et al. Long-term histologic improvement and loss of detectable intrahepatic HCV RNA in patients with chronic hepatitis C and sustained response to interferon-alpha therapy. Ann Intern Med 1997;127:875–81.

16. Lau D T Y, Kleiner D E, Ghany M G, Park Y, Schmid P, Hoofnagle J H. 10-Year follow-up after interferon-alpha therapy for chronic hepatitis C. Hepatology 1998;28:1121–7.

17. Wong J B, Bennett W G, Koff R S, Pauker S G. Pretreatment evaluation of chronic hepatitis C: risks, benefits, and costs. JAMA 1998;280:2088–93.

18. Koff R S. Therapy of hepatitis C: cost-effectiveness analysis. Hepatology 1997;26 (Suppl 1): 152S–5S.

19. Bonkovsky H L, Woolley J M, Consensus Interferon Study Group. Reduction of health-related quality of life in chronic hepatitis C and improvement with interferon therapy. Hepatology 1999;29:264–70.

20. Koff R S. Impaired health-related quality of life in chronic hepatitis C: the how, but not the why. Hepatology 1999;29:277–9.

21. Davis G L, Balart L A, Schiff E R, et al. Treatment of chronic hepatitis C with recombinant alpha-interferon. A multicentre randomized, controlled trial. J Hepatol 1990;11:S31–5.

22. Farrell G C, Bacon B R, Goldin R D. Lymphoblastoid interferon alfa-n1 improves the long-term response to a 6-month course of treatment in chronic hepatitis C compared with recombinant interferon alfa-2b: results of an international randomized controlled trial. Hepatology 1998;27:1121–7.

23. Tong M J, Reddy K R, Lee W M, et al. Treatment or chronic hepatitis C with consensus interferon: a multicenter, randomized, controlled trial. Hepatology 1997;26:747–54.

24. Lee W M. Therapy of hepatitis C: interferon alfa-2a trials. Hepatology 1997;26:(Suppl 1): 89S–95S.

25. Tine F, Magrin S, Craxi A, Pagliaro L. Interferon for non-A, non-B chronic hepatitis. A meta-analysis of randomised clinical trials. J Hepatol 1991;13:192–9.

26. Poynard T, Leroy V, Cohard M, et al. Meta-analysis of interferon randomized trials in the treatment of viral hepatitis C: effects of dose and duration. Hepatology 1996;24:778–89.

27. Poynard T, Bedossa P, Chevallier M, et al. A comparison of three interferon alfa-2b regimens for the long-term treatment of chronic non-A, non-B hepatitis. Multicenter Study Group. N Engl J Med 1995;332:1457–62.

28. Neumann A U, Lam N P, Dahari H, et al. Hepatitis C viral dynamics in vivo and the antiviral efficacy of interferon-alpha therapy. Science 1998;282:103–7.

29. Lam N P, Neumann A U, Gretch D R, Wiley T E, Perelson A S, Layden T J. Dose-dependent acute clearance of hepatitis C genotype 1 virus with interferon alfa. Hepatology 1997;26:226–31.

30. Bonkovsky H L. Therapy of hepatitis C: other options. Hepatology 1997;26 (Suppl 1):152S–5S.

31. Patterson J L, Fernandez-Larsson R. Molecular mechanisms of action of ribavirin. Rev Infect Dis 1990;12:1139–46.

32. Hultgren C, Milich D R, Weiland O, Sallberg M. The antiviral compound ribavirin modulates the T helper (Th) 1/Th2 subset balance in hepatitis B and C virus-specific immune responses. J Gen Virol 1998;79:2381–91.

33. Bodenheimer H C, Lindsay K L, Davis G L, Lewis J H, Thung S N, Seeff L B. Tolerance and efficacy of oral ribavirin treatment of chronic hepatitis C: multicenter trial. Hepatology 1997; 26:473–7.

34. Di Bisceglie A M, Conjeevaram H S, Fried M W, et al. Ribavirin as therapy for chronic hepatitis C: a randomized, double-blind, placebo-controlled trial. Ann Intern Med 1995;123:897–903.

35. Dushieko G M, Mann J, Thomas H, et al. Ribavirin treatment for patients with chronic hepatitis C: results of a placebo-controlled study. J Hepatol 1996;25:591–8.

36. Hoofnagle J H, Lau D, Conjeevaram H, Kleiner D, Di Bisceglie A M. Prolonged therapy of chronic hepatitis C with ribavirin. J Viral Hepatitis 1996;3:247–52.

37. Lai M Y, Kao J H, Yang D M, et al. Long-term efficacy of ribavirin plus interferon alfa in the treatment of chronic hepatitis C. Gastroenterology 1996;111:1307–12.

38. Chemello L, Cavalletto L, Bernardinello E, Guido M, Pontisso P, Alberti A. The effect of interferon alfa and ribavirin combination therapy in naive patients with chronic hepatitis C. J Hepatol 1995;23:8–12.

39. Reichard O, Norkrans G, Fryden A, Braconier J H, Sonnerborg A, Weiland O. Randomised, double-blind, placebo-controlled trial of interferon alpha-2b with and without ribavirin for chronic hepatitis C. Lancet 1998;351:83–7.
40. Gretch D. Diagnostic tests for hepatitis C. Hepatology 1997;26 (Suppl 1):43S–7S.
41. Shiratori Y, Kato N, Yokosuka O, et al. Quantitative assays for hepatitis C virus in serum as predictors of the long-term response to interferon. J Hepatol 1997;27:437–44.
42. Reddy K R, Hoofnagle J H, Tong M J, et al. Racial differences in response to therapy with interferon in chronic hepatitis C. Hepatology 1999;30:787–93.
43. McHutchison J G, Poynard T, Gordon S C, et al. The impact of race on response to anti-viral therapy in patients with chronic hepatitis C. Hepatology 1999;30:302A [abstract].
44. Alberti A, Chemello L, Noventa F, Cavalletto L, De Salvo G. Therapy of hepatitis C: re-treatment with alpha interferon. Hepatology 1997;26(Suppl 1):137S–42S.
45. Davis G L, Esteban-Mur R, Rustgi V, et al. Interferon alfa-2b alone or in combination with ribavirin for the treatment of relapse of chronic hepatitis C. N Engl J Med 1998;339:1493–9.
46. Heathcote E J, Keeffe E B, Lee S S, et al. Re-treatment of chronic hepatitis C with consensus interferon. Hepatology 1998;27:1136–43.
47. Di Marco V, Almasio P L, Vaccaro A, et al. Combined treatment of relapse of chronic hepatitis C with high-dose alfa-2b interferon plus ribavirin for 6 or 12 months. Hepatology 1999;30:303A [abstract].
48. Poynard T, Leroy V, Mathurin P, Cohard M, Opolon P, Zarski J P. Treatment of chronic hepatitis C by interferon for longer duration than six months. Dig Dis Sci 1996;41:99S–102S.
49. Sobesky R, Mathurin P, Charlotte F, et al. Modeling the impact of interferon alfa treatment on liver fibrosis progression in chronic hepatitis C: a dynamic view. Gastroenterology 1999;116:378–86.
50. Shiffman M L, Hofmann C M, Thompson E B, et al. Relationship between biochemical, virological, and histological response during interferon treatment of chronic hepatitis C. Hepatology 1997;26:780–5.
51. Min A D, Jones J L, Lebovics E, et al. Interferon alfa-2b and ribavirin in patients with resistant chronic hepatitis C. Hepatology 1999;30:192A [abstract].
52. Frider B, Findor J A, Perez V, et al. Response to 12-month treatment with interferon alfa-2b plus ribavirin in patients with chronic hepatitis C relapsers or non-reponders to a previous interferon treatment. Hepatology 1999;30:196A [abstract].
53. Alter H J, Congry-Cautilena C, Melpolder J, et al. Hepatitis C in asymptomatic blood donors. Hepatology 1997;26(Suppl 1):29S–33S.
54. Shakil O A, Conry-Cantilena C, Alter H J, et al. Volunteer blood donors with antibodies to hepatitis C virus: clinical, biochemical, virological and histological features. Ann Intern Med 1995;123:330–7.
55. Ryder S D. Progression of liver fibrosis in mild hepatitis C. A prospective paired liver biopsy study. Hepatology 1999;30:316A [abstract].
56. Marcellin P, Levy S, Erlinger S. Therapy of hepatitis C: patients with normal aminotransferase levels. Hepatology 1997;26(Suppl 1):133S–6S.
57. Serfaty L, Chazouillieres O, Pawlotsky J M, Andreani T, Pellet C, Poupon R. Interferon alpha therapy in patients with chronic hepatitis C and persistently normal aminotransferase activity. Gastroenterology 1996;110:291–5.
58. Ideo G, Bellobuono A, Tempini S, Bellati G, Romano L, Zanetti A R. Interferon treatment of chronic hepatitis C patients with normal or near normal alanine aminotransferase levels: might it be harmful rather than useful? Int Hepatol Commun 1996;6:8–15.
59. Areias J, Pedroto I, Freitas T, et al. Hepatitis C virus carriers with normal ALT activity: viremia, genotype and effect of interferon therapy. Gastroenterology 1996;110:A1144.
60. Silverman A L, Piquette E L, Filipiak C L, Neill J S, Bayati N, Gordon S C. Alfa interferon treatment of hepatitis C virus RNA positive patients with normal or near-normal alnine aminotransferase levels. Am J Gastroenterol 1997;92:1783–95.
61. Nordoy I, Krarup H B, Bell H, et al. Interferon-alpha 2b therapy in low-activity hepatitis C: a pilot study. Scand J Gastroenterol 1997;32:1256–60.
62. Rossini A, Ravaggi A, Biasi L, et al. Virological response to interferon treatment in hepatitis C virus carriers with normal aminotransferase levels and chronic hepatitis. Hepatology 1997;26:1012–7.

63. Orito E, Mizokami M, Suzuki K, et al. Interferon-alpha therapy for individuals with normal serum alanine aminotransferase levels before treatment. J Gastroenterol Hepatol 1997;12:58–61.
64. Sangiovanni A, Morales R, Spinzi G, et al. Interferon alfa treatment of HCV RNA carriers with persistently normal transaminase levels: a pilot randomized controlled study. Hepatology 1998;27:853–6.
65. Renault P F, Hoofnagle J H, Park Y, et al. Psychiatric complications of long-term interferon alfa therapy. Arch Intern Med 1987;147:1577–80.
66. Dusheiko G. Side effects of alpha interferon in chronic hepatitis C. Hepatology 1997;26 (Suppl 1):112S–21S.
67. Vinayek R, Shakil A O. Adverse events associated with interferon alfa therapy in patients with chronic viral hepatitis. Viral Hepatitis Rev 1997;3:167–77.
68. Lisker-Melman M, Di Bisceglie A M, Usala S J, Weintraub B, Murray L M, Hoofnagle J H. Development of thyroid disease during therapy of chronic virall hepatitis with interferon alfa. Gastroenterology 1992;102:2155–60.
69. Deutsch M, Dourakis S, Manesis K, et al. Thyroid abnormalities in chronic viral hepatiits and their relationship to interferon alfa therapy. Hepatology 1997;26:206–10.
70. Petrov S. Measurements and application of health-related quality of life in chronic viral hepatitis. Viral Hepatitis Rev 1997;3:253–65.
71. Papo T, Marcellin P, Bernuau J, Durand F, Poynard T, Benhamou J-P. Autoimmune chronic hepatitis exacerbated by alpha-interferon. Ann Intern Med 1992;116:51–3.
72. Shindo M, Di Bisceglie A M, Hoofnagle J H. Acute exacerbation of liver disease during interferon alfa therapy for chronic hepatitis C. Gastroenterology 1992;102:1406–8.
73. Janssen H L A, Brouwer J T, Van der Mast R C, Schalm S W. Suicide associated with alfa-interferon therapy for chronic viral hepatitis. J Hepatol 1994;21:241–3.
74. DiBisceglie A M, Bacon B R, Kleiner D E, Hoofnagle J H. Increase in hepatic iron stores following prolonged therapy with ribavirin in patients with chronic hepatitis C. J Hepatol 1994;21:1109–12.
75. Davis G L. Prediction of response to interferon treatment of chronic hepatitis C. J Hepatol 1994;20:1–3.
76. Gavier B, Martinez-Gonzalez M A, Riezu-Boj J I, et al. Viremia after one month of interferon therapy predicts treatment outcome in patients with chronic hepatitis C. Gastroenterology 1997;113:1647–53.
77. Tong M J, Blatt L M, McHutchison J G, Co R L, Conrad A. Prediction of response during interferon alfa 2b therapy in chronic hepatitis C patients using viral and biochemical characteristics: a comparison. Hepatology 1997;26:1640–5.
78. Shiffman M, Pockros P J, Reddy R K, et al. A controlled, randomized, multicenter, descending dose phase II trial of pegylated interferon alfa-2a vs standard interferon alfa-2a for treatment of chronic hepatitis C. Gastroenterology 1999;116:A1275 [abstract].
79. Heathcote E J, Shiffman M L, Cooksley G, et al. Multinational evaluation of the efficacy and safety of once-weekly peg interferon alfa-2a in patients with chronic hepatitis C with compensated cirrhosis. Hepatology 1999;30:316A [abstract].
80. Kim J L, Morgenstern K A, Lin K A, et al. Crystal strucutre of the hepatitis C virus NS3 protease doman complexed with a synthetic NS4A cofactor peptide. Cell 1996;87:343–55.
81. Love R A, Parge H E, Wickersham J A, et al. The crystal structure of hepatitis C virus NS3 proteinase reveals a trypsin-like fold and a structural zinc-binding site. Cell 1996;87:331–42.
82. Yao N, Hesson T, Cable M, et al. Structure of the hepatitis C virus RNA helicase domain. Nat Struct Biol 1997;4:463–7.
83. Anonymous. Chronic hepatitis C: current disease management. NIDDK Factsheet. Internet site: *www.niddk.nih.gov/health/digest/pubs/chrnhepc/ chrnhepc.htm*

12
HEPATITIS C AND CIRRHOSIS

GIOVANNA FATTOVICH

Servizio Autonomo Clinicizzato di Gastroenterologia
Dipartimento di Scienze Chirurgiche e Gastroenterologiche
Università di Verona, Italy

SOLKO W. SCHALM

Hepatogastroenterology
Erasmus University Hospital Dijkzigt
Rotterdam, The Netherlands

INTRODUCTION

Infection with hepatitis C virus (HCV) affects at least 170 million persons worldwide and is one of the most common causes of cirrhosis and end-stage liver disease. (1) In some areas of the world, more than half of patients presenting with clinical features of cirrhosis have hepatitis C, testing positive for antibody to HCV (anti-HCV) in the absence of evidence of other causes of liver disease. (2, 3) Patients with HCV-related cirrhosis are likely to develop complications such as ascites, jaundice, variceal hemorrhage, hepatic encephalopathy, and hepatocellular carcinoma (HCC). Features predictive of more rapid disease progression include host-related factors such as gender, age, age at infection and virus-related factors such as genotype and viral load, as well as extraneous factors such as source of infection, duration of disease, alcohol consumption, coinfection with other viruses, and as-yet-undefined environmental factors.

The clinical course and long-term prognosis of HCV-related cirrhosis have been the subject of limited longitudinal studies. Major questions about the natural history of hepatitis C include the time required for development of cirrhosis, the incidence of complications, the mortality rate, and the role of host and viral factors in progression. Interferon-α therapy has been reported to prevent or delay progression to HCC in patients with HCV-related cirrhosis independent of the biochemical or virological response to treatment. (4,5) Other studies have shown a benefit of interferon therapy, but only among patients with a long-term remission following treatment. (6) Unfortunately, a sustained response is achieved in a minority of patients with cirrhosis, (7) and the role of interferon therapy in the management of cirrhosis caused by hepatitis C remains controversial.

This chapter will summarize information on the natural history and clinical features of HCV-cirrhosis and review recommendations for management and therapy based upon available information.

PROGRESSION OF HEPATITIS C TO CIRRHOSIS

Rate of Progression

The rate of progression of hepatitis C from acute infection to cirrhosis has been described in several prospective studies on posttransfusion hepatitis. During the first one to two decades of infection, cirrhosis develops in up to 25% of patients. (8–11) In two retrospective analyses, one from Japan (12) and one from the United States, (13) the average time from transfusion to a clinical diagnosis of cirrhosis was 20 years, but the range of values was wide. Examples of rapid progression, with development of cirrhosis within 2 to 5 years of onset of infection have been described, as have examples of slow progression and development of cirrhosis or hepatocellular carcinoma only after 50 years of infection. (9)

Two consensus panel statements published in 1997 provided an estimate that 20 to 25% of patients with hepatitis C develop cirrhosis within the first 20 years of onset of infection. (14,15) Yet in the individual case, predictions are difficult. Findings indicate that the risk of cirrhosis in chronic hepatitis C is partially dependent on the host factors of sex and age at infection. In a study of a large common source outbreak of HCV infection in young women caused by use of HCV-contaminated anti-D immunoglobulin, 376 anti-HCV positive women were identified 17 years after inoculation and underwent medical evaluation and liver biopsy. Only 7 women (2%) had cirrhosis and most were well compensated and asymptomatic. (16) This rate is far lower than the 20 to 25% rate that is usually quoted.

Factors Predictive of Progression of Chronic Hepatitis C to Cirrhosis

In a cross-sectional study of 1157 patients with biopsy-proven chronic hepatitis C for whom the onset of hepatitis C could be dated based upon a history of exposure, factors that were associated with progression to cirrhosis were age at infection of older than 40 years, male sex, and daily alcohol consumption of 50 g or more. (17) The estimated median duration of infection at the time of diagnosis of cirrhosis ranged from as short as 13 years in men infected when they were over age of 40, to as long as 42 years in women who did not drink and were infected before the age of 40 years. Mathematical estimates suggested that only one-third of the patients, typically men who drank alcohol and were infected after the age of 40, would develop cirrhosis within 20 years of onset of infection, and that one-third of patients would not progress to cirrhosis within 50 years of onset.

A separate study conducted on 553 patients with parenterally acquired chronic hepatitis C, including 462 immunocompetent and 91 immunocompromised subjects, confirmed that the variables of age over 40 years at infection and alcohol consumption were independently associated with the development of cirrhosis; in addition, multivariate analysis revealed that a long duration of infection and coinfection with the human immunodeficiency virus (HIV) were also associated with more rapid progression of liver disease. (18)

A number of studies have shown that coinfection with hepatitis B virus (HBV) increases the severity of HCV-related liver disease and promotes histological progression to cirrhosis. (19–21) Similarly, the role of excessive alcohol consumption on disease progression has been confirmed in several studies of hepatitis C. In a retrospective review of liver biopsies from 176 patients with chronic hepatitis C who were stratified for the estimated duration of HCV infection and amount of alcohol consumption (> 40 g/day in women and > 60 g/day in men for > 5 years), the rate of development of cirrhosis was faster in patients who drank excessive amounts of alcohol; 58% being cirrhotic by the second decade as opposed to 10% in the low dose alcohol group. (22)

Overall, these studies have established the importance of host factors (male sex, age above 40 years at infection) and other potentially hepatotoxic exposures (alcohol consumption ≥ 50 g/day and HBV infection) as major risk factors for the occurrence of cirrhosis in HCV-infected patients. Coinfection with HIV also appears to accelerate the progression to cirrhosis, perhaps through modification of host immune factors.

CLINICAL PRESENTATION

Average Age of Onset of HCV-Related Cirrhosis

In several reports on chronic hepatitis C, the age of patients at the time of initial presentation with cirrhosis has averaged 55 years, and men have usually outnumbered women, the male to female ratio ranging from 1.3:1 to 2.3:1. (4,6, 23,24) A consistent finding has been a younger age of presentation among patients with chronic hepatitis C without cirrhosis. In one study, the mean age of patients was 42 years for those without cirrhosis, 55 years for those with cirrhosis, and 66 years for those with hepatocellular carcinoma. (25) In large European collaborative studies on hepatitis C, the average age at the time of diagnosis of compensated cirrhosis was 51 to 60 years and at the time of detection of HCC was 61 to 70 years (Fig. 1). (26,27)

Symptoms of HCV-Related Cirrhosis

Patients with compensated HCV-related cirrhosis typically present with insidious onset of symptoms, such as fatigue, dyspepsia, and upper abdominal discomfort. These symptoms are nonspecific and difficult to measure objectively, factors that make it difficult to determine the prevalence of these symptoms in patients with cirrhosis compared to patients without cirrhosis. Most published studies on the clinical features of chronic hepatitis C have not used validated and standardized means of assessing symptoms and rarely described their frequency. In a European study of 384 patients with compensated cirrhosis due to hepatitis C, only 44% of patients were symptomatic at the time of presentation and diagnosis, and only a minority (16%) were referred to the enrolling center because of these nonspecific symptoms. Symptoms of hepatitis C tend to be mild and are rarely incapacitating, even in the presence of cirrhosis. In many patients with cirrhosis, the diagnosis is made only when elevated aminotransferase levels are discovered on routine blood testing for a health examination or at the time of blood donation. (23) In a cross-section study from the United States

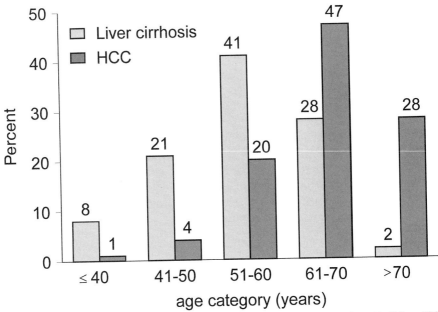

FIGURE I   Age distribution (%) at diagnosis of compensated cirrhosis due to hepatitis C (n = 384) [from EUROHEP] (26) and at diagnosis of HCV-related hepatocellular carcinoma (HCC) (n = 756) (Courtesy of Stroffolini et al., (27) updated)

which included both compensated and decompensated patients, fatigue was the most common symptom (75%), followed by abdominal pain (24%), anorexia (13%), and weight loss (6%). (13) In that study, the frequency and severity of nonspecific symptoms increased with the severity of the cirrhosis.

Physical Examination in HCV-Related Cirrhosis

Hepatomegaly is the most common sign of liver disease in patients newly diagnosed with HCV-related cirrhosis, being detected in 50 to 78% of patients. (13,23,24) Liver firmness is also frequent, being found in 79% of patients with cirrhosis in whom the liver is palpable. (23) Liver firmness is highly predictive for cirrhosis; in a prospective study of 277 patients with chronic liver disease aimed at assessing clinical and noninvasive laboratory features of cirrhosis, liver firmness was an independent predictor of cirrhosis on liver biopsy. (28) Splenomegaly is also common in HCV-related cirrhosis, being detected by physical examination and/or by ultrasonography (spleen > 13 cm in longitudinal diameter) in 25 to 37% of patients. (13,23,24) Peripheral manifestations or stigmata of cirrhosis (vascular spiders and/or palmar erythema) are found in one-third of patients with HCV-related cirrhosis at the time of presentation. (23)

Laboratory Features of HCV-Related Cirrhosis

Laboratory values taken at the time of diagnosis of cirrhosis often show normal values for serum albumin (86 to 90% of patients have normal values), total bilirubin (61 to 75%), and prothrombin time (67 to 84%). Even thrombocytopenia

($\leq 100 \times 10^9$/liter: $\leq 100,000$/mm^3), a sensitive marker for the presence of hypersplenism, is found in only a minority of patients (24 to 28%). (23,24,26) Most patients with cirrhosis have mild to moderate elevations in serum alanine and aspartate aminotransferase (ALT and AST) values. Values of ALT greater than 10 times the upper limit of normal are found in less than 5% of patients. (26) Completely and persistently normal levels of serum aminotransferases are uncommon in HCV-related cirrhosis, (29) although several studies have shown a poor correlation between levels of ALT and histological severity of chronic hepatitis C. (30,31)

α-Fetoprotein levels are mildly elevated in a variable proportion of patients with HCV-related cirrhosis (10 to 43%) without HCC. (13,23) Cryoglobulins, present in low levels, are detectable in appoximately one-third of patients with cirrhosis due to HCV. (32,33)

Clinical Features of Decompensated Cirrhosis Due to Hepatitis C

Once hepatic decompensation occurs, symptoms are usually present, including fatigue, jaundice, ascites, gastrointestinal bleeding, and hepatic encephalopathy. Among 65 patients with HCV-related cirrhosis, the initial episode of clinical decompensation was caused by ascites in 48%, variceal hemorrhage in 21%, encephalopathy in 8%, and jaundice in 6%, and by more than one complication in 17%. (23) In a study of 67 patients from the United States, the most frequent initial complication of cirrhosis was development of ascites. (13) Other symptoms of end-stage liver disease include itching, muscle weakness, wasting, easy bruisability, and peripheral edema.

CLINICAL OUTCOME

There are few longitudinal studies on the natural history of HCV-related cirrhosis. In published series, referral biases in selection of patients and the lack of uniformity in the timing of initiation of follow up makes it difficult to estimate the incidence of hepatocellular carcinoma, decompensation, and mortality in HCV-related cirrhosis. The incidence, course, and predictive factors for these complications need further clarification.

Development of Hepatocellular Carcinoma

Worldwide Incidence of HCC

HCV is a major risk factor for liver cancer worldwide, although the prevalence of anti-HCV among patients with HCC varies considerably by country. Most studies using sensitive methods for detection of anti-HCV indicate that hepatitis C is the main cause of liver cancer in Japan and in many European countries, such as Italy, where HCC is intermediate in incidence; in other regions with a low incidence of HCC, such as the United States and northern Europe, HCV plays a lesser role. (34) Liver cancer associated with HCV infection has been reported to be increasing in both eastern (35) and western (27) countries. The increased trend in the mortality rate from liver cancer in Italy from 4.8 per

100,000 in 1969 to 10.9 in 1994 may reflect the large cohort of subjects infected with HCV via medical exposures such as blood transfusion and use of nondisposable needles and syringes, which were commonly used for medical treatment during the 1950s and 1960s. (27)

Cirrhosis and HCC

Several studies have shown that the risk of HCC in HCV infection correlates with the underlying stage of the liver disease. Thus, cirrhosis is the single major risk factor for HCC and is found in approximately 80% of cases HCC worldwide. (36) The mechanisms by which cirrhosis leads to HCC may be related to prolonged or repeated bouts of liver necrosis and regeneration. Long-term follow up of patients with transfusion-associated hepatitis C have documented the sequential progression from acute hepatitis to HCC through the intermediate stages of mild, moderate, severe chronic hepatitis, and cirrhosis. (10,37)

The EUROHEP Cohort of Compensated Cirrhosis Due to Hepatitis C

The natural history of compensated cirrhosis caused by hepatitis C was assessed in a large cohort study of 384 patients who were followed for an average of 5 years. This study was based on a network of seven European university hospitals participating in a concerted action on viral hepatitis named EURO-HEP. (23) Initially, all patients had Child class A cirrhosis documented by liver biopsy, abnormal serum aminotransferase levels, no history of hepatic decompensation, and lacked clinical and radiological evidence of HCC. Other causes of liver disease were excluded in this cohort, including alcohol abuse, hepatitis B coinfection, and metabolic disorders. The follow-up of this cohort of patients has been updated through 1997 (mean follow-up ± SE: 6.8 ± 0.19 years) evaluating the clinical outcome of 357 Caucasian patients with hepatitis C, excluding the few patients of Asian or African origin or with unknown HCV serology. (26) In this study population, the 5-year cumulative incidence of HCC was 7% (Fig. 2). Similar findings have been reported in a study from the United States evaluating the clinical outcome of a series of 185 patients with HCV-related cirrhosis, in whom the 5-year cumulative incidence of HCC was 8.4%. (25) In another cohort of 103 patients with HCV-related compensated cirrhosis from France, the 4-year cumulative incidence of liver cancer was 11.5%. (24) Studies of patients with HCV-related cirrhosis from Japan have reported higher 5-year cumulative risks for HCC, ranging from 23 to 30%. (4,38)

In the European study, approximately half of patients developing HCC during follow-up did not experience hepatic decompensation before or by the time of diagnosis of liver cancer. (26) These data indicate that HCC usually arises in the clinical setting of compensated cirrhosis which may be silent clinically.

Risk Factors for Development of HCC

Host factors, virus factors, and extraneous factors may play a role in influencing the rate of progression of hepatitis C to liver cancer. In the EUROHEP cohort, prognostic factors for the development of HCC were assessed using Cox regression analysis. This multivariate analysis showed that factors significantly and independently associated with the risk of HCC were age, serum bilirubin

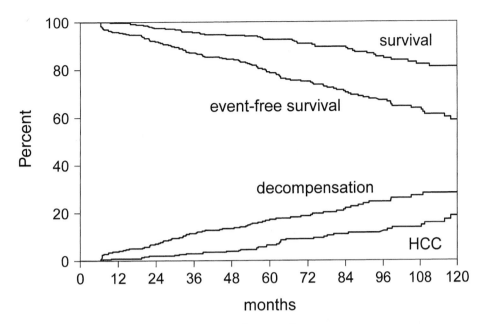

FIGURE 2 Cumulative probability of survival and of survival without liver-related complications and cumulative incidence of hepatocellular carcinoma (HCC) in 357 Caucasian patients with compensated cirrhosis due to HCV. The 5- and 10-year probability of survival was 92 and 81%, respectively, and of event-free survival was 79 and 59%, respectively. The 5- and 10-year rate of HCC was 7 and 19%, respectively. The cumulative incidence of decompensation has been estimated based upon information from 317 of the 357 patients with cirrhosis who remained HCC free; the 5- and 10-year rate of development of decompensation was 17 and 28%, respectively. The number of patients under observation refers to the survival probability. (26)

level, and the presence of peripheral manifestations of liver disease (vascular spiders and/or palmar erythema) at enrollment, parameters which indicate a more advanced stage of cirrhosis. (39) The risk of HCC for patients with four different clinical patterns of baseline characteristics were estimated by mathematical modeling adjusting for age, gender, serum bilirubin, platelet count, and presence of peripheral manifestations of liver disease (Fig. 3, top). (40) The estimated 5-year risk of HCC was relatively low (3%) for the average 50-year-old male with cirrhosis presenting with normal serum levels of bilirubin and platelet counts (example A), and was only slightly higher (7%) for a 60-year-old male with the same baseline features (example B). However, the estimated 5-year risk increased to 15% for a 50-year-old (example C) and to 25% for a 60-year-old man (example D) with cirrhosis and mild elevations in serum bilirubin levels (17 to 51 μmol/liter: 1.0 to 3.0 mg/dl), with a low platelet count (100 to 130 × 10^9/liter: 100,000 to 130,000/mm^3), and with manifestations of spiders and/or palmar erythema on physical examination.

These findings suggest that minor differences in clinical features among patients with compensated cirrhosis can account for the marked differences in the incidence of liver cancer reported in different studies. To best compare the risk of

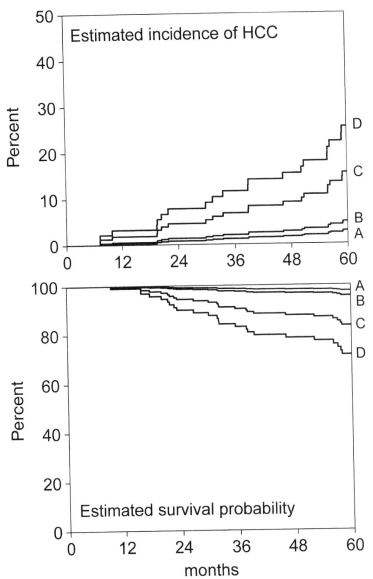

FIGURE 3 (Top) Estimated cumulative incidence of hepatocellular carcinoma (HCC) in patients with compensated cirrhosis due to hepatitis C based upon different baseline characteristics. (A) 50-year-old male with a normal serum bilirubin and platelet count. (B) 60-year-old male with a normal serum bilirubin and platelet count. (C) 50-year-old male with mild elevation in serum bilirubin (between 17 and 51 μmol/liter: 1.0 and 3.0 mg/dl), with a decreased platelet count (between 100 and 130 × 10⁹/liter: 100,000 and 130,000 /mm³), and peripheral manifestations of liver disease (vascular spiders and/or palmar erythema) on physical examination. (D) 60-year-old male with mild elevation in serum bilirubin (between 17 and 51 μmol/liter: 1.0 and 3.0 mg/dl), decreased platelet count (between 100 and 130 × 10⁹/liter: 100,000 and 130,000 /mm³), and peripheral manifestations of liver disease (vascular spiders and/or palmar erythema) on physical examination. The estimated 5-year incidence of HCC was 3% for patient A, 5% for patient B, 15% for patient C and 25% for patient D. (26) (Bottom) Estimated survival probability in patients with compensated cirrhosis due to hepatitis C calculated based upon different baseline characteristics. Curves A–D reflect subgroups as just described. The estimated 5-year survival probability was 97% for patient A, 95% for patient B, 83% for patient C and 71% for patient D. (26)

TABLE I Morbidity and Mortality in 357 Patients with Child A Cirrhosis Caused by Hepatitis C Over a 6.8-Year Mean Follow-Up Period[a]

Outcome	Mean time to occurence (months)	Incidence per 100 persons/years
Hepatocellular carcinoma	62	1.6
Decompensation	46	3.2
Total mortality	67	2.9
Liver-related mortality	66	2.0

[a] Data from EUROHEP cohort. (26)

liver cancer among cohort studies with different periods of follow-up, the incidence of HCC can be expressed as incidence per 100 person years. In the EUROHEP series, the incidence of HCC was 1.6 per 100 person years, and the mean interval from presentation with cirrhosis to the diagnosis of HCC was 62 months (range 7–134 months) (Table I). (26) This incidence is similar to the 1.6 per 100 person years incidence of HCC in a cohort of 185 patients with HCV related cirrhosis followed for a mean period of 4 years in the United States. (25) In another two series of 189 Italian patients and 103 French patients with HCV-related cirrhosis followed for a mean period of 3 years the incidence of HCC was 2.5 (41) and 3.2 (24) per 100 person years, respectively. Studies conducted in Japan have reported an unusually high risk of HCC in untreated patients with compensated HCV-related cirrhosis followed for an average of 5 years in the range of 5.9 (38) to 6.9 (4) cases per 100 person years. These variations in the incidence of HCC may be due to differences in clinical features of patients at entry reflecting different stages of cirrhosis (Table II).

Age of Infection and Risk of HCC

In the subgroup of posttransfusion patients with cirrhosis enrolled in the EUROHEP cohort, the cumulative incidence of HCC was higher in patients who received blood transfusions at or after the age of 50 than in those who had received transfusions at an earlier age (5-year cumulative incidence: 14% vs 2%, respectively, $p = 0.04$). (26) These findings suggest that age, independent of

TABLE II Factors Affecting Prognosis of Compensated Cirrhosis Due to Hepatitis C

Relevant
  Stage of liver disease at presentation
  Age at diagnosis
  Age at infection
  Male sex
  Alcohol intake
  Viral coinfection

Probably not relevant
  Virus genotype

in a cohort of 284 U.S. and Spanish liver transplant recipients. (10) Following liver transplantation, the fibrosis stage was found to increase linearly over time at a median rate of 0.3 (0.004–2.19) per year. Based on these findings, the expected time to graft cirrhosis was estimated to range from 9 to 12 years, with a faster progression observed in recent years when substantial changes in immunosuppression have occurred. Other variables influencing the rate of progression include race, HCV RNA levels at the time of transplantation, and the number of methylprednisolone boluses. This is the first study to assess the long-term histological outcome of HCV-infected immunocompromised liver transplant recipients through statistical modeling and may explain conflicting results on the incidence of graft cirrhosis observed in previous cohorts and the effect of HCV infection on posttransplantation survival. The natural history of HCV disease is highly variable, and periods of follow-up in previous studies have generally not reached the second decade.

Predictive Factors of Disease Severity

Factors influencing disease progression are largely unknown, but likely relate to (i) the intrinsic characteristics of the infecting viral strains, (ii) genetically determined characteristics of the infected individual, and (iii) environmental and/or iatrogenic influences on the infected individual, such as immunosuppression or alcohol consumption (Table II).

TABLE II   Predictors of Disease Severity in Liver Transplantation

Variable	Direction of effect	Strength of data
Genotype	Type 1b → more severe disease	Conflicting
Prettransplantation level of viremia	High viral load → increased fibrosis progression $> 1 \times 10^6$ → decreased patient survival	Single study
Early posttransplantation virological changes	High level of viremia first week → more severe disease High levels of serum/liver HCV RNA → more severe disease	Single study Majority of studies
Early posttransplantation histologic changes	Early recurrence → more progressive disease More severe early recurrence → more severe disease	Consistent
Rejection	More frequent episodes → more severe disease	Majority of studies
Type of immuno- suppression	Cyclosporine vs tacrolimus → no relationship Mycophenolate → increased fibrosis progression	Majority of studies Single study
Amount of immuno- suppression	Methylprednisolone "boluses" → more severe disease Cumulative steroids → more severe disease OKT3 → more severe disease	Consistent Single study Consistent
HLA matching	HLA matching → more severe disease	Conflicting
Race	Non-Caucasians → increased fibrosis progression Non-Caucasians → decreased patient survival	Single study
Year of transplantation	More recent years → increased fibrosis progression	Single study
Viral coinfection	HGV → no relationship HBV → no relationship CMV viremia → more severe disease	Consistent Conflicting Single study
Age	>49 years → more severe disease	Single study

duration of disease, is important in progression of disease and that hepatitis C more rapidly leads to cirrhosis and HCC in older persons.

HCV Genotype and Risk of HCC

The association of HCV genotype and risk of liver cancer is controversial. Studies from Italy (42) and France (24) have reported no association between different HCV genotypes and the risk of HCC, but a second study from Italy indicated a higher risk of HCC among patients with genotype 1b. (43) The effect of the HCV genotype as a risk factor for HCC has been evaluated in a EUROHEP-sponsored, longitudinal cohort study of 255 Caucasian patients with HCV-related compensated cirrhosis followed for a mean period of 7 years at tertiary referral centers in Europe. (44) During follow-up, HCC occurred in 11% of 175 patients infected by genotype 1b, in 12% of 50 patients infected with genotype 2, and in 13% of 30 patients infected by other genotypes, namely 1a and 3a, 4 or 5. By univariate analysis using the Kaplan–Meier method, the cumulative incidence of HCC was similar for patients infected with different HCV genotypes ($p = 0.71$, log rank test) (Table III). In addition, the HCV genotype was not independently associated with development of HCC by multivariate analysis ($p = 0.96$). Thus, most adequately controlled studies indicate no association of HCV genotype and risk of HCC in patients with cirrhosis.

Alcohol and Coinfection with HBV as Risk Factors for HCC

The risk of liver cancer is said to be increased among patients with HCV infection who concomitantly use alcohol. Indeed, in a longitudinal study from Italy conducted in a cohort of 290 patients with cirrhosis, multivariate analysis using the Cox regression showed that age, male sex, previous alcohol abuse, and coinfection with hepatitis B (HBsAg positivity) were independent risk factors for HCC. (45) In a study of 400 Chinese patients with cirrhosis followed for an average of 3 years, the hazard ratio for development of HCC was 3.74 for anti-HCV alone, 4.06 for HBsAg alone, and 6.41 for HCV and HBV coinfection ($p = 0.005$), providing evidence of an independent role and additive interaction of HBV and HCV infection on development of HCC. (46)

A case-control study evaluated the interaction between HCV infection and heavy alcohol intake as well as between HBV infection and alcohol abuse in the development of HCC. (47) Positive interactions between both HCV and HBV

TABLE III Univariate Analysis of the Risk of Hepatocellular Carcinoma in 255 Patients with Child A Cirrhosis Due to Hepatitis C Analyzed by HCV Genotype (Kaplan-Meier Method)[a]

HCV type	5 years (SE)	10 years (SE)	p[b]
1b	0.06 (0.01)	0.19 (0.05)	0.71
2	0.04 (0.03)	0.15 (0.05)	
others[c]	0.04 (0.04)	0.30 (0.13)	

[a] Data from EUROHEP cohort. (26)
[b] Derived from log-rank test.
[c] HCV genotype 1a, 3a, 4, or 5.

infection and heavy alcohol intake were found, suggesting synergism between viral infections and alcohol in the risk of liver cancer.

Development of Hepatic Decompensation

Longitudinal studies provide the optimal approach to evaluate the risk of decompensation for patients with HCV-related cirrhosis. In the EUROHEP cohort study, the 5-year cumulative incidence of an episode of decompensation, either ascites, jaundice, encephalopathy, or variceal bleeding was 17%, the incidence per 100 person years was 3.2, and the mean interval between the time of diagnosis of cirrhosis and the appearance of the first episode of decompensation was 46 months (range 6–137 months) (Fig. 2, Table I). (26) In a prospective cohort study of 112 patients with HCV-related cirrhosis conducted in the United States, the cumulative incidence of decompensation was 22% in 5 years. (48) In a similar study from France of 103 patients with HCV-related compensated cirrhosis, the cumulative incidence of hepatic decompensation was 20% at 4 years. (24) Overall, these findings indicate that a significant proportion of patients with chronic hepatitis C presenting with compensated cirrhosis do not worsen for several years and that hepatic decompensation usually occurs at a relatively late stage in the natural course of the disease.

Longitudinal studies have shown that results of routine laboratory tests that reflect decreased hepatocellular function, such as low serum albumin levels, slight elevations in serum bilirubin, and increases in prothrombin time, are significantly associated with risk of subsequent hepatic decompensation. (25,39)

Mortality From Liver Disease

Survival Rate in Patients with HCV-Related Cirrhosis

The primary cause of mortality among persons with chronic hepatitis C is the development of complications of cirrhosis. In several large series from the United States and Europe, the cumulative rate of death from liver disease in patients with HCV-related cirrhosis varied from 9 to 22% during a mean follow-up of 4 to 5 years. (13,23,25) The variability was probably due to different study designs and initial clinical features of patients, such as whether patients with a history of hepatic decompensation were excluded. The lowest mortality rates have been reported from cohorts of patients starting at early stages of cirrhosis, and in which patients with important cofactors (such as alcohol abuse, HBV co-infection, and metabolic disorders) were excluded. (23)

In a prospective cohort study of HCV-infected patients from Germany, there was a fourfold increase in mortality rate among the 141 patients with cirrhosis documented clinically or by liver biopsy at diagnosis compared with that of a matched general population. (49) In the EUROHEP cohort of 357 patients with cirrhosis who were followed for an average of 6.8 years, the probability of survival was 92% at 5 years, the incidence of liver-related death was 2.0 per 100 person years, and the mean interval between the time of diagnosis of cirrhosis and death from liver disease was 66 months (range 9–180 months) (Fig. 2, Table I). (26) The causes of death included complications of HCC in 35%, liver failure in 26%, gastrointestinal bleeding in 7%, and causes unrelated to liver disease in 32%. Patients followed in this cohort were mostly middle-aged at the time of diagnosis and most did not develop symptoms or complications of liver disease which may explain the high proportion of deaths unrelated to liver disease. There was a linear, although slow, rate of HCC, hepatic decompensation, and liver-related death in this cohort of patients (Fig. 2).

Risk Factors for Mortality in HCV-Related Cirrhosis

In the EUROHEP cohort of patients with compensated cirrhosis, factors associated with poor survival included age, reasons for referral, source of infection, finding of spiders and/or palmar erythema on physical examination, splenomegaly, esophageal varices, increased ratio of AST to ALT, and abnormalities in bilirubin, albumin, platelets, and prothrombin time (Table IV). (23) Reasons for referral to the tertiary medical center correlated with mortality in this cohort of patients probably because this factor correlated indirectly with underlying stage of cirrhosis. Comparison of the clinical and biochemical parameters at enrollment between 130 patients in whom the histological diagnosis of cirrhosis was made during follow-up for chronic hepatitis and 60 patients who were referred because of symptoms revealed that the former group of patients were younger and had less severe liver disease, supporting the concept that cirrhosis was identified at an earlier stage in these patients, which perhaps explains why they have a better prognosis. This bias of referral may explain why mode of transmission of infection may correlate with prognosis in some studies. (25) Survival was worse among patients with HCV-related cirrhosis who had no known risk factors for acquiring hepatitis C, perhaps reflecting a longer duration of liver disease than in patients with a known exposure such as blood transfusion.

In multivariate analysis, risk factors that correlated significantly and independently with prognosis were age, presence of peripheral manifestations of liver disease (vascular spiders and/or palmar erythema), serum bilirubin levels, and platelet count at the time of diagnosis. (23) These are similar to the risk factors for development of HCC and development of decompensation and reflect two major factors: patient age and severity of underlying cirrhosis. The probability of survival for patients with Child A cirrhosis with different baseline clinical characteristics can be estimated by mathematical modeling adjusting for age, gender, serum bilirubin, platelet count, and presence of spiders and/or palmar erythema (Fig. 3, bottom). (40) The estimated 5-year life survival was 98% for a 50-year-old (example A) and 95% for a 60-year-old man (example B) with normal serum bilirubin levels and platelet count. Estimated survival decreased to 83% for the 50-year-old (example C) and 71% for the 60-year-old (example D) who had elevations in serum bilirubin (17 to 51 μmol/liter: 1 to 3 mg/dl), decreased platelet counts (100 to 130 $\times$ 10^9/liter: 100,000 to 130,000/mm^3), and stigmata of liver disease. These findings further indicate that small differences in baseline clinical and biochemical characteristics among patients with well-compensated cirrhosis can account for marked differences in patient outcomes. Such differences may account for the lower 4-year survival rate of 84% reported in a French study of 103 patients with Child class A or B cirrhosis (24) and the rate of 85% reported in a German study of 141 patients

TABLE IV Clinical and Serological Variables of Prognostic Significance for Survival in Univariate Analysis in Patients with Child A Cirrhosis Caused by Hepatitis C[a]

| Variable | No. of patients | Survival probability | | p value |
		5 years (SE)	10 years (SE)	
Age (years) (n = 384)[b]				
≤54	166	0.95 (0.02)	0.83 (0.06)	0.028[c]
>54	218	0.88 (0.03)	0.75 (0.06)	
Referral pattern (n = 384)				
Diagnosis of cirrhosis during follow-up for chronic hepatitis	130	0.94 (0.02)	0.81 (0.07)	0.019[d]
Incidental finding of abnormal aminotransferase levels	119	0.94 (0.02)	0.83 (0.06)	
Diagnosis of cirrhosis made elsewhere previously	75	0.87 (0.04)	0.82 (0.06)	
Symptoms	60	0.85 (0.05)	0.73 (0.09)	
Source of infection (n = 272)				
Blood transfusion	159	0–94 (0.02)	0.94 (0.02)	0.016[c]
Unknown	113	0.89 (0.03)	0.66 (0.09)	
Hepatic stigmata (n = 365)				
Present	113	0.81 (0.04)	0.71 (0.06)	0.001[c]
Absent	252	0.96 (0.01)	0.83 (0.06)	
Splenomegaly (n = 359)				
Present	124	0.85 (0.04)	0.70 (0.08)	0.0062[c]
Absent	235	0.95 (0.02)	0.85 (0.05)	
Esophageal varices (n = 194)				
Present	79	0.77 (0.06)	0.53 (0.12)	0.00001[c]
Absent	115	0.95 (0.02)	0.85 (0.07)	
AST/ALT ratio (n = 367)				
≤ 1	261	0.94 (0.02)	0.87 (0.04)	0.0016[c]
> 1	106	0.85 (0.04)	0.61 (0.09)	
Bilirubin (n = 365)				
≤ 17 µmol/liter (≤ 1.0 mg/dl)	224	0.96 (0.01)	0.86 (0.05)	0.00001[c]
17 to 51 µmol/liter (1.0 to 3.0 mg/dl)	141	0.81 (0.04)	0.67 (0.07)	
Albumin (n = 344)				
≥ 35 g/liter (≥ 3.5 g/dl)	309	0.93 (0.02)	0.80 (0.05)	0.0053[c]
< 35 g/liter (< 3.5 g/dl)	35	0.80 (0.07)	0.64 (0.12)	
Platelets (n = 372)				
≥ 130 × 10^9/liter (≥ 130,000 /mm^3)	186	0.96 (0.02)	0.87 (0.04)	0.0009[c]
< 130 × 10^9/liter (< 130,000 /mm^3)	186	0.86 (0.03)	0.71 (0.07)	
Prothrombin time (n = 343)				
≥ 70%	230	0.93 (0.02)	0.92 (0.02)	0.0033[c]
< 70%	113	0.87 (0.04)	0.53 (0.11)	

[a] Data from Fattovich et al. (23)

[b] Values in parentheses represent the total number of patients in which survival calculation is based as initial data were not available in all patients.

[c] Derived from log-rank test and Breslow test.

[d] Derived by Breslow test.

with different stages of cirrhosis, (49) as well as the lower 5-year survival rate of 83% reported in a study from the United States of 112 patients with biopsy proven or clinically diagnosed cirrhosis. (48)

Genotype and Survival in HCV-Related Cirrhosis

In the large EUROHEP cohort (26) and the studies from France (24) and United States, (48) HCV genotype was not associated with a significant, independent risk of mortality or liver transplantation. These data suggest that genotype of HCV has little or no impact on the course of hepatitis C, particularly once cirrhosis has developed.

Survival after Hepatic Decompensation

Once an episode of decompensation occurs, the prognosis is poor. The 5-year survival rate after the appearance of the first major complication of cirrhosis is only 50%, considerably lower than the survival rate for compensated cirrhosis due to HCV. (23,48) The type of decompensation correlates to some degree with the probability of survival. The lowest survival rates were observed in patients with more than one complication (78 and 50% at 1 and 2 years, respectively) and in patients with encephalopathy (80 and 27% at 1 and 2 years). The highest rate of survival for decompensated patients was in those who presented with ascites (80 and 60% at 1 and 5 years). (26) Such analyses are helpful in guiding management decisions and timing for referral for liver transplantation.

MANAGEMENT

Patients with cirrhosis due to hepatitis C constitute an important therapeutic challenge. Death from liver-related causes has been shown to account for 70% of the mortality in patients with HCV-related cirrhosis (23) compared with only 3% of patients overall with hepatitis C. (50) To lower liver-related mortality in HCV-related cirrhosis, treatment strategies are needed for both compensated and decompensated cirrhosis.

Compensated Cirrhosis

The management of compensated cirrhosis caused by hepatitis C should focus upon both prevention of complications as well as at therapy to induce a biochemical or virological response. Interferon-α has become the standard therapy of chronic hepatitis C, but its role in patients with cirrhosis is still debated. (14, 15) The standard regimen of interferon-α is rarely effective in inducing a long-lasting response in patients with cirrhosis. (7) However, several reports have suggested that a 6 to 12 month course of interferon therapy may reduce the risk of HCC in patients with cirrhosis. (4,5) Other controlled studies have failed to confirm this effect. (39,48,49) Whereas, patients with compensated cirrhosis were routinely included in studies of interferon-α therapy in Europe and North America, these patients were usually excluded in studies from Japan. The Panel that composed the National Institutes of Health Consensus Statement on management of hepatitis C stated that the benefit of interferon therapy for patients with cirrhosis had not been proven, and recommended that patients with cirrhosis be treated largely within the context of randomized controlled trials. Few studies have focused upon patients with cirrhosis, and the role of interferon therapy is still controversial.

Interferon Therapy and Sustained Remission

The sustained response rate for patients with cirrhosis participating in randomized controlled trials assessing standard interferon therapy (3 millions units 3 times per week for 6–12 months) has been consistently low, ranging from 4 to 9%. (7,51–53) A comparative analysis of 80 patients with cirrhosis and 254 patients without cirrhosis from the Benelux study (53) provided some insight in the possible mechanisms of the low rate of response in patients with cirrhosis. An early virological response (HCV RNA falling to less than 1000 copies/ml at 4 weeks) while on therapy occurred in only 21% of patients with cirrhosis compared to 42% of patients without cirrhosis. Furthermore, the rate of subsequent breakthrough in virological response on treatment was 42% for patients with cirrhosis compared to 27% of patients without cirrhosis. The relapse rate after therapy was stopped was similar for patients with or without cirrhosis.

A satisfactory explanation for the low initial response and high rate of breakthrough on therapy in cirrhosis has been lacking. Several studies from Japan have shown that intrahepatic interferon receptor mRNA levels are lower in patients with cirrhosis than those with hepatitis C without cirrhosis (54,55) and that interferon receptor mRNA levels are significantly higher in responders than nonresponders to therapy. (56,57) These studies suggest that progressive fibrosis and diminution of hepatic reserve may diminish the number of interferon receptors on hepatocytes and render patients with cirrhosis relatively resistant to the antiviral effects of interferon-α.

Irrespective of the biological mechanism involved in the low rate of response to interferon-α, higher response rates (14–19%) have been reported in patients with cirrhosis treated with higher doses of interferon, such as 6 million units 3 times per week or 3 million units daily. (58,59) Unfortunately, the side effects of interferon tend to be more severe with higher doses and patients with cirrhosis are more susceptible to the adverse events of interferon therapy.

An univariate analysis of patients with cirrhosis from the Benelux study showed that the HCV genotype was a significant factor affecting the sustained response rate in patients with cirrhosis. Sustained virological responses were 4% for patients with genotype 1 and 10% for those with genotype 2 or 3. (53) These findings suggest that therapy with interferon by itself is unlikely to be very beneficial in patients with hepatitis C and cirrhosis, unless higher doses are given for a longer period than 6 months, particularly in patients with genotype 1.

Interferon and Prevention of Hepatocellular Carcinoma

Despite the low efficacy of interferon in inducing a sustained response, this therapy has been advocated for patients with HCV-related cirrhosis largely because of reports that interferon therapy may prevent development of hepatocellular carcinoma (see also Chapter 15). This concept arose from a prospective study from Japan, (4) but was disputed by two retrospective studies from Europe (6,39) that used multivariate analysis to correct for baseline characteristics

TABLE V   Summary of Seven Studies on the Incidence of Hepatocellular Carcinoma (HCC) among Patients with HCV-related Cirrhosis Treated with Interferon (IFN)-α [a]

Study	Untreated		IFN-treated sustained ALT responders		IFN-treated nonresponders		IFN treated Total	
	No.	No. HCC (%)	No.	No. HCC (%)	No.	No. HCC (%)	No.	No. HCC (%)
Nishiguchi et al. (4)	45	17 (38)	7	0	38	2 (5)	45	2 (4.5)
Mazzella et al. (6)	91	9 (10)	39	0	154	5 (3)	193	5 (2.6)
Fattovich et al. (39)	136	16 (12)	14	0	179	7 (4)	193	7 (3.6)
Serfaty et al. (24)[b]	44	7 (16)	6	1 (16)	53	3 (6)	59	4 (7)
International Interferon-α HCC Study Group et al. (5)	259	48 (18.5)	n.a.	n.a.	n.a.	n.a.	222	21 (9.5)
Niederau et al. (49)[b]	77	13 (17)	2	0	62	3 (5)	64	3 (4.7)
Valla et al. (61)	49	9 (18)	2	n.a.	43	n.a.	45	5 (11)

[a] Average duration of follow-up: 4 years (Nishiguchi et al.), 3 years (Mazzella et al.), 5 years (Fattovich et al.), 3.3 years (Serfaty et al.), 6.5 years (International Interferon-α Hepatocellular Carcinoma Study Group), 4.2 years (Niederau et al.), 3.3 years (Valla et al.).

[b] Courtesy of Serfaty et al., (24) 1998 updated, and Niederau et al., (49) 1998 updated. n.a. = not available.

between untreated and interferon-treated patients. (60) Recently, two retrospective studies further suggested that interferon therapy reduced the subsequent development of HCC; (5,24) other controlled studies, (48,49,61) however, failed to demonstrate a benefit of treatment (Table V).

In view of the discordant results, the EUROHEP cohort of 357 anti-HCV-positive Caucasian patients with cirrhosis was reevaluated by two independent biostatisticians (Personal communication: Hansen B E, Pantalena M). Overall, the 5-year incidence of HCC was higher in the 136 untreated patients (12%) than in the 193 interferon-treated patients with cirrhosis (3.6%). However, when adjustments were made for the differences of age and severity of liver disease in baseline characteristics between treated and untreated patient groups, a beneficial effect of interferon therapy could no longer be demonstrated. These findings suggest that interferon therapy was predominantly offered to patients who were younger, had less severe liver disease, and fewer other comorbidities. Most studies on the incidence of HCC after interferon therapy of patients with HCV-related cirrhosis have used post-hoc analysis of previously collected data from patient cohorts, and the rationale for giving or withholding interferon therapy was not adequately described, suggesting the likelihood of selection bias.

Importantly, in almost all studies that have analyzed the cumulative incidence of HCC in sustained responders and transient responders and nonresponders separately, a lower incidence of HCC was found in sustained responders to treatment (Table V). Thus, a sustained virological and biochemical response to interferon therapy may lower the subsequent risk of HCC in patients with cirrhosis due to HCV. However, this hypothesis awaits confirmation in further large-scale, prospective, randomized, controlled trials utilizing treatments with a higher efficacy in inducing a sustained response.

Interferon and Ribavirin Combination Therapy

Recently, several randomized controlled trials have shown that the combination of interferon-α and ribavirin, an oral nucleoside analogue, increases the sustained virological response rate compared to interferon-α alone in patients with typical chronic hepatitis C. (62–65) These trials of combination therapy included only small numbers of patients with cirrhosis. A meta-analysis of individual patient data from six randomized controlled trials included data on 75 patients with compensated cirrhosis who had completed at least 6 months of therapy and 6 months of follow-up. (66) Patients with cirrhosis were most likely to be males (80%), between the ages of 40 and 60 years (59%), and to have genotype 1 (60%) than patients without cirrhosis. The majority (67%) also were nonresponders to a previous course of interferon-α. No patient enrolled in these studies had decompensated liver disease as defined by a serum bilirubin greater than 34 μmol/liter (2.0 mg/dl), albumin less than 32 g/liter (3.2 mg/dl), abnormal coagulopathy (clotting factors < 35%), or platelet count of less than 50×10^9/liter (50,000/mm^3).

In this group of patients with cirrhosis, combination therapy was more effective than interferon monotherapy in inducing an end-of-treatment biochemical response (combination: 43%, 22/51; interferon alone: 29%, 7/24) as well as sustained response (combination: 22%, 11/51; interferon alone: 4%, 1/24). Most importantly, virological sustained responses occurred only in patients receiving combination therapy (17%, 9/51); none of 24 patients receiving interferon monotherapy remained HCV RNA negative during follow up. The estimated probabilities of a sustained biochemical and virological response derived from a statistical model that corrected for skewed data for subgroups with less than 6–10 patients are given in Fig. 4. The sustained response rate was influenced significantly by virus genotype (genotype 1: 7–10%, genotype 2, 3: 24–33%) but not by status of previous therapy (previously untreated, relapse, or nonresponse). Importantly, results of combination therapy in patients with cirrhosis were at least as good as for 12-month interferon monotherapy in patients with chronic hepatitis C without cirrhosis, which led to the general endorsement of interferon therapy by previous consensus panels. (14,15) These findings indicate that therapy with the combination of interferon-α and ribavirin can be recommended for all patients with compensated cirrhosis due to hepatitis C, as long as there are no contraindications to therapy.

Decompensated Cirrhosis

In patients with decompensated cirrhosis, liver transplantation is the most appropriate approach to management. The 5-year survival rate of patients with end-stage liver disease due to hepatitis C is excellent, averaging 70 to 80%, (67) which is better than the 50% survival rate of patients with decompensated cirrhosis without transplantation. (23,48)

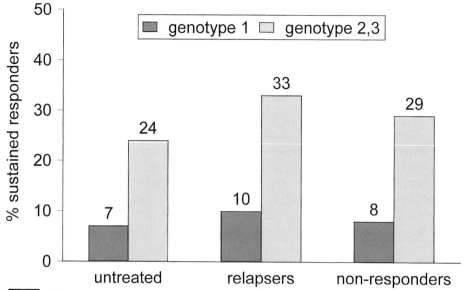

FIGURE 4　Outcomes of therapy with the combination of interferon-α and ribavirin in patients with chronic hepatitis C and cirrhosis. The estimated rate of sustained biochemical and virological responses is given by patient type (previously untreated, relapser, or nonresponder) and genotype. Percentages are derived from a multivariate model constructed with data from 344 patients with chronic hepatitis C, including 75 with cirrhosis. (66)

The role of interferon therapy in patients with decompensated cirrhosis due to hepatitis C has not been adequately assessed, either for virological responses or for effects on survival. There have been anedotal reports of patients with decompensated cirrhosis who had clinical, biochemical, or virological responses to interferon therapy, but for most cases the risks of side effects of therapy outweigh the likelihood of benefits.

In patients with cirrhosis and hepatocellular carcinoma, liver transplantation, hepatic resection, percutaneous ethanol injection, and thermal ablation with radiofrequency are treatment modalities that singly or in combination may improve prognosis. Generally, liver transplantation is an option if the patient is of suitable age, has no other major diseases or limiting medical conditions, and if the tumor is limited in size. In carefully selected patients, 5-year survival after liver transplantation for HCC is similar to that for non-malignant forms of end-stage liver disease. (68)

In the majority of patients with HCV-related cirrhosis and HCC, liver transplantation is not an option. In these patients, hepatic resection and/or local-regional therapies (percutaneous ethanol injection/thermal ablation with radiofrequency) should be considered. In patients with compensated cirrhosis without clinically significant portal hypertension, who present with a single, peripherally located hepatic tumor which is less than 5 cm in diameter and shows no evidence of vascular invasion or metastasis, hepatic resection is probably the optimal approach. (69) In other cases with small tumors, repeated percutaneous ethanol injections has become standard therapy, with survival results similar to those after hepatic resection. (70) More detailed guidelines on treatment options have been provided. (71,72)

CONCLUSION

Hepatitis C virus infection is a common cause of liver disease worldwide and typically progresses to cirrhosis within 20 years of onset in 20 to 25% of patients. The average age at diagnosis of cirrhosis is 55 years and most patients are asymptomatic or complain of only mild nonspecific symptoms such as fatigue. Approximately two-thirds of patients have hepatomegaly and one-third splenomegaly and/or peripheral manifestations of liver disease (vascular spiders or palmar erythema). At the time of diagnosis, laboratory tests usually reveal mild-to-moderate elevations in serum aminotransferases, but normal levels of serum albumin, bilirubin, and prothrombin time (in 60% of patients). Once decompensation occurs, symptoms are more prominent and laboratory test results are usually abnormal. The most frequent form of presentation of decompensation is development of ascites. Longitudinal cohort studies of patients with compensated cirrhosis due to hepatitis C have indicated that the subsequent rates of hepatocellular carcinoma (HCC), hepatic decompensation, and liver-related death are linear over time. The risk of HCC appears to vary geographically; the 4- to 5-year cumulative incidence of HCC being in the range of 7 to 11% (1.6 to 3.2 per 100 person years) in Europe and United States but as high as 30% (6 to 7 per 100 person years) in Japan. The 5-year cumulative incidence of decompensation is approximately 20%. Survival is reasonably good, the 4- to 5-year probability of survival ranging from 84 to 92%. Factors that correlate with prognosis in compensated cirrhosis include severity of the underlying liver disease, older patient age, older age at infection, male sex, concurrent HCV and HBV infection, and excessive alcohol consumption. Most longitudinal studies suggest that the clinical impact of HCV genotype on development of decompensation or HCC is limited. Once decompensation occurs the prognosis is poor (approximately 50% probability of survival at 5 years). The worst survival occurs in patients presenting with more than one complication, and the best in those with ascites alone.

Standard regimens of interferon-α (3 million units 3 times per week for 6 to 12 months) are less effective in inducing a sustained response in patients with cirrhosis (5 to 10%) than in patients without cirrhosis (15 to 25%). The low responsiveness is primarily related to the low initial virological response rate on therapy as well as a high rate of breakthrough. Cumulative evidence suggests that patients with cirrhosis who have a sustained virological response have an improved prognosis, especially for development of HCC. Higher dosages of interferon or the combination of interferon with ribavirin lead to higher sustained response rates (15 to 20%). In view of these improved results, combination therapy can now be recommended in patients with compensated cirrhosis due to hepatitis C. The efficacy of interferon or combination therapy in decompensated cirrhosis is not documented, and its use is limited by poor tolerance and side effects. On the basis of the excellent 5-year survival rates after liver transplantation (70 to 80%), patients with end-stage cirrhosis due to hepatitis C should be considered for liver transplantation.

ACKNOWLEDGMENTS

The authors are grateful for the data and analysis of the EUROHEP group on HCV related cirrhosis, the Benelux Hepatitis C Treatment Study group, and the EUROHEP group on meta-analysis of individual patient data on the combination of interferon-α and ribavrin. In addition, they thank B.E. Hansen (Department of Epidemiology and Biostatistics, Erasmus University Rotterdam, the Netherlands) and M. Pantalena (Servizio Autonomo Clinicizzato di Gastroenterologia, Dipartimento di Scienze Chirurgiche e Gastroenterologiche, University of Verona, Italy) for additional statistical analysis. Participating groups are *The EUROHEP group on cirrhosis type C:* University of Verona, Verona, Italy (G. Fattovich and M. Pantalena); University of Padova, Padova, Italy (P. Bonetti, C. Casarin, G. Diodati, G. Giustina, F. Noventa, and F. Tremolada); University of Palermo, Palermo, Italy (P. Almasio and P. Fuschi); University of Sassari, Sassari, Italy (D. Mura, G. Realdi, A. Solinas, and A. Tocco); Erasmus University Hospital Dijkzigt, Rotterdam, the Netherlands (A. Bhalla, J. T. Brouwer, J. Rai, and S. W. Schalm); University Hospital Gasthuisberg, Leuven, Belgium (J. Basho and F. Nevens); Hôpital Beaujon, Clichy, France (F. Degos and C. Njapoum); St. Mary's Hospital Medical School, London, United Kingdom (R. Galassini and H. Thomas); and University of Milano, Milano, Italy (M. L. Ribero and A. Tagger). *The Benelux Hepatitis C Treatment Study group:* Erasme University Hospital Brussels, Belgium (M. Adler and N. Bourgeois); Centre Hospitalier de Luxembourg, Luxembourg (V. Arendt and J. Weber); University Hospital Liège, Belgium (J. Belaiche, J. Delwaide, and J. Pirotte); St. Joseph Hospital, Gilly and University Hospital St. Luc, Brussels, Belgium (R. Brénard and A. P. Geubel); Academic Medical Center Amsterdam, the Netherlands (C. M. Bronkhorst, R. A. F. M. Chamuleau, H. W. Reesink, P. L. M. Janssen, and F. J. W. ten Kate); Erasmus University Hospital Dijkzigt, Rotterdam, the Netherlands (J. T. Brouwer, B. E. Hansen, R. A. Heijtink, W. C. J. Hop, G. E. M. Kleter, H. G. M. Niesters, and S. W. Schalm); Free University Hospital Brussels, Belgium (P. Buydens and M. L. Hautekeete); Willem Alexander Hospital, Hertogenbosch, the Netherlands (Th. J. M. van Ditzhuysen); Diagnostic Center SSDZ, Delft, the Netherlands (L. J. van Doorn and W. G. V. Quint); University Hospital Gent, Belgium (A. Elewaut, A. E. Elewaut, G. Leroux-Roels, and J. Versieck); University Hospital Antwerpen, Belgium (H. Fierens and P. Michielsen); Gasthuisberg University Hospital Leuven, Belgium (J. Fevery, J. de Groote, F. Nevens, W. van Steenbergen, and S. H. Yap); St. Anne Hospital, Brussels, Belgium (C. de Galocsy); Jolimont Hospital, Haine St. Paul, Belgium (J. Henrion); University Hospital St. Radboud, Nijmegen, the Netherlands (J. P. van Munster); St. Franciscus Hospital, Rotterdam, the Netherlands (J. W. den Ouden); Rode Kruis Hospital, the Hague, the Netherlands (D. Overbosch); Rijnstate Hospital Arnhem, the Netherlands (R. A. de Vries); and Haven Hospital, Rotterdam, the Netherlands (P. J. Wismans). *The EUROHEP group on Meta-analysis of Individual Patient Data on interferon–ribavirin combination therapy:* University of Padova, Padova, Italy (A. Alberti,

L. Cavalletto, and L. Chemello); Niguarda Ca' Granda Hospital, Milan, Italy (A. Bellobuono and G. Ideo); University of Bari, Bari, Italy (M. Milella and G. Pastore); Danderyd Hospital, Danderyd, Sweden (O. Reichard); and Huddinge Hospital, Huddinge, Sweden (R. Schvarcz and O. Weiland).

REFERENCES

1. Alter M J. Epidemiology of hepatitis C. Hepatology 1997;26:62S–5S.
2. Tanaka K, Hirohata T, Koga S, et al. Hepatitis C and hepatitis B in the etiology of hepatocellular carcinoma in the Japanese population. Cancer Res 1991;51:2842–7.
3. De Bac C, Stroffolini T, Gaeta G B, Taliani G, Giusti G. Pathogenic factors in cirrhosis with and without hepatocellular carcinoma: a multicenter Italian study. Hepatology 1994;20:1225–30.
4. Nishiguchi S, Kuroki T, Nakatani S, et al. Randomized trial of effects of interferon-α on incidence of hepatocellular carcinoma in chronic active hepatitis C with cirrhosis. Lancet 1995;346:1051–5.
5. International Interferon-α Hepatocellular Carcinoma Study Group. Effect of Interferon-α on progression of cirrhosis to hepatocellular carcinoma: a retrospective cohort study. Lancet 1998;351:1535–9.
6. Mazzella G, Accogli E, Sottili S, et al. Alpha interferon treatment may prevent hepatocellular carcinoma in HCV-related liver cirrhosis. J Hepatol 1996;24:141–7.
7. Jouet P, Roudot-Thoraval F, Dhumeaux D, Mètreau J M, Le Group Français pour L'Etude du Traitment des Hèpatitis Chroniques NANB/C. Comparative efficacy of interferon alfa in cirrhotic and noncirrhotic patients with non-A, non-B, C hepatitis. Gastroenterology 1994;106:686–90.
8. Hopf U, Moller B, Kuther D, et al. Long-term follow-up of posttransfusion and sporadic chronic hepatitis non-A, non-B and frequency of circulating antibodies to hepatitis C virus (HCV). J Hepatol 1990;10:69–76.
9. Di Bisceglie A M, Goodman Z D, Ishak K G, Hoofnagle J H, Melpolder J J, Alter H J. Long-term clinical and histopathological follow-up of chronic posttrasfusion hepatitis. Hepatology 1991;14:969–74.
10. Tremolada F, Casarin C, Alberti A, et al. Long-term follow-up of non-A, non-B (type C) post-transfusion hepatitis. J Hepatol 1992;16:273–81.
11. Mattsson L, Sonnerborg A, Weiland O. Outcome of acute symptomatic non-A, non-B hepatitis: a 13-year follow-up study of hepatitis C virus markers. Liver 1993;13:274–8.
12. Kiyosawa K, Sodeyama T, Tanaka E, et al. Interrelationship of blood transfusion, non-A, non-B hepatitis and hepatocellular carcinoma: analysis by detection of antibody to hepatitis C virus. Hepatology 1990;12:671–5.
13. Tong M J, El-Farra N S, Reikes A R, Co R L. Clinical outcomes after transfusion-associated hepatitis C. N Engl J Med 1995;332:1463–6.
14. National Institutes of Health Consensus Development Conference Panel statement: management of hepatitis C. Hepatology 1997;26(Suppl 1):2S–10S.
15. Hèpatite C: dèpistage et traitement. Gastroenterol Clin Biol 1997;20:S202–11.
16. Kenny-Walsh E, for the Irish Hepatology Research Group. Clinical outcomes after hepatitis C infection from contaminated anti-D immune globulin. N Engl J Med 1999;340:1228–33.
17. Poynard T, Bedossa P, Opolon P for the OBSVIRC, METAVIR, CLINIVIR and DOSVIRC groups. Natural history of liver fibrosis progression in patients with chronic hepatitis C. Lancet 1997;349:825–32.
18. Pol S, Fontaine H, Carnot F, et al. Predictive factors for development of cirrhosis in parenterally acquired chronic hepatiits C: a comparison between immunocompetent and immunocompromised patients. J Hepatol 1998;29:12–9.
19. Fong T L, Di Bisceglie A M, Waggoner J G, Banks S M, Hoofnagle J H. The significance of antibody to hepatitis C virus in patients with chronic hepatitis B. Hepatology 1991;14:64–7.
20. Fattovich G, Tagger A, Brollo L, et al. Hepatitis C virus infection in chronic hepatitis B virus carriers. J Infect Dis 1991;163:400–2.
21. Weltman M D, Brotodihardjo A, Crewe E B, et al. Coinfection with hepatitis B and C or B, C

and D viruses results in severe chronic liver disease and responds poorly to interferon-α treatment. J Viral Hepatitis 1995;2:39–45.

22. Wiley T E, McCarthy M, Breidi L, McCarthy M, Layden T J. Impact of alcohol on the histological and clinical progression of hepatitis C infection. Hepatology 1998;28:805–9.

23. Fattovich G, Giustina G, Degos F, et al. Morbidity and mortality in compensated cirrhosis C:
a retrospective follow-up study of 384 patients. Gastroenterology 1997;112:463–72.

24. Serfaty L, Aumaître H, Chazouillères O, et al. Determinants of outcome of compensated hepatitis C virus-related cirrhosis. Hepatology 1998;27:1435–40.

25. Gordon S C, Bayati N, Silverman A L. Clinical outcome of hepatitis C as a function of mode of
transmission. Hepatology 1998;28:562–7.

26. EUROHEP: European Concerted Action on HCV-related Cirrhosis. 2000. Updated analysis,
data on file: Fattovich et al. (23)

27. Stroffolini T, Andreone P, Andriulli A, et al. Characteristics of hepatocellular carcinoma in
Italy. J Hepatol 1998;29:944–52.

28. Tinè F, Caltagirone M, Cammà C, et al. Clinical indicants of compensated cirrhosis: a prospective study. In: Dianzani M U, Gentilini P, eds. Chronic Liver Damage. Amsterdam: Elsevier,
1990:187–98.

29. Hoofnagle J H. Hepatitis C: The clinical spectrum of disease. Hepatology 1997;26(Suppl 1):
15S–20S.

30. Haber M M, West A B, Haber A D, Reuben A. Relationship of aminotransferases to liver histological status in chronic hepatitis C. Am J Gastroenterol 1995;90:1250–7.

31. McCormick S E, Goodman Z D, Maydonovitch C L, Sjögren M H. Evaluation of liver histology, ALT elevation, and HCV-RNA titer in patients with chronic hepatitis C. Am J Gastroenterol 1996;91:1516–22.

32. Lunel F, Musset L, Cacoub P, et al. Cryoglobulinemia in chronic liver disease: Role of hepatitis C virus and liver damage. Gastroenterology 1994;106:1291–300.

33. Pawlotsky J M, Roudot-Thoraval F, Simmonds P, et al. Ann Intern Med 1995;122:169–73.

34. Kew M C. Hepatitis C virus and hepatocellular carcinoma in developing and developed countries. Viral. Hepatitis Rev 1998;4:259–69.

35. Okuda K, Fujimoto I, Hanai A, Urano Y. Changing incidence of hepatocellular carcinoma in
Japan. Cancer Res 1987;47:4967–72.

36. Simonetti R G, Cammà C, Fiorello F, Politi F, D'Amico G, Pagliaro L. Hepatocellular carcinoma. A worldwide problem and the major risk factors. Dig Dis Sci 1991;36:962–72.

37. Koretz R L, Abbey H, Coleman E, Gitnick G. Non-A, non-B post-transfusion hepatitis: looking back in the second decade. Ann Intern Med 1993;119:110–5.

38. Chiba T, Matsuzaki Y, Abei M, et al. The role of previous hepatitis B virus infection and heavy
smoking in hepatitis C virus-related hepatocellular carcinoma. Am J Gastroenterol 1996;91:
1195–203.

39. Fattovich G, Giustina G, Degos F, et al. Effectiveness of interferon alpha on incidence of hepatocellular carcinoma and decompensation in cirrhosis type C. J Hepatol 1997;27:201–5.

40. Christensen E. Multivariate survival analysis using Cox's regression model. Hepatology 1987;
7:1346–58.

41. Colombo M, De Franchis R, Del Ninno E, et al. Hepatocellular carcinoma in Italian patients
with cirrhosis. N Engl J Med 1991;325:675–80.

42. Romeo R, Rumi M G, Del Ninno E, Colombo M. Hepatitis C virus genotype 1b and risk of hepatocellular carcinoma. Hepatology 1997;26:1077.

43. Bruno S, Silini E, Crosignani A, et al. Hepatitis C virus genotypes and risk of hepatocellular carcinoma in cirrhosis: a prospective study. Hepatology 1997;25:754–8.

44. Fattovich G, Ribero M L, Pantalena M, et al. Hepatitis C virus genotype and clinical outcome
of compensated cirrhosis type C. Hepatology 1998;28:408A.

45. Benvegnù L, Fattovich G, Noventa F, et al. Concurrent hepatitis B and C virus infection and
risk of hepatocellular carcinoma in cirrhosis. Cancer 1994;74:2442–8.

46. Tsai J F, Jeng J E, Ho M S, et al. Effect of hepatitis C and B virus infection on risk of hepatocellular carcinoma: a prospective study. Br J Cancer 1997;76:968–74.

47. Donato F, Tagger A, Chiesa R, et al. Hepatitis B and C virus infection, alcohol drinking and
hepatocellular carcinoma: a case-control study in Italy. Hepatology 1997;26:579–84.

48. Hu K Q, Tong M J. The long-term outcomes of patients with compensated hepatitis C virus-
related cirrhosis and history of parenteral exposure in the United States. Hepatology 1999;
29:1311–6.

49. Niederau C, Lange S, Heintges T, et al. Prognosis of chronic hepatitis C: results of a large, prospective cohort study. Hepatology 1998;28:1687–95.

50. Seeff L B, Buskell-Bales Z, Wright E C, et al. Long-term mortality after transfusion-associated non-A, non-B hepatitis. N Engl J Med 1992;327:1906–11.

51. Saracco G, Rosina F, Abate M L, et al. Long-term follow-up of patients with chronic hepatitis C treated with different doses of interferon-α 2b. Hepatology 1993;18:1300–5.

52. Saito T, Shinzawa H, Kuboki M, et al. A randomized controlled trial of human lymphoblastoid interferon in patients with compensated type C cirrhosis. Am J Gastroenterol 1994;89:681–6.

53. Brouwer J T, Nevens F, Kleter B, et al. Efficacy of interferon dose and prediction of response in chronic hepatitis C: Benelux study in 336 patients. J Hepatol 1998;28:951–9.

54. Ishimura N, Fukuda R, Fukumoto S. Relationship between the intrahepatic expression of interferon-alpha receptor mRNA and the histological progress of hepatitis C virus-associated chronic liver diseases. J Gastroenterol Hepatol 1996;11:712–7.

55. Mizukoshi E, Kaneko S, Yanagi M, et al. Expression of interferon alpha/beta receptor in the liver of chronic hepatitis C patients. J Med Virol 1998;56:217–23.

56. Fukuda R, Ishimura N, Kushiyama Y, et al. Effectiveness of interferon-alpha therapy in chronic hepatitis C is associated with the amount of interferon-alpha receptor mRNA in the liver. J Hepatol 1997;26:455–61.

57. Morita K, Tanaka K, Saito S, et al. Expression of interferon receptor genes (IFNAR1 and IFNAR2 mRNA) in the liver may predict outcome after interferon therapy in patients with chronic genotype 2a or 2b hepatitis C virus infection. J Clin Gastroenterol 1998;26:135–40.

58. Cooksley W G E. Interferon treatment of chronic hepatitis C with cirrhosis. J Viral Hepatitis 1997;4:85–8.

59. Farrell G, Cooksley W G, Dudley F J, Watson K. Efficacy and tolerance of a 6-month treatment course of daily interferon-alpha 2a for chronic hepatitis C with cirrhosis. The Australian Hepatitis C Study Group. J Viral Hepatitis 1997;4:317–23.

60. Schalm S W, Fattovich G, Brouwer J T. Therapy of hepatitis C: patients with cirrhosis. Hepatology 1997;26(Suppl 1):128S–32S.

61. Valla D C, Chevallier M, Marcellin P, et al. Treatment of hepatitis C virus-related cirrhosis: a randomized, controlled trial of interferon alfa-2b versus no treatment. Hepatology 1999;29:1870–5.

62. Reichard O, Norkrans G, Fryden A, Braconier J-H, Sönnerborg A, Weiland O. Randomized, double-blind, placebo-controlled trial of interferon α-2b with and without ribavirin for chronic hepatitis C. Lancet 1998;351:83–7.

63. Davis G L, Esteban-Mur R, Rustgi V K, et al. Interferon alfa-2b alone or in combination with ribavirin for the treatment of relapse of chronic hepatitis C. N Engl J Med 1998;339:1493–9.

64. McHutchison J G, Gordon S C, Schiff E R, et al. Interferon Alfa-2b alone or in combination with ribavirin as initial treatment for chronic hepatitis C. N Engl J Med 1998;339:1485–92.

65. Poynard T, Marcellin P, Lee S S, et al. Randomised trial of interferon α2b plus ribavirin for 48 weeks or for 24 weeks versus interferon α2b plus placebo for 48 weeks for treatment of chronic infection with hepatitis C virus. Lancet 1998;352:1426–32.

66. Schalm S W, Weiland O, Hansen B E, et al. Interferon-ribavirin for chronic hepatitis C with and without cirrhosis: analysis of individual patient data of six controlled trials. Gastroenterology. 1999;117:408–13.

67. Gane E J, Portmann B C, Naoumov N V, et al. Long-term outcome of hepatitis C infection after liver transplantation. N Engl J Med 1996;334:815–20.

68. Mazzaferro V, Regalia E, Doci R, et al. Liver transplantation for the treatment of small hepatocellular carcinomas in patients with cirrhosis. N Engl J Med 1996;334:693–9.

69. Bruix J, Castells A, Bosch J, et al. Surgical resection of hepatocellular carcinoma in cirrhotic patients: prognostic value of preoperative portal pressure. Gastroenterology 1996;111:1018–22.

70. Livraghi T, Giorgio T, Marin G, et al. Hepatocellular carcinoma in cirrhosis in 746 patients: long-term results of percutaneous ethanol injection. Radiology 1995;197:101–8.

71. Colombo M. Treatment of hepatocellular carcinoma. J Viral Hepatitis 1997;4(Suppl 1):125–30.

72. Llovet J M, Bruix J. Prognostic assessment and medical treatment of advanced hepatocellular carcinoma. In: Arroyo V, Bosch J, Bruguera M, Rodès J, Sànchez Tapias J, eds. Treatment of liver diseases. Barcelona, Spain: Masson, SA, 1999:345–54.

13

HEPATITIS C AND HEPATOCELLULAR CARCINOMA

ADRIAN M. DI BISCEGLIE

Department of Internal Medicine
Saint Louis University School of Medicine
St Louis, Missouri

INTRODUCTION

Hepatocellular carcinoma (HCC) ranks as one of the most common forms of cancer worldwide. Only recently has it been recognized that the hepatitis C virus (HCV) is one of its major causes. Initially, individual case reports had linked long-standing non-A, non-B hepatitis with the development of HCC. With the discovery of HCV as the major cause of non-A, non-B hepatitis and the development of reliable assays for antibody to HCV (anti-HCV), the association of HCC and chronic hepatitis C was strengthened. In studies from Spain and Italy, as many as 60 to 70% of patients with HCC had anti-HCV as the only risk factor for liver cancer. [1,2] Subsequently, studies from all over the world have confirmed this association.

DETERMINATION OF HCV-RELATED HCC

The presence of anti-HCV in a patient with HCC is generally considered adequate evidence that the liver cancer is related to hepatitis C. Currently available, third-generation enzyme immunoassays (EIAs) for anti-HCV have high degrees of sensitivity, although their specificity may not be optimal. Moreover, studies using supplementary tests indicate that most patients with HCC who have anti-HCV detected by EIA can be confirmed as having true antibody reactivity. [3,4] Indeed, most liver cancer patients with anti-HCV are also reactive for HCV RNA. [5] In some cases, HCV RNA may be detectable within liver tissue and even occasionally within the tumor tissue itself. Furthermore, in a small proportion of cases, HCV RNA may be detected in serum in the absence of anti-HCV. The explanation for this latter finding is not clear, but it is consistent with other studies showing that not all patients with chronic HCV infection have anti-HCV detectable in serum.

EPIDEMIOLOGY

Hepatocellular carcinoma is marked by great geographical variations in incidence and associated risk factors. Worldwide, HCC is one of the most common cancers and is particularly common in sub-Saharan Africa, China, and the Far East, where the frequency is as high as 120 cases per 100,000 population each year. (6) The majority of cases in these endemic areas are related to chronic infection with hepatitis B virus (HBV), as shown by the presence of hepatitis B surface antigen (HBsAg) and/or antibody to hepatitis B core antigen (anti-HBc) in serum. In contrast to the high rate of HCC in endemic areas, the incidence of liver cancer is low in developed regions of the world such as the United States and northern Europe and is intermediate in frequency in southern Europe and Japan. Of interest, an increasing incidence of HCC has been reported in the United States and the United Kingdom, the cause of which is believed to be chronic hepatitis C. (7,8) The incidence of HCC in the United States is currently 2.4 per 100,000 persons, and the tumor is more common in men than women, in blacks than in whites, and in older age groups, the peak age of diagnosis being 60–80 years. (8)

Chronic hepatitis C and HCV-related HCC occur worldwide, but the proportion of cases related to HCV varies considerably (Fig. 1). For example, in southern Europe in Italy, Spain, and Portugal, as well as in other isolated countries such as Japan, HCV infection appears to be the most frequent underlying cause of HCC. (6) In the United States, the proportion of patients with HCC who are seropositive for anti-HCV varies by region and ethnic group (Fig. 2). Thus, in Miami, with its high proportion of Hispanic individuals, anti-HCV is commonly associated with HCC, whereas among the predominantly Caucasian patients evaluated in Baltimore, only a small fraction is anti-HCV positive. (9,10) Among patients in the United States of Chinese or African descent as well as native Alaskans, HBV appears to be the most frequent cause of HCC. In addition, a substantial proportion of patients with HCC in the United States have no serological evidence of either HBV or HCV infection.

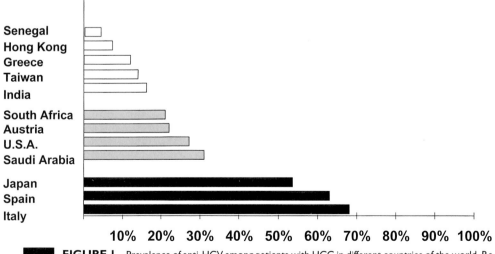

FIGURE I   Prevalence of anti-HCV among patients with HCC in different countries of the world. Reproduced with permission from Di Bisceglie. (6)

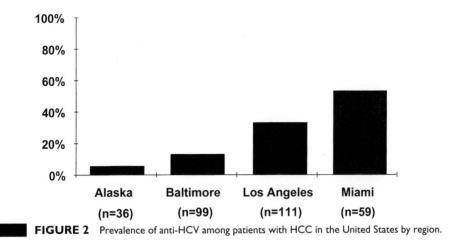

FIGURE 2   Prevalence of anti-HCV among patients with HCC in the United States by region.

NATURAL HISTORY STUDIES

The long-term follow-up of patients with chronic hepatitis C provides the most definitive information on the association of HCV infection and liver cancer. These studies are difficult because HCC rarely appears before 20 to 30 years after onset of infection with HCV. Kiyosawa and colleagues (11) described a cohort of patients with HCV-related HCC in whom the onset of infection could be traced back to a blood transfusion. These patients had been followed over several decades, often undergoing liver biopsy. Many of them demonstrated a stepwise progression in their liver disease from chronic hepatitis, with progressive stages of fibrosis leading to cirrhosis and eventually clinically apparent HCC. The average period between blood transfusion to diagnosis of HCC was 25 years. Similarly, evaluation of a small cohort of patients from the United States with HCV-related HCC showed that the duration of HCV infection from time of presumed exposure to development of HCC ranged from 5 to 30 years with a median of 17.5 years. (12) Comparison of patients with HCV-related to those with HBV-related HCC showed that those with hepatitis C were older at presentation, were likely to be Caucasian, and to have a history of blood transfusion. In a study by Tong and colleagues (13) from Los Angeles, 7 of 131 (5.3%) patients with transfusion-related chronic hepatitis C had HCC when initially referred for evaluation. On follow-up, HCC developed in 7 patients at an average of 3 years after the initial visit. The mean duration between blood transfusion and the development of HCC in this cohort was 28.3 years. Finally, a large cohort of patients from Europe with HCV-related cirrhosis were followed prospectively for the development of HCC. Over a period of 10 years, 15% developed HCC at a rate of approximately 1.5% per year. (14) Similar studies of patients with hepatitis C and cirrhosis from other countries have rates as high as 9% per year in some cohorts. (6)

Overall estimates of progression of disease in chronic hepatitis C indicate that about 20% of all patients with chronic HCV infection develop cirrhosis within 10 to 20 years. (15) Progression to cirrhosis may be influenced by several host factors, such as age at infection, alcohol consumption, and male gender.

TABLE I   **Risk Factors for Hepatocellular Carcinoma in Patients with Chronic Hepatitis C**[a]

Variable	Risk ratio	p value
Age (years)		
<60	1	
>60	2.51	0.003
Gender		
Male	1	
Female	0.78	>0.2
Histologic staging score		
F1 or F2	1	
F3 or F4	2.34	0.049
Histologic activity score		
<10	1	
>10	2.27	0.029
Alanine aminotransferase level (U/liter)		
<100	1	
>100	1.59	0.144
Platelet count		
>140,000/mm^3	1	
<140,000/mm^3	1.70	0.173
α-Fetoprotein level (ng/ml)		
<20	1	
>20	1.27	>0.2
Interferon therapy		
Untreated	1	
Treated	0.53	0.041

[a]Reproduced from Imai et al. (17) with permission.

Once cirrhosis is present, HCC develops at a rate between 1.5 and 9% per year. (14,16) Thus over a period of 20 years, the risk of developing HCC has been estimated at approximately 5% in individuals infected with HCV. Risk factors for the development of HCC among patients with hepatitis C include age, gender, alcohol use, severity of the cirrhosis, and possibly coinfection with hepatitis B. Relative risks associated with these factors among a large cohort of carefully evaluated patients with HCV-related HCC from Japan are listed in Table I. (17)

MECHANISMS OF HEPATOCARCINOGENESIS

Mechanisms by which HCV infection results in HCC are not well defined. Clearly, cirrhosis plays a central role as the majority of cases of HCV-related HCC occur in the presence of cirrhosis or at least severe architectural distortion. This association suggests that inflammation associated with chronic hepatitis C and the recurrent bouts of liver injury and hepatic regeneration that underlie the development of cirrhosis also predispose to HCC. This association is less firm for chronic hepatitis B, where HCC not infrequently occurs in the absence of cirrhosis, particularly among children or young adults. Cases of HCC in patients with hepatitis C without cirrhosis have been reported. (18)

Cirrhosis is well known to represent a major risk factor for the development of HCC. (19) As many as 10% of patients dying with cirrhosis are found to have an unsuspected HCC at autopsy. This is borne out in transplant studies where between 3 and 6% of explanted livers are found to contain unsuspected HCC. Diseases causing cirrhosis with the highest risk of HCC are chronic viral hepatitis (including hepatitis C), alcoholic liver disease, hemochromatosis, and α_1-antitrypsin deficiency. (16) The risk may be lower in cirrhosis due to Wilson's disease, primary biliary cirrhosis, and autoimmune hepatitis. Nevertheless, HCC has been well documented to occur in all forms of cirrhosis, and the rate of HCC in these conditions may relate more to other risk factors, such as gender, age, and duration of disease.

The mechanisms by which cirrhosis leads to HCC are not known. While inflammation, injury, and regeneration may all play a role, investigators have implicated the dysplastic nodules commonly seen in cirrhosis as being important precursors to HCC. (19) These dysplastic nodules have the appearance of large (>1 cm) cirrhotic nodules macroscopically, whereas microscopically they have features of dysplasia, particularly a change to small cells with large nuclei. Borzio and colleagues (20) studied a cohort of patients of cirrhosis, among whom 32 had dysplastic nodules. During follow-up, HCC developed in 8 (25%) of these nodules and elsewhere in the liver in an additional 3 (9%) cases. The origin of dysplastic nodules is disputed. They may represent cirrhotic nodules that have outgrown surrounding companions; alternatively, they may represent clonal proliferation of a single transformed hepatocyte arising between other cirrhotic nodules. (19)

HCV itself has been suggested to have direct carcinogenic potential, although its genome does not become integrated within the host chromosomes as occurs with HBV. (18) In particular, the HCV core protein has been implicated as being possibly carcinogenic (Table II). (20–25) There also may be viral factors associated with a high risk of developing HCC. In several reports, HCV genotype 1b has been associated with a higher risk of HCC than other genotypes. HCV genotype 1b has also been linked, although inconsistently, with more severe and rapidly progressive liver disease. (14) These studies linking genotype with HCC, however, did not address the role of a cohort effect; thus, most persons infected with HCV more than 20 years previously were infected with genotype 1. (26) Studies from Japan, Europe, and the United States have shown that

TABLE II Evidence Suggesting a Direct Carcinogenic Role for HCV Core Protein

Reference	Evidence
Moriya et al. (21)	HCV core transgenic mice develop HCC
Ray et al. (22)	Core protein suppresses apoptosis
Yasui et al. (23)	Core protein trafficks through the nucleus
Ray et al. (24)	Core protein transforms rat embyro fibroblasts
Kim et al. (25)	Core protein acts as a trans suppressor

other genotypes, such as genotype 3, have been introduced more recently than genotype 1.

HCV-related HCC has been suggested to be multicentric in origin more often than HBV-related cancer, as well as to recur more frequently following resection. The validity of these observations has yet to be confirmed.

COFACTORS FOR DEVELOPMENT OF HCC

Several factors have been suggested to increase the risk of developing HCC among those with chronic HCV infection, including alcohol ingestion, coinfection with HBV, and the presence of porphyria cutanea tarda. (14,17,26–29) Alcohol is thought to have independent carcinogenic properties, and alcohol consumption has been clearly linked to several forms of cancer, including carcinoma of the pancreas, esophagus, pharynx, and larynx. Alcoholic liver disease (in particular cirrhosis) is a well-known risk factor for HCC, and alcohol consumption has been reported to increase the risk of HCC among patients with cirrhosis due to hepatitis C. (27) The mechanisms by which these cofactors might operate are not known. One possibility is that alcohol ingestion hastens the progression of liver disease and that the duration and severity of cirrhosis are the primary factors leading to HCC. Coinfection with HBV has also been linked to an increased risk of HCC among patients with chronic hepatitis C, and coinfection also appears to lead to more severe liver injury than with hepatitis C alone. Kew and colleagues (28) found that South African patients infected with both HBV and HCV had a more than tenfold higher relative risk of developing HCC than those with HCV alone (Table III).

The association of porphyria cutanea tarda with HCC has been reported by several groups of investigators. Salata and co-workers (29) described a cohort of 83 patients with porphyria cutanea tarda in Spain of whom 13 had HCC (15.6%). The role of HCV infection among these cases was not known as this study was published before the discovery of HCV, but hepatitis C has subsequently been shown to be a major cause or association with porphyria cutanea tarda. The mechanism by which porphyria might promote development of HCC is not known. Other forms of acute and chronic porphyria are associated with an increased risk of developing HCC. Furthermore, porphyria cutanea tarda is often associated with iron overload and the increased hepatic iron content may increase the risk of HCC as occurs in hereditary hemochromatosis. In several

TABLE III   Hepatitis B Virus Infection as a Cofactor with HCV for Development of HCC[a]

HBsAg	Anti-HCV	Cases	Controls	Relative risk	95% CI
Negative	Negative	69	197	1.0	
Negative	Positive	39	15	6.6	2.7–15.7
Positive	Negative	103	18	23.3	9.2–59.4
Positive	Positive	20	1	82.5	8.9–761.8

[a] Adapted from Kew et al. (28) with permission.

reports, increased hepatic iron has been implicated as a risk factor for HCC, even in the absence of hereditary hemochromatosis. (30)

Other as yet unknown cofactors may exist that increase the risk of HCC in chronic hepatitis C. Infection with the hepatitis G virus (or GB virus-C) does not appear to constitute a risk factor for HCC. (31–33)

DIAGNOSIS AND SCREENING

HCC typically presents clinically at an advanced stage, once the tumor is large enough to cause worsening of liver disease, right upper quadrant pain, or weight loss. At this stage, there are few therapeutic options available. If, however, HCC is detected at an earlier stage, either by routine or screening abdominal ultrasound examination or by determination of serum α-fetoprotein level, the tumor may be amenable to curative resection. Regular screening ultrasound and/or α-fetoprotein testing is often recommended for patients with chronic hepatitis C, even though a clear survival benefit has yet to be shown. Patients with the highest risk for HCC are those with established cirrhosis. Because HCC rarely develops in patients without cirrhosis, routine screening using ultrasound or α-fetoprotein might best be limited to patients with cirrhosis, either documented by liver biopsy or suggested by patterns of biochemical laboratory tests. In patients with established cirrhosis, resection may not be an option even if the HCC is small and confined to a single lobe. These patients can also be considered for liver transplantation or some form of minimally invasive ablation such as transcutaneous alcohol injection, intraarterial embolization, or radiofrequency thermal ablation. Of these options, liver transplantation has been associated with the best survival rates and should be considered where tumors are small (less than 5 cm) and few (less than three). Unexpected HCC may also be discovered at the time of liver transplantation for advanced cirrhosis due to hepatitis C. (34,35)

PREVENTION OF HCC

Prevention of HCV-related HCC might be accomplished by prevention of primary infection with HCV (either by vaccination or other public health interventions), by prevention of development of cirrhosis in patients already infected with HCV, or by prevention of development of cancer in patients with advanced fibrosis or cirrhosis due to HCV. Primary prevention is an elusive goal at present, as effective vaccines for HCV have yet to be developed; even with a vaccine, several decades are needed before such interventions will decrease the rate of HCC. Thus, in hepatitis B, where an effective vaccine became available in the early 1980s, HCC did not even begin to decrease until over a decade after the initiation of wide-scale vaccination programs. (36) No such vaccine is available for HCV, and prevention approaches are limited to use of other public health measures, including screening of blood transfusions for anti-HCV, inactivation of HCV in plasma products, and education of persons in high-risk groups regarding modes of transmission. As a consequence of such programs, the number of new cases of HCV infection in the United States has decreased considerably in recent years. (37) However, the number of new cases of HCC related to HCV infection acquired in the last several decades is expected to increase for some time to come, given the long natural history of HCV infection.

Prevention of progression of hepatitis C to cirrhosis and progression of cirrhosis to liver cancer should also help prevent the development of HCC. Nonspecific measures include avoidance of cofactors for worsening of chronic hepatitis C and HCC, such as alcohol and hepatitis B. Thus, patients with chronic hepatitis C should be counseled to avoid alcohol and should be vaccinated against HBV if they have not already been exposed. Iron overload may also predispose to development of worsening fibrosis in chronic hepatitis C. For this reason, patients should be assessed with noninvasive tests for iron status and have routine iron stains done on liver biopsies. Patients with hepatitis C and iron overload (with 3+ staining on a scale of 0 to 4+ on liver biopsy) should undergo phlebotomy. Similar patients with porphyria cutanea tarda should be treated adequately with phlebotomy therapy to reestablish a normal iron status.

The goal of antiviral therapy of hepatitis C is to eradicate the viral infection and arrest the liver disease. Patients who have cleared HCV RNA following a course of treatment with interferon and remained negative in follow-up generally show a marked improvement in the degree of necroinflammatory changes and mild-to-moderate decreases in the amount of hepatic fibrosis on liver biopsy. Thus, if the development of HCC is dependent on ongoing necrosis and regeneration, improvement in these features following therapy may be expected to decrease the risk of HCC.

Published results on the effects of interferon therapy on ultimate rates of HCC in chronic hepatitis C have been somewhat contradictory. Most trials of interferon therapy have reported results of 6 to 12 months follow up of treatment only, which is too short to assess the effects of treatment on the development of cirrhosis or HCC. An exception to this was reported by Nishiguchi et al. (38) who conducted a randomized control trial in 90 patients with cirrhosis due to hepatitis C with a follow-up period of 2 years after treatment Patients were treated with interferon alone at standard doses for a period of 6 months. Compared to controls, treated patients developed HCC at a significantly lower rate than those who were not treated. Thus, after nearly 5 years of follow-up, 4.4% of treated patients compared to 38% of controls had developed HCC. Furthermore, the decreased risk of HCC occurred independent of whether there was a sustained loss of HCV RNA with treatment. Similar findings have been reported in retrospective analyses of larger cohorts of patients treated in Europe and Japan (Table IV). (14,17,38–44) Most of these studies, however, were not prospectively designed, and treated patients and controls were not matched or randomly assigned to be treated or not. A retrospective analysis of a large cohort from Italy, in which there was a careful adjustments for known risk factors for HCC, subsequently failed to detect a significant benefit of interferon therapy on the morbidity of patients with compensated cirrhosis due to hepatitis C. (40) Thus, HCC developed less commonly among patients who were treated with interferon, but treated patients tended to be younger and to have less severe cirrhosis than untreated controls. When risk factors were controlled for in the analysis, the 5-year estimated probability of developing HCC was 2.1% among 193 treated patients and 2.7% among untreated controls.

A surprising observation from many of the retrospective analyses of inter-

TABLE IV   Rates of Development of Hepatocellular Carcinoma in Patients with Chronic Hepatitis C Treated with Interferon-α

| Author | Year | Development of hepatocellular carcinoma | | |
		Untreated	Sustained responders	Non-responders
Nishiguchi et al. (38)	1995	17/45 (38%)	0/7 (0%)	2/38 (5%)
Mazzella et al. (39)	1996	16/136 (12%)	0/14 (0%)	7/179 (4%)
Fattovich et al. (40)	1997	9/91 (10%)	0/39 (0%)	5/154 (3%)
Imai et al. (17)	1998	19/144 (13%)	1/151 (0.6%)	27/268 (10%)
Kasahara et al. (41)	1998	—	5/313 (16%)	41/709 (6%)
Miyajima et al. (42)	1998	—	0/63 (0%)	12/150 (8%)
Ikeda et al. (43)	1999	67/452 (15%)	7/606 (1%)	21/585 (3%)
Overall		128/868 (14.7%)	13/1193 (1.0%)	115/2083 (5.5%)

[a] Summary of seven studies on the incidence of HCC in patients with hepatitis C and cirrhosis comparing treated and untreated patients as well as patients with and without a sustained virological response. Nonresponders included patients who had a transient response and relapse.

feron treatment of patients with cirrhosis was that the decrease in the risk of HCC associated with interferon treatment occurred independently of whether there was a successful outcome of therapy. This effect of interferon treatment may reflect the fact that patients selected for treatment have less severe liver disease than those who are not treated and therefore have a lesser likelihood of developing HCC. This issue is not likely to be resolved in the absence of a prospective randomized, suitably controlled trial of antiviral therapy in patients at greatest risk of developing HCC. More recently, the combination of interferon and ribavirin appears to have eclipsed interferon alone as the mainstay of therapy in chronic hepatitis C. No data are available yet about the potential impact of this combination therapy on the subsequent risk of HCC.

CONCLUSION

Chronic infection with HCV is a well-established risk factor for the development of HCC and in many areas of the world is the most common etiological factor in the development of liver cancer. Hepatitis C appears to cause HCC as a result of chronic or recurrent bouts of hepatocellular necrosis and hepatic inflammation and regeneration, but the virus may also be directly carcinogenic as a result of the effects of HCV protein products on normal growth, apoptosis, repair, and cellular signaling pathways. The risk of developing HCC in patients with hepatitis C relates to the duration and severity of the disease as well as cofactors such as age, male gender, iron overload, porphyria, coinfection with hepatitis B, and alcohol use. The risk of HCC is probably less than 5% overall during the first 20 to 30 years of hepatitis C, but this risk increases greatly once cirrhosis is present. Among patients with compensated cirrhosis due to hepatitis C, the risk of HCC is 1 to 4% per year. The prevention of HCC can be expected by primary prevention of HCV infection and also by secondary prevention in patients already infected with this virus by avoidance of alcohol, correction of iron overload, prevention of hepatitis B coinfection, and successful treatment of hepatitis C with antiviral therapy. Because patients with cirrhosis due to hepatitis C can be identified as being at risk of HCC, they can be screened regularly to detect HCC at an early, potentially treatable stage and may also be candidates for therapy with interferon-α with or without ribavirin in an attempt to decrease the risk of hepatic malignancy.

REFERENCES

1. Colombo M, Kuo G, Choo Q L, et al. Prevalence of antibodies to hepatitis C virus in Italian patients with hepatocellular carcinoma. Lancet 1989;2:1006–8.
2. Bruix J, Barrera J M, Calvet X, et al. Prevalence of antibodies to hepatitis C virus in Spanish patients with hepatocellular carcinoma and hepatic cirrhosis. Lancet 1989;2:1004–6.
3. Colombo M, Rumi M G, Donato M F, et al. Hepatitis C antibody in patients with chronic liver disease and hepatocellular carcinoma. Dig Dis Sci 1991;36:1130–1.
4. Mangia A, Vallari D S, Di Bisceglie A M. Use of confirmatory assays for diagnosis of hepatitis C viral infection in patients with hepatocellular carcinoma. J Med Virol 1994;43:125–8.
5. Bukh J, Miller R H, Kew M C, Purcell R H. Hepatitis C virus RNA in southern African Blacks with hepatocellular carcinoma. Proc Natl Acad Sci U S A 1993;90:1848–51.
6. Di Bisceglie A M Hepatitis C and hepatocellular carcinoma. Hepatology 1997;26:34S–8S.
7. Taylor-Robinson S D, Foster G R, Arora S, Hargreaves S, Thomas H C. Increase in primary liver cancer in the UK, 1979–94. Br Med J 1997;350:1142–3.
8. El-Serag H, Mason A. Rising incidence of hepatocellular carcinoma in the United States. N Engl J Med 1999;340:745–50.
9. Hasan F, Jeffers L J, de Medina M, et al. Hepatitis C-associated hepatocellular carcinoma. Hepatology 1990;12:589–91.
10. Di Bisceglie A M, Klien J, Choo Q, et al. Role of chronic viral hepatitis in hepatocellular carcinoma in the United States. Am J Gastroenterol 1991;86:335–8.
11. Kiyosawa K, Sodeyama T, Tanaka E, et al. Interrelationship of blood transfusion, non-A, non-B hepatitis and hepatocellular carcinoma: analysis by detection of antibody to hepatitis C virus. Hepatology 1990;12:671–5.
12. Di Bisceglie A M, Simpson L H, Lotze M T, Hoofnagle J H. Development of hepatocellular carcinoma among patients with chronic liver disease due to hepatitis C viral infection. J Clin Gastroenterol 1994;19:222–6.
13. Tong M J, El-Farra N S, Reikes A R, Co R L. Clinical outcomes after transfusion-associated hepatitis C. N Engl J Med 1995;332:1463–6.
14. Fattovich G, Giustina G, Degos F, et al. Morbidity and mortality in compensated cirrhosis type C: a restrospective follow-up study of 384 patients. Gastroenterology 1997;112:463–72.
15. National Institutes of Health Consensus Development Conference Panel Statement: management of hepatitis C. Hepatology 1997;26:2S–10S.
16. Mandelli C, Fraquelli M, Fargion S, et al. Comparable frequency of hepatocellular carcinoma in cirrhosis of different etiology. Eur J Gastroenterol Hepatol 1994;6:1129–34.
17. Imai Y, Kawata S, Tamura S, et al. Relation of interferon therapy and hepatocellular carcinoma in patients with chronic hepatitis C. Ann Intern Med 1998;129:94–9.
18. De Mitri MS, Poussin K, Baccarini P, et al. HCV-associated liver cancer without cirrhosis. Lancet 1995;345:413–5.
19. Theise N D. Cirrhosis and hepatocellular neoplasia: more like cousins than like parent and child. Gastroenterology 1996;111:526–8.
20. Borzio M, Bruno S, Roncalli M, et al. Liver cell dysplasia is a major risk factor for hepatocellular carcinoma in cirrhosis; a prospective study. Gastroenterology 1998;108:812–6.
21. Moriya K, Fujie H, Shintani Y, et al. The core protein of hepatitis C virus induces hepatocellular carcinoma in transgenic mice. Nat Med 1998;4:1065–7.
22. Ray R B, Meyer K, Ray R. Suppression of apoptotic cell death by hepatitis C virus core protein. Virology 1996;226:176–82.
23. Yasui K, Wakita T, Tsukiyama-Kohara K, Funahashi S I. The native form and maturation process of hepatitis C virus core protein. J Virol 1998;72:6048–55.

24. Ray R B, Lagging L M, Meyer K, Ray R. Hepatitis C virus core protein cooperates with ras and transforms primary rat embryo fibroblasts to tumorigenic phenotype. J Virol 1996;70:4438–43.

25. Kim D W, Suzuki R, Harada T, Saito I, Miyamura T. Trans-suppression of gene expression by hepatitis C viral core protein. Jpn J Med Sci Biol 1994;47:211–20.

26. Benvegnu L, Pontisso P, Cavalletto D, Noventa F, Chemello L, Alberti A. Lack of correlation between hepatitis C virus genotypes and clinical course of hepatitis C virus—related cirrhosis. Hepatology 1997;25:211–5.

27. Yamauchi M, Nakahara M, Maezawa Y, Satoh S, Nishikawa F, Ohata M. Prevalence of hepatocellular carcinoma in patients with alcoholic cirrhosis and prior exposure to hepatitis C. Am J Gastroenterol 1993;88:39–43.

28. Kew M C, Yu M C, Kedda M, Coppin A, Sarkin A, Hodkinson J. The relative roles of hepatitis B and C viruses in the etiology of hepatocellular carcinoma in southern African Blacks. Gastroenterology 1997;112:184–7.

29. Salata H, Cortes J M, de Salamanca R E, et al. Porphyria cutanea tarda and hepatocellular carcinoma—Frequency of occurence and related factors. J Hepatol 1985;1:477–87.

30. Turlin B, Juguet F, Moirand R, et al. Increased liver iron stores in patients with hepatocellular carcinoma developed on a noncirrhotic liver. Hepatology 1995;22:446–50.

31. Kao J, Chen P, Lai M, et al. GB virus-C/hepatitis G virus infection in an area endemic for viral hepatitis, chronic liver disease, and liver cancer. Gastroenterology 1997;112:1265–70.

32. Tagger A, Donato F, Ribero M L, et al. A case-control study on GB virus C/hepatitis G virus infection and hepatocellular carcinoma. Hepatology 1997;26:1653–7.

33. Lightfoot K, Skelton M, Kew M C, et al. Does hepatitis GB virus-C infection cause hepatocellular carcinoma in black Africans? Hepatology 1990;26:740–2.

34. Mor E, Kaspa R, Sheiner P, Schwartz M. Treatment of hepatocellular carcinoma associated with cirrhosis in the era of liver transplantation. Ann Intern Med 1998;129:643–53.

35. Miller W J, Baron R L, Dodd G D, Federle M P. Malignancies in patients with cirrhosis: CT sensitivity and specificity in 200 consecutive transplant patients. Radiology 1994;193:645–50.

36. Chang M, Chen C, Lai M, et al. Universal hepatitis B vaccination in Taiwan and the incidence of hepatocellular carcinoma in children. N Engl J Med 1997;336:1855–9.

37. Alter M J, Mast E E. The epidemiology of viral hepatitis in the United States. Gastroenterol Clin North Am 1994;23:437–51.

38. Nishiguchi S, Kuroki T, Nakatani S, et al. Randomized trial of effects of interferon-α on incidence of hepatocellular carcinoma in chronic active hepatitis C with cirrhosis. Lancet 1995;346:1051–5.

39. Mazzella G, Accogli E, Sottili S, et al. Alpha interferon treatment may prevent hepatocellular carcinoma in HCV-related liver cirrhosis. J Hepatol 1996;24:141–7.

40. Fattovich G, Giustina G, Degos F, et al. Effectiveness of interferon alfa on incidence of hepatocellular carcinoma and decompensation in cirrhosis type C. J Hepatol 1997;27:201–5.

41. Kasahara A, Hayashi N, Mochizuki K, et al. Risk factors for hepatocellular carcinoma and its incidence after interferon treatment in patients with chronic hepatitis C. Hepatology 1998;27:1394–402.

42. Miyajima I, Sata M, Kumashiro R, et al. The incidence of hepatocellular carcinoma in patients with chronic hepatitis C after interferon treatment. Oncol Rep 1998;5:201–4.

43. Ikeda K, Saitoh S, Arase Y, et al. Effect of interferon therapy on hepatocellular carcinogenesis in patients with chronic type C hepatitis: a long-term observation study of 1,643 patients using statistical bias correction with proportional hazard analysis. Hepatology 1999;29:1124–30.

44. International Interferon Hepatocellular Carcinoma Study Group, Brunetto M, Oliveri F, Koehler M, Zahm F, Bonino F. Effect of interferon on progression of cirrhosis to hepatocellular carcinoma: a retrospective cohort study. Lancet 1998;351:1535–9.

14
HEPATITIS C AND LIVER TRANSPLANTATION

MARINA BERENGUER AND TERESA L. WRIGHT

Department of Veterans Affairs Medical Center
University of California
San Francisco, California

INTRODUCTION

The hepatitis C virus (HCV) has major implications in liver transplantation, not only in the number of infected recipients but also in the number at risk with serious recurrent disease leading to graft failure and retransplantation. Cirrhosis secondary to HCV infection, alone or in combination with alcohol, has become the leading indication for liver transplantation among adults, accounting for approximately half of transplantations in many centers. (1) There is a real concern that the high prevalence of HCV in the general U.S. population (1.8%) will result in an increased need for liver transplantation as progressive liver disease develops in a subset. (2) Given the lack of a universally effective antiviral therapy, it is expected that the demand on the already limited donor organ supply will continue to rise.

Recurrent infection, defined as the presence of virus in serum, is universal in those with pretransplantation infection. (3) Short-term, severe graft dysfunction is rare. (4–6) However, recurrent histologic disease occurs in at least 50% of HCV-infected recipients within 1–2 years of follow-up. Progressive liver injury therefore may ultimately result in reduced graft and patient survival compared with patients transplanted for nonviral causes. (6–10) Strategies to prevent or reduce the effect of HCV infection after liver transplantation are therefore desirable. In contrast to hepatitis B virus (HBV) infection, where the hepatitis B immune globulin has proven to be beneficial, effective prophylactic therapies are not available for HCV. Treatment of posttransplant HCV disease with interferon (11,12) or ribavirin (13,14) as single agents have been met with limited success. Ribavirin and interferon combination therapy appears a promising alternative. (15)

In order to ensure that liver transplantation continues to be an appropriate option for HCV-infected patients with end-stage liver disease, the following are necessary: (i) that effective therapy is developed to modify the natural history of HCV-related liver disease prior to transplantation in such a way that transplantation can be delayed or even obviated; (ii) that the number of organ donors is increased; (iii) that recurrent HCV infection is prevented, possibly by the use of immunotherapy or antivirals in the perioperative period; (iv) that recurrent disease is treated effectively if and when it occurs; and (v) that the management of recurrent HCV disease is improved, particularly regarding immunosuppression.

PRETRANSPLANTATION EVALUATION

Liver transplantation should be considered a therapeutic option when the course of the disease is sufficiently advanced that median-term survival is unlikely without this intervention. While this assumption has been demonstrated clearly for decompensated HCV-related end-stage liver disease, data confirming the benefits of transplantation over traditional management are less conclusive for compensated HCV cirrhotic patients. (16,17) The prognosis of compensated HCV-related cirrhosis has been assessed in two studies. In the first one, (16) the 5-year survival of 384 European-compensated HCV cirrhotic patients was 91%. Hepatic decompensation and hepatocellular carcinoma were observed in 18 and 7%, respectively. In the second study, (17) the 4-year survival of 103 HCV cirrhotic patients was 84%, with a 4-year risk of hepatic decompensation and of hepatocellular carcinoma of 20 and 11.5%, respectively. Thus, in the absence of controlled trials assessing the efficacy of liver transplantation, the 5-year outcome of compensated HCV cirrhotic patients favors observation in absence of transplantation. With the exponential rise in waiting time for liver transplantation, (18) decisions must be made in advance, limiting further the ability to choose the appropriate time point for patient referral.

Two approaches can be used in an attempt to decrease the mortality in these patients. The first is to use effective antiviral therapy in order to reduce clinical disease progression and need of transplantation. The second is to enlarge the pool of potential donors by including those who are anti-HCV positive. Although the first approach has not met with success in the past, use of anti-HCV positive donors may represent a solution in time of organ shortage.

Antiviral Therapy

Interferon alone or in combination with ribavirin has been used to suppress viral replication in cirrhotic patients. Combination therapy appears more effective than interferon alone in achieving sustained virological clearance, but the response is lower than in noncirrhotic patients. (19) Data regarding its effect in disease progression are scarce. Studies suggest a possible beneficial effect of interferon in patients with compensated cirrhosis in reducing the incidence of hepatocellular carcinoma (17,20,21) and other complications of end-stage liver disease, (17) even among those without virological response. Additional data are needed to confirm these preliminary results. Cirrhotic patients should thus be included in studies evaluating the benefits of antiviral therapy in preventing the development of complications and ultimately in reducing the need for transplantation. There have been anecdotal case reports of the use of interferon in decompensated HCV cirrhotic patients, as these patients have been typically excluded from randomized trials. Interferon is poorly tolerated in this setting and could potentially precipitate worsening hepatic function. Enrollment in a clinical trial should be considered whenever possible. Treatment outside clinical trials should be undertaken with caution.

HCV-Positive Organ Donors

The use of hepatitis C-positive organ donors becomes a potential way of improving the shortage of suitable donors. The reported prevalences of anti-HCV enzyme immune analysis (EIA 2) and of HCV RNA polymerase chain reaction (PCR) in cadaver organ donors in the United States are 4.2% (range 2.3–8.3%) and 2.4% (range 0.8–4.2%), respectively. (22) Organs from anti-HCV (RIBA 2)- and PCR-positive donors transmit infection almost universally. In contrast, organs from anti-HCV recombinant immunoblotting assay (RIBA 2)-positive PCR-negative donors transmit infection at a rate of only 50%. (22) Thus, approximately 50% of anti HCV-positive donors are not viremic and hence harbor a reduced chance of transmitting infection. PCR is, however, labor-intensive and time-consuming and is not a suitable screening method for donors. Discarding all anti-HCV organs would eliminate transmission, but would also lead to a waste of almost 2% of organs, which, albeit seropositive, lack true infection. Furthermore, the question concerning the suitability of organs from these donors largely depends on the prognosis of recipients receiving HCV-infected grafts. Data regarding this issue remain controversial (23) and may be related to differences in (i) the type of organ transplanted, (ii) assessment of disease severity (histologically versus biochemically), (iii) assessment of infection in the donor (serologically versus virologically), and (iv) duration of follow-up. Documentation of progressive liver disease in a substantial proportion of patients with recurrent HCV infection raises serious concern about the suitability of anti-HCV-positive organs for uninfected liver transplant candidates. An alternative option is the use of anti-HCV-positive organs for candidates who are already HCV infected. Superinfection in that setting has been described, (24) but the medium-term outcome of anti-HCV-positive recipients receiving HCV-infected grafts seems to be similar to that of anti-HCV-positive recipients receiving anti-HCV-negative grafts. (25,26) In addition, data from the immunocompetent population, where rates of disease progression are similar in patients with a high likelihood of superinfection such as intavenous drug users and those at low risk of superinfection such as those following transfusion, further suggest that the natural history of superinfected liver transplant recipients will not differ from that of the HCV-infected patient receiving an organ from an anti-HCV-negative donor. Further studies are, however, needed to evaluate the long-term impact of HCV superinfection. Until these data become available, seropositive donors should only be used in life-threatening situations, situations that will likely continue to increase. The consequences of superinfection with HCV should be evaluated carefully.

POSTTRANSPLANTATION INFECTION

Source of Infection

When the patient is infected at the time of transplantation, persistent HCV infection after transplantation is the rule. (3) In these circumstances, a rapid and sharp decline in viral load occurs immediately after removal of the infected liver, followed by a progressive increase in serum HCV RNA starting 72 hr after liver transplantation (27) to reach levels 10- to 20-fold higher than those detected prior to transplantation. (28–30)

The virus may be acquired in those without evidence of viral infection prior to transplantation from contaminated blood and organ donors and by nosocomial acquisition of virus during the hospitalization. (3) Routine donor screening with specific serologic tests for HCV and improvements in surgical techniques are likely the reasons for the drop in *de novo* acquisition of HCV infection following transplantation, which currently ranges from 0 to 5%. (29)

Natural History

Orthotopic liver transplantation provides a unique opportunity to study the natural history of HCV infection for the following reasons: (i) the exact timing of the infection is known as opposed to the immunocompetent patient where the timing of initial infection is often difficult to determine accurately as acute infection is typically subclinical and (ii) multiple liver biopsies are usually available, which facilitates the study of the histological evolution of HCV-associated liver disease. However, the presence of a substantial number of unmeasured or unknown variables influencing disease progression represents a limitation of this model.

The estimation of the natural history of HCV-related liver damage following liver transplantation and the factors associated with disease severity may help with the (i) identification of patients before transplantation who are at risk for severe recurrence, (ii) selection of patients who are most likely to benefit from therapy, and (iii) management of recipients with severe HCV disease through rational modification of immunosuppression.

The natural history of HCV infection in liver transplant recipients has been investigated by several centers. (5,6,8–10,31,32) Results, however, are difficult to compare, mainly due to differences in length of follow-up, ranging from 1 to 12 years, and a lack of uniformity in defining recurrent hepatitis C. Recurrent "HCV infection" defined as the presence of viremia by virological testing should be differentiated from recurrent "HCV disease" in which there is histologic evidence of liver injury. Uniform criteria should be adopted to define both concepts in order to compare data from different centers.

Defining HCV infection posttransplantation by serological means has limitations as these typically lack sensitivity. (33) New second- and third-generation assays are more sensitive, as titers of antibodies to C22, C25, NE1, and NE2 are less affected by immunosuppression. (34) Indeed, a positive RIBA-2 result is a reasonably good marker of viremia in the transplant population, and indeterminate RIBA-2 results (defined by a single reactive band pattern), found frequently among immunocompromised patients, often indicate HCV infection in this setting. In addition, defining recurrent disease biochemically as opposed to histologically also has limitations, as liver function tests, while indicative of liver disease, lack specificity and are not correlated with either viremia or histologic disease severity. (6,8)

Viremia is often but not always associated with disease. (28) Evidence of histologic hepatitis has been reported to vary from 48 to 100% of viremic liver

TABLE I HCV Infection Following Liver Transplantation: Median-Term Natural History Studies

Author	End points	No. biopsies (bx) n (range)	Histologic hepatitis	Follow-up (range)	Patient survival	Control group survival
Feray et al. (5) HCV group = 79, Control group = 106	Histologic severity; patient and graft survival	Mean bx/patient: n = 5 (2–12)	Actuarial rates of hepatitis at 1, 2, and 4 years: 57, 62, and 72%	HCV group: 46 months (12–84 months) Control: 55 months (1–86 months)	95, 90, and 80% at 1, 2, and 5 years	98, 96, and 89% at 1, 2, and 5 years
Gane et al. (6) HCV group = 149, Control group = 623	Histologic severity; patient and graft survival	Mean bx/patient: n = 4 (1–12)	Last biopsy: 12% normal (20 months), 54% mild hepatitis (35 months), 27% moderate (35 months), 8% cirrhosis (51 months)	36 months (1–138 months)	79, 74, and 70% at 1, 3, and 5 years	75, 71, and 69% at 1, 3, and 5 years
Boker et al. (31) HCV group = 71 Control group = 474	Patient and graft survival	n = 95	Inflammatory changes: 88% Fibrosis: 24%	Reinfected group: 33 ± 30 months De novo HCV group: 92 ± 32 months	67, 62, and 62% at 2, 5, and 10 years	62, 57, and 52% at 2, 5, and 10 years
Charlton et al. (32) HCV group = 166 Control group = 509	Patient and graft survival	NA[a]	NA	HCV: 60 months Control: 62 months	70% at 6 years	At 6 years: cholestatic 90%, alcoholic 65%
Prieto et al. (8) HCV group = 81	Histologic severity; patient and graft survival	n = 202	Last biopsy: hepatitis in 97% (moderate/severe in 64%). Actuarial rate of cirrhosis: 3.7 and 28% at 1 and 5 years	Mean histological follow-up: 32 ± 17 months	95, 91, and 84% at 2, 3, and 5 years	NA
Feray et al. (9) HCV group = 652	Histologic severity; patient and graft survival	Mean bx/patient: n = 3	Actuarial rate of hepatitis: 68 and 80% at 3 and 5 years. Actuarial rate of cirrhosis: 5 and 10% at 3 and 5 years	42 ± 28 months	75 and 70% at 3 and 5 years	NA
Berenguer et al. (10) HCV group = 284	Histologic severity and fibrosis progression; patient and graft survival	Mean bx/patient: n = 3	Fibrosis progression/year: 0.3 (0.004–2.19). Actuarial rate of cirrhosis at 5 years: 10 and 31% in U.S. and Spanish centers	Mean histological follow-up: 31 ± 21 months	83% at 5 years	NA

[a]None available.

transplant recipients (Table I). (4,6,8–10) Differences in time of histologic assessment and lack of protocol biopsies may explain this wide range. In order to describe accurately the natural history of HCV infection following liver transplantation, protocol liver biopsies need to be performed in all patients, a routine that is rarely followed in transplant centers. (8) Rather, patients are usually biopsied when clinically indicated, which may in turn bias the spectrum of liver disease. Concerns about the long-term outcome of HCV-infected liver transplant recipients are becoming increasingly apparent as more reports of chronic hepatitis progressing to graft cirrhosis, graft failure, and need for retransplantation are documented. (6,8–10) One study showed that moderate chronic hepatitis developed in 27% of patients after a median of 35 months, which progressed to cirrhosis in 8% after a median of 51 months. (6) In another study, (8) where protocol biopsies were performed annually during the first 5 years posttransplantation, histologic hepatitis, which was present in 97% of patients in the most recent biopsy, was moderate or severe in 64%. The actuarial rate of HCV cirrhosis increased from 3.7% at 1 year posttransplantation to 28% at 5 years.

Despite these reports, hepatitis C continues to be considered a good indication for liver transplantation as graft and patient survival are similar to those of uninfected controls. (6,9,31,32) How to reconcile these findings is problematic but may be related to (i) the selection of the control group, (ii) the presence of several unmeasured or unaccounted pre- and/or posttransplantation confounding variables, and (iii) insufficient numbers of patients or inadequacy of follow-up to measure the full effect of recurrent HCV disease. Selecting the most appropriate control group is essential as there is a wide variation in outcomes depending on the initial diagnosis, with patients with cholestatic liver disease doing the best and patients with hepatocellular carcinoma doing the worst. Alcoholics are only an appropriate control group for comparison if HCV infection is carefully excluded from the alcohol group. Patients with hepatocellular carcinoma should be either excluded from the analysis or matched on specific tumor features known to influence the posttransplantation outcome. (35) In addition, the presence of confounding variables such as Child's Pugh, United Network for Organ Sharing (UNOS) status, donor age, HCV RNA levels, and type and amount of immunosuppression, which may alter the outcome, are either unidentified or unmeasured and hence not controlled for in many studies. After adjusting for these factors, data from the UNOS suggest that HCV infection adversely affects both patient and graft survival. (7) Patient survival at 5 years was only 65% in those undergoing liver transplantation for HCV infection whereas it reached 80% in patients undergoing transplantation for cholestatic or autoimmune liver disease. Patients with alcoholic liver disease have comparable results to the HCV group at 2 years. (7)

Finally, the typical chosen end points, such as mortality, are unlikely to develop frequently within short and medium durations of follow-up. As a consequence, studies measuring the full effect of HCV infection on the posttransplantation outcome will most likely require a longer duration of follow-up, and are thus difficult to carry out. Intermediate end points, such as histological disease progression, used previously in the immunocompetent population, (36) have been applied to predict the time required for the development of graft cirrhosis

Viral factors, such as genotype and HCV RNA levels posttransplantation, have been proposed to affect the rate of progression, but no universal agreement has been reached. Viral factors may be important in the pathogenesis of disease either directly, through as yet undefined viral-induced injury, or indirectly, through differential immune response associated with one viral strain but not with another.

Several (6,9,37) but not all studies (10,32,38) have implicated genotype 1, particularly subtype 1b, in causing a more aggressive posttransplantation course when compared to non-1 genotypes. Factors explaining these discrepancies include differences in (i) genotype distribution of the study population, (ii) genotyping methods, (iii) type and amount of immunosuppression, (iv) duration of histological follow-up, and (v) the definition and methods of assessing disease severity.

Circulating HCV RNA levels following liver transplantation are often 10- to 20-fold higher than levels prior to transplantation. (28–30) As has been true for studies of immunocompetent individuals with HCV disease, cross-sectional studies of liver transplant recipients have failed to show a correlation between serum HCV RNA levels and disease severity (28–30). Thus, the mechanism of liver injury is more likely due to a host immune response to the infection than to a direct cytopathic effect of the virus. Indeed, some patients have very high levels of virus with no histologic evidence of hepatitis, (28) suggesting the presence of a "healthy carrier state," as has been described in immunocompetent patients with HCV infection. (39) In contrast to cross-sectional studies, longitudinal studies have shown an association between early HCV RNA titers and the subsequent development of chronic hepatitis. (29,40) A strong correlation was observed between the first determination of intrahepatic HCV RNA at the time of acute hepatitis and the risk of subsequent progression to chronic active hepatitis. Intrahepatic HCV RNA levels declined with time despite progression to severe liver disease. This decline paralleled the decrease in the amount of immunosuppression. (40) Because liver injury continued to occur in those individuals who were presumably "immune reconstituted" as immunesuppression was reduced, chronic liver damage in this setting is likely to be immune mediated. The central role of the host immune response in HCV-related disease severity is further supported by the observation of a marked and aberrant intrahepatic expression of molecules involved in antigen recognition, together with the evidence of intercellular and vascular adhesion molecules involved in regulating the recruitment and activation of cytotoxic T cells in patients with severe posttransplant hepatitis C. (41) Finally, data (10,32) suggest that high HCV RNA levels at the time of transplantation as an important predictive factor of severe posttransplantation disease (10) and poor posttransplantation outcome. (32)

The degree of viral genetic heterogeneity has been associated with progressive liver disease in both immunocompetent (42) and immunocompromised patients. Findings are conflicting and may be related to differences in (i) the definition of genetic heterogeneity (complexity vs diversity), (ii) methods for measuring genetic heterogeneity, (iii) region of the genome analyzed, (iv) the method used to quantify the severity of posttransplantation disease severity, and (iv) the number of clones sequenced. Studies performed to date in the transplant population have included very few patients (43–45) and do not demonstrate a clear relationship between dominance of certain viral species and disease severity. Further examination of this issue is necessary.

Coinfection with HGV does not seem to influence the posttransplantation course of HCV disease. (46) Coinfection with other hepatotropic viruses such as HBV may influence histologic disease severity, but results are conflicting. (9, 47) Although no effect was found in an initial study, (47) coinfected patients appeared to have a milder histological course than patients infected only with HCV. (9) Although viral interactions could explain this phenomenon, the passive transmission of antibodies against HCV in coinfected patients receiving HBIg during the pre-HCV era is a more likely explanation. Cytomegalovirus (CMV) viremia has been reported to be associated with an increased risk of severe recurrent HCV disease. (48) Reasons for this association are unknown but likely relate to the induction of immune deficiencies, release of tumor necrosis factor by CMV, or the existence of cross-reactive immunological responses.

The role of host factors in disease severity and progression following liver transplantation is also under investigation. The natural history of HCV infection is truncated in immunosuppressed transplant recipients when compared to immunocompetent patients, (10,49) suggesting a role of immunosuppression in disease progression. Although evidence is accumulating that the amount of immunosuppression (i.e., grams of methylprednisolone, cumulative steroids, OKT3 use) is linked to disease severity, (8,50–52) it has been difficult to associate a particular type of immunosuppressive regimen with a worse outcome. (6, 10,53) Accurate assessment of the role played by immunosuppression in the progression of HCV-related liver disease has also been complicated by the development of new immunosuppressive agents of varying potency and changes in immunosuppressive regimens in individual patients over time.

Some (54) but not all studies (6) have suggested that HLA-B sharing between the donor and the recipient promotes the recurrence of viral hepatitis in liver transplant recipients, probably by facilitating a more efficient major histocompatibility complex (MHC)-restricted HCV antigen presentation. Racial difference has also been implicated in HCV-related disease progression posttransplantation, with Caucasians appearing to do better than other races. (10,32) Additional studies are needed to confirm these preliminary results and to evaluate HLA typing of different ethnicities. Age was also found as a predictor of disease severity following transplantation, with patients older than 49 years doing worse than those younger. (9)

Necroinflammatory activity and fibrosis staging observed in early liver biopsies after transplantation have been associated with a subsequent development of severe liver disease. (8,40,55) In contrast, the rate of progression prior to transplantation and that observed after transplantation suggests that variables present at the time of transplantation and those related to posttransplantation management are more important in influencing disease progression than genetic or viral variables unique to the individual. (10)

The identification of patients with a high risk of severe outcome posttransplantation is desirable as these patients can be targeted for intervention. To this point, no single or combination of variables is capable of predicting accurately which individual will develop serious disease posttransplantation and which individual will not. HCV RNA levels prior to and/or early following transplantation, severe and early acute hepatitis, and strong immunosuppression appear currently to be three variables associated most consistently with poor outcome, but further analysis is required to confirm these findings.

Pathology

The histopathological features of recurrent HCV disease include many of the features seen in nonimmunocompromised patients, such as portal-based mononuclear cell infiltrates, lymphoid aggregates, fatty changes, bile duct damage, and patchy parenchymal lymphocytic aggregates, as well as features that appear to be unique to the transplant recipient, such as progressive fibrosis and marked periportal and parenchymal inflammation with hepatocyte necrosis. (4) Early liver changes seen in the acute phase of hepatitis include weak lobular inflammation with scattered apoptotic bodies and minimal cell swelling. This lesion progresses within 2–4 weeks to a more fully developed hepatitis, with portal and lobular inflammation of varying degrees in association with hepatocyte necrosis and midzonal macrovesicular steatosis. Mononuclear inflammatory infiltrates in the portal triads may form lymphoid aggregates. Atypical histological findings, including marked ductal injury, venulitis, profound cholestasis, bile duct proliferation, and perivenular ballooning of hepatocytes, are also seen in patients with recurrent HCV infection, mimicking other entities such as rejection, obstruction, or ischemia. Interpretation of allograft biospies is facilitated considerably by knowledge of the date of transplantation. "Nonhepatitis biopsy findings" are typically seen earlier in time than "acute and chronic hepatitis findings," which are rarely seen within the first month posttransplantation. Exclusion of other etiological factors such as CMV hepatitis, obstruction, ischemia, or hepatotoxic drugs may require serologic, immunohistochemical, radiological, and endoscopic studies or drug discontinuation, respectively.

HCV infection can occasionally (4–9%) result in progressive liver dysfunction characterized by profound intrahepatic cholestasis with fibrosis and progressive hyperbilirubinemia, (56) a pattern originally described in patients with recurrent severe hepatitis B infection. These patients typically progress to graft loss and death within 1 to 2 years from transplantation. Histological features include progressive lobular inflammation and necrosis with bridging and confluent necrosis associated with severe cholestasis and centrilobular hepatocellular drop out.

Other Complications of Posttransplantation HCV Infection

Some of the usual complications of a liver transplant have been shown to occur with a higher incidence among HCV-infected recipients. These complications could in turn adversely affect the outcome of these patients. (32) In particular, a higher incidence of major infections, mainly fungal and viral infection, has been reported in HCV-infected patients as compared to uninfected controls. (32,57) The role of HCV infection on renal function has been assessed in one study, (58) and while there were no differences in serum blood urea nitrogen, creatinine, or creatinine clearance between HCV-infected recipients and controls, the percentage of patients with more than 1 g of proteinuria per 24 hr was higher if they were infected with HCV.

TREATMENT

Although short-term survival is sufficiently good to warrant continued transplantation of this group of patients, the potential seriousness of this disease prompts a continuous search for more potent antiviral agents, rational assessment of the efficacy of current therapy, evaluation of the optimal immunosuppressive regimen, and assessment of the suitability of HCV-related graft cirrhosis as an indication for liver retransplantation. While preventing HCV recurrence is the major end point, there is currently no suitable intervention to prevent HCV recurrence. This is in contrast to the prevention of HBV reinfection where hepatitis B immune globulin has been shown to be highly beneficial.

There are four potential alternative and /or complementary approaches (Table III): (i) preemptive antiviral therapy pretransplantation with the goal of

TABLE III Hepatitis C Following Liver Transplantation: Therapeutic Approaches

Author (number)	Type of study[a]	Type, dose, and duration of therapy	End point	Virological benefit	Histological benefit
Wright et al. (11) (n = 18)	UC	Interferon (3 MU 3 times weekly) for 6 months	Treatment of CHC[b]	Yes	No
Feray et al. (12) (n = 14)	C, NR	Interferon (3 MU 3 times weekly) for 6 months	Treatment of CHC	Yes	No
Gane et al. (13) (n = 30)	R	Interferon (3 MU 3 times weekly) vs ribavirin (1.200 mg/day) for 6 months	Treatment of CHC	Yes (interferon group)/no (ribavirin group)	No
Singh et al. (60) (n = 18)	UC	Interferon (3 MU 3 times weekly) for up to 18 months	Treatment of CHC	NA	NA
Sheiner et al. (61) (n = 71)	C, R	Interferon (3 MU 3 times weekly) for 6 months	Post-OLT[c] prophylaxis	No	Yes
Singh et al. (62) (n = 24)	C, R	Interferon (3 MU 3 times weekly) for 6 months	Post-OLT prophylaxis	No	No
Bizollon et al. (15) (n = 21)	UC	Interferon (3 MU 3 times weekly) and ribavirin (1.200 mg/day) for 6 months followed by ribavirin monotherapy	Treatment of CHC	Yes	Yes
Mazaferro et al. (63) (n = 21)	UC	Interferon (3 MU 3 times weekly) and ribavirin (1.200 mg/day)	Post-OLT prophylaxis	Yes	Yes

[a] UC, uncontrolled; C, controlled; R, randomized; NR, nonrandomized.
[b] Chronic hepatitis C.
[c] Liver transplantation.

suppressing viral replication in order to reduce the risk of aggressive recurrent HCV disease; (ii) treatment of disease when and if it does occur; (iii) early post-transplantation antiviral therapy before occurrence of histologic damage in an attempt to prevent progression of HCV-related graft disease; and (iv) changes in patient management, as some variables such as immunosuppression have been associated with more severe disease.

Preemptive Therapy before Liver Transplantation

A potential benefit for antiviral therapy in HCV-infected patients considered for liver transplantation is the reduction in levels of viremia, which may in turn influence the posttransplantation course. Interferon alone or in combination with ribavirin has been used to suppress viral replication in cirrhotic patients. (19) Studies of the kinetics of HCV have suggested that the effect of interferon, at least in genotype 1 infection, is dose dependent and directly antiviral with a rapid HCV decline starting the first day of therapy. (59) If previous findings are confirmed, antiviral therapy early before transplantation could become a way to improve long-term survival of these patients. The main difficulty with this approach, however, is that the timing of antiviral therapy is unknown as the waiting time for transplantation varies greatly across centers.

Treatment of HCV-Related Graft Disease

Treatment of recurrent HCV disease with interferon or ribavirin in monotherapy has thus far been disappointing (Table III), but initial results from combination therapy with interferon and ribavirin are encouraging. Interferon alone, at a dose of 3 MU, thrice weekly for 6 months, has failed to clear serum HCV RNA, despite normalization of ALT values in a subset of treated patients (0–28%). (11,12) Furthermore, relapse after discontinuing treatment is almost the rule, and histologic improvement is minor. In addition, there has been concern about using interferon in solid organ transplant recipients because interferon can upregulate the expression of HLA class I and II antigens, which may in turn increase the risk of allograft rejection. Prolonged interferon therapy has been described in one uncontrolled small study (60) in which patients were treated for a mean of 21 months with an apparent enhanced response rate, which unfortunately was only assessed by biochemical but not virological end points.

Ribavirin monotherapy has also been evaluated in liver transplant recipients, with biochemical improvement observed in many patients, but virological clearance achieved in none. (13,14) Biochemical relapse was universal after cessation of therapy and no histological improvement was observed. The main side effect was hemolysis, which resolved after the cessation of therapy. One randomized trial (13) has compared 12 months of ribavirin versus interferon monotherapy in 31 liver transplant recipients. Although ribavirin was superior in achieving biochemical response (85% vs 43%, $p < 0.05$), only patients treated with interferon had a reduction in HCV RNA levels.

Combination therapy is the most recent approach with promising results. (15) In a nonrandomized pilot study, Bizollon et al. (15) assessed the safety and efficacy of combination therapy with ribavirin and interferon for the treatment of recurrent hepatitis C. Twenty-one patients with early documented recurrent HCV hepatitis were treated with interferon-α (3 MU/thrice weekly) and ribavirin (1000 mg/day) for 6 months and then maintained on ribavirin monotherapy until the end of the study. All patients normalized ALT and 50% cleared HCV RNA from serum at the end of the combination treatment period. Although viremic, the remaining patients experienced a 50% reduction in viral load. Only 1 patient had a biochemical relapse during the 6-month period on ribavirin alone, despite the reappearance of serum HCV RNA in 50% who had initially cleared HCV RNA. Most importantly, all but 1 patient who tolerated the drug showed an improvement in liver histology. Safety and tolerability were satisfactory, with reversible hemolytic anemia being the most common side effect. No patient experienced graft rejection. This favorable outcome is noteworthy because all patients had high HCV RNA levels (mean value of 125 Meq/ml) and 92% were infected with HCV genotype 1, features classically associated with a lack of response to therapy. Maintenance therapy with ribavirin is likely important to avoid relapse, as all 3 patients who stopped ribavirin because of adverse events had a biochemical relapse in association with histological deterioration. Whether maintenance therapy could be discontinued in patients who have responded virologically remains to be determined.

Early Posttransplantation Antiviral Therapy

A final approach is the use of either interferon alone (61,62) or in combination with ribavirin (63) early after liver transplantation in an attempt to prevent HCV disease recurrence. In one study, (61) 86 recipients were randomized within 2 weeks after transplantation to receive either interferon alone ($n = 38$) or placebo ($n = 48$) for 1 year. While patient and graft survival at 2 years did not differ between groups and the rate of virus persistence was not affected by treatment, histologic disease recurrence was observed less frequently in interferon-treated patients (8 of 30 evaluable at 1 year) than in those who were not treated (22 of 41; $p = 0.01$). In a second controlled trial, (62) 24 recipients were randomized at 2 weeks posttransplantation to receive interferon or placebo for 6 months. Both the incidence of histologic recurrence and its severity did not differ between groups. Interferon, however, delayed the development of HCV hepatitis, which occurred at a median of 408 days after transplantation in the treated group versus 193 days in the untreated group ($p = 0.05$). No difference in graft or patient survival was observed.

In a case series, (63) 21 recipients were treated with interferon-α and ribavirin starting in the third posttransplantation week. After a median follow-up of 12 months, 4 patients (19%) had developed acute recurrent hepatitis C, but only 1 (5%) had evolved to chronic active hepatitis, despite the presence of viremia in 59% of patients.

Management of Immunosuppression

Choosing the best induction and maintenance immunosuppression regimen for this patient population is probably an important problem faced by hepatologist and surgeons. Treatment of rejection episodes also raises concerns, particularly when there are doubts between rejection and recurrent hepatitis C. The majority of studies have found no differences in patient and/or graft survival in recipients treated with cyclosporine-based versus those treated with tacrolimus-based induction regimens. (6,32) Prospective trials are underway to assess this issue. The more severe liver disease described in patients treated with a high number of methylprednisolone boluses and/or OKT3 (50–52) suggests that rejection treatment should be less aggressive in these patients. Additionally, when doubts exist between rejection and hepatitis C as a result of atypical histological findings, serial biopsies should be performed. Features more suggestive of HCV infection include lymphoid aggregates, fatty changes, and sinusoidal dilatation, whereas those more suggestive of rejection include endotheliitis, bile duct necrosis, and a mixed portal inflammatory infiltrate (eosinophils and neutrophils as well as mononuclear cells). (4) Although proposed previously as a means to differentiate the two entities, a therapeutic trial with a short course of steroids may be detrimental in the long term and thus is not recommended at the present time. If data supporting the presence of both entities exist, treatment with corticosteroids may be attempted.

RETRANSPLANTATION

One of the challenges faced by surgeons and hepatologists is the decision to retransplant a patient who has developed HCV-related end-stage liver disease of the first graft. The reported outcome of retransplantation for these patients has been generally poor. (64) Surgery was associated with high mortality, with sepsis being the main cause of death, particularly in patients with concomitant renal failure. Successful retransplantation has been performed before renal failure develops. In these patients, the rate of disease recurrence appears to be similar to that seen in the original allograft. (65) Larger studies are needed to answer these questions. The increasing shortage of organ donors that accompanies the growing number of patients in need of a first transplantation will have severe consequences on the candidacy of patients being considered for retransplantation.

CONCLUSION

HCV disease is a common indication for liver transplantation, accounting for 25–50% of all indications in most transplant centers. Despite uncertainties regarding posttransplantation disease-progression rates, there is a consensus emerging that recurrent HCV infection results in liver failure in a significant, although currently unmeasured, proportion of patients and that the time course over which this progression occurs is shorter than in the immunocompetent population. As the disease process moves into its second decade, it can be anticipated that future morbidity and liver-related mortality are likely to increase.

Whether progression is enhanced by definable factors is not yet fully established, but HCV RNA levels pretransplantation and/or early following transplantation, as well as potent immunosuppression, appear to influence the posttransplantation course. Strategies to prevent or reduce the effect of HCV infection after liver transplantation are therefore desirable. Our ability to intervene in this disease is, however, limited. The main obstacles are the difficulty in predicting the outcome for the individual patient and the lack of effective therapy. In contrast to hepatitis B, where hepatitis B immune globulin has had a positive effect, therapeutic strategies aimed at preventing the recurrence of HCV have had limited efficacy. Both interferon and ribavirin, when given as single agents, rarely result in sustained viral clearance. However, administration of both drugs given in combination either to prevent disease or to treat recurrence when it occurs appears more promising. The inability of currently available antiviral therapy to eliminate HCV in the liver transplant setting suggests that indefinite treatment designed to suppress the effects of the virus may be necessary. The feasibility of such an approach will depend on the demonstration of a reduction in histologic disease progression or improved graft and patient survival. Toxicity, cost, and resistance issues should be addressed before this approach is feasible. Ultimately, the development of potent antivirals given either before or after liver transplantation may change the course of posttransplantation disease and hopefully obviate the need for liver transplantation in those with advanced HCV disease.

REFERENCES

1. Annual report of the U.S. Scientific Registry for Tranplant Recipients and the Organ Procurement and Transplantation Network-Transplant Data: 1988–1994. Richmond, VA: United Network for Organ Sharing, and the Division of Organ Transplantation, Bureau of Health Resources Development.
2. Alter M J. Epidemiology of hepatitis C in the West. Semin Liver Dis 1995;15:5–14.
3. Wright T L, Donegan E, Hsu H, et al. Recurrent and acquired hepatitis C viral infection in liver transplant recipients. Gastroenterology 1992;103:317–22.
4. Ferrell L, Wright T, Roberts J, et al. Hepatitis C viral infection in liver transplant recipients. Hepatology 1992;16:865–76.
5. Feray C, Gigou M, Samuel D, et al. The course of hepatitis C virus infection after liver transplantation. Hepatology 1994;20:1137–43.
6. Gane E, Portmann B, Naoumov N, et al. Long-term outcome of hepatitis C infection after liver transplantation. N Engl J Med 1996;334:815–20.
7. Detre K. Liver transplantation for chronic viral hepatitis. Presented at A.A.S.L.D. Single Topic Conf., Reston, VA, 1995.
8. Prieto M, Berenguer M, Rayón M, et al. High incidence of allograft cirrhosis in hepatitis C virus genotype 1b infection following transplantation: relationship with rejection episodes. Hepatology 1999;29:250–6.
9. Feray C, Caccamo L, Alexander G J M, et al. European Collaborative Study on factors influencing the outcome after liver transplantation for hepatitis C. Gastroenterology 1999;117:619–25.
10. Berenguer M, Ferrell L, Watson J, et al. HCV-related fibrosis progression following liver transplantation: increase in recent years. J Hepatol 2000 (in press).
11. Wright T L, Combs C, Kim M, et al. Interferon alpha therapy for hepatitis C virus infection following liver transplantation. Hepatology 1994;20:773–9.
12. Feray C, Samuel D, Gigou M, et al. An open trial of interferon alfa recombinant for hepatitis C after liver transplantation: antiviral effects and risk of rejection. Hepatology 1995;22:1084–9.
13. Gane E J, Lo S K, Riordan S M, et al. A randomized study comparing ribavirin and interferon

alfa monotherapy for hepatitis C recurrence after liver transplantation. Hepatology 1998;27: 1403–7.

14. Cattral M S, Hemming A W, Wanless I R, et al. Outcome of long-term ribavirin therapy for recurrent hepatitis C after liver transplantation. Transplantation 1999;67:1277–80.

15. Bizollon T, Palazzo U, Ducerf C, et al. Pilot study of the combination of interferon alfa and ribavirin as therapy of recurrent hepatitis C after liver transplantation. Hepatology 1997;26: 500–4.

16. Fattovitch G, Giustina G, Degos F, et al. Morbidity and mortality in compensated cirrhosis type C: a retrospective follow-up study of 384 patients. Gastroenterology 1997;112:463–72.

17. Serfarty L, Aumaître H, Chazouillères O, et al. Determinants of outcome of compensated hepatitis C virus-related cirrhosis. Hepatology 1998;27:1435–40.

18. UNOS: Reported deaths on the OPTN waiting list, 1988 to 1994. UNOS update 1996;12:25.

19. Liang T J. Combination therapy for hepatitis C infection. N Engl J Med 1998;339:1549–50.

20. International Interferon-α Hepatocellular Carcinoma Study Group. Effect of interferon-α on progression of cirrhosis to hepatocellular carcinoma: a retrospective cohort study. Lancet 1998; 351:1535–9.

21. Kasahara A, Hayashi N, Mochizuki K, et al. Risk factors for hepatocellular carcinoma and its incidence after interferon treatment in patients with chronic hepatitis C. Hepatology 1998;27: 1394–402.

22. Pereira B J, Wright T L, Schmid C H, Levey A S. A controlled study of hepatitis C transmission by organ transplantation. Lancet 1995;345:484–7.

23. Bouthot B A, Murthy B V R, Schmid C H, et al. Long-term follow-up of hepatitis C virus infection among organ transplant recipients: implications for policies on organ transplantation. Transplantation 1997;63:849–53.

24. Laskus T, Wang L F, Rakela J, et al. Dynamic behavior of hepatitis C virus in chronically infected patients receiving liver graft from infected donors. Virology 1996;220:171–6.

25. Testa G, Goldstein R M, Netto G, et al. Long-term outcome of patients transplanted with livers from hepatitis C-positive donors. Transplantation 1998;65:925–9.

26. Vargas H E, Laskus T, Wang L F, et al. Outcome of liver transplantation in hepatitis C virus-infected patients who received hepatitis C virus-infected grafts. Gastroenterology 1999;117: 149–53.

27. Fukomoto T, Berg T, Ku Y, et al. Viral dynamics of hepatitis C early after orthotopic liver transplantation: Evidence for rapid turnover of serum virions. Hepatology 1996;24:1351–4.

28. Chazouilleres O, Kim M, Combs C, et al. Quantitation of hepatitis C virus RNA in liver transplant recipients. Gastroenterology 1994;106:994–9.

29. Gretch D, Bacchi C, Corey L, et al. Persistent hepatitis C virus infection after liver transplantation: clinical and virological features. Hepatology 1995;22:1–9.

30. Gane E, Naoumov N, Qian K, et al. A longitudinal analysis of hepatitis C virus replication following liver transplantation. Gastroenterology 1996;110:167–77.

31. Boker K H W, Dalley G, Bahr M J, et al. Long-term outcome of hepatitis C virus infection after liver transplantation. Hepatology 1997;25:203–10.

32. Charlton M, Seaberg E, Wiesner R, et al. Predictors of patient and graft survival following liver transplantation for hepatitis C. Hepatology 1998;28:823–30.

33. Donegan E, Wright T, Roberts J, et al. Detection of hepatitis C after liver transplantation. Four serologic tests compared. Am J Clin Pathol 1995;104:673–9.

34. Lock A S F, Chien D, Choo Q-L, et al. Antibody response to core, envelope and nonstructural hepatitis C virus antigens: comparison of immunocompetent and immunosuppressed patients. Hepatology 1993;18:497–502.

35. Figueras J, Jaurrieta E, Valls C, et al. Survival after liver transplantation in cirrhotic patients with and without hepatocellular carcinoma: a comparative study. Hepatology 1997;25:1485–9.

36. Poynard T, Bedossa P, Opolon P. Natural history of liver fibrosis progression in patients with chronic hepatitis C. Lancet 1997;349:825–32.

37. Feray C, Gigou M, Samuel D, et al. Influence of genotypes of heapatitis C virus on the severity of recurrent liver disease after liver transplantation. Gastroenterology 1995;108:1088–96.

38. Zhou S, Terrault N, Ferrell L, et al. Severity of liver disease in liver transplantation recipients with hepatitis C virus infection: relationship to genotype and level of viremia. Hepatology 1996; 24:1041–6.

39. Prieto M, Olaso V, Verdu C, et al. Does the healthy hepatitis C virus carrier state really exist? An analysis using polymerase chain reaction. Hepatology 1995;22:413–7.

40. DiMartino V, Saurini F, Samuel D, et al. Long-term longitudinal study of intrahepatic hepatitis C virus replication after liver transplantation. Hepatology 1997;26:1343–50.

41. Asanza C G, Garcia-Monzon C, Clemente G, et al. Immunohistochemical evidence of immunopathogenetic mechanisms in chronic hepatitis C recurrence after liver transplantation. Hepatology 1997;26:755–63.

42. López-Labrador F X, Ampurdanès S, Giménez-Barcons M, et al. Relationship of the genomic complexity of hepatitis C virus with liver disease severity and response to interferon in patients with chronic HCV genotype 1B infection. Hepatology 1999;29:897–903.

43. Yun Z, Barkholt L, Sonnenberg A. Dynamic analysis of hepatitis virus polymorphism in patients with orthotopic liver transplantation. Transplantation 1997;64:170–2.

44. Sullivan D G, Wilson J J, Carithers R L Jr, et al. Multigene tracking of hepatitis C virus quasispecies after liver transplantation: correlation of genetic diversification in the envelope region with asymptomatic or mild disease patterns. J Virol 1998;72:10036–43.

45. Pessoa M G, Bzowej N H, Berenguer M, et al. Evolution of hepatitis C (HCV) quasispecies in patients with severe cholestatic hepatitis following liver transplantation. Hepatology 1999 (in press).

46. Berenguer M, Terrault N A, Piatak M, et al. Hepatitis G virus infection in patients with hepatitis C virus infection undergoing liver transplantation. Gastroenterology 1996;111:1569–75.

47. Huang E, Wright T L, Lake J, et al. Hepatitis B and C coinfections and persistent hepatitis B infections: clinical outcome and liver pathology after transplantation. Hepatology 1996;23:396–404.

48. Rosen H, Chou S, Corless C, et al. Cytomegalovirus viremia. Risk factor for allograft cirrhosis after liver transplantation for hepatitis C. Transplantation 1997;64:721–6.

49. Pol S, Fontaine H, Carnot F, et al. Predictive factors for development of cirrhosis in parenterally acquired chronic hepatitis C: a comparison between immunocompetent and immunocompromised patients. J Hepatol 1998;29:12–9.

50. Sheiner P A, Schwartz M E, Mor E, et al. Severe or multiple rejection episodes are associated with early recurrence of hepatitis C after orthotopic liver transplantation. Hepatology 1995;21:30–4.

51. Rosen H R, Shackleton C R, Higa L, et al. Use of OKT3 is associated with early and severe recurrence of hepatitis C after liver transplantation. Am J Gastroenterol 1997;92:1453–7.

52. Berenguer M, Prieto M, Córdoba J, et al. Early development of chronic active hepatitis in recurrent hepatitis C virus infection after liver transplantation: association with treatment of rejection. J Hepatol 1998;28:756–63.

53. Casavilla F A, Rakela J, Kapur S, et al. Clinical outcome of patients infected with hepatitis C virus infection on survival after primary liver transplantation under tacrolimus. Liver Transplant Surg 1998;4:448–54.

54. Manez R, Mateo R, Tabasco J, et al. The influence of HLA donor-recipient compatibility on the recurrence of HBV and HCV hepatitis after liver transplantation. Transplantation 1994;59:640–2.

55. Rosen H R, Gretch D R, Oehlke M, et al. Timing and severity of initial hepatitis C recurrence as predictors of long-term liver allograft injury. Transplantation 1998;65:1178–82.

56. Schluger L, Sheiner P, Thung S, et al. Severe recurrent cholestatic hepatitis C following orthotopic liver transplantation. Hepatology 1996;23:971–6.

57. Singh N, Gayowski T, Wagener M M, Marino I R. Increased infections in liver transplant recipients with recurrent hepatitis C virus hepatitis. Transplantation 1996;61:402–6.

58. Kendrick E A, McVicar J P, Kowdley K V, et al. Renal disease in hepatitis C-positive liver transplant recipients. Transplantation 1997;63:1287–93.

59. Neuman A U, Lam N P, Dahari H, et al. Dose-dependent acute clearance of hepatitis C genotype 1 virus with interferon-alpha therapy. Science 1998;282:103–7.

60. Singh N, Gayowski T, Wannstedt C F, et al. Interferon-alpha therapy for hepatitis C virus recurrence after liver transplantation: long-term response with maintenance therapy. Clin Transplant 1996;10:348–51.

61. Sheiner P, Boros P, Klion F M, et al. The efficacy of prophylactic interferon alfa-2b in preventing recurrent hepatitis C after liver transplantation. Hepatology 1998;28:831–8.

62. Singh N, Gayowski T, Wannstedt C, et al. Interferon-α for prophylaxis of recurrent viral hepa-
    titis C in liver transplant recipients. Transplantation 1998;65:82–6.
63. Mazzaferro V, Regalia E, Pulvirenti A, et al. Prophylaxis against HCV recurrence after liver
    transplantation. Effect of interferon and ribavirin combination. Transplant Proc 1997;29:
    519–21.
64. Sheiner P A, Schluger L K, Emre S, et al. Retransplantation for recurrent hepatitis C. Liver
    Transplant Surg 1997;3:130–6.
65. Rosen H, O'Reilly P, Shackleton C, et al. Graft loss following liver transplantation in patients
    with chronic hepatitis C. Transplantation 1997;62:1773–6.

15

MIXED CRYOGLOBULINEMIA AND OTHER EXTRAHEPATIC MANIFESTATIONS OF HEPATITIS C VIRUS INFECTION

VINCENT AGNELLO

*Lahey Clinic, Burlington, Massachusetts
and The Edith Norse Rogers Memorial Veterans Affairs Hospital
Bedford, Massachusetts*

INTRODUCTION

Mixed cryoglobulinemia is a systemic vasculitis with clinical manifestations ranging from palpable purpura to severe vasculitis involving vital organs, particularly the kidneys. This often benign-appearing but deceptive and potentially life-threatening disease has been shown to be strongly associated with hepatitis C virus infection (HCV). The specific concentration of the virus in the cryoglobulins and the detection of HCV in the palpable purpura lesions have strongly implicated the virus in the etiology of the disease. This chapter reviews the background, current knowledge of the pathogenesis, therapy, and hypotheses on the etiologic role of HCV in mixed cryoglobulinemia. In addition, a wide array of other putative extrahepatic manifestations of HCV, most of which are uncertain associations without evidence of involvement of HCV in the pathogenesis, are discussed.

MIXED CRYOGLOBULINEMIA

Historical Perspective

Cryoglobulins, proteins that reversibly precipitate from serum on cooling (Fig. 1A), were first described by Wintrobe and Buell in a patient with multiple myeloma over 65 years ago (1) and first termed *cryoglobulins* by Lerner and Watson in 1947. (2) In 1962, Lospalluto and colleagues (3) first delineated cryoglobulinemias that resulted from IgM rheumatoid factor (RF) reactivity with IgG. In 1966, Meltzer and colleagues (4) first used the term *mixed cryoglobulins* for these IgG, IgM RF cryoglobulins and described the clinical syndrome consisting of purpura, arthralgia, and weakness that was associated with mixed cryoglobulins. Two of the nine patients studied had primary Sjögren syndrome, and this is the reason that this primary disease was not an exclusion for essential cryoglobulinemia in some subsequent studies. Studies performed by Franklin's group and by others implicated the cryoglobulin components in the immune complex-mediated vascular and glomerular lesions that occur in many patients with mixed cryoglobulinemia. The Meltzer–Franklin syndrome, as it is now called, was also called *essential mixed cryoglobulinemia* to distinguish it from similar mixed cryoglobulinemia secondary to a variety of infectious, autoimmune, and malignant diseases.

The high prevalence of hepatocellular disease in patients with essential mixed cryoglobulinemia suggested that a hepatotropic virus may be the etiologic agent for the disease. Studies in the early 1970s implicated the hepatitis B virus in essential mixed cryoglobulinemia, but it is now established that the hepatitis B virus is present in relatively few patients with the disease. (5) The development of serologic testing for HCV led to investigation of a role for HCV in essential mixed cryoglobulinemia. Following the initial report by Pasqual and co-workers in 1990, (6) the high prevalence of HCV infection with mixed cryoglobulinemia has been documented extensively (reviewed in reference 7). Studies were predominantly from southern Europe, and the prevalence of HCV infection ranged from 30 to 98%; the association has been documented in the United States as well. (8–10)

A striking historical note is that 20 years before the discovery of HCV it was discovered that monoclonal RF from different patients with essential mixed cryoglobulinemia was identical as determined by typing with an antibody that reacted with an epitope in the antigen-combining site of the RF called a "cross-idiotype." (11,12) Hence, the monoclonal RF in these patients was highly restricted rather than arising randomly from the entire antibody repertoire and suggested that the monoclonal RF in different individuals arose from stimulation with the same antigen. This cross-idiotype was dubbed "WA" after the patient whose monoclonal RF was used to raise the original typing antiserum. (12) Another striking historical note is that the first use of interferon-α for the therapy of HCV infection was in the treatment of essential mixed cryoglobulinemia, although unbeknownst to the investigators. (13) Ninety percent of the patients treated were later determined to have had HCV infection. (14)

Classification, Detection, and Characterization of Cryoglobulins

Classification

The biochemical classification of cryoglobulinemia that is currently widely used, formulated by Brouet and colleagues, (15) defined three types of cryoglobulins based on the characterization of cryoglobulins from 86 patients with various diseases, most with manifestations of immune complex disease. Type I cryoglobulins consisted of a single isotype of monoclonal immunoglobulins or free light chains. Type II cryoglobulins consisted of a mixture of immunoglobulin isotypes with a monclonal component processing antibody activity toward polyclonal IgG. The monoclonal components were predominantly IgM. Type II cryoglobulins consisted of a mixture of polyclonal immunoglobulins of various isotypes; most of these were also the complexes of polyclonal IgG and poly-

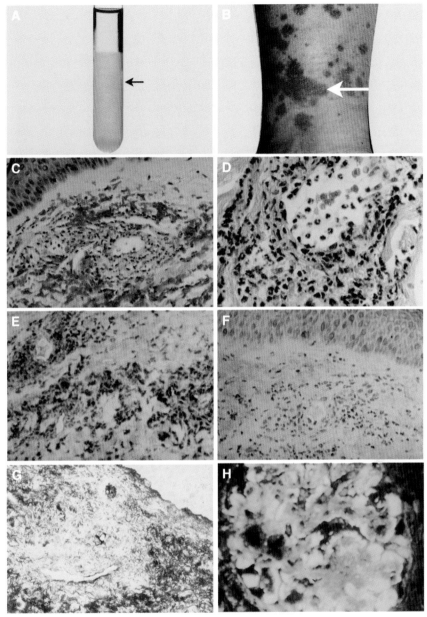

FIGURE I (A) Serum of a patient with type II cryoglobulinemia after 48 hr at 4°C. Cryoglobulins (arrow) are shown before centrifugation. (B) The typical palpable purpura lesion in a patient with type II cryoglobulinemia is shown. A and B are reprinted from Sakil and DiBisceglie (29) with permission. (C–G) Serial sections of a skin biopsy specimen from a patient with type II cryoglobulinemia and HCV infection. (C) Hematoxylin and eosin stain shows classic leukocytoclastic vasculitis. (D) Higher power view of C shows disruption of the vessel wall and extravasation of blood. (E) Demonstration of the virion form of HCV (brown staining) using antisense HCV riboprobe. (F) Staining for the putative replicative form of HCV using a HCV sense riboprobe. No replicative form of the virus was found. (G) Staining for IgM (red) showing perivascular deposition. IgG showed similar distribution (not shown). C, E–G: magnification ×500; D: ×1250. C and E are reprinted from Agnello and Abel (38) with permission. (H) Patient with type II cryoglobulinemia and membranoproliferative glomerulonephritis; glomerulus stained with fluorescein-labeled anti-IgM shows heavy lumpy deposits of IgM (green staining), magnification ×250.

███ **TABLE I** **Classifications of Cryoglobulinemia**

Biochemical
  Type I   Single monoclonal immunoglobulin
  Type II   Polyclonal IgG and monoclonal IgM rheumatoid factor
  Type III   Polyclonal IgG and polyclonal IgM rheumatoid factor
Clinical
  Secondary mixed cryoglobulinemia: Primary disease present
  Essential mixed cryoglobulinemia: No primary disease present.

clonal RF that were mainly IgM. Although three types were described, strict criteria for classification were not delineated, resulting in ambiguity in the correlation of mixed cryoglobulins with clinical noninfestations. (16) A simplified version of Brouet classification of cryoglobulinemia, as well the clinical classification, is given in Table I.

Detection

It is essential that proper methods of collecting and processing samples are used to detect cryoglobulinemia in serum as cryoglobulins are easily lost by improper handling. Blood must be drawn in prewarmed syringes, clotted at 37°C for 1 hr, and serum separated by centrifugation at 37°C. The serum is removed and stored at 4°C for a minimum of 72 hr. Delays in transport, refrigeration of the sample before processing, and processing at room temperature will result in loss of cryoglobulins.

There are no interlaboratory standards for processing or measuring cryoglobulins. From 1 to 10 ml of serum is used, refrigerated from 72 hr to 2 weeks, and measured either by volume (cryocrit) or by determining the amount of protein in the washed cryoprecipitate. Regardless of the methodology used, concentrations of cryoglobulins are markedly higher for type II than for type III.

Characterization

There is no standardized methodology for determining the immunoglobulin composition of cryoglobulins. The presence of various classes of immunoglobulins is usually determined by immunodiffusion using immunoglobulin class-specific antiserum. The presence of monoclonal immunoglobulins is determined by immunoelectrophoresis, immunofixation, or immunoblotting, with increasing sensitivity; complete identification of 157 samples was obtained in 98% of the samples by immunoblotting, 54% by immunofixation, and 28% by immunoelectrophoresis. (17) Microheterogeneity of monoclonal immunoglobulins was observed by immunoblotting and immunofixation in 13 and 6% of cases studied, respectively.

An unusual pattern of complement activation that involves only the early components C1, C4, and C2 is frequently found in sera of patients with mixed cryoglobulinemia, particularly those with type II cryoglobulinemia. *In vitro* studies with isolated type II cryoglobulins has demonstrated that this pattern is due to the C4 binding protein, which preferentially binds to the assembled early components on the IgM to block further activation of the complement cascade. (18) A similar pattern of early complement component activation has been demonstrated *in vitro* using monoclonal RF from type II cryoglobulins and aggregated IgG. (19) However, C3 has been demonstrated in glomerular deposits in membranoproliferative glomerulonephritis lesions in type II cryoglobulinemia, and C3 serum levels have been reported to correlate inversely with the severity of nephritis. (20) In addition, cryoglobulins from these patients have been shown to activate C3. (18)

The presence of complement components in mixed cryoglobulins was documented in early studies (21); however, characterization of complement proteins in mixed cryoglobulins was not reported nor has the relationship of complement components in the cryoglobulins to the pattern of complement depletion in the serum been reported. Serum complement levels are determined in evaluating mixed cryoglobulinemia; however, characterization of complement components in cryoglobulins is not routinely done in the analysis of cryoglobulins.

Two cross-idiotypes were identified in type II cryoglobulins: WA, the predominant cross-idiotype present in 80%; and PO, a minor cross-idiotype present in 7%. (12,22) The immunologically defined WA cross-idiotype appears to be a conformational epitope, requiring both heavy and light chains, that is located in or near the site of antigen binding, as anti-WA cross-idiotype antibody blocks the binding of WA monoclonal RF to IgG. (23) From protein sequence and light and heavy chain cross-idiotype analysis, WA mRF appears to be derived predominantly from germ-line VkIIIb and Vh1 genes with little somatic mutation. (24)

A third monoclonal RF cross-idiotype, BLA, which was not detected in type II cryoglobulins, has been shown to be relevant because it demonstrated that RF-binding sites can bind non-IgG antigen in addition to IgG. (25) The RF bearing this cross-idiotype reacted with IgG but also reacted with DNA nucleoprotein. Both antigens blocked the binding of the anti-cross-idiotype antiserum to BLA mRF. Hence the BLA cross-idiotype defined a group of cross-reactive RF and provided the rationale for suspecting cross-reactivity with non-IgG antigen among monoclonal RF bearing the WA cross-idiotype that predominates in type II cryoglobulins.

Prevalences

Reported prevalences of mixed cryoglobulinemia may vary widely because of the lack of standardization in the measurement of cryoglobulins and the method of selecting patients for study. Prevalences of type II cryoglobulinemia appear to be higher when the presence of palpable purpura is one of the main clinical features of the selected populations, (5) whereas lower prevalences are detected where the presence of mixed cryoglobulins in the serum (26) or clinical liver disease is used for selection. (27) Analysis is confounded further by the heterogeneity of mixed cryoglobulins that were originally defined as having a RF IgM component. Most studies now include cryoglobulins characterized for mixed isotypes of immunoglobulins but not for RF activity.

The prevalence of mixed cryoglobulinemia among unselected HCV-infected patients has not been determined. Among French patients with chronic hepati-

████ **TABLE II   Clinical Manifestations in 1033 Patients with Essential Mixed Cryoglobulinemia**[a]

Purpura	82%
Arthralgia	42%
Weakness	45%
Liver involvement	42%
Renal involvement	34%
Peripheral neuropathy	26%
Raynaud's phenomenon	22%
Sicca syndrome	6%
Female sex	66%
Mean age	52.5 years

[a] Reprinted from Agnello (28) with permission.

tis C, the prevalence is 54%. (27) The prevalence of type II cryoglobulinemia among patients with chronic hepatitis C is 34% in Italy (5) and 20% in France. (27) The higher prevalence in southern Europe is a subject of speculation; an epidemic of HCV infection after World War II may be responsible. Among Italian patients selected for essential mixed cryoglobulinemia, the prevalence of type II cryoglobulinemia was 81 to 91%. (5,14)

Clinical Manifestations

It has become apparent since the initial description of the Meltzer–Franklin syndrome that the clinical manifestations of mixed cryoglobulinemia vary markedly and, in addition, remission of disease can occur spontaneously. A review of 1033 patients with essential mixed cryoglobulinemia is shown in Table II (28); 654 of these cases were from the Italian multicenter study, in which 80% were seropositive for HCV. (5)

Palpable purpura (Fig. 1B) (29) was the most prominent clinical manifestation of mixed cryoglobulinemia, confirming the original observation of Meltzer and colleagues (4); however, the triad of palpable purpura, fatigue, and weakness that characterized the Meltzer series was found in less than 50% of the patients in Table II, and in the Italian multicenter study, the prevalence was even lower (28%) but was more prevalent in type II than type III cryoglobulinemia. The prevalence of renal involvement (34%) was also lower in the Italian multicenter study (22%). The vasculitis associated with mixed cryoglobulinemia ranges from the benign cutaneous vasculitis responsible for the palpable purpura that occurs in almost all of these patients to life-threatening vasculitis involving vital organs. Although the association of mixed cryoglobulinemia with vasculitis of small- and medium-sized vessels has been established since the mid-1970s, the pathogenesis has not been well delineated.

Renal disease in mixed cryoglobulinemia was three times more prevalent in patients with type II than in those with type III cryoglobulinemia, occurred mainly in older patients, was associated with decreased levels of C4 component of complement, and did not correlate with palpable purpura. (5) In approximately 25% of patients with renal involvement, the first manifestation was acute nephrotic syndrome, however, the majority had an indolent disease that did not progress to end-stage renal disease despite persistent renal dysfunction. Overall, nephrotic syndrome occurred in approximately 45% of patients. Arterial hypertension accompanies the onset of renal disease in 80% of patients. (30) In one study of the natural history of the disease, 37% of patients developed membrane proliferative glomerulonephritis over an 8- to 17-year follow-up and 50% died of renal insufficiency. (31) A more recent study found a similar 10-year survival rate after renal biopsy diagnosis (49%), but only 14% of patients developed chronic uremia. A third of the deaths in the 10 years following diagnosis were due to renal failure; the remainder were due to extrarenal complications. (30) An increased risk for death or end-stage renal failure was associated with older age, recurrent purpura, high cryoglobulin concentrates, low levels of serum C3, and high serum creatinine. (32) Purpura, arthritis, or neuropathy was present in only one-half of patients with mixed cryoglobulinemia, HCV infection, and membranoproliferative glomerulonephritis. (33)

The prevalence of liver involvement in Table II (42%) was similar to that for patients with essential mixed cryoglobulinemia in the Italian multicenter study (39.5%). However, in the latter study the prevalence of liver involvement at the onset of purpura was considerably lower (15%) but increased with duration of disease. Although the consensus prevalence for peripheral neuropathy in essential mixed cryoglobulinemia is 26% (Table II), there is a wide range of reported prevalences. (5) In one study, 82% of patients with essential mixed cryoglobulinemia had peripheral neuropathy using the criteria of abnormal nerve conduction studies. (34) The prevalence of sicca syndrome was 6%; however, some patients with primary Sjögren syndrome were included in the studies reviewed. In the Italian multicenter study the prevalence was 3.8%, after connective tissue disease and primary syndrome were excluded. (5)

Cutaneous Vasculitis

Cutaneous vasculitis has been classified as an immune complex-mediated leukocytoclastic (LCV) based on studies in which only a small fraction of cases demonstrated the classic finding of LCV. (4,15,35,36) HCV has been demonstrated in cutaneous vasculitis lesions with antigens demonstrated in the vessel walls and perivascular spaces using monoclonal antisera to structural and nonstructural HCV antigens; the HCV antigens colocalized with IgG and IgM. (37) In a second study using *in situ* hybridization, (38) the viral form of HCV RNA was detected in leukocytoclastic lesions in patients with type II cryoglobulinemia in the same perivascular localizations as IgG and IgM (Fig. 1C–1G). Evidence suggested that the colocalization of HCV, IgG, and IgM in the lesion resulted in the *in situ* formation of complexes of HCV, IgG, and monoclonal RF. One possible mechanism is that after an as yet uncharacterized initial event triggering the activation of vascular endothelial cells and infiltration of neutrophils and leading to vessel wall damage, complexes of HCV, IgG, and monoclonal RF deposit in the perivascular tissues as a result of cooling of the blood and stasis from increased hydrostatic pressure in lower extremities.

A discrepancy between the two studies on HCV in cutaneous vasculitis lesions was that using immunohistochemical methodology that is threefold less sensitive than *in situ* hybridization methodology, the HCV antigen was found localized within and between endothelial cells in normal skin of the patients, (37) whereas in the *in situ* hybridization study normal skin was completely negative and HCV was detected only in the lesions. (38)

Membranoproliferative Glomerulonephritis

Membranoproliferative glomerulonephritis is the major type of glomerulonephritis in mixed cryoglobulinemia and occurs predominantly in type II cryoglobulinemia secondary to HCV infection. Several lines of evidence have implicated mixed cryoglobulins in the pathogenesis of membranoproliferative glomerulonephritis. Using immunofluorescence analysis (Fig. 1H), glomerular deposits have been shown to contain IgG, IgM, and the C3 component of complement. (39) The IgM in the deposits has been shown to have RF activity. (20) By idiotype analysis, the IgM in the glomerular deposits corresponded to the monoclonal RF in the serum. (40) By electron microscopy, glomerular deposits have been shown to have crystalloid structures that occur in tubular and annular shapes. (41) These structures are thought to be IgG–monoclonal RF complexes as similar structures have been seen in the serum cryoglobulins, and recombination studies of monoclonal RF and IgG have reproduced these structures. (42) Concentration of cryoglobulins in glomerular capillaries induced by the filtration process has been proposed as the mechanism for deposition of the immune complexes that mediate the glomerulonephritis. (39) Results of studies on IgG3 cryoglobulins in MRL-Ipr/Ipr mice are consistent with this mechanism, as deposition of the IgG3 in the glomeruli was sufficient to induce the nephritis. (43)

More recently, D'Amico (30) has proposed, based on studies of injected human type II cryoglobulinemia in mice, (44) that affinity of the monoclonal IgMK RF for the glomerular mesangium is involved in deposition of the cryoglobulin in membranoproliferative glomerulonephritis. *In vitro* studies (45) suggest that cryoglobulin deposition in the mesangium is due to the IgMK affinity for fibronectin, a known constituent of the mansangial matrix.

There have been relatively few studies on the pathogenesis of membranoproliferative glomerulonephritis associated with HCV infection; in eight patients with these lesions and HCV infection, five had type II cryoglobulinemia and seven had serum RF. (9) Immunofluorescence studies of the glomerular lesions were consistent with mixed cryoglobulinemia and, in electron microscopy studies, three of four renal biopsy specimens showed the crystalloid structure characteristic of cryoglobulins. Neither HCV antigens nor HCV RNA was detected in the glomerular lesions; however, the methodology used was not reported.

There have been two reports of detection of HCV antigen in glomerular immune deposits in patients with HCV infection and membranoproliferative glomerulonephritis using monoclonal antisera to HCV antigens. (46,47) The HCV core antigen was detected in 2 of 6 biopsies (46) and both structural and nonstructural antigens were detected in 8 of 12 biopsies. (47) The validity of these results is in question because the RF-binding artifact of the intact monoclonal antibodies was not specifically excluded. (48) In preliminary studies, HCV RNA was not detected in the glomerular immune deposits in 13 renal biopsy specimens studied using an *in situ* hybridization assay. (28) In five cases of membranoproliferative glomerulonephritis, only the viral form of HCV was found in the proximal tubule endothelial cells. These preliminary findings suggest that, in contrast to cutaneous vasculitis, intact virion is not detected in the immune complex deposits in membranoproliferative glomerulonephritis lesions in type II cryoglobulinemia.

Peripheral Neuropathy

There are conflicting reports on the presence of immune complex vasculitis in peripheral nerve lesions (5,34); however, only a small number of cases have been studied by immunofluorescence. There are no published reports on HCV in the pathogenesis of peripheral neuropathy lesions in mixed cryoglobulinemia. In an unpublished report of studies on eight nerve biopsy samples from patients with essential mixed cryoglobulinemia and peripheral neuropathy, no HCV RNA could be detected in the lesions by *in situ* hybridization assay. Six of the cases have type II and two had type III cryoglobulinemia. Seven of the biopsy samples showed histological evidence of vasculitis; immunofluorescence studies were performed in only one patient in whom large amounts of IgM, trace IgG and no C3 were found in the vessel wall deposits (Ábel G, Cacoub P, Maisonbe T, Musset L, Agnello V: unpublished observation). Hence, preliminary studies of peripheral neuropathy lesions in patients with essential mixed cryoglobulinemia, like those of MPGN, failed to demonstrate HCV by *in situ* hybridization.

Hepatitis

The histology of hepatitis in patients with essential mixed cryoglobulinemia is similar to that seen in chronic hepatitis C. (5) However, the prevalence of minimal and mild hepatitis is greater, and the prevalence of cirrhosis is decreased compared with patients selected for chronic hepatitis C with or without cryoglobulinemia. (5) The lymphocytic infiltrate in the liver in chronic hepatitis C contains predominantly T cells (49); however, the lymphoid aggregates or nodules, which are a feature of HCV infection of the liver, contain B cells. These nodules are more prevalent in type II cryoglobulinemia, where they occur more frequently as pseudofollicle (50) composed predominantly of monoclonal B cells. In both chronic hepatitis C and hepatitis associated with patients with type II mixed cryoglobulinemia, progression from the minimal/mild activity group to the moderate/severe/cirrhosis activity group seems to be associated with a loss of lymphoid nodules. (50,51)

Bone Marrow and Lymphoid Involvement

Monoclonal B cells have also been detected in the bone marrow in patients with type II cryoglobulinemia; 22 of 39 cases were shown to have discrete infiltrates of monoclonal IgMk B cells that had strong Bc1-2 and weak Ki-67 expression (52) similar to the B cells found in the liver. (50) In another study, both bone marrow and sera were positive for HCV by reverse transcriptase polymerase chain reaction (RT-PCR) in all 15 patients with mixed cryoglobulinemia and HCV infection; however, the methodology employed could not determine whether marrow cellular elements were infected. (53)

The detection of HCV in peripheral blood mononuclear cells (PBMC) has been widely reported, and the consensus is that the virion form of the virus (positive strand) is present in PBMC, but that detection of the replicative from (negative strand) is controversial. Early studies were uniformly flawed because of the false priming that occurred with routine RT-PCR, resulting in the detection of negative-strand HCV in the presence of positive-strand HCV. A well-controlled, well-documented quantitative study using a high strand-specific (Tth-based) method of RT-PCR (54) found no evidence of HCV replication in PBMC from 10 human and 5 chimpanzee subjects. However, it appears that negative strand HCV can be detected in very small numbers of PBMC using "tagged" RT-PCR methodology (55) or a Tth-based strand-specific assay (56) in the setting of immunosuppression induced by either drug (55) or HIV. (56)

Lymphocytes that infiltrate liver and marrow in patients with mixed cryoglobulinemia and HCV infection have been classified as low-grade malignant cells. (57–59) Although these findings suggest a malignant process, only 5–10% of patients with essential mixed cryoglobulinenia (EMC) developed frank malignancy in long-term follow-up. (15,35) In a preliminary report, the bone marrow showed B cells morphologically consistent with those found in chronic lymphocytic leukemia/small lymphocytic lymphoma. After an 8.5-year follow-up, 17 cases showed clinical overt non-Hodgkin's lymphoma in 101 of 123 cases with type II cryoglobulinemia. In two cases studied extensively, B cells were shown to arise from a minor B-cell population present in the initial bone marrow and not the predominant monoclonal B-cell population. (60) Hence, at least a portion of the malignancies in type II cryoglobulinemia arise stochastically.

In an earlier study, all four cases of Waldenstrom's macroglobulinemia were positive for HCV (8); two of the four cases produced WA mRF. This finding suggests that the malignancy in these cases arose from the population of monoclonal B cells producing the WA monoclonal RF found in the cryoglobulins and would support the hypothesis that malignancies in type II cryoglobulinemia arise as a result of malignant transforming mutational events occurring in the setting of an antigen-driven benign proliferation process. (28,50)

Therapy

In the conventional approach to therapy of patients with mixed cryoglobulinemia, patients with apparently benign manifestations of disease, mild palpable purpura, arthralgias, and fatigue are usually not treated or are treated symptomatically with nonsteroidal anti-inflammatory drugs, whereas those with significant organ system involvement are treated with glucocorticoids, cytotoxic immunosuppressives, or plasmapheresis, alone or in combination. Treatment protocols have been based largely on uncontrolled observations, and only studies of small number of patients have been published. The consensus on conventional therapy is that combination therapy can induce short- to medium-term remission, that each of the treatments alone is poorly effective, and that all of the protocols are ineffective in inducing long-range remission.

The first use of interferon-α therapy for essential mixed cryoglobulinemia was apparently based on the rationale that the disease was a low-grade malignancy and that the antiproliferative action of the drug may be effective. These studies by Bonomo et al. (13) and Casato et al. (61) are notable for two reasons: (1) the unconventional regimen of 3 million units (MU) interferon-α daily for 3 months followed by 3 MU thrice weekly and (2) the high response rate (77%) and the prolonged remission.

Casato and colleagues (14) reported a 12-year prospective study on a high dose of interferon therapy (234 to 849 MU) of 31 consecutive patients with type II cryoglobulinemia and HCV infection that included patients treated in the initial studies. (13,61) The prevalence of complete response was 62% with a median response of 33 months. The prevalence of normalization of transaminase levels was 100%. Relapses of elevated aminotransferases occurred in 100 and 8% of patients receiving less than or greater than 621 MU, respectively. The only pretherapy parameter that correlated with complete response was a solitary anti-C-22 antibody pattern. There was no correlation with HCV genotype, NS5a gene mutations, liver histology, or HLA-DR phenotype.

There are three controlled therapeutic trials of patients with mixed cryoglobulinemia and HCV infection, two testing interferon-α and methylprednisolone therapy. In a randomized crossover-controlled trial, 20 patients with mixed cryoglobulinemia and HCV infection without renal disease (58% were type II) were treated with interferon-α 2 MU daily for 1 month, then every other day for 5 months, and the results were compared with a 6-month period without therapy. During the treatment period, all patients had a significant improvement of purpura, but not neuropathy, accompanied by a decrease in cryoglobulins and serum transaminases. HCV RNA in 2 of 15 patients decreased to undetectable levels after therapy. (62)

In a prospective, randomized controlled study of 53 patients with HCV-associated type II cryoglobulinemia and a 75% prevalence of renal disease, 60% of the 27 patients treated with 3 MU interferon-α thrice weekly for 6 months, in comparison to controls, had significant improvement in cutaneous vasculitis and renal disease accompanied by decreased cryoglobulins and a decease of HCV RNA to undetectable levels. In all patients, the disease relapsed within 6 to 13 months following therapy. (63)

In another randomized controlled study of 65 patients with type II mixed cryoglobulinemia and HCV infection, combination therapy with natural interferon, 3 MU three times weekly, and methylprednisolone, 16 mg daily for 1 year, was compared with treatment with interferon alone, methylprednisolone alone, and untreated patients. The combination therapy had a slightly greater and more rapid response rate than interferon alone (71% compared with 67%) compared with a response rate of 22% with prednisolone alone and a 13% spontaneous remission in the control group. By the end of the follow-up period, however, the sustained remission rate was essentially the same (25% versus 33%). Considering that HCV RNA levels rose significantly with prenisone and that the relapse rate after 3 months was not different, the marginal effects of combined therapy do not warrant the use of this protocol. It was also noted that lower HCV RNA levels were predictive of response to therapy. (64)

Trials on interferon–ribavirin combination therapy in mixed cryoglobulinemia have not as yet been reported.

Pathogenesis

Chronic Immune Complex Stimulation

The oldest and most widely held hypothesis is that RF in mixed cryoglobulinemia results from the chronic stimulation of the immune system by complexes consisting of IgG bound to antigens of an infectious agent. Supporting this hypothesis is that the production of RF by circulating immune complexes is well established from animal model studies and RF production is common in chronic immune complex disease, such as rheumatoid arthritis, systemic lupus erythematosus, and subacute bacterial endocarditis. However, although this hypothesis explains the high prevalence of RF in chronic hepatitis C (65) and the development of type III cryoglobulinemia adequately, it does not explain the development of type II cryoglobulinemia, as in the chronic immune complex disease the RF is polyclonal and monoclonal RF occurs rarely.

The French prospective study of patients with chronic hepatitis and type II cryoglobulinemia provided evidence that with prolonged stimulation of polyclonal RF, B cells could lead to monoclonal RF in some patients and type III cryoglobulins could transform to type II cryoglobulins. (27) It is also possible that only a portion of patients with HCV infection are genetically predisposed to developing type II cryoglobulins and develop type II cryoglobulinemia without first developing type III cryoglobulinemia.

Low-Grade Malignancy

A low-grade malignant lymphoproliferative disorder has been postulated as the etiology of type II cryoglobulinemia. The presence of a monoclonal population of B cells in type II cryoglobulins, the occurrence of type II cryoglobulins in patients with lymphoid malignancies, and the presence of malignant-appearing lymphoplasmacytoid cells in the liver and bone marrow of patients with essential mixed cryoglobulinemia (57) have been cited as supporting evidence for this hypothesis. In long-term follow-up studies, however, few patients with type II cryoglobulinemia have developed malignancy. Moreover, the hypothesis does not explain the development of type III cryoglobulinemia.

HCV Infection of B Cells

It has been postulated that both polyclonal and monoclonal B-cell proliferation result from infection of these cells with HCV. (66,67) Although HCV has been widely detected in peripheral blood monocytes in patients with mixed cryoglobulinemia and HCV infection, replication of HCV in any cell other than hepatocytes is highly controversial (see Section II,D,5). Although HCV is not an oncogenic virus, experimental evidence shows that HCV nonstructural protein NS3 and the HCV core protein can transform cells *in vitro*. (68,69) There have not been any reports of the detection of HCV in the malignant cells of patients with mixed cryoglobulinemia progressing to frank malignancy. Although the controversial association of HCV infection with non-Hodgkin's lymphoma has been reported, HCV has not been detected in non-Hodgkin's lymphoma cells in these patients. (70,71)

Chronic Stimulation of B Cells by HCV Complexed to Very Low Density Lipoprotein (VLDL)

Studies have provided evidence for a new hypothesis on the etiology and pathophysiology of mixed cryoglobulinemia secondary to HCV infection. The hypothesis is that the WA monoclonal RF is produced as a result of direct chronic stimulation of a specific population of B cells in the liver by a complex of HCV and a VLDL. The main findings supporting this hypothesis have been the selective concentration of HCV with WA monoclonal RF and VLDL in the cryoglobulins, the possible LDL receptor mediation of HCV endocytoses, a threefold increased risk of developing essential mixed cryoglobulinemia among HCV-infected patients who carry the apolipoprotein (apo) E2 allele, (28) and the demonstration that hepatic lymphoid follicles in patients with type II cryoglobulinemia consist predominantly of monoclonal IgMk B cells that are CD5$^+$, strongly Bcl-2$^+$, and weakly Ki-67$^+$. (50) A corollary of this hypothesis is that monoclonal RF may provide a protective effect against hepatitis in some patients with cryoglobulinemia. The greatly reduced prevalence of cirrhosis reported in patients with type II cryoglobulinemia (5) provides indirect evidence for this hypothesis. The proposed mechanism for the protective effect of WA monoclonal RF is that complexes of HCV–VLDL secreted by infected hepatocytes stimulate B cells in the liver of patients with type II cryoglobulinemia to produce WA monoclonal RF that blocks the spread of HCV infection of hepatocytes mediated by LDL receptors.

OTHER EXTRAHEPATIC MANIFESTATIONS

Twenty-seven extrahepatic disease manifestations, mainly of the autoimmune type, have been reported to be associated with HCV infection (Table III). The

TABLE III Extrahepatic Disease Manifestation of HCV Infection Other Than Mixed Cryoglobulinemia

Sialadenitis
Porphyria cutanea tarda
Membranoproliferative
Membranous glomerulonephritis
Sjögren's syndrome
Lichen planus
Autoimmune thyroiditis
Antiphospholipid syndrome
Idiopathic thrombocytopenia purpura
Idiopathic pulmonary fibrosis
Mooren corneal ulcers
Uveitis
Rheumatoid arthritis
Systemic lupus erythematosus
Dermatomyositis
Polymyositis
CREST syndrome
Fibromyalgia
Polyarteritis nodosa
Waldenstrom's macroglobulinemia
Non-Hodgkin's lymphoma
Diabetes mellitus
Aplastic anemia
Guillain-Barré syndrome
Behcet's syndrome
Hypertrophic cardiomyopathy
IgA deficiency

validity of most of these associations is doubtful. In most instances, relatively few cases have been reported, and there is a patient selection bias that produces false associations, especially in endemic regions where coincidental disease is more likely to be observed. This patient selection bias was illustrated in the early reports that found high prevalences: 48–88% among patients positive for antiliver/kidney microsomal (LKM) autoantibodies in Italy, France, and Germany. When prevalences of these autoantibodies were studied in HCV–infected patients, prevalences of 3–5% were found. (72)

In general, there is a lack of studies of unselected large numbers of patients with HCV infection in determining the prevalence of extrahepatic manifestations. Despite these concerns, there does appear to be a strong association of HCV infection with sialadenitis and porphyria cutanea tarda (which is discussed in another chapter). Although the evidence is contradictory for the association of membranoproliferative glomerulonephritis without mixed cryoglobulinemia and sparse for the association of membranous glomerulonephritis, there are pathophysiologic bases for these associations. In addition, there is a high prevalence of a variety of autoantibodies associated with HCV infection, predominantly without clinical manifestations. These observations are further confounded by increased prevalences of autoantibodies with female gender and advanced age.

Sialadenitis

High prevalences of salivary gland lesions have been reported in patients with chronic hepatitis C; lymphocytic capillaritis was found in 49% and lymphocytic adenitis in 57 to 80%. (65,73,74) These patients, however, differed from patients with Sjögren's syndrome by the lower female sex prevalence (30% versus 100%), absence of serum antinuclear antibodies (0% versus 90%), lower association with HLA DR 3 (38% versus 87%), milder histopathology (80% grade, I and II versus 80% grades II–IV), and clinical symptoms (only 30% had xerostomia and none had xerophthalmia). This distinction was confirmed by a study of 48 patients who had Sjögren's syndrome without mixed cryoglobulinemia and who were all positive for SSA/Ro; none had HCV infection. HCV is common only in patients with Sjögren's syndrome associated with mixed cryoglobulinemia, which itself is a major extrahepatic manifestation of HCV infection. (75)

Studies in transgenic mice expressing HCV envelope genes found sialadenitis that had features similar to the lesions in humans and also showed no gender prevalence and antinuclear autoantibodies were negative. (76) Despite some technical concerns and reservations regarding the nonphysiologic overexpression of envelope proteins in this animal model, results suggest that the HCV virus may be directly involved in sialadenitis rather than triggering an autoimmune process.

Glomerulonephritis

Membranoproliferative glomerulonephritis in the absence of cryoglobulinemia in HCV infection has been suspected but not proven and currently remains controversial. (77) A reported exclusion of cryoglobulinemia based on negative serologic studies is problematic because of the marked variability in cryoglobulin testing (see Section II,B,2). Moreover, renal biopsy studies excluding the crystalloid structures characteristic of cryoglobulins and RF in the glomerular immune deposits are generally lacking. Considering the broad humoral immune response to HCV antigens and the chronicity of the infection, a wide variety of immune complexes may be present that do not contain RF or cryoprecipitate but may have nephrotoxicity. Hence, it is plausible to have membranoproliferative glomerulonephritis in the absence of cryoglobulins.

Membranous glomerulonephritis is uncommon in HCV infection, but in contrast to membranoproliferative glomerulonephritis, these lesions are not associated with cryoglobulinemia, rheumatoid factors, or hypocomplementemia. In the few patients with these lesions that have been reported, there have not been sufficient studies to determine the role, if any, of HCV or HCV antigens.

Autoantibodies

A variety of autoantibodies occur with HCV infection, usually in low titers. Anti-GOR antibodies directed to a host protein cloned from plasma of an HCV-infected chimpanzee are the most prevalent, detected in 80% of infected patients. (78) In a retrospective study of patients in the United States with elevated aminotransaminases and positive HCV serology, the prevalence of autoantibodies was measured compared to patients with alcohol-induced liver disease and controls with no liver disease. (79) Prevalences were: antinuclear antibodies (ANA), 14%; antismooth muscle antibodies (SMA), 66%; rheumatoid factor, 70%; and antiliver/kidney microsomal, 2%. Autoantibody titers were mostly low except for RF titers, which were moderate to high. Prevalences were similar for males and females. In a prospective study of French patients with chronic hepatitis C, the prevalence of autoantibodies was: ANA, 13%; SMA, 13%; RF, 70%; anti-LKM1, 3%; antithyroglobulin, 1%; and antithyroid, 1%. Antimitochondrial and anti-RO/SSA autoantibodies were not detected. (65)

From these studies it appears that autoantibodies, particularly RF, are prevalent in chronic hepatitis C; however, age-matched controls were absent in both studies, the duration of disease was not known, and there have been no studies of earlier stages of disease. In contrast to these studies, a study of HCV-infected patients in Ireland did not find an increase prevalence of autoantibodies, except for RF, which was present in 14% of patients compared to 3% in the general population. (80) Patients in the study were predominantly women who were infected from HCV-contaminated anti-D antibodies; the mean of duration of disease was well defined: 15.1 years. The study on this cohort suggests that genetic factors may be important in the association of autoantibodies with HCV infection, but also raises the possibility that the duration of disease greater than 15 years is responsible for the reported high prevalences of RF in chronic hepatitis C.

The reported prevalences of antithyroid antibodies in HCV infection are controversial. (81–83) Antithyroid antibody and clinical thyroid disease occurred only in females and correlated with increased age. The prevalence of clinical thyroid disease was only a fraction of the prevalence of thyroid autoantibodies. Considering the female predilection for autoimmune thyroiditis and a prevalence of thyroid antibodies in 15–24% of normal women above the age of 60, (82) the significance of the reported prevalence of thyroid antibodies and thyroid dysfunction in chronic hepatitis C is questionable.

Therapy with interferon induces reversible antithyroid antibodies and dysfunction *de novo* mainly in female patients with chronic hepatitis without pre-existing thyroid abnormalties. (83) Other studies have found that a positive microsomal antibody test at the onset of interferon therapy was a risk factor for thyroid dysfunction. (84)

There is an increased prevalence of anticardiolipin antibodies in patients with HCV infection compared to healthy blood donors. (85) These antibodies have the characteristics of anticardiolipin antibodies associated with viral infection: low titer, absence of thrombotic events, and absence of thrombocytopenia and anti β_2-glycoprotein I, a cofactor of anticardiolipin associated with clinical manifestations of these antibodies. Another antibody population with no apparent pathologic effects are the IgM antibodies in patients with HCV infection and type II cryoglobulinemia that reacts with mimotopes of the CD4-like lymphocyte activation gene-3 (LAG-3) human protein. (86)

Most autoantibodies in HCV infection are distinct from those associated with "autoimmune" disease. This is illustrated by the difference in clinical presentation between autoimmune hepatitis type 2 that is not associated with HCV infection but with anti-LKM1 and HCV infection with anti-LKM1. The former patients are predominantly young females with marked elevations of ALT and high anti-LKM1 titers who respond to immunosuppression therapy but not interferon; these patients are frequently HLA DR 3 positive. In contrast, the latter patients are older without gender bias and have mildly elevated ALT and low anti-LMK1 titers and respond to interferon therapy but not immunosuppression. (72)

CONCLUSION

There is ample circumstantial evidence that HCV is involved in the etiology and pathogenesis of mixed cryoglobulinemia, but the mechanism involved in the proliferation of B cells that results in the production of both polyclonal RF and monoclonal RF remains to be determined. There is no convincing evidence that HCV produces a productive infection of lymphocytes that results in RF production and other autoantibodies. In fact, the mechanism involved in the production of monoclonal RF is undoubtedly different from the mechanism(s) involved in the production of the wide array of other autoantibodies associated with HCV infection. These autoantibodies appear to resemble the physiologic type that accompanies many viral infections. Studies that have shown that autoantibodies associated with HCV infection are distinct from those found in autoimmune hepatitis and the low incidence of clinical autoimmune disease in HCV infection underscore the point that HCV infection does not directly cause autoimmune disease.

Thus far, investigations into the role of HCV in the pathogenesis of mixed cryoglobulinemia have been rudimentary. In particular, the precise role of the virus in the pathogenesis of the renal disease, the major cause of morbidity and mortality in this disease, remains to be delineated. Whether HCV and HCV antigens are directly involved in mediating the immune complex glomerular lesions or only indirectly involved as a result of stimulating the production of monoclonal rheumatoid factors is the key question to be answered.

REFERENCES

1. Wintrobe M M, Buell M V. Hyperproteinemia associated with multiple myeloma, with report of a case in which extraordinary hyperproteinemia was associated with thrombosis of retinal veins and symptoms suggesting Reynaud's disease. Bull Johns Hopkins Hosp 1933;52:156–65.
2. Lerner A B, Watson C J. Studies of cryoglobulins; Unusual purpura associated with the presence of a high concentration of cryoglobulin (cold precipitable serum globulin). Am J Med Sci 1947;214:410–5.
3. Lospalluto J, Dorward B, Miller W Jr, Ziff M. Cryoglobulinemia based on interaction between a gamma macroglobulin and 7S gamma globulin. Am J Med 1962;32:142–7.
4. Meltzer M, Franklin E C, Elias K, McCluskey R T, Cooper N. Cryoglobulinemia: a clinical and laboratory study. II. Cryoglobulins with rheumatoid factor activity. Am J Med 1966;40:837–56.
5. Monti G, Galli M, Invernizzi F, et al. Cryoglobulinemias: a multi-centre study of the early clinical and laboratory manifestations of primary and secondary disease. GISC. Italian Group for the Study of Cryoglobulinemias. Q J Med 1995;88:115–26.
6. Pascual M, Perrin L, Giostra E, Schifferli J A. Hepatitis C virus in patients with cryoglobulinemia type II (letter). J Infect Dis 1990;162:569–70.
7. Agnello V, Romain P L. Mixed cryoglobulinemia secondary to hepatitis C virus infection. Rheum Dis Clin North Am 1996;22:1–21.
8. Agnello V, Chung R T, Kaplan L M. A role for hepatitis C virus infection in type II cryoglobulinemia. N Engl J Med 1992;327:1490–5.
9. Johnson R J, Gretch D R, Yamabe H, et al. Membranoproliferative glomerulonephritis associated with hepatitis C virus infection. N Engl J Med 1993;328:465–70.
10. Levey J M, Bjornsson B, Banner B, et al. Mixed cryoglobulinemia in chronic hepatitis C infection: a clinicopathologic analysis of 10 cases and review of recent literature. Medicine 1994;73:53–67.
11. Agnello V, Joslin F G, Kunkel H G. Cross idiotypic specificity among monoclonal IgM antiglobulins. Scand J Immunol 1972;1:283.
12. Kunkel H G, Agnello V, Joslin F G, Winchester R J, Capra J D. Cross-idiotypic specificity among monoclonal IgM proteins with anti-g-globulin activity. J Exp Med 1973;137:331–42.
13. Bonomo L, Casato M, Afeltra, A, Caccavo D. Treatment of idiopathic mixed cryoglobulinemia with alpha interferon. Am J Med 1987;83:726–30.
14. Casato M, Agnello V, Pacillo, L P, et al. Predictors of long-term response to high-dose interferon therapy in type II cryoglobulinemia associated with hepatitis C virus infection. Blood 1997;90:3865–73.
15. Brouet J C, Clauvel J P, Danon, F, Klein M, Seligmann M. Biologic and clinical significance of cryoglobulins: a report of 86 cases. Am J Med 1974;57:775–88.
16. Agnello V. Mixed cryoglobulinemia after hepatitis C virus: more and less ambiguity. Ann Rheum Dis 1998;57:701–2.
17. Musset L, Diemert M C, Taibi F, et al. Characterization of cryoglobulins by immunoblotting. Clin Chem 1992;38:798–802.
18. Gigli I. Complement avtivation in patients with mixed cryoglobulinemia. In: Ponticelli C, Minetti L, D'Amico G, eds. Antiglobulins, cryoglobulins, and glomerulonephritis. Dordrecht, The Netherlands: Martinus Nijhoff, 1986;135–46.
19. Circolo A, Barnes J L, Agnello V. Inhibition of complement activation by anti-cross-idiotype antibodies. FASEB J 1988;2:A1647.
20. Maggiore Q, Bartolomeo F, L'Abbate A, et al. Glomerular localization of circulating antiglobulin activity in essential mixed cryoglobulinemia with glomerulonephritis. Kidney Int 1982;21:387–94.

21. Hanauer L B, Christian C L. Studies of cryoproteins in systemic lupus erythematosus. J Clin Invest 1967;46:400–8.
22. Agnello V, Zhang Q X, Abel G, Knight G B. The association of hepatitis C virus infection with monoclonal rheumatoid factors bearing the WA cross-idiotype: implications for the etiopathogenesis and therapy of mixed cryoglobulinemia. Clin Exp Rheum 1995;13(Suppl 13):S101–4.
23. Agnello V, Barnes J L. Human rheumatoid factor cross-idiotypes I: WA and BLA are heat-labile conformational antigens requiring both heavy and light chains. J Exp Med 1986;164:1809–14.
24. Gorevic P D, Frangione B. Mixed cryoglobulinemia cross-reactive idiotypes: implications for the relationship of MC to rheumatic and lymphoproliferative diseases. Semin Hematol 1991;28:79–94.
25. Agnello V, Arbetter A, Ibanez de Kasep G, Powell R, Tan E M, Joslin F. Evidence for a subset of rheumatoid factors that cross-react with DNA-histone and have distinct cross-idiotype. J Exp Med 1980;151:1514–27.
26. Cacoub P, Fabiani F L, Musset L, et al. Mixed cryoglobulinemia and hepatitis C virus. Am J Med 1994;96:124–32.
27. Lunel F, Musset L, Cacoub P, et al. Cryoglobulinemia in chronic liver diseases: the role of hepatitis C virus and liver damage. Gastroenterology 1994;106:1291–300.
28. Agnello V. The etiology and pathophysiology of mixed cryoglobulinemia secondary to hepatitis C virus infection. Springer Semin Immunopathol 1997;19:111–29.
29. Shakil A O, Di Bisceglie A M. Vasculitis and cryoglobulinemia related to hepatitis C. N Engl J Med 1994;331:1624.
30. D'Amico G. Renal involvement in hepatitis C infection: Cryoglobulinemic glomerulonephritis. Kidney Int 1998;54:650–71.
31. Invernizzi F, Galli M, Serino G, et al. Secondary and essential cryoglobulinemias. Frequency, nosological classification and long-term follow-up. Acta Haematol 1983;70:73–82.
32. Tarantino A, Campise M, Banfi G, et al. Long-term predictors of survival in essential mixed cryoglobulinemic glomerulonephritis. Kidney Int 1995;47:618–23.
33. Johnson R J, Wilson R, Yambe H, et al. Renal manifestations of hepatitis C virus infection. Kidney Int 1994;46:1255–63.
34. Ferri C, LaCivita L, Cirafis C, et al. Peripheral neuropathy in mixed cryoglobulinemia: clinical and electrophysiologic investigations. J Rheumatol 1992;19:889–95.
35. Gorevic P D, Kassab H J, Levo Y, et al. Mixed cryoglobulinemia: clinical aspects and long-term follow-up of 40 patients. Am J Med 1980;69:287–308.
36. Cattaneo R, Fenini M G, Facchetti F. The cryoglobulinemic vasculitis. Ric Clin Lab 1986;16:327–33.
37. Sansonno D, Cornacchiulo V, Iacobelli A R, Di Stefano R, Lospalluti M, Dammacco F. Localization of hepatitis C virus antigens in liver and skin tissues of chronic hepatitis C virus-infected patients with mixed cryoglobulinemia. Hepatology 1995;21:305–12.
38. Agnello V, Abel G. Localization of hepatitis C virus in cutaneous vasculitic lesions in patients with type II mixed cryoglobulinemia using in situ hybridization. Arthritis Rheum 1997;40:2007–15.
39. D'Amico G, Colasanti G, Ferrario R, Sinico R A. Renal involvement in essential mixed cryoglobulinemia. Kidney Int 1989;35:1004–14.
40. Sinico R A, Winearls C G, Sabadini E, Fornasieri A, Castiglione A, D'Amico G. Identification of glomerular immune deposits in cryoglobulinemia glomerulonephritis. Kidney Int 1988;34:109–16.
41. Cordonnier D, Martin H, Groslambert P, Micouin C, Chenais F, Stoebner P. Mixed IgG-IgM cryoglobulinemia with glomerulonephritis. Immunochemical fluorescent and ultrastructural study of kidney and in vitro cryoprecipitate. Am J Med 1975;59:867–72.
42. Stoebner P, Renversez J C, Groulade J, Vialtel P, Cordonnier D. Ultrastructural study of human IgG IgM crystalcryoglobulins. Am J Clin Pathol 1978;71:404–10.
43. Reininger L, Berney T, Shibata T, Spertini F, Merino R, Izui S. Cryoglobulinemia induced by a murine IgG3 rheumatoid factor: skin vasculitis and glomerulonephritis arise from distinct pathogenic mechanisms. Proc Natl Acad Sci U S A 1990;87:10038–42.
44. Fornasieri A, Li M, Armelloni S, et al. Glomerulonephritis induced by human IgMκ-IgG cryoglobulins in mice. Lab Invest 1993;69:531–40.
45. Fornasieri A, Armelloni S, Bernasconi P, et al. High binding of immunoglobulin Mκ rheumatoid

factor from type II cryoglobulins to cellular fibronectin: a mechanism for induction of in situ immune complex glomerulonephritis. Am J Kidney Dis 1996;27:476–83.

46. Yamabe H, Inuma H, Osawa H, et al. Glomerular deposition of hepatitis C virus in membrano-proliferative glomerulonephritis. Nephron 1996;72:741.

47. Sansonno D, Gesualdo L, Manno C, Schena F P, Dammacco F. Hepatitis C virus-related proteins in kidney tissue from hepatitis C virus-infected patients with cryoglobulinemic membrano-proliferative glomerulonephritis. Hepatology 1997;25:1237–44.

48. Agnello V. Immune complexes in hepatitis C (letter). Hepatology 1997;26:1687–8.

49. Scheuer P J, Krawczynski Dhillon A P. Histopathology and detection of hepatitis C virus in liver. Springer Semin Immunopathol 1997;19:27–45.

50. Monteverde A, Ballare M, Pileri S. Hepatic lymphoid aggregates in chronic hepatitis C and mixed cryoglobulinemia. Springer Semin Immunopathol 1997;19:99–110.

51. Agnello V, Abel G, Zhang Q X, Knight G B, Muchmore El. Detection of widespread hepatocyte infection in chronic hepatitis C. Hepatology 1998;28:573–84.

52. Monteverde A, Sabattini E, Poggi S, et al. Bone marrow findings further support the hypothesis that essential mixed cryoglobulinemia type II is characterized by a monoclonal B-cell proliferation. Leuk Lymphoma 1995;2:119–24.

53. Galli M, Zehender G, Monti G, et al. Hepatitis C virus RNA in the bone marrow of patients with mixed cryoglobulinemia and in subjects with noncryoglobulinemic chronic hepatitis type C. Infect Dis 1995;171:672–5.

54. Lanford R E, Chavez D, Chisari F V, Sureau C. Lack of detection of negative-strand hepatitis C virus RNA in peripheral blood mononuclear cells and other extrahepatic tissues by the highly strand-specific rTth reverse transcriptase PCR. Virology 1995;69:8079–83.

55. Muratori L, Gibellini D, Lenzi M, et al. Quantification of hepatitis C virus-infected peripheral blood mononuclear cells by *in situ* reverse transcriptase-polymerase chain reaction. Blood 1996;88:2768–74.

56. Laskus T, Radkowski M, Wang L, Sook J L, Vargas H, Rakela J. Hepatitis C virus quasi species in patients infected with HIV-1. Correlation with extrahepatic viral replication. Virology 1998;248:164–71.

57. Monteverde A, Rivano M T, Allegra G C, et al. Essential mixed cryoglobulinemia, type II: a manifestation of a low-grade malignant lymphoma? Clinical-morphological study of 12 cases with special reference to immunohistochemical findings in liver frozen sections. Acta Haematol 1988;79:20–5.

58. Mussini C, Mascia M T, Zanni G, Curci G, Bonacorsi G, Artusi T. A cytomorphological and immunohistochemical study of bone marrow in the diagnosis of essential mixed type II cryoglobulinemia. Haematologica 1991;76:389–91.

59. Pozzato G, Mazzaro C, Crovatto M et al. Low-grade malignant lymphoma, hepatitis C virus infection and mixed cryoglobulinemia. Blood 1994;84:3047–53.

60. Ballare M, De Vita S, Bertoncelli M C, Pivetta B, Biocchi M, Pileri S. Clinical, pathological and molecular differences between the bone marrow lymphoproliferation and the overt B-cell lymphomas in patients with the type II mixed cryoglobulinemia and the HCV infection. Abstr. 4th Intern Meet HCV Relat Virus, Kyoto, Jpn, 1997:222.

61. Casato M, Lagana B, Antonelli G, Dianzani F, Bonomo L. Long-term results of therapy with interferon-α for type II essential mixed cryoglobulinemia. Blood 1991;78:3142–7.

62. Ferri C, Marzo E, Longombardo G. Interferon alfa and mixed cryoglobulinemia patients: A randomized crossover-controlled trial. Blood 1993;81:1132–6.

63. Misiani R, Bellavita P, Fenili D, et al. Hepatitis C virus infection in patients with essential mixed cryoglobulinemia. Ann Intern Med 1992;117:573–7.

64. Dammacco F, Sansonno D, Han J H, et al. Natural interferon-α versus its combination with 6-methyl-prednisolone in therapy of type II mixed cryoglobulinemia: A long term, randomized, controlled study. Blood 1994;84:3336–43.

65. Pawlotsky J M, Roudot-Thoraval F, Simmonds P, et al. Extrahepatic immunologic manifestations in chronic hepatitis C and hepatitis C virus serotypes. Ann Intern Med 1995;122:169–73.

66. Ferri C, Monti M, LaCivita L, Longombardo G, Greco F, Pasero G, Gentilini P, Bombardieri S, Zignego AL. Infection of peripheral blood mononuclear cells by hepatitis C virus in mixed cryoglobulinemia. Blood 1993;82:3701–4.

67. Sansonno D, DeVita S, Iacobelli A R, et al. Clonal analysis of intra hepatic B cells from HCV-

infected patients with and without mixed cryoglobulinemia. Immunology 1998;160:3594–601.

68. Ray R B, Lagging L M, Meyer K, et al. Transcriptional regulation of cellular and viral promotors by the hepatitis C virus core protein. Virus Res 1995;37:209–20.

69. Ray R B, Lagging L M, Meyer K, et al. Hepatitis C virus core protein cooperates with ras and transforms primary rat embryo fibroblast to tumorigenic phenotype. J Virol 1996;70:4438–43.

70. De Vita S, Sasonno D, Dolcetti R, et al. Hepatitis C virus within a malignant lymphoma lesion in the course of type II mixed cryoglobulinemia. Blood 1995;86:1887–92.

71. Ascoli V, Lo Coco F, Artini M, et al. Extranodal lymphomas associated with hepatitis C virus infection. Am J Clin Pathol 1998;109:600–9.

72. Strassburg C P, Obermayer-Straub P, Manns M P. Autoimmunity in hepatitis C and D virus infection. J Viral Hepatitis 1996;3:49–59.

73. Haddad J, Deny P, Gotheil C M, et al. Lymphocytic sialadenitis of Sjögren's syndrome associated with chronic hepatitis C virus liver disease. Lancet 1992;339:321–3.

74. Pirisi M, Scott C, Fabris C, et al. Mild sialadenitis: a common finding inpatients with hepatitis C virus infection. Scand J Gastroenterol 1994;29:940–2.

75. King P D, McMurray R W, Becherer P R. Sjögren's syndrome without mixed cryoglobulinemia is not associated with hepatitis C virus infection. Am J Gastroenterol 1994;89:1047–50.

76. Kioke K, Moriya K, Ishibashi K, et al. Sialadenitis histologic resembling Sjögren syndrome in mice transgenic for hepatitis C virus envelope genes. Proc Natl Acad Sci U S A 1997;94:233–6.

77. Stehman-Breen C, Wilson R, Johnson R J. Is there a hepatitis C-associated membranoproliferative glomerulonephritis? Am J Kidney Dis 1997;30:189–90.

78. Mishiro S, Hoshi Y, Takeda K, et al. Non-A, non-B hepatitis specific antibodies directed at host-derived epitope: implication for an autoimmune process. Lancet 1990;336:1400–3.

79. Clifford B D, Donahue D, Smith L, et al. High prevalence of serologic markers of autoimmunity inpatients with chronic hepatitis C. Hepatology 1995;21:613–9.

80. Sachithanandan S, Fielding J F. Autoimmune disease is not a feature of hepatitis C infection in Ireland. J Clin Gastroenterol 1997;25:522–4.

81. Tran A, Quaranta J F, Benzaken S, et al. High prevalence of thyroid autoantibodies in a prospective series of patients of patients with chronic hepatitis C before interferon therapy. Hepatology 1993;18:253–7.

82. Boadas J, Rodriguez-Espinosa J, Enriquez J. Prevalence of thyroid autoantibodies is not increased in blood donors with hepatitis C infection. Hepatology 1995;22:611–5.

83. Marazuela M, García-Buey L, González-Fernández B, García-Monzón C, Arranz A, Borque M J, Moreno-Otero R. Thyroid autoimmune disorders in patients with chronic hepatitis C before and during interferon-α therapy. Clin Endocrinol 1996;44:635–42.

84. Watanabe U, Hashimoto E, Hisamitsu T, et al. The risk factor for development of thyroid disease during interferon α therapy for chronic hepatitis C. Am J Gastroenterol 1994;89:399–403.

85. Cacoub P, Musset L, Amoura Z, et al. Anticardiolipin, anti-beta2-glycoprotein I, and antinucleosome antibodies in hepatitis C virus infection and mixed cryoglobulinemia. Multivirc Group. J Rheumatol 1997;24:2139–44.

86. Mecchia M, Casato M, Rosalba T, et al. Nonrheumatoid IgM in human hepatitis C virus-associated type II cryoglobulinemia recognize mimotopes of the CD4-like LAG-3 protein. J Immunol 1996;157:3727–36.

16

HEPATITIS C VIRUS AND HUMAN IMMUNODEFICIENCY VIRUS COINFECTION

MARC GHANY
Liver Diseases Section, Digestive Diseases Branch
National Institute of Diabetes and Digestive and Kidney Diseases, National Institutes of Health
Bethesda, Maryland

DARYL T.-Y. LAU
Division of Gastroenterology and Hepatology
University of Texas
Galveston, Texas

INTRODUCTION

The hepatitis C virus (HCV) and human immunodeficiency virus (HIV-1) share similar routes of transmission and have a similar propensity to cause chronic infection. For these reasons, coinfection with HCV and HIV is not uncommon in high-risk individuals, such as injection drug users, patients with hemophilia, and, to a lesser extent, persons with multiple sexual partners and children born to HCV–HIV coinfected mothers. Until recently, hepatitis C was not considered to be a major clinical problem in HIV-infected individuals. However, as a result of highly reactive antiretroviral therapy (HAART), survival has increased in HIV-infected patients and the contribution of HCV to morbidity and mortality is likely to become significant. Evidence also indicates that the course of HCV infection is more severe in HIV-positive patients, although the reasons for this are not clear. This chapter focuses on the interaction between HCV and HIV, defining the prevalence of the problem, the role of HIV infection in the natural course of HCV infection, and current treatment options available for coinfected individuals.

EPIDEMIOLOGY OF HCV AND HIV COINFECTION

Prevalence of HCV Infection

The prevalence of antibody to HCV (anti-HCV) in the general United States population is estimated to be 1.8% of whom 74% have detectable HCV RNA in serum. [1,2] These findings indicate that approximately 2.7 million Americans have chronic HCV infection. A similar prevalence of anti-HCV reactivity is found in most other countries of the world, although enclaves of high prevalence exist, e.g., in Zaire and Egypt, where rates of up to 40% are reported. (3) Worldwide, an estimated 170 million persons are infected with HCV. (2) The groups at greatest risk for hepatitis C are persons with direct percutaneous exposures such as recipients of blood or blood products and injection drug users who share contaminated needles. Thus, hemophiliacs who received factor concentrates prepared before 1986, which were not heat inactivated, have a prevalence of anti-HCV exceeding 90%. (4–6) Similar high rates are found among injection drug users. (7,8) Transmission of hepatitis C by sexual contact appears to be rare, and rates of anti-HCV among men who have sex with men have ranged from 2 to 12%. (9)

Prevalence of HIV Infection

The prevalence of anti-HIV in the general U.S. population is probably less than 1%. Anti-HIV is detected in up to 0.8% of Job Corps entrants and 0.1% of applicants for military service. (10) These rates are considerably lower than those for anti-HCV, probably because HCV has been present in the population for longer and there is more widespread awareness of HIV and modes of its spread. High-risk groups for HIV infection include recipients of blood and blood products (prepared before routine screening tests were introduced), injection drug users, children born to HIV-infected mothers, and persons with multiple sexual partners. Prevalence rates of anti-HIV among injection drug users vary widely. In a survey of 6429 persons entering drug treatment centers in the United States during 1997, the median prevalence rate was 14.8%, which may be an underestimate because only injection drug users enrolling in treatment programs were studied. (10) HIV infection is more likely than HCV to be spread by sexual contact. Among 53,656 individuals attending sexually transmitted diseases (STD) clinics in the United States, the median prevalence of anti-HIV was 3.9% and was highest among men who have sex with men (19.3%). (10) Heterosexual transmission probably accounts for a large proportion of persons infected by HIV in other parts of the world. There are an estimated 30 million HIV-infected individuals worldwide. (10)

Prevalence of HIV-HCV Coinfection

Because HCV and HIV share similar routes of transmission, it is not surprising to find coinfection in high-risk individuals. The prevalence of coinfection varies according to the risk. Groups at highest risk for coinfection include individuals who receive multiple transfusions with blood or blood products, such as persons with hemophilia, as well as injection drug users and persons who have multiple sexual partners.

Hemophilia

The highest rates of HCV-HIV coinfection are reported in persons with hemophilia, the majority of whom acquired HCV from the infusion of contaminated clotting factor concentrates during the 1970s and early 1980s. Because clotting factor concentrates were prepared from pools of donor plasma, most recipients were infected at time of first exposure. The prevalence of HCV in individuals who received nonheat-treated factor concentrates during the last two decades ranges from 60 to 95%. This figure is similar to the prevalence of HIV infection in individuals transfused with clotting factor concentrates before 1985, prior to the implementation of donor screening and viral inactivation procedures. (11) Since 1985, the prevalence of HIV infection in persons with hemophilia has fallen, but the prevalence of anti-HCV has remained elevated, probably because reliable screening tests for anti-HCV were not available until mid-1992. The prevalence of anti-HCV in the populations of persons with hemophilia has been found to correlate with a history of use of clotting factor concentrates, older age, anti-HBc seropositivity, and anti-HIV seropositivity. (5) The frequency of anti-HIV in treated persons with hemophilia varies widely from 25 to 60% and may be reflective of different usage of concentrates or a low prevalence of HIV in the donor population.

In populations of persons with hemophilia, almost all anti-HIV-positive patients are also anti-HCV positive. This association suggests that both infections were acquired by the same route. Since the introduction of screening for anti-HIV and anti-HCV, together with viral inactivation procedures and the availability of recombinant clotting factor, the rates of both HIV and HCV infection are reported to be declining in persons with hemophilia.

Injection Drug Use

The prevalence of anti-HCV in injection drug users is similar to the prevalence in persons with hemophilia. Among drug users, the prevalence of anti-HCV is generally higher than that of anti-HIV, which suggests that HCV is transmitted more easily than HIV or that reinfection occurs because of a lack of protective antibodies. Van Ameijden et al. (7) tested serum from 305 male injection drug users who denied a history of having sex with men for anti-HIV, anti-HBc, and anti-HCV. Anti-HIV was detected in 31%, antibodies to hepatitis B in 68%, and anti-HCV in 65% of the drug users. Notably, 99% of HIV-positive subjects had serological evidence of HBV, HCV, or both, suggesting that HCV may be transmitted more efficiently by anti-HIV-positive than anti-HIV-negative persons or that HCV is more likely to progress to a chronic infection among HIV-positive persons. The major risk factor for the development of anti-HCV was a history of recent injection use and, for HIV, recent injection use and borrowing of injection equipment. Similar findings were reported in a cross-sectional study by Bolumar et al. (12) in which 1056 active injection drug users were tested for antibodies to HCV, HIV, and HBV. The seroprevalence of anti-HCV was 86%. Of those injection drug users with less than 1 year of addiction, 69% were HCV seropositive compared with 41% for HBV and 14% for HIV. These findings indicate that HCV infection is acquired rapidly after the initiation of injection drug use.

Sexual Transmission

HCV appears to be transmitted sexually much less efficiently than HIV. As a consequence, the prevalence of HCV–HIV coinfection in individuals whose only risk factor is sexual exposure is significantly lower than that of persons with hemophilia and injection drug users. The seroprevalence of anti-HCV was examined in a group of 61 patients followed to determine the rate of heterosexual transmission of HIV. (13) Of the 61 couples that were followed, 30 partners were at risk because of sexual contact alone, of whom 12 (40%) became infected with HIV and none with HCV. Thirty-one couples were at risk because of both injection drug use and sexual exposure, of whom 16 (52%) became infected with HIV and 25 (80%) with HCV. Thus, injection drug use appeared to be the major cause of spread among partners. In a cross-sectional study, the prevalence of serological markers for HCV, HBV, and HIV infection and syphilis was determined in 1257 persons who were attending a sexually transmitted diseases clinic and who denied injection drug use. Of these, 122 (9.7%) had anti-HCV and 44 (3.5%) had anti-HIV. (14) Thus the rate of HCV infection was high in this sexually active population, but the role of sexual transmission remained in question because of possible underreporting of injection drug use.

Eyster et al. (15) reported on the frequency of transmission of HCV and HIV in a cohort of 234 female sexual partners of 231 men with hemophilia. The prevalence of anti-HCV among partners of anti-HCV-positive men was 3% (5 of 194). In contrast, the prevalence of anti-HIV among sexual partners of anti-HIV-positive men was 13% (25 of 196). Thus, sexual spread of HIV appeared to be much more common than that of HCV. Of note, transmission of HCV to the spouse did not occur in the absence of concurrent HCV–HIV coinfection in the index patient with hemophilia. Furthermore, HIV coinfected men appeared to be five times more likely to transmit both viruses than HCV infection alone. When a single virus was transmitted to a female sexual partner by a coinfected male, it was more often HIV (18 of 164) than HCV (2 of 164). (15) Thus, sexual transmission of HCV was low but was more common in the presence of concurrent HIV infection.

Maternal–Infant Transmission

Hepatitis C can be transmitted from an HCV-infected mother to her newborn; reported rates of transmission range from 0 to 22%. (16–18) Higher rates of maternal–infant transmission are reported from mothers who are viremic and have high titers of HCV RNA. In one study, no child developed HCV infection from anti-HCV-positive mothers who were HCV RNA negative or who had HCV RNA levels below 10^5 viral copies/ml. (17)

The role of HIV coinfection in vertical transmission of HCV is controversial. HIV coinfection in the mother has been associated with higher rates of maternal–infant transmission with an overall relative risk of 3.2. (18,19) Other studies have reported that vertical transmission of HCV in HIV-positive mothers is infrequent. (20,21) Discrepancies in the reported rates may reflect differences in study size, maternal viral carriage rates, viral genotypes, differences in the rigor of follow-up of children of infected mothers, and lack of standardization of PCR testing for HCV RNA. The potential mechanism(s) by which HIV coinfection increases the risk of perinatal transmission of HCV is believed to be due to higher titers of HCV RNA among coinfected mothers. In contrast, HCV is not known to facilitate the vertical transmission of HIV, although one report has suggested that it may. (22) In summary, the rate of vertical transmission of HCV is low in the absence of HIV coinfection and high maternal levels of HCV RNA.

NATURAL HISTORY OF HEPATITIS C AMONG HIV INFECTED PATIENTS

The natural history of HCV infection in the immune-competent host is variable. Probably less than 30% of cases of acute hepatitis C are symptomatic and icteric, with the remainder being subclinical. (23) The rate of chronicity is high, approximately 75% of acutely infected individuals develop chronic infection. Most patients with chronic hepatitis C have a mild hepatitis as assessed by symptoms, aminotransferase levels, and liver histology, and progression can be slow unless other cofactors such as alcohol are present. Twenty-five percent of individuals, however, will progress to cirrhosis and end-stage liver disease within the first few decades of infection, which is reflected in the statistic that hepatitis C is now the leading indication for liver transplantation in adults in the United States. The average time of progression to cirrhosis is generally accepted to range from 20 to 40 years. (24) Factors associated with an increased rate of progression include excessive alcohol consumption, older age at acquisition of infection, elevated intrahepatic iron, male sex, and HIV coinfection.

The natural history of hepatitis C in the immune-compromised person is also not well defined. Simultaneous HIV infection is believed to alter the natural history of HCV infection. Three early studies suggested that patients with concurrent HCV and HIV infection have an increased incidence of liver failure compared to patients with HCV alone. (25–27) Martin et al. (25) reported on a series of 97 patients with non-A, non-B hepatitis, of whom three had HIV coinfection: all three coinfected patients but only 8 (9%) HIV-negative patients developed hepatic decompensation within 3 years of presentation and diagnosis. Eyster et al. (26) found that 8 (9%) of 91 persons with hemophilia and HIV–HCV coinfection developed liver failure during follow-up compared to none of 58 followed for the same period who had HCV alone (age-adjusted relative risk = 3.2; $p = 0.03$). Telfer et al. (27) reported that the relative risk of developing liver failure was 21 in hemophiliacs coinfected with HCV and HIV compared to hemophiliacs with HCV infection alone. These earlier findings were substantiated in a study by Soto et al. (28) In addition, several case reports suggest that the simultaneous acquisition of HIV and HCV may increase the rate of HCV-related liver failure. More recent work suggests that the rate of progression of fibrosis in HCV–HIV coinfected patients is higher compared to patients infected with HCV only. A group of 122 coinfected individuals were compared to 122 controls with HCV only and were matched for age, sex, alcohol consumption, age at acquisition of HCV infection, duration, and route of HCV infection. Coinfected patients had more advanced liver fibrosis (60% vs 47%, respectively) as well as more disease activity (47% vs 30%, respectively) compared to control patients. Using a model that assumes absence of fibrosis at time of infection and that progression of fibrosis is constant, the authors predicted an expected time to cirrhosis of 26 years in HIV-positive patients and 34 years in non-HIV-infected patients. In multivariate analysis, a low CD4 count , alcohol, and age at acquisition of HCV infection were associated with a higher rate of progression of liver fibrosis in coinfected individuals. (29)

A contribution of HIV coinfection to a more rapid progression of chronic hepatitis C has not been found in all studies of HCV–HIV coinfection, particularly in cross-sectional analyses. Wright et al. (8) reported on a cohort of

512 HIV-positive, predominantly noninjection drug-using, male homosexuals of whom 224 had AIDS. (8) On retrospective testing, 12% had anti-HCV. HCV coinfection did not appear to influence the survival of HIV-infected patients with or without manifestations of AIDS. All deaths were caused by infectious or malignant complications of AIDS; only one patient had evidence of liver disease and this patient was anti-HCV negative. (8) Similarly, Quan et al. (30) reported on a group of 226 patients with HIV infection who were predominantly injection drug users and in whom the prevalence of anti-HCV was 8%. Despite the coexistence of HIV and HCV infection, liver disease appeared to be mild and HCV infection did not appear to increase the severity of HIV infection.

Differences in the outcome of liver disease among HIV–HCV coinfected patients in these various studies have not been well explained. Possible explanations include referral bias (whether to an infectious disease or a hepatology clinic) in the cohorts, differences in the average duration of HCV infection, or differences in the timing of the two infections, whether HIV or HCV infection occurred first. Thus, the frequency of significant liver disease among HIV-positive persons with hemophilia as opposed to injection drug users may relate to the fact that persons with hemophilia probably acquired hepatitis C early in childhood, whereas injection drug users are exposed later in life as adults. Accordingly, when first in contact with HIV, injection drug users probably had hepatitis C for a shorter period than persons with hemophilia. Clearly, these factors may interact and may actually reflect other known prognostic features, such as age, gender, alcohol use, other drug toxicities, and opportunistic infections. (31)

Prior to the availability of nucleoside analogues and protease inhibitor therapy, opportunistic infections may have been the major cause of liver disease in HIV–infected persons. In the current HIV treatment era, patients may live longer and the consequences of HCV infection become more obvious. In addition, the toxicity of drugs used to treat HIV infection may now play a role in causing morbidity and mortality from liver disease. Fulminant hepatic failure in patients with HIV infection is more likely to be due to hepatitis A or B or drug toxicity than to hepatitis C, the acute phase of which does not appear to be worsened by HIV infection. However, HIV infection may cause a greater proportion of patients with acute HCV infection to develop chronic infection. Thus, HIV coinfection appears to worsen the prognosis of chronic hepatitis C and leads to more rapid development of cirrhosis and end-stage liver disease. The role of HIV infection in promoting hepatocellular carcinoma has not been evaluated but deserves prospective evaluation.

PATHOGENESIS

The mechanism(s) by which HIV coinfection hastens the development of cirrhosis and end-stage liver disease due to HCV is not known. Indeed, the pathogenesis of HCV infection even in immune competent individuals is not well understood, and evidence supports both a cytopathic mechanism and an immune-mediated mechanism of liver injury. The findings of injured and degenerating hepatocytes without adjacent inflammation in liver biopsies, higher HCV RNA levels in patients with more severe disease, and a parallel fall in aminotransferase levels with clearance of HCV RNA during treatment all support a cytopathic mechanism. However, there is also evidence that links a humoral and a cellular immune response to hepatocellular injury in HCV infection. Lymphoid aggregates in portal areas that contain activated B cells suggest an active local humoral response. The demonstration of rigorous T-cell proliferative responses to HCV antigens in individuals who resolve acute infection and the isolation of HCV-specific cytotoxic $CD8^+$ T cells from liver and/or peripheral blood in a significant proportion of patients with chronic HCV infection suggest that cellular responses are important in the pathogenesis of liver injury in hepatitis C (see Chapter 8).

The pathogenesis of liver cell injury may be more complex in persons with HIV–HCV coinfection. Progressive immunodeficiency leads to higher levels of HCV viremia, which may be the cause of the more severe and rapidly progressive disease. Eyster et al. (32) measured HCV RNA levels in serial serum samples from 17 HCV–HIV coinfected and from 17 HCV-positive but HIV-negative patients with hemophilia who were carefully matched for age. Before HIV seroconversion, serum levels of HCV RNA were similar in the two groups. During the first 2 years after development of anti-HIV, mean HCV RNA levels increased 10-fold, from 0.28 to 2.84 million copies/ml. During subsequent follow-up, HCV RNA levels increased approximately 3-fold in subjects who remained HIV negative, compared to 58-fold among those who were HIV positive. The overall rate of increase in HCV RNA levels was 8-fold faster in HIV-positive than HIV-negative patients with hemophilia. Thus, immunosuppression appeared to cause progressive elevations in serum HCV RNA levels.

Consequently, levels of HCV RNA in HIV-infected persons average 10 to 100 times (1–2 logs) higher than levels in non-HIV coinfected individuals. At these levels, HCV may be directly cytopathic. Nevertheless, it has been difficult to attribute worsening of liver disease directly to changes in levels of viral replication. In most cross-sectional studies, little or no correlation is found between viral titers and severity or liver disease. In a retrospective, cross-sectional study by Ghany et al., (33) 100 patients with hemophilia were tested for anti-HCV and anti-HIV, and levels of HCV RNA were carefully quantitated by the branched DNA signal amplification method in all anti-HCV-positive patients. A total of 79% had anti-HCV and 42% had anti-HIV. There was no significant difference in HCV RNA levels between anti-HIV-positive and -negative patients with hepatitis C, even though HCV RNA levels were significantly higher in those anti-HIV-positive patients with CD4 counts below $200/mm^3$. Although there was an inverse correlation between HCV RNA levels and CD4 counts, there was no association of HCV RNA and ALT levels. (33) Results of liver biopsies were not reported as this cohort had hemophilia. Similar results showing a lack of correlation of aminotransferase and HCV RNA levels have been reported by two other groups of investigators. (34,35) Other mechanisms of hepatic injury may be important in HIV-infected patients with hepatitis C, such as altered cytokine profiles leading to an increase in proinflammatory signals and promotion of fibrogenesis. Furthermore, the role of drug toxicity associated with HAART treatment of HIV, as well as opportunistic infections in the worsening of liver disease, needs to be evaluated further.

DIAGNOSIS

The diagnosis of chronic hepatitis C in HIV-infected patients can be problematic. Diagnosis of HCV infection is usually made by the detection of anti-HCV by an enzyme immunoassay (either EIA-2 or EIA-3) and a positive result confirmed by supplemental testing for anti-HCV by recombinant immunoblot assay (RIBA-2 or RIBA-3) or testing for HCV RNA in serum by PCR. The EIA-2 and RIBA-2 assays employ four recombinant antigens, whereas the EIA-3 and RIBA-3 systems employ five. Patients with immune deficiencies may lose antibody to one or several HCV antigens, leading to a false-negative test. Thus, testing for anti-HCV may fail to detect infection in some individuals and underestimate the prevalence of HCV infection in HIV-positive cohorts. Lok et al. (36) have shown a decrease in antibody titer to the C-100 and C-33-c antigens of HCV in immunosuppressed kidney and bone marrow transplant recipients. Thus, if anti-HCV testing is negative, direct testing for HCV RNA by PCR is needed to reliably exclude hepatitis C as a cause of liver injury in the HIV-positive patient.

False-negative results may be less of a problem with third-generation assays for anti-HCV (EIA-3 and RIBA-3). Samples that react with only one antigen in the immunoblot assay are called "indeterminate" and require further testing. Indeterminate results appear to be more common among anti-HIV-positive than -negative patients. Marcellin and co-workers (37) evaluated indeterminate RIBA-2 reactions in both HIV-positive and -negative cohorts. Indeterminate results were more common in HIV-positive (38 of 167; 23%) than HIV-negative (48 of 318; 15%) subjects ($p < 0.05$). Most HIV-infected individuals with an indeterminate RIBA test were viremic when tested by PCR, whereas HIV-negative persons with an indeterminate RIBA pattern were usually not HCV RNA positive. (37)

Genotypes of HCV in HIV-Infected Patients

The genotype distribution of HCV has been evaluated in several cohorts of HIV–HCV coinfected patients. In a study from the United States, Eyster et al. (38) found that HCV genotype 3a was the most prevalent, present in 41% in their cohort, followed by genotypes 1a (31%) and 1b (13%). Over a 10-year period of follow-up, the predominant HCV genotype appeared to change in 58% of subjects and occurred more commonly among HIV-positive than -negative subjects. No consistent pattern of change in genotype was detected. Interestingly, genotypes changed in one-third of patients during the period that they were receiving virus-inactivated clotting factor concentrates, arguing against reinfection as a cause for the change in genotype. Nucleotide sequencing confirmed the change in genotype in two patients. Persons with hemophilia have multiple exposures to HCV and are therefore likely to be infected with multiple strains and genotypes of virus. The patterns of apparent change in genotype are complex and probably merely reflect changes in the predominant genotypes from period to period rather than actual episodes of reinfection or mutation of HCV strains. The clinical significance of the predominant genotype among persons with hemophilia has not been clearly defined. It is well known that patients with genotypes 2 and 3 are more likely to respond to antiviral therapy. Clinical differences in outcome of disease based on genotype has not been documented consistently. Nevertheless, at least one study has reported an association between HCV genotype 1b and the progression to AIDS and death in a cohort of men with hemophilia. (39) The association of progression of HIV with genotype 1b was largely independent of age at seroconversion and changes in CD4 cell count. It is difficult to explain these associations and they need to be confirmed in other populations.

HISTOLOGY

There is little published data on liver histology in HIV–HCV coinfected individuals. In small studies, the histological features of hepatitis C among HIV-infected persons have been similar to those reported in chronic hepatitis C. In larger studies, more hepatic inflammation and a greater degree of fibrosis have been reported in dually infected persons, but surprisingly, no patients had cirrhosis. (40,41) In an Italian study of liver biopsy histology from 160 patients with hepatitis C, of whom 68 also had HIV infection, there were no differences in inflammatory scores between HIV-positive and -negative patients. (42) In contrast, HIV-positive patients with CD4 counts less than 400 had a significantly lower grade of portal inflammation and piecemeal necrosis. In a liver biopsy and autopsy series, Bierhoff et al. (43) described a significantly higher rate of granulocytic cholangitis and centrilobular fibrosis in HIV-positive than in -negative patients with hepatitis C. These are features not commonly described in patients with typical hepatitis C without HIV coinfection. In that study, the rate of cirrhosis in HIV–HCV coinfected and the HCV only infected patients undergoing liver biopsy was the same (18%). However, in the autopsy series, the rate of cirrhosis reported was considerably higher in coinfected patients. No cases of cirrhosis were seen in HIV-positive patients without HCV infection. (43) Thus, histological features of chronic hepatitis appear similar in HIV-positive and -negative patients.

TREATMENT OF HEPATITIS C IN HIV INFECTED PATIENTS

The currently recommended therapy of chronic hepatitis C is a 24- to 48-week course of the combination of interferon-α (3 million units thrice weekly) and ribavirin (1000 or 1200 mg daily). This regimen has been shown to result in a long-term loss of HCV RNA and improvements in the underlying liver disease in 35 to 45% of patients. (44,45) The addition of ribavirin increases the sustained response rate significantly, by at least threefold. Interferon-α alone yields a long-term response rate of only 5–10% when given for 24 weeks and 15–20% when given for 1 year.

Studies of interferon-α and combination therapy with ribavirin have largely been performed in patients with typical chronic hepatitis C and without immune deficiencies or HIV infection. The role of these therapies in patients with HIV is currently unclear. Several small studies of interferon monotherapy have been carried out in HIV coinfected patients, but there have been no studies of combination therapy in this group (see Table I). Because of the increasing survival rate among persons with HIV infection and the increasing evidence that hepatitis C can be progressive in coinfected patients, therapies for the HCV infection are needed.

Most studies of antiviral therapy for HIV–HCV coinfected patients have been done in persons who acquired the infections through injection drug use rather than clotting factor concentrations. Part of this is due to the difficulty in performing liver biopsies in patients with hemophilia, making the evaluation of long-term responses to treatment difficult.

In a multicenter, open labeled study, Soriano and colleagues (41) from Spain treated 119 patients with chronic hepatitis C with interferon-α, 90 of whom had HIV–HCV coinfection. Interferon was given in a dose of 5 million units three times weekly for 3 months, and those patients who responded during this period were continued on a reduced dose of 3 million units three times weekly for 9 more months, a total treatment period of 1 year. The end-of-treatment combined biochemical and virological response was the same in coinfected patients as in HIV-negative patients with hepatitis C, occurring in 26 (29%) HIV-positive patients as compared to 10 (34%) HIV-negative patients ($p = 0.67$). However, 12 months after stopping therapy, the relapse rate was higher (31%) in the coinfected group compared to the group with hepatitis C alone (12.5%). A retrospective, multivariate analysis of predictive factors for an end-of-treatment response revealed that a CD4 count of greater than $500 \times 10^6/\text{mm}^3$ and a baseline HCV RNA level below 10^7 viral copies/ml were most closely associated with a response. The drop out rate for HIV coinfected patients was high (11%), mostly due to lack of follow-up. During interferon therapy, $CD4^+$ lymphocyte counts fell markedly in 10 patients and remained low in 3 even after stopping interferon. One patient developed an AIDS-defining event. Thus, this study indicated that patients with HCV–HIV coinfection can respond to standard therapy with interferon-α but that the long-term sustained response rate is lower (18%) compared to patients without HIV infection (31%).

In a second study by Boldorini et al. (40) from Italy, 24 injection drug users with hepatitis C were treated with interferon-α. Twelve patients were HIV positive and 12 were negative. Interferon-α was given three times weekly in a dose of 6 million units for 6 months followed by a dose of 3 million units for an additional 6 months. A sustained response was defined by a normal serum ALT level (biochemical response) and absence of HCV RNA (virological response) 6 months or more after stopping therapy. Sustained biochemical responses occurred in 4 (33%) HIV coinfected patients compared to 6 (50%) HIV-negative patients. Importantly, only 1 of the coinfected patients (8%) had a sustained virological response compared to 6 (50%) of the HIV-negative patients with hepa-

███ **TABLE I** **Analysis of Treatment Trials in HCV and HIV Coinfected Patients**

Reference	Group	No. treated HIV/HCV	Total IFN dose (MU)[b]	End of treatment response (%)[c]	Sustained response (%)[d]
Soriano et al. (41)	IDU[a]	80	504	33	30
Marcellin et al. (48)	IDU	20	216	30	15
Mauss et al. (46)	Not reported	17	360–780	47	62
Pol et al. (49)	IDU	16	216	19	0
Marriot et al. (47)	IDU	14	1404	33	44
Boldorini et al. (40)	IDU	12	648	Not reported	8
Areias et al. (50)	IDU	10	216	40	20

[a] Injection drug use.
[b] Million units.
[c] Normal ALT and HCV RNA negative by PCR at end of treatment.
[d] Normal ALT and HCV RNA negative by PCR 6 months following end of treatment.

titis C. Histological features at follow-up confirmed the poor rate of response among HIV coinfected patients. Average histological activity index scores did not change in HIV-positive patients, but decreased significantly (in piecemeal and parenchymal necrosis scores) in the HIV-negative group. No information was given about toxicity or CD4 counts during and after interferon therapy.

There have been two other small studies of interferon therapy in HIV coinfected patients, both using interferon for 12 months. (46,47) The sustained virological response in both studies was 29%, which is similar to what is found in HIV-negative patients with hepatitis C. Neither report mentioned significant toxicity of interferon or problems with CD4 counts or progression of HIV infection.

There have been no reports on the use of the combination of interferon-α with ribavirin among HIV-positive patients. One difficulty with this therapy is that ribavirin causes a dose-related hemolysis, which is exacerbated by the myelosuppressive actions of interferon. On average, hemoglobin levels decrease by 2–4 g/dl, generally starting after 2 weeks and reaching a nadir at 3 to 6 weeks of therapy. In some patients, the decrease in hemoglobin is marked and leads to symptomatic anemia, which is a major reason for dose modification and early discontinuation of therapy (especially in women). Among HIV-infected patients this may be particularly problematic because of the use of HAART and other agents that cause hemolysis or bone marrow suppression. Furthermore, the addition of two other agents for a 24- to 48-week period is a considerable challenge in patients who are already taking three to five antiretroviral medications. Nevertheless, the favorable results with combination therapy and the long-term loss of HCV RNA and remission of disease that can occur with interferon therapy argue for use of combination therapy in patients with HIV coinfection. The major issue is how to regulate other antivirals during the course of interferon and ribavirin therapy. Protease inhibitors for HIV have been reported to lead to a transient increase in HCV RNA and ALT levels during treatment, but no cases of hepatic failure have been reported. (51)

CONCLUSION

HCV and HIV share similar modes of transmission and it is not surprising that certain groups have a high rate of HIV-HCV co-infection. These groups are injection drug users and recipients of blood or blood products made before the introduction of routine screening for HCV and HIV and the use of viral-inactivation procedures. Among injection drug users, 65% to 90% have anti-HCV, 0% to 38% have anti-HIV, and up to one-third have both antibodies. Among persons with hemophilia, born before 1986, 70% to 90% have anti-HCV, 40% to 45% have anti-HIV and a large proportion have both. Hepatitis C appears to be somewhat more severe among HIV co-infected persons than in persons with hepatitis C alone and progression of disease to cirrhosis can occur more rapidly. Therapy of hepatitis C in HIV infected patients is difficult, because these patients frequently have other major medical problems and are taking other medications that make combination treatment of interferon-α and ribavirin difficult. Nevertheless, several small studies have suggested that patients with HIV infection and adequate CD4 counts respond to therapy of hepatitis C at a rate that is similar to that among patients without HIV infection. Studies of the combination of interferon-α and ribavirin in HIV infected patients are needed, particularly focused upon management of the multiple antiviral agents during the period of therapy.

REFERENCES

1. Alter M J, Kruszon-Moran D, Nainan O V, et al. The prevalence of hepatitis C virus infection in the United States 1988 through 1994. N Engl J Med 1999;341:556–62.
2. Alter M J. Epidemiology of hepatitis C. Hepatology 1997;26(Suppl 1):62S–5S.
3. Abdel-Wahab M F, Zakaria S, Kamel M, et al. High seroprevalence of hepatitis C infection among risk groups in Egypt. Am J Trop Med Hyg 1994;51:563–7.
4. Brettler D B, Alter H J, Dienstag J L, Forsberg A D, Levine P H. Prevalence of hepatitis C virus antibody in a cohort of hemophilia patients. Blood 1990;76:254–6.
5. Makris M, Preston F E, Triger D R, et al. Hepatitis C antibody and chronic liver disease in haemophilia. Lancet 1990;335:1117–9.
6. Rumi M G, Colombo M, Gringeri A, Mannucci P M. High prevalence of antibody to hepatitis C virus in multitransfused hemophiliacs with normal transaminase levels. Ann Intern Med 1990;112:379–80.
7. Van Ameijden E J, Van den Hoek J A, Mientjes G H, Coutinho R A. A longitudinal study on the incidence and transmission patterns of HIV, HBV and HCV infection among drug users in Amsterdam. Eur J Epidemiol 1993;9:255–62.
8. Wright T L, Hollander H, Pu X, et al. Hepatitis C in HIV-infected patients with and without AIDS: prevalence and relationship to patient survival. Hepatology 1994;20:1152–5.
9. Dienstag J L. Sexual and perinatal transmission of hepatitis C. Hepatology 1997;26(Suppl 1): 66S–70S.
10. Centers for Disease Control and Prevention. National HIV prevalence surveys, 1997 summary. Atlanta, GA: Centers for Disease Control and Prevention, 1998:1–25.
11. Goedert J J, Kessler C M, Aledort L M, et al. A prospective study of human immunodeficiency virus type 1 infection and the development of AIDS in subjects with hemophilia. N Engl J Med 1989;321:1141–8.
12. Bolumar F, Hernandez-Aguado I, Ferrer L, Ruiz I, Avino M J, Rebagliato M. Prevalence of antibodies to hepatitis C in a population of intravenous drug users in Valencia, Spain, 1990–1992. Int J Epidemiol 199;25:204–9.

13. Wyld R, Robertson J R, Brettle R P, Mellor J, Prescott L, Simmonds P. Absence of hepatitis C virus transmission but frequent transmission of HIV-1 from sexual contact with doubly-infected individuals. J Infect 1997;35:163–6.

14. Thomas D L, Cannon R O, Shapiro C N, Hook E W 3rd, Alter M J, Quinn T C. Hepatitis C, hepatitis B, and human immunodeficiency virus infections among non-intravenous drug-using patients attending clinics for sexually transmitted diseases. J Infect Dis 1994;169:990–5.

15. Eyster M E, Alter H J, Aledort L M, Quan S, Hatzakis A, Goedert J J. Heterosexual co-transmission of hepatitis C virus (HCV) and human immunodeficiency virus (HIV). Ann Intern Med 1991;115:764–8.

16. Ohto H, Terazawa S, Sasaki N, et al. Transmission of hepatitis C virus from mothers to infants. The Vertical Transmission of Hepatitis C Virus Collaborative Study Group. N Engl J Med. 1994;330:744–50.

17. Giacchino R, Picciotto A, Tasso L, Timitilli A, Sinelli N. Vertical transmission of hepatitis C. Lancet 1995;345:1122–3.

18. Thomas D L, Villano S A, Riester K A, et al. Perinatal transmission of hepatitis C virus from human immunodeficiency virus type 1-infected mothers. Women and Infants Transmission Study. J Infect Dis 1998;177:1480–8.

19. Zanetti A R, Tanzi E, Paccagnini S, et al. Mother-to-infant transmission of hepatitis C virus. Lombardy Study Group on Vertical HCV Transmission. Lancet 1995;345:289–91.

20. Manzini P, Saracco G, Cerchier A, et al. Human immunodeficiency virus infection as risk factor for mother-to- child hepatitis C virus transmission; persistence of anti-hepatitis C virus in children is associated with the mother's anti-hepatitis C virus immunoblotting pattern. Hepatology 1995;21:328–32.

21. Lam J P, McOmish F, Burns S M, Yap P L, Mok J Y, Simmonds P. Infrequent vertical transmission of hepatitis C virus. J Infect Dis 1993;167:572–6.

22. Hershow R C, Riester K A, Lew J, et al. Increased vertical transmission of human immunodeficiency virus from hepatitis C virus-coinfected mothers. Women and Infants Transmission Study. J Infect Dis 1997;176:414–20.

23. Hoofnagle J H. Hepatitis C: the clinical spectrum of disease. Hepatology 1997;26(Suppl 1):15S–20S.

24. Seeff L B. Natural history of hepatitis C. Hepatology 1997;26(Suppl 1):21S–8S.

25. Martin P, Di Bisceglie A M, Kassianides C, Lisker-Melman M, Hoofnagle J H. Rapidly progressive non-A, non-B hepatitis in patients with human immunodeficiency virus infection. Gastroenterology 1989;97:1559–61.

26. Eyster M E, Diamondstone L S, Lien J M, Ehmann W C, Quan S, Goedert J J. Natural history of hepatitis C virus infection in multitransfused hemophiliacs: effect of coinfection with human immunodeficiency virus. The Multicenter Hemophilia Cohort Study. J Acquired Immune Defic Syndr 1993;6:602–10.

27. Telfer P, Sabin C, Devereux H, Scott F, Dusheiko G, Lee C. The progression of HCV-associated liver disease in a cohort of haemophilic patients. Br J Haematol 1994;87:555–61.

28. Soto B, Sanchez-Quijano A, Rodrigo L, et al. Human immunodeficiency virus infection modifies the natural history of chronic parenterally-acquired hepatitis C with an unusually rapid progression to cirrhosis. J Hepatol 1997;26:1–5.

29. Benhamou, Y, Bochet M, Di Martino V, et al. Liver fibrosis progression in human immunodeficiency virus and hepatitis C virus coinfected patients. Hepatology 1999;30:1054–58.

30. Quan C M, Krajden M, Grigoriew G A, Salit I E. Hepatitis C virus infection in patients infected with the human immunodeficiency virus. Clin Infect Dis 1993;17:117–9.

31. Pol S, Lamorthe B, Thi N T, et al. Retrospective analysis of the impact of HIV infection and alcohol use on chronic hepatitis C in a large cohort of drug users. J Hepatol 1998;28:945–50.

32. Eyster M E, Fried M W, Di Bisceglie A M, Goedert J J. Increasing hepatitis C virus RNA levels in hemophiliacs: relationship to human immunodeficiency virus infection and liver disease. Multicenter Hemophilia Cohort Study. Blood 1994;84:1020–3.

33. Ghany M G, Leissinger C, Lagier R, Sanchez-Pescador R, Lok A S. Effect of human immunodeficiency virus infection on hepatitis C virus infection in hemophiliacs. Dig Dis Sci 1996;41:1265–72.

34. Beld M, Penning M, Lukashov V, et al. Evidence that both HIV and HIV-induced immunodeficiency enhance HCV replication among HCV seroconverters. Virology 1998;244:504–12.

35. Thomas D L, Shih J W, Alter H J, et al. Effect of human immunodeficiency virus on hepatitis C virus infection among injecting drug users. J Infect Dis 1996;174:690–5.

36. Lok A S, Chien D, Choo Q L, et al. Antibody response to core, envelope and nonstructural hepatitis C virus antigens: comparison of immunocompetent and immunosuppressed patients. Hepatology 1993;18:497–502.

37. Marcellin P, Martinot-Peignoux M, Elias A, et al. Hepatitis C virus (HCV) viremia in human immunodeficiency virus- seronegative and -seropositive patients with indeterminate HCV recombinant immunoblot assay. J Infect Dis 1994;170:433–5.

38. Eyster M E, Sherman K E, Goedert J J, Katsoulidou A, Hatzakis A. Prevalence and changes in hepatitis C virus genotypes among multitransfused persons with hemophilia. The Multicenter Hemophilia Cohort Study. J Infect Dis 1999;179:1062–9.

39. Sabin C A, Telfer P, Phillips A N, Bhagani S, Lee C A. The association between hepatitis C virus genotype and human immunodeficiency virus disease progression in a cohort of hemophilic men. J Infect Dis 1997;175:164–8.

40. Boldorini R, Vigano P, Monga G, et al. Hepatic histology of patients with HIV infection and chronic hepatitis C treated with interferon. J Clin Pathol 1997;50:735–40.

41. Soriano V, Garcia-Samaniego J, Bravo R, et al. Interferon alpha for the treatment of chronic hepatitis C in patients infected with human immunodeficiency virus. Hepatitis-HIV Spanish Study Group. Clin Infect Dis 1996;23:585–91.

42. Guido M, Rugge M, Fattovich G, et al. Human immunodeficiency virus infection and hepatitis C pathology. Liver 1994;14:314–9.

43. Bierhoff E, Fischer H P, Willsch E, et al. Liver histopathology in patients with concurrent chronic hepatitis C and HIV infection. Virchows Arch 1997;430:271–7.

44. McHutchison J G, Gordon S C, Schiff E R, et al. Interferon alfa-2b alone or in combination with ribavirin as initial treatment for chronic hepatitis C. N Engl J Med 1998;339:1485–92.

45. Poynard T, Marcellin P, Lee S S, et al. Randomized trial of interferon alpha 2b plus ribavirin for 48 weeks or for 24 weeks versus interferon alpha2b plus placebo for 48 weeks for treatment of chronic infection with hepatitis C virus. International Hepatitis Interventional Therapy Group (IHIT). Lancet 1998;352:1426–32.

46. Mauss S, Klinker H, Ulmer A, et al. Response to treatment of chronic hepatitis C with interferon alpha in patients infected with HIV-1 is associated with higher CD4+ cell count. Infection 1998;26:16–9.

47. Marriott E, Navas S, del Romero J, et al. Treatment with recombinant alpha-interferon of chronic hepatitis C in anti-HIV-positive patients. J Med Virol 1993;40:107–11.

48. Marcellin P, Boyer N, Arejas J, Erlinger S, Benhamou J P. Comparison of efficacy of alpha interferon in former intravenous drug addicts with chronic hepatitis C with or without HIV infection. Gastroenterology 1994;106:A938.

49. Pol S, Trinh Thi N, Thiers V, et al. Chronic hepatitis C of drug users: influence of HIV infection. Hepatology 1995;22:340A.

50. Areias J, Pedroto I, Barrias S, Maros P, Freitas T, Saraiva A M. Pilot study of interferon alpha 2b treatment of chronic hepatitis C in patients coinfected with the human immunodeficiency virus. Hepatology 1994;20:162A.

51. Rutschmann O T, Negro F, Hirschel B, Hadengue A, Anwar D, Perrin L H. Impact of treatment with human immunodeficiency virus (HIV) protease inhibitors on hepatitis C viremia in patients coinfected with HIV. J Infect Dis 1998;177:783–5.

17
HEPATITIS C AND RENAL DISEASE

STEVEN ZACKS AND MICHAEL W. FRIED
Division of Digestive Diseases and Nutrition
University of North Carolina, School of Medicine
Chapel Hill, North Carolina

INTRODUCTION

Hepatitis C has a special relationship to renal disease. Hepatitis C virus (HCV) infection is more common in patients with kidney disease than in the general population and chronic hepatitis C is an important cause of morbidity and mortality of patients with renal disease, on chronic dialysis and after renal transplantation. In addition, hepatitis C is a cause of kidney disease (see Chapter 15). The common occurrence of hepatitis C in patients with kidney disease is largely due to the frequent use of blood and blood products in persons with end-stage kidney disease and to the multiple invasive medical procedures to which these patients are exposed. Hepatitis C is more difficult to diagnose as well as to manage in patients with kidney disease, largely because of effects of renal disease and its therapy on general health, the immune system, and bone marrow. Unfortunately, there have been few studies of the natural history and therapy of hepatitis C in kidney disease patients, which makes conclusions regarding hepatitis C in this population difficult.

This chapter reviews the prevalence and incidence of HCV infection, the clinical features and natural history of hepatitis C, and recommendations for management and therapy in patients with renal disease, patients on chronic dialysis, and patients undergoing renal transplantation.

EPIDEMIOLOGY OF HEPATITIS C IN KIDNEY DISEASE PATIENTS

Prevalence of Hepatitis C

As soon as serological tests for antibody to HCV (anti-HCV) became available in the early 1990s, seroepidemiological studies of hepatitis C in renal disease patients were initiated. These studies demonstrated a wide range in prevalence of anti-HCV in hemodialysis patients, ranging from as low as 5% to as high as 50%. (1) The reported prevalence varied widely between countries and between dialysis centers within countries (Table I). (2–14) Some of the variation in prevalence was due to the sensitivity and specificity of the different generations of enzyme immunoassay (EIA) used. Thus, second-generation EIAs identified a higher rate of anti-HCV among dialysis and renal failure patients than first-generation

TABLE I   **Prevalence of Anti-HCV in Dialysis Patients**

Reference	Prevalence of anti-HCV by EIA2[a] % (total n)	Detectable HCV RNA among EIA2-positive patients (%)
Hemodialysis		
Chauveau et al. (France) (2)	47 (110)	83
Chan et al. (Hong Kong) (3)	22 (51)	73
Kuhns et al. (USA) (4)	25 (63)	75
Fabrizi et al. (Italy) (5)	48 (104)	46
Golan et al. (Israel) (6)	30 (76)	N/A
Dussol et al. (France) (7)	25 (923)	N/A
Huraib et al. (Saudi Arabia) (8)	68 (1147)	N/A
Elzouki et al. (Libya) (9)	21 (153)	N/A
Todorov et al. (Bulgaria) (10)	66 (79)	N/A
Al-Wakeel et al. (Saudi Arabia) (11)	28 (65)	N/A
Peritoneal dialysis		
Golan et al. (Israel) (6)	7 (44)	N/A
Ng et al. (Taiwan) (12)	30 (101)[b]	N/A
Gladziwa et al. (Germany) (13)	5 (333)	N/A
Dussol et al. (France) (7)	8 (61)	N/A
Lee et al. (Singapore) (14)	2 (155)	N/A
Al-Wakeel et al. (Saudi Arabia) (11)	6 (18)	N/A

[a] Second-generation enzyme immunoassay.
[b] First-generation EIA.

EIAs. (15) Among 27,086 patients surveyed in the National Surveillance of Dialysis Associated Diseases in the United States conducted by the Centers for Disease Control and Prevention (CDC) in 1994, the prevalence of anti-HCV using second-generation EIA was 8.1%. (16) In subsequent years, the seroprevalence of anti-HCV increased to 10.4% and then declined to 9.3% by 1997. (17) Within the United States, there was great variability in the prevalence of HCV infection among dialysis centers with 40 or more patients, ranging from 0 to 51%.

Prevalence rates of HCV infection are also markedly different between patients on continuous ambulatory peritoneal dialysis (CAPD) and hemodialysis. In a study from Taiwan, the prevalence of anti-HCV was 5.9% in CAPD patients and 46.7% in hemodialysis patients. (18) Another study found that the prevalence of anti-HCV in hemodialysis patients was nine times the prevalence in CAPD patients and was increased proportionally to the length of time on dialysis. (19) The difference in prevalence between modes of dialysis was associated with transfusion history, although it is also possible that patients selected for the rigorous regimen of CAPD represent a different patient population than those maintained on hemodialysis. (19)

There is little information on the prevalence of HCV in patients with renal disease before starting dialysis. An Italian study reported a prevalence of anti-HCV of 13% in persons starting dialysis compared to a prevalence of 1.3% among local blood donors. These findings suggest that the high prevalence of HCV infection in patients with renal failure may be due in part to factors other than nosocomial infection during dialysis. Transfusions prior to blood product

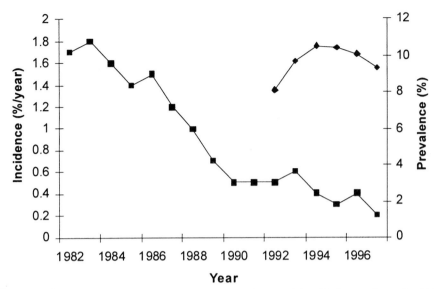

FIGURE 1 Changes in the incidence of non-A, non-B hepatitis (■) and in the prevalence of anti-HCV (♦) between 1982 and 1997. (19)

screening, hospitalizations, and procedures that occurred while renal disease developed and progressed may be the source of infection in these patients. (20) In addition, hepatitis C is a cause of glomerulonephritis, and 13% may represent that proportion of cases of renal failure in Italy due to HCV infection.

Incidence of Hepatitis C

The incidence of acute infection with hepatitis C and the prevalence of chronic HCV infection in dialysis patients in the United States appear to be leveling off or even decreasing (Fig. 1). (16,21) The lack of universal reporting and wide variation in the incidence between individual centers makes it difficult to determine trends in incidence accurately. Among the member nations of the European Dialysis and Transplantation Association, the prevalence of anti-HCV in dialysis patients fell from 21% in 1992 to 17% in 1993. The possible decline in prevalence and incidence of infection in the United States and decline in prevalence in Europe may be attributable to the reduction of transfusion-associated HCV infection as well as to the expanded use of infection control measures to prevent nosocomial transmission within dialysis units. (15)

Transmission of Hepatitis C to Dialysis Staff

The high rate of hepatitis B virus (HBV) markers among staff members in dialysis units suggests, by analogy, that hepatitis C may also be increased among dialysis staff as a result of patient-to-staff transmission and frequent handling of blood products. However, several serological surveys have found a 0% prevalence of anti-HCV in dialysis staff. (11,22–24) Two Italian studies, in contrast, reported rates of anti-HCV of 5.5 and 6.7% in staff members, rates that were considerably higher than the general population in Italy. In the CDC study of

United States dialysis centers, the prevalence of anti-HCV among staff members was 1%, and during an 18-month follow-up period, no cases of acute hepatitis C were identified. (22) These findings suggest that the occupational spread of HCV infection in dialysis units in the United States is uncommon and that dialysis staff are not at high risk of acquiring hepatitis C. To say that acquisition of hepatitis C by staff is rare, however, is not to say that it cannot or does not happen; strict application of universal blood precautions needs to stay a high priority in dialysis units.

Risk Factors for Transmission of Hepatitis C in Renal Failure Patients

Risk Factors for Transmission of Hepatitis C

Patients with chronic renal failure have several risk factors for HCV infection (Table II). Before the availability of testing for anti-HCV, transfusions of blood and blood products were probably the most common cause of spread of HCV infection. The role of transfusions in the spread of hepatitis C was shown in a cross-section study from Saudi Arabia in which 74% of patients with anti-HCV on either hemodialysis or intermittent peritoneal dialysis had a history of blood transfusion. (11) Regardless, the presence of anti-HCV in a proportion of hemodialysis patients who never received blood transfusions indicates that nosocomial infection also occur. (22) Exposure to blood or blood-contaminated equipment during hemodialysis rather than actual blood transfusions may be an important cause of transmission of hepatitis C in dialysis patients.

Studies of dialysis units for hepatitis B in the 1970s demonstrated the potential for contamination of dialysis equipment and immediate environment with blood. (23) In those studies, visual splashing of blood was observed. Furthermore, the hepatitis B surface antigen was found on hemodialysis equipment. These findings suggest by analogy that hemodialysis machines may become contaminated with HCV. (24) Because the duration of hemodialysis is a clear risk factor for acquisition of anti-HCV, contamination of dialysis equipment may account for the high rate of HCV infection in some dialysis units, estimated to be as high as 10% per year. (25) Fortunately, increased attention to the use of universal precautions has led to a reduction in the incidence of HCV infection in patients on hemodialysis. (26)

Hemodialysis versus CAPD

The method of dialysis is also a risk factor for the acquisition of chronic hepatitis C. There has been a consistently lower prevalence of HCV infection found among CAPD compared to hemodialysis patients. In a study from Singapore, the prevalence of anti-HCV was 6.5% among 155 CAPD patients, com-

TABLE II   Factors Associated with HCV Infection in Dialysis Patients

Transfusion
Nosocomial (patient to patient)
Method of dialysis (hemodialysis as opposed to CAPD)
Previous history of injection drug use

pared to 28% among hemodialysis patients in the same center. In addition, the majority of anti-HCV positive CAPD patients (7 of the 10) had a history of transient hemodialysis exposure. In that study, duration of dialysis and history of transfusion were not associated with the presence of anti-HCV.

There are several reasons why hepatitis C may be less common in patients receiving CAPD than hemodialysis. The lower blood transfusion requirement of CAPD patients, the absence of extracorporeal circulation of blood, and the performance of CAPD in isolation from other patients probably reduce the risk of nosocomial transmission. Additional evidence that isolation reduces transmission comes from studies demonstrating that home hemodialysis patients have a lower prevalence of anti-HCV than patients receiving hemodialysis at specialized centers. (27–29) Hemodialysis centers with a high prevalence of HCV infection also have a high incidence of infection. Furthermore, patients receiving hemodialysis at the same center tend to be infected with the same HCV genotypes, (26) providing further support that routine dialysis techniques may contribute to the acquisition of this disease.

Mode and Vehicle of Transmission of Hepatitis C in Dialysis Patients

The risk of HCV transmission in hemodialysis patients may vary by the type and size of the inoculum during exposure, the concentration of the virus in the inoculum, and the route of transmission. Considering the risk factors for HCV infection, patient-to-patient transmission of HCV via contaminated equipment within hemodialysis units is the most likely route of transmission. Other types of transmission appear rare, such as patient-to-staff and staff-to-patient transmission. Among dialysis center staff who sustained a needle-stick injury from anti-HCV positive patients, between 2.7 and 10% become infected. (30,31) Without such obvious injuries, transmission to health care workers is uncommon. Furthermore, there is little evidence of spread of hepatitis C from infected health care workers to patients, with no instances having been reported in several years of surveillance. (32)

In contrast, patient-to-patient transmission via contaminated equipment appears to be a major cause of transmission of hepatitis C. This occurs when there is lack of strict adherence to universal blood precautions. A study in Spain reported a 7% incidence of HCV infection among dialysis patients, most of which was attributed to lapses in sterile technique. (33) Small outbreaks of hepatitis C in dialysis units have been linked to the sharing of heparin vials and to the failure to change gloves between patients with and without known HCV infection. Physical proximity of infected and noninfected patients appears to increase the risk of transmission, which may account for the clustering of infected patients within the hemodialysis center environment. (34) Sharing dialysis machines between infected and noninfected patients is also associated with an increased risk of infection (35) and the incidence of infection is reported to be lower in centers that use dedicated machines for patients with anti-HCV. (36)

Hemodialysis Membranes and Hepatitis C

During hemodialysis, the dialysis membrane is believed to act as a physical barrier to HCV. (37) The diameter of the HCV particle is estimated to be between 40 and 60 nm, which is far larger than the size of pores in even the most permeable of dialyzer membranes. However, breakdown in the integrity of the membrane could lead to the passage of virus into the dialysate. There is debate on whether some dialyzer membrane materials (cellulose, cellulose-diacetate, polysulfone, and polyacrilonitrile) are better than others in preventing cross of HCV into the dialysate. In some studies, HCV RNA could not be found in dialysates, regardless of the type of membrane. (38) In another study, HCV RNA was detectable in the dialysate when apparently intact polyacrilonitrile membranes were used but not when cellulose membrane dialyzers were used for HCV-infected patients. (39) The difference in results between the studies may be explained by the differences in sensitivity of the polymerase chain reaction (PCR) assays used to detect HCV RNA. In addition, viral RNA detected by PCR may be fragments of genomic material not encapsidated in virions and not infectious. Studies of the most clinically meaningful end point, the prevalence of anti-HCV in hemodialysis patients stratified by the type of dialyzer membrane used, have failed to find an association between HCV infection and type of membrane. (15)

Reuse of Dialyzers and Hepatitis C

The possible role of reprocessed dialyzers in the spread of hepatitis C in dialysis units is also controversial. In some studies of dialysis centers that used reprocessed dialyzers, the lowest rates of anti-HCV were found in centers that reprocessed dialyzers of HCV-infected patients separately from those of noninfected patients. Low rates of infection were also found in centers that did not reprocess dialyzers used on HCV-infected patients. (36) In another study, nonreusable dialyzers were associated with a 63.5% reduction in the relative risk of hepatitis C, although the difference from the control group was not statistically significant. Thus, firm conclusions concerning the advisability of reusing dialyzers cannot be established at this time.

Isolation of HCV-Infected Hemodialysis Patients

Because HCV is similar to HBV in its mode of transmission and frequency in dialysis units, the argument has been made that patients with chronic HCV infection should be isolated from patients without HCV in a manner similar to that for HBV-infected dialysis patients. In one study, reverse isolation of patients who were negative for anti-HCV led to an 84% reduction in the relative risk of acquisition of anti-HCV. These data were not prospectively acquired with control of other methods of prevention of transmission in a dialysis center. Furthermore, patient isolation is costly and may be particularly cost-ineffective in dialysis centers with a low prevalence of anti-HCV. In a prospective study of HCV patients dialyzed on dedicated machines, no new infections developed within the dialysis center over 25 months. (40)

Arguments against the need for isolation of anti-HCV positive dialysis patients include the fact that HCV is less infectious than hepatitis B and is rapidly inactivated by environmental exposure at room temperature. Furthermore, anti-HCV testing is not sensitive, missing those HCV-infected patients who do not produce anti-HCV as well as newly infected patients who have not yet developed antibody. These patients would remain a source of infection unless PCR techniques for HCV RNA were used routinely, procedures that would markedly increase the already high costs of hemodialysis. (15) Finally, anti-HCV does not confer immunity and some patients with antibody do not have chronic infection but have recovered. These patients would be dialyzed with other dialysis patients with chronic HCV infection and would be susceptible to reinfection. (41) Patients with chronic infection would also be susceptible to superinfection with another strain or genotype of HCV. The presence of multiple genotypes and subtypes of HCV and the antigenic variability of the virus have made vaccine development difficult, and the lack of effective immune serum globulin makes prospects for active or passive prophylaxis after HCV exposure unlikely in the near term. (42) These features of hepatitis C make it important to practice strict universal blood precautions and methods of prevention of spread of HCV for all patients on dialysis, regardless of anti-HCV status.

Other Risk Factors in Spread of Hepatitis C

Renal failure patients may have other risk factors for acquiring hepatitis C, including having multiple sexual partners and using injection drugs. Chronic hepatitis C can also cause chronic renal disease, which is another reason for a high rate of anti-HCV among patients with renal failure on hemodialysis. Limited data also suggest that the prevalence of HCV infection is lower in women than in men with renal failure and that males have higher serum levels of virus. (15) The presence of high levels of HCV may be an independent risk factor for spread of the infection by nonparenteral means. Patients with renal failure and on hemodialysis need to be counseled on the risk of hepatitis C and how to best prevent spread to family members and intimate contacts.

NATURAL HISTORY AND COURSE OF HEPATITIS C

HCV appears to have a modest effect on mortality in renal failure patients. In a large cohort study comparing HCV-infected patients to controls, the relative risk of death due to liver disease or infection was 2.39 [95% with a confidence interval (CI) of 1.28–4.48]. (43) Another cohort study of patients with renal failure showed that the crude relative risk of death comparing HCV-positive to -negative patients was not significant (0.93 with a 95% CI of 0.54–1.58). After adjusting for age, transplantation, time on dialysis, and race, the relative risk of death comparing HCV-infected patients to HCV-negative patients increased to a modestly significant level (1.78 with a 95% CI of 1.01–3.14). (44) Additional studies are needed to assess the impact of HCV infection on this population.

Histologial, Biochemical, and Virological Correlates of Anti-HCV Positivity

HCV RNA and Chronic Hepatitis in Patients with Renal Disease

In a survey of hemodialysis patients in France, 84% of patients with anti-HCV were found to have HCV RNA detectable in blood. Among those undergoing liver biopsy, 78% had histological evidence of chronic hepatitis. (45) However, only 26% of patients with biopsy-proven hepatitis and HCV RNA in serum had elevations in serum aminotransferase levels. In studies from the United States and France, more than 75% of patients with anti-HCV detected by EIA had HCV RNA detectable by PCR (46) compared to 94% of patients who were positive by a third-generation recombinant immunoblot assay (RIBA). Surprisingly, in one study, no home hemodialysis or CAPD patient had detectable HCV RNA, despite the fact that 2 of 23 were anti-HCV positive by a second-generation EIA. (44) Differences in the prevalence of viremia in antibody-positive patients may arise from the different sensitivities and specificities of the tests used. In addition, a 2-year study of a cohort of 38 patients with chronic hepatitis C on dialysis demonstrated that some patients have intermittent viremia. (47)

HCV Genotypes

In a northern Italian population of hemodialysis patients, 2a was the most common and 1b the second most common genotype. There was no difference in clinical characteristics or serum aminotransferase levels of patients with different genotypes. The distribution of genotypes was similar between different dialysis units participating in the cross-sectional study. Interestingly, the distribution of genotypes differed from the distribution of genotypes among patients with community-acquired hepatitis C in whom genotype 1b was the most common. (48) Other regions of the world have reported different distributions of genotypes in renal failure patients, with 1b being the predominant genotype in studies from Austria, France, and Korea. (49)

Occult HCV in Peripheral Blood Mononuclear Cells

Several studies have suggested that HCV can infect peripheral blood mononuclear cells. In a study of 67 Austrian patients with renal failure, 6 patients had detectable HCV RNA in peripheral blood mononuclear cells, but only 3 had anti-HCV and HCV RNA in serum, 2 had HCV RNA without antibody, and 1 had neither anti-HCV nor HCV RNA detectable in serum. While the specificity of the virological testing may be questioned, these findings have several implications. First, testing for anti-HCV may have serious limitations in surveying for HCV infection among renal failure patients. Second, peripheral blood mononuclear cells may be a reservoir of HCV that may lead to clinically apparent infection only after immunosuppression is instituted after transplantation. (50)

TREATMENT OF HEPATITIS C IN PATIENTS WITH RENAL DISEASE

Interferon-α with or without ribavirin is now the standard therapy of patients with chronic hepatitis C. The role of interferon therapy in patients with renal disease and hepatitis C, however, has yet to be defined. The metabolism of interferon is not dependent on renal function and, therefore, dose and regimen of interferon treatment need not be altered in patients with renal disease because of altered pharmacokinetics. (51) Rather, issues with interferon therapy in patients with renal disease are low rate of response and high rate of side effects.

Studies of Interferon Monotherapy

A summary of results from published studies on interferon therapy in patients with renal disease is given in Table III. (52–63) The majority of patients had

TABLE III Treatment of Hepatitis C in Patients with Renal Failure[a]

Reference	n	Interferon dose (× 10⁶ units thrice weekly)	Interferon type	Duration (weeks)	Response
Süleymanlar et al. (52)	3	4.5	2a	16	All HCV RNA +ve at end of treatment
Koenig et al. (53)	37	5	2b	16	15 HCV RNA −ve at end of treatment 8 −ve 2 months later
Djordjevi et al. (54)	6	3	2b 2b	12	2 ALT normal 6 months after treatment 2 HCV RNA −ve months after treatment
Taltavull et al. (55)	10	3 3	Lymphoblastoid	48	8 ALT normal 3 months after treatment
Rostaing et al. (56) (posttransplant)	15	3	2b	24	0 HCV RNA −ve 1 month after treatment 1 lost graft function
Özyilkan et al. (57)	13	3	2a	26	9 ALT normal 3 months after treatment 3 biopsies better 6 months after treatment
Raptopoulou-Gigi et al. (58)	19	3	2b	24	12 ALT normal 14 months after treatment 12 HCVRNA −ve 14 months after treatment
Yasumura et al. (59) (posttransplant)	6	6	α	28 weeks (on average)	3 ALT normal 1 month after treatmeat 1 HCVRNA −ve 18 months after treatment 1 elevated creatinine—not treated
Rodrigues et al. (60)	7	3	2b	24	1 HCV RNA −ve 11 months after treatment
Pol et al. (61)	19	3	2b	24	12 HCV RNA −ve 6 months after treatment
Simsek (62)	17	3	2b	24	15 ALT normal at end of treatment 5 histological improvement 10 ALT normal 3 months after treatment

[a] Adapted from Diego and Roth. (63) Note that criteria for response were not uniform.

improvement in alanine aminotransferase (ALT) levels, serum HCV RNA levels, and liver histology while on therapy. (15) A course of interferon-α in a dose of 3 million units (MU) given three times weekly led to fall of ALT levels into the normal range in 62 to 100% of patients and clearance of HCV RNA in 62 to 77% as detected by either branched DNA signal amplification (bDNA) or PCR techniques. Unfortunately, the majority of patients relapsed when therapy was stopped, and sustained virological response rates were disappointingly low in studies in which these results were available. In addition to the low sustained response rates, side effects of interferon were often problematic, leading to early discontinuation of therapy in 30 to 40% of patients and dose reduction in a further 26 to 67%. (61,64–67)

One study reported an end-of-treatment virological response rate of 100% and a sustained virological response rate of 92%. (65) Most other studies have not been as encouraging. In a study of 37 patients treated with interferon-α 2b in a dose of 5 MU thrice weekly for 4 months, only 23 patients were able to complete therapy of whom 15 had an end-of-treatment virological response. However, within 2 months, 7 of the 15 relapsed. (68) In 10 renal failure patients treated with either interferon-α 2b or lymphoblastoid interferon for a year, only 7 patients were able to complete therapy of whom only 1 had no detectable HCV RNA in follow-up. (69) In a small study of 6 hemodialysis patients treated with 6 months of interferon-α 2b, 4 of the 6 relapsed biochemically within 6 months of completing treatment. Because testing for HCV RNA was not available, virological response rates were not reported. (70)

Because renal failure patients have a reduced survival without transplantation and interferon is both poorly tolerated and expensive, the value of treating patients with renal failure and hepatitis C has been questioned. (70) Interferon may benefit renal failure patients with a recent onset of infection, low levels of viremia, genotypes 2 and 3, low levels of hepatic iron, and minimal fibrosis (71) and may be of greatest value in patients who are being considered for renal transplantation. (70) The major limitation to the use of interferon monotherapy has been the low sustained response rates seen in these immunologically compromised patients. As more effective and better tolerated antiviral agents are developed, the risk–benefit ratio will be altered so that treatment of patients with renal failure will be more cost-effective.

Combination Therapy

The combination of interferon-α with ribavirin, an oral nucleoside analogue, has been shown to increase the sustained virological response rate compared to interferon alone in patients with hepatitis C who have normal renal function. Unfortunately, ribavirin is cleared by the kidneys, is not dialyzed during conventional hemodialysis, and causes a dose-dependent hemolytic anemia, which makes it contraindicated in patients with renal failure. The renal clearance of ribavirin leads to rapid rises in serum levels, which can induce severe hemolysis and life-threatening anemia in patients with reduced creatinine clearance. Additional studies are required to determine the optimal use of interferon-α and other antiviral agents for patients with end-stage renal disease.

HEPATITIS C IN RENAL TRANSPLANT PATIENTS

Epidemiology of Hepatitis C in Renal Transplant Patients

Prevalence of Hepatitis C in Renal Transplant Recipients

In 1997, a total of 34,766 patients were on waiting lists for renal transplantation in the United States. (43) Kidney transplantation has been shown to improve the long-term outcome for patients with renal failure, but the shortage of organs for transplantation has limited its use. Compared to continuation of dialysis, renal transplantation is associated with an increased relative risk of death in the first month (2.43), but a marked decrease in relative risk (0.36) by 12 months after transplantation. (72) Infectious diseases and comorbidities can have a significant impact on the outcome of renal transplantation. Hepatitis C is now the leading cause of posttransplant chronic liver disease (73) and cirrhosis is the third leading cause of death in long-term renal allograft recipients. (69) A survey of renal transplant centers in the United States showed that 89% of transplant groups were accepting HCV-infected patients for kidney transplantation. Of the centers transplanting HCV-infected patients, 37% required that the patients have no histological evidence of progressive liver disease. (74)

The prevalence of anti-HCV among renal transplant recipients has ranged from 11 to 49%. (43) The majority of patients with anti-HCV were also positive at the time of transplantation. Of course, HCV infection can occur *de novo* after transplantation as a result of exposure to blood or blood transfusions or via the renal graft. The incidence of *de novo* HCV infection after renal transplantation was only 3% in a study of patients from 1989 to 1994. (75) In a large serological study of 716 kidney donors, 13 (1.8%) were found to be anti-HCV positive by first-generation EIA. (76) Of the 29 patients who received organs from these donors, 14 (48%) developed hepatitis after an average of 3.8 months. If the donor had circulating HCV RNA, 100% of recipients acquired HCV RNA and 70% developed anti-HCV posttransplant. (76) In other studies, the use of renal grafts from anti-HCV positive donors resulted in infection as shown by testing for HCV RNA in 0 to 100% of recipients. (77,78)

The wide variation in the incidence of *de novo* infections after renal transplantation may be due in part to the different techniques used to perfuse the renal graft at the time of harvesting. Perfusion of grafts with preservative can reduce the viral levels by as much as 99%, whereas slush preservation without perfusion does not change the viral level within the graft. (79) Another source of variation in the rate of viremia in transplant recipients is the sensitivity of the assays used to detect HCV RNA and the difficulty of establishing the diagnosis of hepatitis C in the posttransplant situation. (80,81)

Use of Renal Grafts from HCV-Infected Donors

Despite the risk of HCV transmission, the use of kidneys from anti-HCV-positive donors may be appropriate in some situations. Because of the shortage of kidney donors, the refusal to use kidneys from anti-HCV-positive donors would deny transplantation to many patients. Among 20 recipients of kidneys from HCV RNA-positive donors who were followed prospectively, only 6 developed elevated serum aminotransferase levels. (46) Furthermore, the HCV status of the kidney donor was not associated with a decrease in 5-year patient and graft survival. (46) However even if the risk of clinically important liver disease is low, it may be unacceptable to risk HCV infection in a noninfected renal transplant recipient when there is still the potential for continued dialysis and future transplantation with a noninfected organ. What does appear reasonable is to transplant kidneys from anti-HCV positive donors into renal failure patients who themselves are HCV RNA positive. This approach would maximize potential donors at little increase in risk for the recipient. A cost–benefit analysis and a cohort study suggest that transplanting HCV-positive patients with grafts from HCV-positive donors is an acceptable practice. (82,83) However, because HCV infection does not confer immunity to reinfection, patients who are anti-HCV positive but do not have HCV RNA should probably not receive kidneys from HCV-infected donors. (79)

Effects of HBV Coinfection

In a study from France, the prevalence of coinfection with HCV and HBV in a cohort of renal transplant patients was 3.5%, although the serological definition of coinfection was not stated explicitly. Patients with coinfection had a higher frequency of hepatitis compared to patients infected with HCV alone. Cirrhosis was present more often in coinfected patients than in renal transplant patients with HCV infection alone (22.2% versus 7.7%). (84) Similar results were reported from Taiwan in patients who were positive for both anti-HCV and hepatitis B surface antigen. The risks of chronic liver disease, cirrhosis, and decompensated liver disease were greater in coinfected patients than in patients with anti-HCV alone. (85)

Impact of HCV on Outcomes of Renal Transplantation

Effect of HCV Infection on Short-Term Outcome of Renal Transplantation

The impact of HCV infection on the outcome of renal transplantation is only partially and incompletely defined. HCV is the leading cause of posttransplant liver disease and may be a significant cause of morbidity and mortality in transplant patients, (86) although some studies suggest that the presence of anti-HCV does not have a significant impact on patient survival. In one study, after 4 years of follow-up, only 34% of patients developed chronic hepatitis, 7.6% cirrhosis, and 1.3% hepatic failure. (87) Another study suggested that the 1-year survival in HCV-positive renal transplant recipients was slightly decreased compared to renal transplant recipients without HCV, but the difference was not statistically significant (80% versus 90%, $p = 0.263$). The 1-year graft survival was also slightly lower at 76% in HCV-infected patients compared to 85% in HCV-negative patients, but this difference was also not statistically significant ($p = 0.37$). (88) Other studies have suggested that the presence of anti-HCV in renal transplant patients does have an effect on outcome; the relative risk of death among anti-HCV-positive patients was 3.3 compared to antibody-negative patients. The higher risk of death persisted for 6 months after transplant. (43)

Reasons for Differences in Effects of HCV Infection on Renal Transplantation

Differences between the cohort studies of the outcome of HCV renal transplant patients may be partially due to selection bias. The severity of pretransplant liver disease is associated with the risk of posttransplant death, and variations in the severity between studies may be one explanation for the differences in patient outcome. (89) One can speculate that centers who perform pretransplant liver biopsies and exclude those patients with more severe stages of hepatitis C may have less liver-related mortality in HCV-infected patients following transplant. A randomized trial allocating patients between dialysis and transplantation could address the issue of selection bias, but, for obvious reasons, cannot be accomplished.

Some of the debate about the course of postrenal transplant HCV infection is fueled by differences in the end points followed in patients after transplantation. Over 50% of anti-HCV-positive renal transplant patients who underwent liver biopsy in one series had histological evidence of hepatitis or cirrhosis. (90) Presence of detectable viremia and duration of transplant were both associated with a worse histological grade of hepatitis, as measured by the histology activity index score. (91) Female sex, advanced age at transplantation, and histological evidence of significant hepatitis were each associated with a higher likelihood of progression to cirrhosis. (92) In another series, 59 posttransplant patients with anti-HCV positivity underwent 64 liver biopsies, which revealed normal liver histology in 8, chronic hepatitis in 45, cirrhosis in 1, and a variety of non-specific changes in the remainder. (76) In that study, all patients with normal ALT levels had normal histology. Approximately 97% of anti-HCV-positive patients who were tested had HCV RNA detectable in serum.

Other studies, using different end points, have suggested that HCV infection has little impact on patient outcomes after renal transplantation. In a study with an average follow-up of 6 years, there was no difference in patient or graft survival in HCV-positive patients compared to controls, although 42% of the HCV-infected patients developed hepatitis posttransplant. (93) A retrospective cohort study comparing patients with and without chronic HCV-induced liver disease over a 10-year period did not find any difference in patient or graft survival. Interestingly, there was a higher incidence of CMV disease in patients with biopsy-proven liver disease. (94,95)

Effects of HCV Infection on Long-Term Outcome of Renal Transplantation

With longer follow-up after transplantation, however, differences in outcome between HCV-infected and noninfected patients have become more apparent. In a series of 83 anti-HCV-positive patients, 5 developed severe liver disease and 3 received liver transplants between 24 and 120 months after renal transplantation. (90) In a large, multicenter study from France, survival after renal transplantation was decreased significantly in anti-HCV-positive compared to anti-HCV-negative patients at 10 years after transplantation. The difference in mortality was not apparent at 5 years and only appeared after the first decade. (96) Among anti-HCV-positive patients, liver disease was the leading cause of death, whereas none of the anti-HCV-negative patients died of liver disease. (97)

HCV Infection and Graft Rejection

HCV infection may be associated with an increased risk of graft rejection. (70,98) One explanation for this is that patients with hepatitis C are more likely to receive lower doses of immunosuppressive drugs, which might result in higher rates of acute rejection. Hepatitis C may also increase the risk of rejection by affecting the regulation of major histocompatibility complex class II antigen expression in the renal graft. (46) While early graft survival appears to be similar in anti-HCV-positive and -negative renal transplant recipients, ultimately graft survival may be diminished. After 59 months of follow-up, the incidence of rejection was not significantly different comparing HCV-positive and -negative patients. Graft survival was not significantly different comparing 62 anti-HCV-positive patients followed for a mean of 72 months to HCV-negative controls. (93) In patients with a median follow-up of 9 years, graft survival also was not significantly different. (99) However, in a more recent study, a significantly higher proportion of anti-HCV-positive patients experienced renal graft loss compared with uninfected controls after 10 years of follow-up: graft survival 20 years after transplantation was 36% in anti-HCV-positive patients versus 64% in controls. (96) Another study found a significant proportion of HCV-infected patients experienced graft loss by 10 years (51% for anti-HCV patients versus 37% for controls). (97) The cause of graft loss was not stated in these studies.

Immunosuppression and HCV Infection

Postrenal transplant immunosuppression may alter the course of HCV infection. In one study, HCV viral titers rose within 20 to 30 days after transplantation. Similarly, titers rose within days after treatment with antilymphocyte therapy for rejection. There were no differences in serum aminotransferase levels between patients receiving tacrolimus and those receiving cyclosporine, although the two groups were small. (95) In another study, the prevalence of hepatitis in HCV-infected patients at an average of 60.8 months after renal transplantation was 80%. (100) The severity of hepatitis was associated with a longer duration of immunosuppression. (101) Abnormal serum aminotransferase levels were found in 20% of anti-HCV-positive patients posttransplantation, whereas the prevalence of hepatitis as detected by liver biopsy was 45%. (76)

Several lines of evidence suggest that immunosuppressive medications increase the risk of the progression of chronic viral disease and may account for a more rapid progression of liver disease after renal transplantation. First, renal transplant patients with hepatitis B surface antigen have a higher prevalence of liver disease and incidence of death compared to hepatitis B patients on dialysis. (102) Second, immunosuppressed transplant patients infected with the human immunodeficiency virus develop acquired immunodeficiency syndrome within 1.5 to 2 years compared to 7 to 8 years in nonimmunosuppressed patients. (103) Third, there is a higher incidence of liver disease in anti-HCV positive patients who receive antilymphocyte preparations as part of their immunosuppression compared to patients who do not. (104) Fourth, serum HCV RNA levels increase after transplantation. (89) Finally, HCV-infected patients with hypogammaglobulinemia appear to have an accelerated course of liver disease. (105)

HCV-Related Glomerulonephritis after Renal Transplantation

Hepatitis C is known to cause several forms of systemic vasculitis, including cryoglobulinemia and glomerulonephritis. The possibility that HCV infection could lead to glomerulonephritis in the graft after renal transplantation has been investigated in several patient cohorts. Posttransplant membranous glomerulonephritis was identified in 12 of 399 renal transplant patients, of whom 3 (25%) had concomitant HCV infection. (68) In the same study, another 12 patients had membranoproliferative glomerulonephritis, of whom 7 (78%) had hepatitis C. The prevalence of HCV in the cohort of 399 patients was 29% (117 patients) and the prevalence of membranoproliferative glomerulonephritis was significantly higher in the HCV-positive compared to the HCV-negative group. Despite the higher prevalence of renal disease, survival and graft survival were similar. (76) Patients with type I membranoproliferative glomerulonephritis tended to have either circulating cryoglobulins or hypocomplementemia, suggesting a link among HCV, immune activation, and renal disease. (106)

HCV Serology after Transplantation

Antibody to HCV persists after transplantation. The sensitivity of third-generation EIAs in detecting anti-HCV in posttransplant patients on immunosuppression who were reactive for HCV RNA was 95% with a specificity of 95%. The positive predictive value of finding anti-HCV reactivity was 93% and the negative predictive value of its absence was 96%. Patients who were anti-HCV positive but lacked circulating RNA may have cleared virus or may have had low levels of HCV RNA below the detectability of the PCR assay. Importantly, after renal transplantation, occasional patients will have HCV RNA detectable by PCR in the absence of anti-HCV. (107) In a more recent series, HCV RNA was detectable in 2 to 9% of transplanted patients who were anti-HCV negative by second-generation EIA testing. (108,109) Thus, patients with liver disease after renal transplantation should be tested for HCV RNA even in the absence of anti-HCV positivity to exclude hepatitis C as the cause.

It remains unclear whether there is a significant difference in patient or graft survival between HCV-positive and -negative patients after transplantation. For this reason, intensive pretransplant screening for HCV and liver disease will be time-consuming and costly, yet have little or no impact on the transplant outcome. (110) At present, it is reasonable to offer renal transplantation to HCV-positive patients, provided that their liver disease is not advanced. For this reason, liver biopsy may be useful to accurately assess the extent of liver disease as a part of the pretransplant evaluation. (111) However, there is little evidence to suggest that information from liver biopsy improves posttransplant outcomes over and above information that can be derived from a careful clinical and laboratory evaluation. Policies on using liver biopsy and criteria for excluding patients with advanced liver disease vary by transplant center and are difficult to standardize.

Treatment of Hepatitis C after Transplantation

Therapy of hepatitis C after renal transplantation is problematic in respect to both safety and efficacy. In several small studies using interferon-α in doses of 3 million units given three times weekly for 6 months, approximately 50% of treated patients developed graft rejection. (53,108,112) Indeed, when recombinant interferon-α 2b was used for prophylaxis against cytomegalovirus infection after renal transplantation, even low doses of interferon were associated with steroid-resistant vascular rejection. (113) Despite these findings, not all studies of interferon therapy have reported a high rate of rejection. In one study, treatment led to a virological response in 16% and an incidence of rejection of only 3%. (114) Another study reported a 37.5% incidence of renal deterioration while on interferon therapy for hepatitis C. Half of the patients experiencing a decline in renal function lost their grafts and required hemodialysis, and withdrawal of interferon did not halt the progression of renal disease. (115) In renal transplant patients who received interferon and experienced renal insufficiency, large tubulointerstitial lesions consisting of edema, expansion of peritubular capillaries, and diffuse tubular flattening were seen beneath a thick capsule, suggesting that interferon may have intrinsic renal toxicity in the absence of acute rejection. (113) These findings are consistent with reports of proteinuria, membranoproliferative glomerulonephritis, crescentic glomerulonephritis, acute interstital nephritis, hemolytic-uremic syndrome, focal segmental glomerulosclerosis, and acute renal failure seen in patients treated with high doses of interferon for malignancy. Based on this high incidence of rejection and the potential for other nephrotoxicity, renal transplantation is generally considered as a contraindication to treatment with interferon.

CONCLUSION

Hepatitis C is the most common cause of liver disease in the dialysis patient. The prevalence of chronic hepatitis C determined by anti-HCV testing in this population ranges from 6 to 38%. Using second-generation EIA assays, the prevalence of anti-HCV among patients participating in the 1997 National Surveillance of Dialysis Associated Diseases in the United States was 9.3%. Polymerase chain reaction testing for HCV RNA has shown that the prevalence of chronic HCV infection can be as high as 20 to 30% of dialysis patients.

The causes and source of infection in patients with chronic renal failure on hemodialysis are multiple. Before the introduction of routine screening of blood donors for anti-HCV, blood transfusions were an important risk factor for the acquisition of hepatitis C. Other potential sources of infection include exposure to contaminated equipment and nosocomial routes such as patient-to-patient exposure. The risk of infection appears to correlate with the duration of hemodialysis and the number of transfusions. Interestingly, dialysate and buffers have been shown to be virus free even when used in hepatitis C-infected patients.

The natural history of chronic hepatitis C infection in patients with renal failure is not well characterized. Although persistent elevations in ALT levels occur in 12 to 50% of dialysis patients, the frequency of persistently normal ALT levels in HCV-infected dialysis patients appears to be higher than in HCV-infected patients without renal failure. Overt liver disease and liver failure occur rarely. The degree of inflammation in liver biopsies of renal failure patients is usually mild. Thus, progressive liver disease may be less common in patients with advanced renal disease, but further studies are required to assess the true impact of hepatitis C infection in this high-risk population.

The impact of hepatitis C infection on morbidity and mortality of patients with end-stage renal disease remains poorly defined. Initial studies have failed to show a significant increase in mortality among HCV-infected hemodialysis or renal transplant patients within the first 5 years following transplantation. In contrast, studies with an extended follow-up of renal transplant recipients suggest that hepatitis C infection may affect patient and graft survival during the second decade. Further studies are required to identify the mechanisms of infection of patients with end-stage renal disease and to define better treatment strategies for these patients before and after kidney transplantation.

REFERENCES

1. Huang C C. Hepatitis in patients with end-stage renal disease. J gastroenterol Hepatol 1997; 12(Suppl.):S236–41.
2. Chauveau P, Courouce A M, Lemarec N, et al. Antibodies to hepatitis C virus by second generation test in hemodialysed patients. Kidney Int 1993;43:S149–52.
3. Chan T M, Lok A S F, Cheng I K P, Chan R T. Prevalence of hepatitis C virus infection in hemodialysis patients: A longitudinal study comparing the results of RNA and antibody assays. Hepatology 1993;17:5–8.
4. Kuhns M, De Medina M, McNamara A, et al. Detection of hepatitis C virus RNA in hemodialysis patients. J Am Soc Nephrol 1994;4:1491–7.
5. Fabrizi F, Lunghi G, Guarnori I, et al. Virological characteristics of hepatitis C virus infection in chronic hemodialysis patients: a cross-sectional study. Clin Nephrol 1995;44:49–55.
6. Golan E, Korzets Z, Cristal-Lilov A, Ben-Tovim T, Bernheim J. Increased prevalence of HCV antibodies in dialyzed Ashkenazi Jews—a possible ethnic predisposition. Nephrol, Dial, Transplant 1996;11:684–6.
7. Dussol B, Berthezène P, Brunet P, Roubicek C, Berland Y. Hepatitis C virus infection among chronic dialysis patients in the south of France: A collaborative study. Am J Kidney Dis 1995; 25:399–404.
8. Huraib S, Al-Rashed R, Aldrees A, Aljefry M, Arif M, Al-Faleh F A. High prevalence of and risk factors for hepatitis C in hemodialysis patients in Saudi Arabia: a need for new dialysis strategies. Nephrol, Dial, Transplant 1995;10:470–4.
9. Elzouki A N Y, Bushala M, Tobji R S, Khfaifi M. Prevalence of anti-hepatitis C virus antibodies and hepatitis C virus viraemia in chronic hemodialysis patients in Libya. Nephrol, Dial, Transplant 1995;10:475–6.
10. Todorov V, Boneva R, Ilieva P, Doichinova T, Donchev M. High prevalence of hepatitis C virus infection in one dialysis center in Bulgaria. Nephron 1998;79:222–3.
11. Al-Wakeel J, Malik G H, Al-Mohaya S, et al. Liver disease in dialysis patients with antibodies to hepatitis C virus. Nephrol, Dial, Transplant 1996;11:2265–8.
12. Ng Y Y, Lee S D, Wu S C, Yang W C, Chiang S S, Huang T P. Antibodies to hepatitis C virus in uremic patients on continuous ambulatory peritoneal dialysis. J Med Virol 1991;35:263–6.
13. Gladziwa U, Schlipkoter V, Lorbeer B, Cholmakow K, Roggendorf M, Sieberth H G. Prevalence of antibodies to hepatitis C virus in patients on peritoneal dialysis: a multicenter study. Clin Nephrol 1993;40:46–52.
14. Lee G S L, Roy D K, Fan F Y, Thanaletchumi K, Woo K T. Hepatitis C antibodies in patients on peritoneal dialysis: Prevalence and risk factors. Peritoneal Dial Int 1996;16(Suppl 1):S424–28.
15. Murthy B V R, Pereira B J G. A 1990s perspective of hepatitis C, human immunodeficiency virus, and tuberculosis infections in dialysis patients. Semin Nephrol 1997;17:346–63.
16. Tokars J, Alter M J, Favero M S, Moyer L A, Miller E, Bland L. National surveillance of hemodialysis associated diseases in the United States. ASAIO J 1994;40:1020–31.
17. Centers for Disease Control. National surveillance of dialysis-associated diseases in the United States. Atlanta, GA: CDC, 1997.
18. Huang C C, Wu M S, Lin D Y, Liaw Y F. The prevalence of hepatitis C virus antibodies in patients treated with continuous ambulatory peritoneal dialysis. Peritoneal dialysis Int 1992;12: 31–5.
19. Chan T M, Lok A S F, Cheng I K P. Hepatitis C infection among dialysis patients: A comparison between patients on maintenance hemodialysis and continuous ambulatory peritoneal dialysis. Nephrol, Dial, Transplant 1991;6:944–7.

20. Fabrizi F, Locatelli F. Hepatitis C virus infection in dialysis and clinical nephrology. Int J Artif Organs 1995;18:235–44.

21. Tokars J I, Miller E R, Alter M J, Arduino M J. National surveillance of dialysis-associated diseases in the United States, 1997. National Center for Infectious Diseases, Centers for Disease Control and Prevention, Atlanta, GA: 1997.

22. Niu M T, Coleman P J, Alter M J. Multicenter study of hepatitis C virus infection in chronic hemodialysis patients and hemodialysis center staff members. Am J Kidney Dis 1993;22:568–73.

23. Anonymous. Experimental studies on environmental contamination with infected blood during hemodialysis. A report by a working party set up by the Medical Research Council Sub-committee on Hepatitis in Renal and Associated Units. J Hyg 1975;74:133–48.

24. Favero M S, Maynard J E, Petersen N J, et al. Hepatitis-B antigen on environmental surfaces. Lancet 1973;2(7483):1455.

25. Hardy N M, Sandroni S, Danielson S, Wilson W J. Antibody to hepatitis C virus increases with time on dialysis. Clin Nephrol 1992;38:44–8.

26. Jadoul M, Cornu C, Van Ypersele de Strihou C, Universitaires Cliniques St-Luc Collaborative Group. Universal precautions prevent hepatitis C virus transmission: A 54 month follow-up of the Belgian multicenter study. Kidney Int 1998;53:1022–5.

27. Pascual J, Teruel J L, Mateos M. Nosocomial transmission of hepatitis C virus (HCV) infection in a hemodialysis (HD) unit during two years of prospective follow up. J Am Soc Nephrol 1992; 3:386.

28. Barril G, Traver J A. Prevalence of hepatitis C virus in dialysis patients in Spain. Nephrol, Dial, Transplant 1995;10(Suppl 6):78–80.

29. Bruguera M, Vidal L, Sanchez-Tapias J M, Costa J, Revert L, Rodes J. Incidence and features of liver disease in patients on chronic hemodialysis. J Clin Gastroenterol 1990;12:298–302.

30. Kiyosawa K, Sodeyama T, Tanaka E, et al. Hepatitis C in hospital employees with needlestick injuries. Ann Intern Med 1991;115:367–9.

31. Mitsui T, Iwano K, Masuko K, et al. Hepatitis C virus infection in medical after needlestick accident. Hepatology 1992;16:1109–14.

32. Loureiro A, Macedo G, Pinto T. Hepatitis C virus infection in haemodialysis patients: lessons from epidemiology and prophylaxis. Nephrol, Dial, Transplant 1995;10(Suppl 6):83–7.

33. Forns X, Fernández-Llama P, Pons M, et al. Incidence and risk factors of hepatitis C infection in haemodialysis unit. Nephrol, Dial, Transplant 1997;12:736–40.

34. Da Porto A, Adami A, Susanna F, et al. Hepatitis C virus in dialysis units: a multicenter study. Nephron 1992;61:309–10.

35. Brugnano R, Francisci D, Quintaliana G, et al. Antibodies against hepatitis C virus in hemodialysis patients in the central Italian region of Umbria: Evaluation of some risk factors. Nephron 1992;61:263–5.

36. Dos Santos J P, Loureiro A, Cendoroglo Neto M, Pereira B J. Impact of dialysis room and reuse strategies on the incidence of HCV infection in hemodialysis units. Nephrol, Dial, Transplant 1996;11:2017–22.

37. Yuasa T, Ishikawa G, Manabe S, Sekiguchi S, Takeuchi K, Miyamura T. The particle size of hepatitis C virus estimated by filtration through microporous regenerated cellulose fibre. J Gen Virol 1991;72:2021–4.

38. Hubmann R, Zazgornik J, Gabriel C, Garbeis B, Blauhut B. Hepatitis C virus-does it penetrate the hemodialysis membrane? PCR analysis of hemodialysis ultrafiltrate and whole blood. Nephrol, Dial, and Transplant 1995;10:541–2.

39. Lombardi M, Cerrai T, Dattolo P, et al. Is the dialysis membrane a safe barrier against HCV infection? Nephrol, Dial, Transplant 1995;10:578–9.

40. Blumberg A, Zehnder C, Burckhardt J J. Prevention of hepatitis C infection in haemodialysis units. A prospective study. Nephrol, Dial, Transplant 1995;10:230–3.

41. Jadoul M. Transmission routes of HCV infection in dialysis. Nephrol, Dial, Transplant 1996; 11(Suppl 4):36–8.

42. Marian F. Hepatitis C after needlestick injuries. Ann Intern Med 1992;116:345.

43. Pereira B J, Natov S N, Bouthot B A, et al. Effects of hepatitis C infection and renal transplantation on survival in end-stage renal disease. The New England Organ Bank Hepatitis C Study Group. Kidney Int 1998;53:1374–81.

44. Stehman-Breen C O, Emerson S, Gretch D, Johnson R J. Risk of death among chronic dialysis patients infected with hepatitis C virus. Am J Kidney Dis 1998;32:629–34.

45. Pol S, Romeo R, Zins B, et al. Hepatitis C virus RNA in anti-HCV-positive hemodialyzed patients: significance and therapeutic implications. In: Viral hepatitis and liver disease. Nishioka K, Suzuki H, Mishiro S, Ota T, eds., Tokyo: Springer-Verlag, 1994:489–90.

46. Roth D. Hepatitis C virus: the nephrologist's view. Am J Kidney Dis 1995;25:3–16.

47. Couroucé A, Bouchardeau F, Chauveau P, et al. Hepatitis C virus infection in haemodialysed patients: HCV-RNA and anti-HCV antibodies (third generation assays). Nephrol, Dial, Transplant 1995;10:234–9.

48. Fabrizi F, Lunghi G, Pagliari B, et al. Molecular epidemiology of hepatitis C virus infection in dialysis patients. Nephron 1997;77:190–6.

49. Hofman H. Genotypes and virus load in patients with hepatitis C infection. Infection 1995;23:133–7.

50. Oesterreicher C, Hammer J, Koch U, et al. HBV and HCV genome in peripheral blood mononuclear cells in patients undergoing chronic hemodialysis. Kidney Int 1995;4:1967–71.

51. Hirsch M S, Tolkoff-Rubin N E, Kelly A P, Rubin R H. Pharmacokinetics of human and recombinant leucocyte interferon in patients with chronic renal failure who are undergoing hemodialysis. J Infect Dis 1983;148:335.

52. Süleymanlar I, Sezer T, Isitan F, Yakupoglu G, Süleymanlar G. Efficacy of interferon alpha in acute hepatitis C in patients on chronic hemodialysis. Nephron 1998;79:353–4.

53. Koenig P, Vogel W, Umlauft F, et al. Interferon treatment for chronic hepatitis C virus infection in uremic patients. Kidney Int 1994;45:1507–9.

54. Djordjevi V, Kostic S, Stefanovi V. Treatment of chronic hepatitis C with interferon alpha in patients on maintenance hemodialysis. Nephron 1998;79:229–31.

55. Taltavull T C, Baliellas C, Sesé E, et al. Interferon may be useful in hemodialysis patients with hepatitis C virus chronic infection who are candidates for kidney transplant. Transplant Proc 1995;27:2229–30.

56. Rostaing L, Izopet J, Baron E, et al. Preliminary results of treatment of chronic hepatitis C with recombinant interferon alpha in renal transplant patients. Nephrol, Dial, Transplant 1995;10 (Suppl 6):93–6.

57. Özyilkan E, Simsek H, Uzunalimoglu B, Telatar H. Interferon treatment of chronic active hepatitis C in patients with end-stage chronic renal failure. Nephron 1995;71:156–9.

58. Raptopoulou-Gigi M, Spaia S, Garifallos A, et al. Interferon-2b treatment of chronic hepatitis C in haemodialysis patients. Nephrol, Dial, Transplant 1995;10:1834–7.

59. Yasumura T, Nakajima H, Hamashima T, et al. Long-term outcome of recombinant INF-α treatment of chronic hepatitis C in kidney transplant recipients. Transplant Proc 1997;29:784–6.

60. Rodrigues A, Morgado T, Areias J, et al. Limited benefits of INF-α therapy in renal graft candidates with chronic viral hepatitis B or C. Transplant Proc 1997;29:777–80.

61. Pol S, Thiers V, Carnot F, et al. Efficiency of alpha-2b interferon in the treatment of HCV infection in hemodialyzed patients. Hepatology 1994;20:160A.

62. Simsek H. Interferon-alpha treatment of haemodialysis patients with chronic viral hepatitis and its impact on kidney transplantation. Nephrol, Dial, Transplant 1996;11:912–3.

63. Diego J M, Roth D. Treatment of hepatitis C infection in patients with renal disease. Curr Opin Nephrol Hypertens 1998;7:557–62.

64. Ellis M E, Alfurayh O, Halim M A, et al. Chronic non-A, non-B hepatitis complicated by end stage renal failure treated with recombinant inteferon alpha. J Hepatol 1993;18:210–6.

65. Raptopoulou-Gigi M, Spaia S, Garifallos A, et al. Interferon-alpha-2b treatment of chronic hepatitis C in hemodialysis patients. Nephrol, Dial, Transplant 1995;10:1834–7.

66. Okuda K, Hayashi H, Yokozeki K, Kondo T, Kashima T, Irie Y. Interferon treatment for chronic hepatitis C in haemodialysis patients: Suggestions based on a small series. J Gastroenterol Hepatol 1995;10:616–20.

67. Pol S, Thiers V, Carnot F, et al. Effectiveness and tolerance of interferon-α 2b in the treatment of chronic hepatitis C in haemodialysis patients. Nephrol, Dial, Transplant 1996;11(Suppl 4):58–61.

68. Koenig P, Umlarift F, Lhotta K, et al. Treatment of hmodialysis patients suffering from chronic HCV-infection with interferon alpha. J Am Soc Nephrol 1993;4:361.

69. Casanovas-Taltavull T, Baliellas C, Sesé E, et al. Interferon may be useful in hemodialysis patients with hepatitis C virus chronic infection who are candidates for kidney transplant. Transplant Proc 1995;27:2229–30.

70. Djordjevi V, Kosti S, Stefanovi V. Treatment of chronic hepatitis C with interferon alpha in patients on maintenance hemodialysis. Nephron 1998;79:229–31.

71. Rodrigues A, Morgado T, Areias F. Limited benefits of INF-α therapy in renal graft candidates with chronic viral hepatitis B or C. Transplant Proc 1997;29:770–80.

72. Port F, Wolfe R, Mauger E, Berling D, Jiang K. Comparison of survival probabilities for dialysis patients vs. cadaveric renal transplant recipients. JAMA 1993;270:1339–43.

73. Pereira B J G. Hepatitis C infection and post-transplantation liver disease. Nephrol, Dial, Transplant 1995;10(Suppl 1):58–67.

74. Schweitzer E J, Bartlett S T, Keay S, Hadley G A, Cregar J, Stockdreher D D. Impact of hepatitis B or C infection on the practice of kidney transplantation in the United States. Transplant Proc 1993;25:1456–7.

75. Cisterne J M, Rostaing L, Izopet J, et al. Epidemiology of HCV infection: disease and renal transplantation. Nephrol, Dial, Transplant 1996;11(Suppl 4):46–7.

76. Berthoux F. Hepatitis C virus infection and disease in renal transplantation. Nephron 1995; 71:386–94.

77. Roth D, Fernandez J A, Babischkin S, et al. Detection of hepatitis C virus infection among cadaver organ donors: evidence for low transmission of disease. Ann Intern Med 1992;117: 470–5.

78. Pereira B J G, Milford E L, Kirkman R L, et al. Prevalence of hepatitis C virus RNA in organ donors positive for hepatitis C antiobody and in the recipients of their organs. N Engl J Med 1992;327:910–5.

79. Zucker K, Cirocco R, Roth D, et al. Depletion of hepatitis C virus from procured kidneys using pulsatile perfusion preservation. Transplantation 1994;57:832–40.

80. Pirson Y, Goffin E. Hepatitis C infection in renal transplant patients: new insights and unanswered questions. Nephrol, Dial, Transplant 1996;11(Suppl 4):42–5.

81. Pereira B J G, Levey A S. Hepatitis C virus infection in dialysis and renal transplantation. Kidney Int 1997;51:981–99.

82. Kiberd B A. Should hepatitis C-infected kidneys be transplanted in the United States? Transplantation 1994;57:1068–72.

83. Morales J M, Campistol J M, Castellano G, et al. Transplantation of kidneys from donors with hepatitis C antibody into recipients with pre-transplantation anti-HCV. Kidney Int 1995;47: 236–40.

84. Pouteil-Noble C, Maiza H, Donia A, et al. Comparison of isolated infection by hepatitis C (HCV) or by hepatitis B (HBV) viruses and of coinfection by HCV-HBV in 1098 renal transplant patients. Transplant Proc 1997;29:791–2.

85. Chen K-S, Lo S-K, Lee N, Leu M-L, Huang C-C, Fang K-M. Superinfection with hepatitis C virus in hemodialysis patients with hepatitis B surface antigenemia: its prevalence and clinical significance in Taiwan. Nephron 1996;73:158–64.

86. Pereira B J G, Levey A S. Hepatitis C virus infection in dialysis and renal transplantation. Kidney Int 1997;51:981–99.

87. Huang C C, Liaw Y F, Lai M K, Chu S H, Chuang C K, Huang J Y. The clinical outcome of hepatitis C virus antibody-positive renal allograft recipients. Transplantation 1992;53:763–5.

88. Askari H, Abidi S, Abbas K, et al. Early experience of renal transplantation in hepatitis C patients. Transplant Proc 1995;27:2600–1.

89. Pereira B J G, Wright T L, Schmid C H, Levey A S, New England Organ Bank Hepatitis C Study Group. The impact of pretransplantation hepatitis C infection on the outcome of renal transplantation. Transplantation 1995;60:799–805.

90. Morales J M, Munoz M A, Castellano G, et al. Impact of hepatitis C in long-functioning renal transplants: a clinicopathological follow-up. Transplant Proc 1993;25(1 pt 2):1450–3.

91. Hestin D, Hussenet F, Frimat L, et al. Hepatitis C after renal transplantation: histopathological correlations. Nephrol, Dial, Transplant 1996;11(Suppl 4):52–3.

92. Rao K V, Anderson W R, Kasiske B, Dahl A C. Value of liver biopsy in the evaluation and management of chronic liver disease in renal transplant recipient. Am J Med 1993;94:241–50.

93. Haem J, Berthoux P, Mosnier J F, et al. Clear evidence of the existence of of healthy carriers of hepatitis C virus among renal transplant recepients. Transplantation 1996;62:699–704.

94. Roth D, Fernandez J A, Burke G W, Esquenazi V, Miller J. Detection of antibody to hepatitis C virus in renal transplant recipients. Transplantation 1991;51:396–400.
95. Roth D, Zucker K, Cirocco R. A prospective study of hepatitis C virus infection in renal allograft recipients. Transplantation 1996: 61:886–9.
96. Hanafusa T, Ichikawa Y, Kishikawa H, et al. Restrospective study on the impact of hepatitis C virus infection on kidney transplant patients over 20 years. Transplantation 1998;66:471–6.
97. Mathurin P, Mouquet C, Poynard T, et al. Impact of hepatitis B and C on kidney transplantation outcome. Hepatology 1999;29:257–263.
98. Ponz E, Campistol J M, Bruguera M, et al. Hepatitis C virus infection among kidney transplant recipients. Kidney Int 1991;40:748–51.
99. Ynares C, Johnson H K, Kerlin T, Crowe D, MacDonell R, Richie R. Impact of pretransplant hepatitis C antibody status upon long-term patient and renal allograft survival—a 5- and 10-year follow-up. Transplant Proc 1993;25:1466–8.
100. Haem J, Berthoux P, Cécillon S, Mosnier J F, Pozzetto B, Berthoux F. HCV liver disease in renal transplantation: a clinical and histological study. Nephrol, Dial, Transplant 1996;11 (Suppl 4):48–51.
101. Hestin D, Hussenet F, Frimat L, et al. Hepatitis C after renal transplantation: histopathological correlations. Nephrol, Dial, Transplant 1996;11(Suppl 4):52–3.
102. Harnett J D, Zeldis J B, Parfey P S, et al. Hepatitis B in dialysis and transplant patients. Transplantation 1987;44:369–76.
103. Rubin R H, Tolkoff-Rubin N E. Infection: The new problems. Transplant Proc 1989;21:1440–5.
104. Roth D, Fernandez J, Demattos A, et al. The impact of hepatitis C virus (HCV) on the potential renal allograft recipient. J Am Soc Nephrol 3,878 [abstract].
105. Bjoro K, Froland S, Yun Z, Samdal H, Haaland T. Hepatitis C infection in patients with primary hypogammaglobulinemia after treatment with contaminated immunoglobulin. N Engl J Med 1994;331:1607–11.
106. Hammoud H, Haem J, Laurent B, et al. Glomerular disease during HCV infection in renal transplantation. Nephrol, Dial, Transplant 1996;11(Suppl 4):54–5.
107. David-Neto E, Abdallah K A, Bassit L, et al. Anti-HCV antibody is sensitive but not sufficient to detect HCV active infection in renal transplanted patients: the role of PCR for HCV-RNA. Transplant Proc 1997;29:781–2.
108. Chan T M, Lok A S F, Cheng I K P, Ng I O L. Chronic hepatitis C after renal transplantation: treatment with interferon. Transplantation 1993;56:1095–8.
109. Lau J Y N, Davis G L, Brunson M E, et al. Hepatitis C virus infection in kidney transplant recipients. Hepatology 1993;18:1027–31.
110. Knoll G A, Tankersley M R, Lee J Y, Julian B A, Curtis J C. The impact of renal transplantation on survival in hepatitis-C positive end-stage renal disease patients. Am J Kidney Dis 1997;29:608–14.
111. Goffin E, Pirson Y, Van Ypersele de Strihou C. Implications of chronic hepatitis B or C infection for renal transplant candidates. Nephrol, Dial, Transplant 1995;10(Suppl 6):88–92.
112. Mancini C, Gaeta A, Lorino G, et al. Alpha interferon therapy in patients with hepatitis infection undergoing organ transplantation. Transplant Proc 1989;21(1 pt 2):2429–30.
113. Rostaing L, Modesto A, Baron E, Cisterne J M, Chabannier M H, Durand D. Acute renal failure in kidney transplant patients treated with interferon alpha 2b for chronic hepatitis C. Nephron 1996;74:512–6.
114. Yasumura T, Nakajima H, Hamashima T, et al. Long-term outcome of recombinant INF treatment of chronic hepatitis C in kidney transplant recipients. Transplant Proc 1997;29:784–6.
115. Coroneos E, Petrusevska G, Varghese F, Truong L D. Focal segmental glomerulosclerosis with acute renal failure associated with interferon therapy. Am J Kidney Dis 1996;28:888–92.

18
CHRONIC HEPATITIS C AND PORPHYRIA CUTANEA TARDA

JOSEPH R. BLOOMER

The Liver Center
University of Alabama at Birmingham
Birmingham, Alabama

INTRODUCTION

The name porphyria cutanea tarda (PCT) was originally given by Waldenstrom in 1937 to a disorder in which patients typically presented in adulthood with cutaneous lesions in areas of sun exposure. (1) It is the most common porphyria with clinical expression in the United States, although the exact prevalence is unknown. More than 70% of cases are acquired or sporadic in type, without evidence of genetic transmission. (2) Approximately 20% of patients inherit the disorder in an autosomal dominant pattern, termed familial PCT. PCT has also been caused by toxic exposure to chlorinated organic compounds, the most notable being an outbreak in Turkey in the 1950s in people who ingested grain that had been treated with hexachlorobenzene. (2)

The predominant clinical manifestation is the development of bullous lesions and erosions following minor trauma to the skin (Fig. 1). (3) This is caused by increased skin fragility. Lesions occur in areas exposed to the sun, with the dorsal aspects of the hand being involved most frequently. However, acute photosensitivity is uncommon. When the blisters break, they heal slowly and leave atrophic scars and milia in areas of pigment change. Hypertrichosis occurs on the face. With chronic disease, the skin may take on a sclerodermoid appearance, and there may be scarring alopecia and chloracne. Recurrent abdominal pain is not a feature of PCT, and patients do not have acute porphyric attacks.

Skin lesions in PCT are caused by the photoactive properties of hydrophilic porphyrins, which accumulate in skin tissue. (4) This causes damage to the lysosomes in cells, and skin lesions are due in part to the release of proteolytic enzymes from the lysosomes. Complement activation and stimulation of collagen biosynthesis may also be important factors in the development of skin changes.

PCT is frequently associated with alcoholism, use of estrogens, and ingestion of iron-containing compounds. (2) These are considered to be factors that precipitate the disease in susceptible individuals. Since 1992, several studies have also demonstrated a striking increase in the prevalence of chronic hepatitis C (HCV) in patients with PCT (Table I). (5–16) This has been most notable in southern European countries, where HCV is found in more than 70% of patients with PCT. The prevalence in other countries is variable but is still increased compared to the general population.

TABLE I Prevalence of Chronic Hepatitis C (HCV) in Porphyria Cutanea Tarda (PCT)

Country of study	Patients with PCT	% with HCV	First author and reference
Italy	74	76	Fargion et al. (5)
Italy	23	91	Ferri et al. (6)
Spain	100	75	Herrero et al. (7)
Spain	62	62	DeCastro et al. (8)
France	124	21	Lamoril et al. (9)
Netherlands	38	18	Siersema et al. (10)
Germany	106	8	Stolzel et al. (11)
Ireland	20	10	Murphy et al. (12)
Australia	112	23	Gibson et al. (13)
New Zealand	25	0	Salmon et al. (14)
Japan	20	85	Tsukazaki et al. (15)
United States	70	56	Bonkovsky et al. (16)

In the United States, the prevalence of HCV has been shown to be 56% in 70 unselected patients with PCT. (16) The presence of HCV was documented by a positive test for hepatitis C antibody and RNA. In this study, the mean age of patients who had HCV was lower than those without HCV (45 years versus 51 years), and a higher proportion were male (82% versus 26%). The two groups did not differ in the type or severity of skin lesions, and the total urinary porphyrin excretion also did not differ (mean for the entire population was 4300 mcg for 24 hr). In 23% of the patients there was evidence of familial PCT. This occurred in both groups of patients. Alcohol use was also found in both groups but was significantly more frequent in patients with HCV (97% versus 50%). (16)

LIVER DISEASE IN PCT

Irrespective of whether HCV is present, patients with clinically overt PCT usually have biochemical and histological evidence of liver disease (Fig. 2). (17–19) Approximately two-thirds of the patients have an elevation of the serum transaminase level at the time diagnosis is made, commonly between two and four times the upper limit of normal. Liver biopsy specimens have red autofluorescence when exposed to ultraviolet light due to the accumulation of uroporphyrin, and the presence of needle-like cytoplasmic inclusions indicates that uroporphyrin crystals have formed. (17–19) Steatosis and iron overload are common, and iron stains demonstrate hemosiderosis in hepatocytes, Kupffer cells, and lobular necroinflammatory aggregates. Uroporphyrin crystals appear to colocalize with hemosiderin deposits, and transmission electron microscopy has shown the crystals to be surrounded by ferritin clusters. (20)

Liver biopsy specimens from patients with both PCT and HCV have also shown changes similar to those in specimens from patients with HCV alone. (8) These include lymphoid follicles, acidophilic bodies, portal inflammation, bile duct damage, periportal and lobular necrosis, and fibrosis. In one study, serum

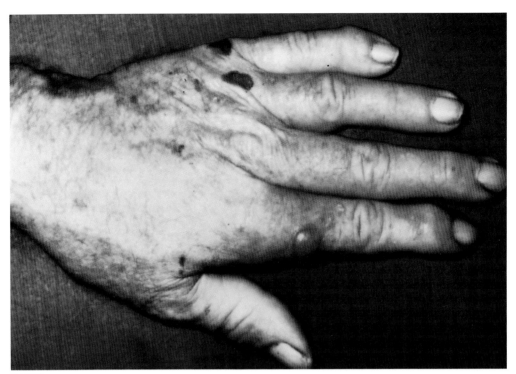

FIGURE 1   The cardinal clinical manifestation in PCT is the development of bullous lesions and erosions in sun-exposed areas of skin following minor trauma. The dorsal aspects of the hand are involved most frequently. Lesions occur because of increased skin fragility and heal slowly, leaving atrophic scars and milia. Reproduced from Rank et al., (3) by permission of the publisher.

THE LIVER IN PORPHYRIA CUTANEA TARDA

Fluorescence

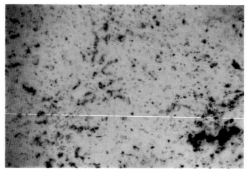

Siderosis

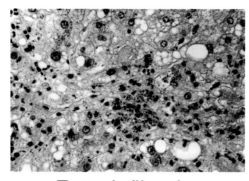

Fatty Infiltration

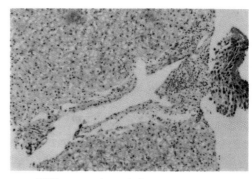

Fibrosis; Hepatoma

FIGURE 2 Histological abnormalities that commonly occur in liver biopsy specimens from patients with active PCT include red autofluorescence on exposure to ultraviolet light due to the presence of uroporphyrin, siderosis, and steatosis. Variable degrees of necrosis and fibrosis may be present, and hepatocellular carcinoma may develop in patients with long-standing untreated PCT. Liver biopsy specimens from patients with PCT who have HCV in addition show features consistent with HCV.

transaminase levels were significantly higher in patients with both HCV and PCT. Taken together with the liver biopsy findings in the patients, the authors concluded that HCV infection makes a significant contribution to liver disease activity in PCT when present. (8)

An autopsy study from Czechoslovakia in 1972 indicated that patients with long-standing PCT may progress to cirrhosis and develop hepatocellular carcinoma. (21) Because this study was carried out prior to the discovery of the hepatitis C virus, the role of HCV cannot be determined. A more recent study from the Netherlands found the incidence of hepatocellular carcinoma to be 13% in 38 patients with PCT who were followed for 2 to 18 years (mean 10 years). (10) Factors that appeared to be related to an increased risk of hepatocellular carcinoma were a long symptomatic period before the start of treatment and the presence of chronic active hepatitis and/or advanced fibrosis or cirrhosis in liver biopsy specimens. There was no difference in the prevalence of HCV in patients with hepatocellular carcinoma (20%) compared to those without (18%). Thus hepatocellular carcinoma may develop in the patient with PCT irrespective of whether HCV is contributing to the liver damage.

BIOCHEMICAL FEATURES OF PCT

The biochemical hallmark of PCT is the increased excretion of uroporphyrin (octacarboxylic porphyrin) and hepatocarboxylic porphyrin in urine. The diagnosis is made in the patient with clinically active disease by measuring the urine excretion of these compounds (typically greater than 1000 mcg/24 hr). The increased accumulation and excretion of these porphyrins reflect their hepatic overproduction due to an acquired (sporadic PCT) or genetic (familial PCT) deficiency of uroporphyrinogen decarboxylase (UROD) activity, the fifth enzyme in the heme biosynthetic pathway.

UROD catalyzes the conversion of uroprophyrinogen to coproporphyrinogen by the sequential removal of the carboxylic groups of the four acetic acid side chains (Fig. 3). The human enzyme has a molecular mass of approximately 46 kDa, and its crystal structure reveals a homodimer with one active site. (22) A single UROD gene is located in chromosome region 1p34 and contains 10 exons. The availability of UROD cDNA and genomic sequences has permitted mutations in PCT to be identified. Genetic heterogeneity (many different mutations) has been documented in familial PCT, (23) whereas no mutations have been found in patients with sporadic PCT. (24) The manner in which a deficiency of hepatic UROD develops in patients with sporadic PCT remains unclear. Currently, it is thought that an inhibitor of UROD is formed by the oxidation of uroporphyrinogen to nonporphyrin products. This is an iron-dependent process, which may be enhanced by the induction of cytochrome P450s (2) (Fig. 4). There may also be a cytochrome P450IA2-mediated increase in the oxidation rate of uroporphyrinogen to uroporphyrin, which cannot be used as a substrate by UROD. (2)

Hepatic UROD activity returns to normal in patients with sporadic PCT whose disease is placed in clinical remission by treatment with phlebotomy. (25, 26) During recovery there is a significant inverse correlation between hepatic

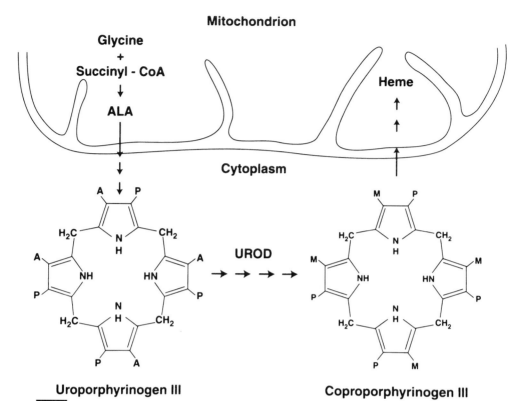

Uroporphyrinogen III   **Coproporphyrinogen III**

FIGURE 3   Liver tissue from a patient with active PCT has a deficiency of uroporphyrinogen decarboxylase (UROD) activity. UROD, the fifth enzyme in the heme biosynthetic pathway, catalyzes the conversion of uroporphyrinogen to coproporphyrinogen by the sequential removal of the carboxylic groups
of the four acetic acid side chains. As a consequence of this enzyme deficiency, uroporphyrin accumu-
lates and is excreted in excessive amounts in urine.

UROD activity and both hepatic and urine porphyrin levels. (26) These observations further establish the central role of deficient hepatic UROD activity
in the pathogenesis of PCT. Nevertheless, most patients with familial PCT, in
which there is a 50% deficiency of UROD activity in the liver and other heme-
forming tissues, are asymptomatic and do not excrete excessive amounts of uroporphyrin. Thus, the decrease in UROD activity must be pronounced, on the
order of 75%, before porphyrin formation is increased to a level that causes
clinical disease. (27) Precipitating factors appear to be necessary for this to occur, even in familial PCT.

   HCV by itself does not affect the level of hepatic UROD activity. Hepatic
UROD activity in patients with HCV who do not have PCT has not differed
from those in normal controls, and the activity in patients with both disorders
has not differed from those in patients with PCT alone. (26) There also appears
to be no correlation between the degree of liver damage and the level of hepatic
UROD activity in either patients with PCT or non-PCT control groups. (26) Patients with HCV alone may have increased excretion of coproporphyrin in the
urine. (28) However, this is a nonspecific condition termed secondary porphyri-

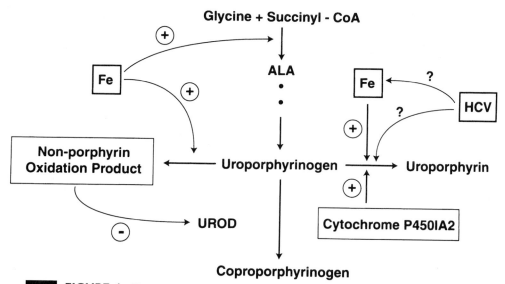

FIGURE 4 The heme biosynthetic pathway is illustrated through the step catalyzed by UROD in which uroporphyrinogen is converted to coproporphyrinogen. Hepatic UROD activity is decreased in active PCT. Iron may cause oxidation of uroporphyrinogen to uroporphyrin, which cannot be used as a substrate for UROD, and is a critical factor in the formation of a nonporphyrin oxidation product from uroporphyrinogen that may inhibit UROD. Iron may also cause an increased production of uroporphyrinogen by enhancing the first step in the heme biosynthetic pathway. The mechanism by which HCV may be a precipitating factor in PCT is unknown. Potentially this could occur through an effect on iron metabolism in the liver or by independently enhancing the oxidation of uroporphyrinogen to uroporphyrin. HCV by itself does not inhibit UROD activity.

nuria that occurs in a variety of hepatobiliary disorders. It probably reflects a diversion of some coproporphyrin excretion from bile to urine.

Iron metabolism is usually abnormal in patients with active PCT, as indicated by increased transferrin saturation and elevated ferritin levels, and the presence of hepatic hemosiderosis. (2,19) Thus, iron most likely has a key role in the pathogenesis of PCT. Iron may increase the production of uroporphyrin by enhancing the rate at which uroporphyrinogen is oxidized, by playing a critical role in the formation of the nonporphyrin inhibitor of hepatic UROD activity, and by affecting the initial step of hepatic heme biosynthesis (29) (Fig. 4).

Studies from Great Britain, the Netherlands, and Australia have shown that 40 to 50% of patients with PCT carry the C282Y mutation in the hemochromatosis gene, (30–32) with 10 to 20% being homozygous. In Italian patients the H63D mutation has been found to be increased. (33) A study from the United States has shown that 42% of patients with PCT carry the C282Y mutation (15% homozygous) and that 31% carry the H63D mutation (8% homozygous). (16) These reports establish an increased prevalence of the hemochromatosis gene mutations in patients with PCT and suggest a mechanism by which some patients have abnormal iron metabolism. Presumably, the C282Y mutation causes hepatic iron accumulation, which promotes the development of PCT in the susceptible individual. The relationship of the H63D mutation to PCT is less clear, as the Italian study found no relationship between the presence of the mutation and the iron status of the patients. The authors suggested that the H63D mutation might produce a subtle abnormality of iron metabolism which escapes detection by standard tests, and that the mutation might have a synergistic effect with HCV and/or alcohol intake to produce clinically manifest PCT. (33)

The C282Y mutation in the hemochromatosis gene and HCV are independent cofactors for PCT, at least in Australian patients. (32) In that study, the mean transferrin saturation and serum ferritin concentration were similar in PCT patients who were either homozygous or heterozygous for the C282Y mutation and greater in both groups than in healthy controls. HCV was present in seven of the patients (26%), none of whom carried the C282Y mutation. Nevertheless, patients with HCV also had elevated transferrin saturation and serum ferritin concentrations.

Elevated serum iron and/or ferritin levels are found in approximately 40% of patients with HCV. (34,35) However, increased hepatic iron is found in only 10 to 15% of patients when assessed by direct measurement, (34,35) although a French study found increased hepatic iron in 42% of patients when this was assessed histologically after Perls' staining. (36) In that study, the prevalence of the C282Y mutation did not differ in patients with or without iron overload (12% vs 9%). These findings suggest that the viral infection per se or other unidentified factors may promote abnormal iron metabolism in some patients with HCV.

ROLE OF HCV IN PCT

Several studies have shown that the prevalence of HCV is increased in patients with PCT. However, it is clear that HCV is neither necessary nor sufficient for the development of PCT. Most patients with HCV do not have clinical or biochemical evidence of PCT. The abnormality in porphyrin metabolism that usually occurs is secondary coproporphyrinuria, which is seen in a variety of hepatobiliary diseases and other disorders. Conversely, many patients with PCT do not have HCV. If there is an important role for HCV in the development of PCT, it is as a precipitating factor, as is the case with alcoholism and the use of estrogens. Central to the development of PCT is a metabolic predisposition to the hepatic overproduction of uroporphyrin, through a deficiency of UROD enzyme activity and other factors. It is against this background that HCV may be a precipitating factor.

As noted in the preceding section, HCV does not alter the activity of hepatic UROD, (26) which is deficient in patients with active PCT. HCV also does not appear to increase the rate of synthesis or degradation of hepatic heme. Thus, there is no evidence that HCV has a direct effect on the hepatic metabolism of heme, of which biosynthetic pathway the porphyrins are intermediates.

One possibility is that HCV promotes hepatic iron overload, which appears to be critical to the development of PCT in the susceptible individual. (2) Indeed, some patients with HCV have hepatic iron overload, (34–36) which is independent of mutations in the hemochromatosis gene. (32,36) Excess hepatic iron may promote the hepatic overproduction of uroporphyrin by several different mechanisms as noted in the preceding section. HCV may also cause stored iron to be released in a form that catalyzes the production of reactive oxygen species, which are critical to the inactivation of hepatic UROD. (2)

Another possibility is that HCV promotes oxidative stress in hepatocytes independent of iron. Evidence for increased hepatic lipid peroxidation in HCV has been presented, (37,38) but this has not been compared in patients with and without PCT. Plasma levels of ascorbic acid, which modulates chemically induced uroporphyrin accumulation in experimental animals, are low in patients with PCT, but the decrease is not related to HCV. (39)

There have been no consistent data indicating that specific viral parameters of HCV are associated with the development of PCT. PCT occurs with all genotypes of the virus, and in some studies the genotype pattern has been similar to that observed in nonporphyric HCV patients. (9,40) The development of PCT also does not correlate with the level of HCV RNA in blood. (41) Nevertheless, it is possible that the nonspecific effects of chronic viral illness are factors in the precipitation of PCT. An association has also been suggested between PCT and infection with the human immunodeficiency virus and hepatitis B virus. (42–44)

Finally, the increased prevalence of HCV in PCT could occur because alcoholism is associated with both conditions, providing a link between the two. Some studies have found there to be increased alcohol use in patients with concomitant PCT and HCV compared to either condition alone, (16) whereas others have not. (9)

MANAGEMENT OF PCT IN PATIENTS WITH HCV

In light of the association between the two disorders, any patient with PCT should be evaluated for HCV by testing for antibody to hepatitis C (Fig. 5). Likewise, any patient with HCV who has fragile skin with blisters and erosions in sun-exposed areas should be evaluated for PCT by measuring the urine excretion of uroporphyrin. Because a significant fraction of patients with PCT may carry hemochromatosis gene mutations, with 10 to 20% being homozygous, it is also reasonable to test for these mutations.

Patients with active PCT should be told to stop ingesting alcohol and iron-containing compounds, and the use of estrogens should be discouraged. Foods rich in iron should be restricted. They should protect themselves from the sun, wearing hats and long-sleeved shirts when it is necessary to be outdoors, and using opaque sunscreens. The wavelength of light that initiates skin damage in PCT (400 to 410 nm; soret band) is not filtered by window class, and precautions must also be taken when driving a car.

Because HCV may be a precipitating factor of PCT in the susceptible individual, it is tempting to start with therapy of HCV in patients in whom both disorders are present. Indeed, a few case reports have documented the remission of PCT in patients treated with interferon. (45,46) However, it is prudent to proceed first with phlebotomy therapy in order to remove excess hepatic iron, (47) particularly as there is evidence that hepatic iron overload reduces the response to interferon in HCV. (48) The liver typically contains an excess of 2–4 g of iron, and the amount of phlebotomy needed will therefore be on the

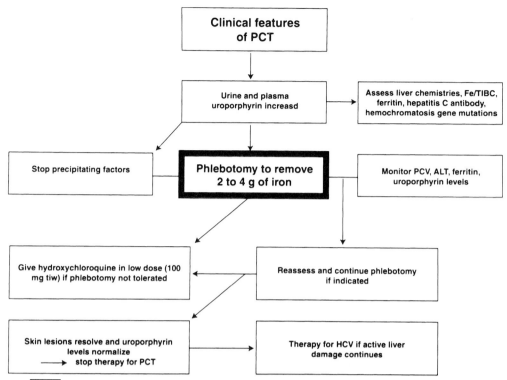

FIGURE 5 Scheme for evaluation and management of a patient with active PCT. In a patient with concomitant HCV, the present recommendation is to treat the patient first with phlebotomy to remove hepatic iron before proceeding with therapy for the HCV.

order of 4 liters of blood or greater. Phlebotomy is done until the patient develops mild anemia or the serum ferritin level and transferrin saturation indicate iron depletion has been achieved. The effect of phlebotomy on porphyrin metabolism can be assessed by measuring the plasma porphyrin level and/or the urine excretion of uroporphyrin. After phlebotomy is completed, urine excretion of uroporphyrin will continue to decrease toward normal, and more than 90% of the patients will have normal levels within 12 months. Clinically the patient will have a decrease in skin fagility and no longer develop bullous lesions. Pigment changes and hirsutism may take longer to clear, and sclerodermoid changes may not resolve for several years. If the patient is intolerant of phlebotomy, hydroxychloroquine can be tried at a low dose, starting at 100 mg thrice weekly. For the rare patient who has chronic renal failure requiring hemodialysis, administration of erythropoietin in combination with small volume phlebotomy may be successful in achieving remission. (49)

Once phlebotomy has been completed, consideration should be given to therapy for HCV, especially if there continues to be active hepatocellular damage as assessed by measurement of the serum ALT (alanine aminotransferase) level. Combination therapy with interferon and ribavirin is probably the regimen of choice, although ribavirin potentially may increase hepatic iron levels through its well-known complication of hemolysis, which increases enteral iron absorption. (50) Thus PCT may potentially be activated when combination therapy is used. Until data are available regarding this possibility, patients who are treated with combination therapy for HCV after PCT is in remission should be monitored closely by observing new skin lesions and by measuring plasma and/or urine uroporphyrin levels.

CONCLUSION

Several studies have shown an increased prevalence of HCV in patients with PCT, with variability depending on the country in which the study was performed. In the United States, the prevalence is on the order of 50–60%. However, HCV is neither necessary nor sufficient to cause PCT. Rather, it is probably one of several precipitating factors that may bring out the disease in the patient who has a metabolic predisposition to the hepatic overproduction of uroporphyrin. The mechanism by which HCV may precipitate PCT in the susceptible individual remains undetermined. One possibility is that HCV alters hepatic iron metabolism. Hepatic iron overload is common in patients with PCT, and iron appears to play a key role in the pathogenesis of this disorder. Other possibilities are nonspecific effects of the chronic viral illness or that HCV promotes oxidative stress in hepatocytes independent of iron. Specific viral parameters of HCV, such as genotype and viral level, do not appear to be important.

The initial management of the patient with PCT who has concomitant HCV should be phlebotomy in order to remove iron from the liver. Once phlebotomy has been completed, therapy of HCV may be considered. Because ribavirin causes hemolysis and therefore has the potential to cause relapse or worsen disease in the patient with PCT by altering iron metabolism, the patient should be monitored appropriately if combination therapy is used.

REFERENCES

1. Waldenström J. Studien über Porphyrie. Acta Med Scand 1937;82:1–254.
2. Elder G H. Porphyria cutanea tarda. Semin Liver Dis 1998;18:67–75.
3. Rank J M, Straka J G, Bloomer J R. Porphyria. In: Kaplowitz N, ed. Liver and biliary diseases. Baltimore, MD: Williams & Wilkins, 1996:535–48.
4. Poh-Fitzpatrick M B. Pathogenesis and treatment of photocutaneous manifestations of the porphyrias. Semin Liver Dis 1982;2:164–76.
5. Fargion S, Piperno A, Cappellini M D, et al. Hepatitis C virus and porphyria cutanea tarda: evidence of a strong association. Hepatology 1992;16:1322–6.
6. Ferri C, Baichi U, LaCivita L, et al. Hepatitis C virus-related autoimmunity in patients with porphyria cutanea tarda. Eur J Clin Invest 1993;23:851–5.
7. Herrero C, Vincente A, Bruguera M, et al. Is hepatitis C virus infection a trigger of porphyria cutanea tarda? Lancet 1993;341:788–9.
8. DeCastro M, Sanchez J, Herrera J F, et al. Hepatitis C virus antibodies and liver disease in patients with porphyria cutanea tarda. Hepatology 1993;17:551–7.
9. Lamoril J, Andant C, Bogard C, et al. Epidemiology of hepatitis C and G in sporadic and familial porphyria cutanea tarda. Hepatology 1998;27:848–52.
10. Siersema P D, ten Kate F J W, Mulder P G H, Wilson J H P. Hepatocellular carcinoma in porphyria cutanea tarda: frequency and factors related to its occurrence. Liver 1992;12:56–61.

11. Stolzel U, Kostler E, Koszka C, et al. Low prevalence of hepatitis C virus infection in porphyria cutanea tarda in Germany. Hepatology 1995;21:1500–3.

12. Murphy A, Dooley S, Hillary J B, Murphy G M. HCV infection in porphyria cutanea tarda. Lancet 1993;341:1534–5.

13. Gibson P R, Ratanaike S, Blake D, et al. Porphyria cutanea tarda and hepatitis C. Med J Aust 1995;162:54.

14. Salmon P, Oakley A, Rademaker M, et al. Hepatitis C virus infection and porphyria cutanea tarda in Australia/Asia. Arch Dermatol 1996;132:91.

15. Tsukazaki N, Watanabe M, Irifune H. Porphyria cutanea tarda and hepatitis C virus infection. Br J Dermatol 1998;138:1015–7.

16. Bonkovsky H L, Poh-Fitzpatrick M, Pimstone N, et al. Porphyria cutanea tarda, hepatitis C, and HFE gene mutations in North America in the U.S.A. Hepatology 1998;27:1661–9.

17. Cortes J M, Oliva H, Paradinas F J, Hernandez-Guio C. The pathology of the liver in porphyria cutanea tarda. Histopathology 1980;4:471–85.

18. Rank J M, Straka J G, Bloomer J R. Liver in disorders of porphyrin metabolism. J Gastroenterol Hepatol 1990;5:573–85.

19. Lefkowitch J H. Disorders of iron overload: pathology. In: Bloomer J R, Goodman Z D, Ishak K G, eds. Clinical and pathological correlations in liver disease: approaching the next millennium. Washington, DC: Armed Forces Institute of Pathology, 1998:296–302.

20. Siersema P D, Rademakers L H P M, Cleton M I, et al. The difference in liver pathology between sporadic and familial forms of porphyria cutanea tarda: The role of iron. J Hepatol 1995;23:259–67.

21. Kordac V. Frequency of occurrence of hepatocellular carcinoma in patients with porphyria cutanea tarda in long-term followup. Neoplasma 1972;19:135–9.

22. Whitby F G, Phillips J D, Kushner J P, Hill C P. Crystal structure of human uroporphyrinogen decarboxylase. EMBO J 1998;17:2463–71.

23. Mendez M, Sorkin L, Rossetti M V, et al. Familial porphyria cutanea tarda: characterization of seven novel uroporphyrinogen decarboxylase mutations and frequency of common hemochromatosis alleles. Am J Hum Genet 1998;63:1363–75.

24. Garey J R, Franklin K F, Brown D A, et al. Analysis of uroporphyrinogen decarboxylase complementary DNA's in sporadic porphyria cutanea tarda. Gastroenterology 1993;105:165–9.

25. Elder G H, Urquhart A J, De Salamanca R, et al. Immunoreactive uroporphyrinogen decarboxylase in the liver in porphyria cutanea tarda. Lancet 1985;1:229–32.

26. Moran M J, Fontanellas A, Brudieux E, et al. Hepatic uroporphyrinogen decarboxylase activity in porphyria cutanea tarda patients: the influence of virus C infection. Hepatology 1998;27:584–9.

27. Elder G H. Porphyria cutanea tarda: a multifactorial disease. Recent Adv Dermatol 1990;8:55–69.

28. Cribier B, Rey D, Uhl G, et al. Abnormal urinary coproporphyrin levels in patients infected by hepatitis C virus with or without human immunodeficiency virus. A study of 177 patients. Arch Dermatol 1996;132:1448–52.

29. Bonkovsky H L. Disorders of iron overload: Clinical. In: Bloomer J R, Goodman Z D, Ishak K G, eds. Clinical and pathological correlation in liver disease: approaching the next millennium. Washington, DC: Armed Forces Institute of Pathology, 1998:303–29.

30. Roberts A G, Whatley S D, Morgan R R, et al. Increased frequency of the hemochromatosis Cys282Tyr mutation in porphyria cutanea tarda. Lancet 1997;349:321–3.

31. Santos M, Clevers H C, Marx J J. Mutations of the hereditary hemochromatosis candidate gene HLA-H in porphyria cutanea tarda. N Engl J Med 1997;336:1327–8.

32. Stuart K A, Busfield F, Jazwinska E C, et al. The C282Y mutation in the hemochromatosis gene (HFE) and hepatitis C virus infection are independent cofactors for porphyria cutanea tarda in Austrialian patients. J Hepatol 1998;28:404–9.

33. Sampietro M, Piperno A, Lupica L, et al. High prevalence of the His63Asp HFE mutation in Italian patients with porphyria cutanea tarda. Hepatology 1998;27:181–4.

34. Di Bisceglie A M, Axiotis C A, Hoofnagle J H, Bacon B R. Measurements of iron status in patients with chronic hepatitis. Gastroenterology 1992;102:2108–13.

35. Riggio O, Montagnese F, Fiore P, et al. Iron overload in patients with chronic viral hepatitis: how common is it? Am J Gastroenterol 1997;92:1298–301.

36. Hezode C, Cazeneuve C, Coue O, et al. Hemochromatosis Cys 282Tyr mutation and liver iron overload in patients with chronic active hepatitis . Hepatology 1998;27:306.
37. Farinati R F, Cardin R, DeMaria N, et al. Iron storage, lipid peroxidation and glutathine turnover in chronic anti-HCV positive hepatitis. J Hepatol 1995;22:449–56.
38. Kageyama F, Kobayashi Y, Kawaski T, et al. Enhanced hepatic lipid peroxidation in chronic hepatitis C. Hepatology 1997;26:148A.
39. Sinclair P R, Gorman N, Shedlofsky S I, et al. Ascorbic acid deficiency in porphyria cutanea tarda. J Lab Clin Med 1997;130:197–201.
40. Sampietro M, Fracqnzani A L, Corbetta N, et al. HCV type 1b in patients with chronic liver diseases and porphyria cutanea tarda. Hepatology 1995;22:350A.
41. Cribier B, Petiau P, Keller F, et al. Porphyria cutanea tarda and hepatitis C viral infection: a clinical and virological study. Arch Dermatol 1995;131:801–4.
42. Blauvelt A, Harris H R, Hogan D J, et al. Porphyria cutanea tarda and human immunodeficiency virus infection. Int J Dermatol 1992;31:474–9.
43. Gregory N, DeLeo V A. Clinical manifestations of photosensitivity in patients with human immunodeficiency virus infection. Arch Dermatol 1994;130:630–3.
44. Navas S, Bosch O, Castillo J, et al. Porphyria cutanea tarda and hepatitis C and B viruses infection: a retrospective study. Hepatology 1995;21:279–84.
45. Siegel L B. Porphyria cutanea tarda remission. Ann Intern Med 1994;121:308–9.
46. Okano J, Horie Y, Kawasaki H, Kondo M. Interferon treatment of porphyria cutanea tarda associated with chronic hepatitis type C. Hepato-Gastroenterology 1997;44:525–8.
47. Epstein J H, Redeker A G. Porphyria cutanea tarda: a study of the effect of phlebotomy. N Engl J Med 1968;279:1301–5.
48. Bonkovsky H L, Banner B F, Rothman A L. Iron and chronic viral hepatitis. Hepatology 1997;25:759–68.
49. Anderson K E, Goeger D E, Carson R W, et al. Erythropoietin for the treatment of porphyria cutanea tarda in a patient on long-term hemodialysis. N Engl J Med 1990;322:315–7.
50. Di Bisceglie A M, Bacon B R, Kleiner D E, Hoofnagle J H. Increase in hepatic iron stores following prolonged therapy with ribavirin in patients with chronic hepatitis C. J Hepatol 1994;21:1109–12.

19

HEPATITIS C VIRUS INFECTION AND ALCOHOL

JAMES EVERHART * **AND DAVID HERION**[+]

Epidemiology and Clinical Trials Branch, Division of Digestive Diseases and Nutrition
[+]*Liver Diseases Section, National Institute of Diabetes and Digestive and Kidney Diseases, National Institutes of Health*
Bethesda, Maryland

INTRODUCTION

In developed countries, alcohol and hepatitis C virus (HCV) infection are the two leading causes of cirrhosis and end-stage liver disease. (1–4) In areas of the world where chronic hepatitis B infection is uncommon, cirrhosis of the liver would be rare if not for the effects of alcohol and HCV infection. Which is the leading cause depends primarily on the proportion of the population exposed to each factor. (5) For example, in a country such as Italy with high per capita alcohol consumption and alcoholism, alcohol may be found to be the leading cause. (2) Given the importance of these two risk factors for liver disease, it is not surprising that much attention has been focused on their relationship. (6–8) This chapter discusses the following issues: the characteristics of alcohol use and alcohol-related problems; alcohol consumption and the risk of liver injury with alcohol; the increased risk of HCV infection with increasing alcohol consumption; the association of viral measurements with alcohol consumption; the proportion of cirrhosis among alcoholics that can be attributed to HCV infection; the increased risk of chronic liver disease and hepatocellular carcinoma (HCC) with increasing alcohol consumption among persons infected with HCV; joint effects of HCV infection and alcohol in the pathogenesis of liver fibrosis; and the effects of alcohol on treatment outcomes in HCV infection.

CHARACTERISTICS OF ALCOHOL USE

Definition of Alcohol Dependence and Abuse

People who have psychosocial, legal, financial, and other behavioral problems in conjunction with alcohol use are generally described as alcoholic. Indeed, the majority of the damage and cost of excessive alcohol use is psychological and social rather than from organ toxicity. This damage predominates among persons who meet criteria for alcohol disorders as defined by the American Psychiatric Association in its diagnostic and statistical manual. *Alcohol dependence*

363

is a cluster of cognitive, behavioral, and physiologic symptoms, which indicate that a person continues to drink despite significant alcohol-related problems, including physical problems such as liver disease. *Alcohol abuse* is characterized as repetitive patterns of drinking in harmful situations with adverse consequences, including an impaired ability to fulfill responsibilities or negative effects on social and interpersonal functioning and health. Alcohol abuse is seen more often early in the drinking history of alcoholics. When criteria for dependence are met, this more serious diagnosis supersedes the diagnosis of abuse. Alcohol intoxication is an acute condition that is characterized by clinically significant maladaptive behavior or psychotic changes shortly after alcohol ingestion and is accompanied by physical signs such as slurred speech and unsteady gait. (9)

No alcohol-related psychiatric disorder is defined by the amount of alcohol consumed. There is, however, a strong relationship between dependence and both average daily intake and consumption of large amounts at one time. Results from the United States National Health Interview Survey found a risk of dependence of less than 3% with less than one drink per day, 12% at two to three drinks per day, and 50% with six or more drinks per day. (10) At each level of daily intake, persons who consumed five or more drinks on at least one occasion were at higher risk than persons who consumed fewer than five drinks. In fact, persons who reported an average of less than one drink per day but had drunk five or more drinks at one time had a higher prevalence of alcohol dependence than persons who averaged three or more drinks per day but never had five or more drinks. Similar results regarding alcohol dependence have been found in other national surveys. (11)

Quantification of Alcohol Intake

Alcohol consumption is usually quantified as the amount of ethanol consumed per day or week on a regular basis. This amount is determined from the percentage alcohol times the volume in milliliters times the density of ethanol (0.8 g/ml). Thus a standard bottle of wine with 12% alcohol by volume contains 67 g of ethanol (700 ml $\times$ 0.12 ml ethanol per ml $\times$ 0.8 g/ml). A typical glass of wine, drink with spirits, or standard bottle of beer contains 11–15 g of ethanol. A carefully obtained lifetime drinking history can reproducibly categorize persons by several categories of total amount of alcohol consumed. (12–15) Improvement in validity of the alcohol history has come with careful preparation of trained interviewers, one-on-one interviews, and use of an isolated room, plus a confidential, nonpressured interview in which alcohol history is the focus. Although a history can be obtained reproducibly, there is not much information on the accuracy of the history. Even among motivated subjects, recalled consumption has been reported to capture only 60–70% of consumption recorded from diaries. (16,17) Also, the degree of underreporting may increase with the amount of actual consumption. (16)

Most studies of risk of liver disease and drinking quantify intake by an average daily amount consumed, usually in grams. An extra dimension is provided by quantifying total lifetime consumption in kilograms of ethanol, but this measure is strongly associated with age and lacks the ease with which average daily consumption can be converted into the readily understandable number of drinks per day. Studies have not evaluated the risk of chronic liver disease in association with excess alcohol consumption related to binge drinking, which can be assessed according to the frequency of consumption of a large number of drinks, such as at least five. Just as binge drinking is strongly associated with alcohol dependence, the physiologic effects of intermittent high hepatic exposure to ethanol might be as important to the development of disease as a relatively constant high daily intake. To this point, none of the studies of HCV and alcohol have addressed binge drinking as a risk factor for liver disease.

ALCOHOL CONSUMPTION AND RISK OF LIVER INJURY

HCV infection and excessive alcohol consumption are independent risk factors for chronic liver disease, i.e., each appears to be able to cause liver injury without the other factor being present. (18) Knowledge of how alcohol causes liver injury and the risk and severity of liver disease among drinkers is critical for understanding the importance of drinking on the risk of liver disease in persons infected with HCV.

Most studies have indicated an increasing risk of cirrhosis with increasing levels of alcohol consumption. A meta-analysis of studies did not find a minimum level of alcohol consumption at which there was no increased risk. (19) At a daily consumption of 25 g, the meta-analysis derived at least a 40% increase in risk of cirrhosis over nondrinkers. However, the large majority of studies did not exclude infections with hepatitis C or other hepatic risk factors that are more common in drinkers. Studies that have examined the risk of cirrhosis after excluding patients with HCV and HBV have also found an increasing risk of cirrhosis with increasing alcohol consumption. However, results were not consistent regarding a minimum threshold for alcohol consumption and cirrhosis. A large hospital-based case-control study from Italy found that patients who regularly drank up to 50 g of alcohol per day had twice the risk of cirrhosis as abstainers, with a somewhat higher risk for women. (20) In contrast, two prospective population-based studies found the minimum daily consumption needed to cause chronic liver disease as roughly three drinks or 45 g or more per day in men and somewhat lower in women. (21,22)

It is uncertain what cofactors, such as binge drinking and type of beverage, might increase the risk of chronic liver disease. Other drinking patterns, such as nonmeal drinking, may also increase the risk of liver disease. (22) A number of studies have indicated that women are at a greater risk of alcohol-related chronic liver disease at the same level of consumption as men. (20)

ASSOCIATION OF DRINKING AND HCV INFECTION

Persons who drink have a higher prevalence of HCV infection than persons who do not drink and that prevalence increases with the amount drunk. (23) This relationship was examined in the third National Health and Nutrition Examination Survey, a population-based evaluation of health and nutritional status among the noninstitutionalized U.S. population conducted in the years 1988–1994. (24,25) One advantage of this survey was its complex sample design that allowed estimates for the U.S. population. Among the many measures incorporated into this study were a second-generation enzyme-linked immunoassay (EIA) for antibody to HCV (anti-HCV) with confirmation by dot-blot immunoassay (HCV MATRIX) (Abbott Laboratories), alcohol consumption history, and serum alanine aminotransferase (ALT) activity on 16,443 adult participants. Three hundred eighty-six of these participants were positive for anti-HCV, which equaled an estimated 3.7 million United States adults. Participants were categorized according to their self-reported usual drinking pattern: non-drinkers had fewer than 12 drinks in their lifetime, past drinkers had at least 12 drinks in their lifetime but fewer than 12 in the previous year, and current drinkers were categorized as consuming fewer than 7 drinks per week, 7–14 drinks per week, and more than 14 drinks per week. About 20% of persons seropositive for HCV reported drinking an average of more than 2 alcoholic drinks per day, which was nearly four times the proportion of uninfected persons (Table I). Expressed another way, over 7% of persons who reported more than 2 drinks per day were seropositive for HCV. Likewise, a disproportionate number of heavy drinkers and alcoholics have infection with HCV.

Similar results have been reported from other areas of the developed world. For example, of 201 consecutive patients admitted to a Swedish hospital for alcohol detoxification, 14% had evidence of infection. (26) Similarly, of 100 male patients consecutively admitted to a veterans administration alcoholic rehabilitation program, 23% had antibody to HCV. (27) In a direct comparison of persons without known viral hepatitis risk factors conducted at a New York Veterans Administration facility, anti-HCV seropositivity was present in 0 (out of 77 tested) nonalcoholic general medicine clinic patients, 3% (1/33) of alcoholic general medicine clinic patients, and 10% (9/87) of alcoholic patients admitted for detoxification. (28)

It is uncertain why heavy drinkers are more likely to be infected with HCV. It is possible that differences in alcohol consumption reflect other behavioral differences between HCV-infected and noninfected individuals. Heavy drink-

TABLE I   U.S. Prevalence among Adults of Antibody to Hepatitis C Virus (Anti-HCV) and Level of Alcohol Consumption during the Previous 12 Months in the Third National Health and Nutrition Examination Survey (1988–1994)

	Anti-HCV positive Million (% of total)	Anti-HCV negative Million (% of total)	Prevalence of anti-HCV[a]
Total Anti-HCV positive	3.7 (100%)	169.4 (100%)	2.1%
Drinking status			
Never	0.3 (8.9%)	24.2 (14.3%)	1.2%
Not current	1.1 (29.6%)	53.7 (31.7%)	2.0%
<7 per week	0.8 (22.3%)	63.8 (37.7%)	1.2%
7–14 per week	0.6 (15.3%)	16.2 (9.5%)	3.5%
>14 per week	0.8 (20.8%)	9.9 (5.8%)	7.4%
Unknown amount	0.1 (3.1%)	1.7 (1.0%)	5.6%

[a] Percentages affected by rounding.

ers, particularly alcoholics, are more likely to have used injection drugs and have had other exposures to the virus. (28–32) Attempts to account for such exposures may not be completely successful. (28) In addition to greater exposure, heavy drinkers also have a greater susceptibility to infection, (33–35) perhaps due to a reduction in immune function. (36–38) Whether suppression of immune function is due entirely to alcohol or is related to malnutrition is uncertain. Immune suppression related to alcohol consumption is discussed further in the following section.

ALCOHOL AND CHARACTERISTICS OF HCV INFECTION

The ability to recover from HCV infection, as defined by the presence of anti-HCV without HCV RNA, does not appear to be impaired significantly by heavy alcohol consumption. Thus the proportion of anti-HCV-positive problem drinkers who have detectable viremia is similar to that in other clinical populations, ranging between approximately 75 and 85%. (26,27,39–41) High levels of virus have been associated with alcohol consumption in most, (42–45) but not all, studies. (41,46) Furthermore, the correlation of ethanol consumption with viral levels accounts for little of the differences in levels. However, in some individuals, particularly alcohol abusers, virus levels do appear to fluctuate with periods of drinking and abstinence. (41,43) One study reported a decline in the viral level over 4 months corresponding to a marked reduction in alcohol intake from a mean of 73 to 11 g/day in 12 patients. (44) Genotype distribution appears to differ little between drinkers and nondrinkers, (45) although a higher proportion of nonserotypable strains has been reported among alcoholic patients. (47) A higher degree of HCV quasispecies complexity has been reported among alcoholics than in nonalcoholics with compensated cirrhosis. (48)

CIRRHOSIS ATTRIBUTABLE TO HCV INFECTION IN ALCOHOLICS

Calculation of Attributable Fraction of Cirrhosis Due to HCV and Alcohol

Because HCV infection is common in heavy drinkers, it can be assumed that some of the chronic liver disease attributed to excessive drinking in studies published before the availability of testing for anti-HCV was caused by HCV rather than alcohol. This effect became apparent shortly after the discovery of HCV. (49) For certain groups of heavy alcohol users it is possible to estimate the proportion of liver disease due to HCV infection by knowing the prevalence of HCV infection and the relative risk of liver disease in HCV-infected versus noninfected persons. The resulting attributable fraction is the proportion of liver disease in alcoholic patients that could have been prevented theoretically if infection with HCV were not present. (50) Ideally, incidence rates of disease for exposed and unexposed individuals are needed to calculate the attributable fraction (AF), but an estimate can be obtained from prevalence in cross-sectional studies:

$$AF = \frac{RR - 1}{[RR + (1/P_0) - 1]}, \tag{1}$$

where RR is the relative risk of cirrhosis, approximated here by the prevalence ratio of liver disease in alcoholics with HCV divided by the prevalence in those without HCV, and P_0 is the proportion of alcoholics with HCV. In a case-control study, where the proportion of the population with HCV is not known, the alternative formula is

$$AF = \frac{(OR - 1)P_1}{OR}, \tag{2}$$

where OR is the odds ratio and P_1 is the proportion with liver disease who have HCV.

Summary of Studies of Attributable Risk

Table II summarizes studies of liver disease in alcoholics in which the attributable fraction could be calculated. (26,27,39,51–54) The attributable fraction

TABLE II Proportion of Cirrhosis (Attributable Fraction) among Alcoholics Attributable to Hepatitis C Virus (HCV) Infection

Reference	Study description	Prevalence of chronic liver disease by HCV status	Percentage of study population infected with HCV	Fraction attributable to HCV infection
Befrits et al. (26)	201 chronic alcoholics admitted to Swedish hospital for detoxification	HCV+ = 20.8% HCV− = 7.0%	14.4%	22.1%
Parés et al. (51)	140 patients who consumed >80 g/day ethanol >5 years	HCV+ = 75% cirrhotic HCV− = 33% cirrhotic using EIA1 and RIBA confirmation	24.3%	23.6%
Coelho-Little et al. (27)	100 U.S. male veterans in alcoholic rehabilitation program	HCV+ = 73.9% HCV− = 29.9%	23.0%	25.3%
Quintela et al. (52)	180 alcoholic patients admitted to internal medicine department	HCV+ = 92% cirrhotic HCV− = 39% cirrhotic	7.8%	10.0%
		Cirrhosis odds ratio for HCV	Percentage of cases infected with HCV	
Mendenhall et al. (53)	350 male veteran cases with alcoholic liver disease and 126 alcoholic controls without liver disease	7.5 by EIA1 8.3 with RIBA confirmation	27% by EIA1 10% with RIBA confirmation	23.3% 8.8%
Shimizu et al. (54)	39 heavy drinkers with cirrhosis and 121 without liver disease	13.0 by RIBA	36% by RIBA	33.2%
Zignego et al. (39)	50 alcoholics with cirrhosis and 22 alcoholic controls without liver disease	5.6 by RIBA2	36%	30%

varied in these studies largely according to the prevalence of HCV in the population. Such variability could be seen in a large case-control study among U.S. veterans. (53) With the prevalence of HCV infection based on nonspecific first-generation EIA, the attributable fraction was 23%, but only 9% based on positive RIBA, which was present in less than 40% of EIA1-positive patients. Because of a high rate of false-positive results of anti-HCV by EIA1 in alcoholics, perhaps due to hyperglobulinemia, less credence should be attached to studies of the relationship of alcohol in which the diagnosis of HCV was based primarily or exclusively on EIA1. (55)

INTERACTION OF ALCOHOL AND HCV FOR RISK OF LIVER INJURY

Calculation of Interactions between Risk Factors for Liver Disease

It is important to know whether the cooccurrence alcohol and HCV infection increases the risk of liver disease more than would be expected from the effect of either alone. The potential joint effect of alcohol and HCV on liver disease can be conceptualized through the epidemiological concept of interaction. (56) The following table defines the risk of cirrhosis according to the presence of HCV and alcohol exposure. For simplicity, alcohol is considered at only two levels: abstinence and at a defined level of consumption. The risk of developing cirrhosis, R, is shown for the four combinations of the two risk factors:

	No HCV infection	HCV infection
No alcohol	R_{00}	R_{01}
Alcohol	R_{10}	R_{11}

In a simple biologic model for the joint effect of the two risk factors, the average risk will follow an additive pattern when there is no interaction. (56) This means that the sum of the differences of the risks given alcohol (R_{10}) and HCV (R_{01}) exposure alone and the risk in the absence of both exposures (R_{00}) will equal the difference in risk given both alcohol and HCV exposure (R_{11}) and the risk in the absence of both exposures (R_{00}). Additive risk corresponds to

$$(R_{11} - R_{00}) = (R_{01} - R_{00}) + (R_{10} - R_{00}) \tag{3}$$

or

$$R_{11} - R_{01} - R_{10} + R_{00} = 0. \tag{4}$$

If this sum is greater than 0, then additive interaction is considered present. In many studies, relative risks (RR) of exposed to unexposed are compared. Dividing by R_{00} gives

$$R_{11}/R_{00} - R_{01}/R_{00} - R_{10}/R_{00} + R_{00}/R_{00} = RR_{11} - RR_{01} - RR_{10} + 1 = 0. \tag{5}$$

Again, if this sum is greater than 0, then additive interaction is considered present. If a study is designed to exclude other known causes of liver disease, then R_{00} approaches 0 and interaction is present when

$$R_{11} - R_{01} - R_{10} > 0. \tag{6}$$

If the question of interest is whether a level of alcohol consumption that is insufficient to cause cirrhosis by itself ($R_{10} = 0$) will increase the risk of cirrhosis in HCV-infected individuals, then additive interaction is defined simply as

$$R_{11} - R_{01} > 0. \tag{7}$$

This same equation holds if $R_{00} = R_{10} > 0$. If relative risks are measured, then additive interaction is present when

$$RR_{11}/ RR_{01} > 1 \tag{8}$$

Considerations of Interactions between HCV and Alcohol

Hypothetical associations of HCV and alcohol with and without interactions are shown in Fig. 1. In uninfected persons, assuming that other known causes of cirrhosis have been excluded, the risk of cirrhosis (R_{00}) is 0 in abstainers, 1%

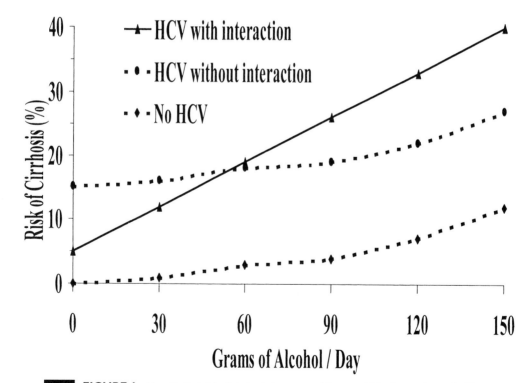

FIGURE 1   Hypothetical risk of cirrhosis (percentage) for no additive interaction and additive interaction of hepatitis C infection (HCV) and alcohol.

with 30 g per day, and then increases by 2–3% with each 30 g per day increase in alcohol (R_{10}). This projection is consistent with reports on risk of cirrhosis. (21,22) In the absence of an additive interaction, persons infected with HCV have a risk of cirrhosis that is 15% higher than uninfected persons, regardless of level of consumption. With an additive interaction, there would be a 5% risk difference for alcohol abstainers and increasing difference with increasing levels of consumption: 11% at 30 g per day, 16% at 60 g per day, and on up to 28% at the highest consumption level. The effects of abstinence on risk of cirrhosis would be markedly different for these two models. In the absence of an additive interaction, for the large majority of drinkers who consume less than 60 g per day (four to five drinks per day), abstinence would have little effect on the risk of cirrhosis in patients with HCV. The risk of cirrhosis would be lowered by no more than 3% from 18 to 15%. Without interaction, at least 33 HCV-infected patients would need to stop drinking to prevent one case of cirrhosis. However, with an additive interaction, the effect of abstinence on HCV-infected persons who drink 60 g per day would be to lower the risk by 14% from 19 to 5%. With this degree of additive interaction, only 7 patients infected with HCV would need to stop drinking to prevent one case of cirrhosis.

At this point, we do not have the information needed to determine which pattern in Fig. 1 is closer to the truth or whether the pattern may vary from population to population. No examination of this relationship has had a large enough sample size and been free from significant problems in variable measurements and study design. One problem common to most studies is not separating heavy from moderate drinkers. Without splitting these groups, one cannot exclude the possibility that an increased risk of liver disease could be due to heavy consumption. Another problem is more subtle. Most studies report histological findings from liver biopsies from centers known for the management of liver disease. It is possible that persons who drink and have severe HCV-related liver disease are more likely to be evaluated at such centers than persons with a similar degree of liver disease who do not drink. Persons who drink are also more likely to undergo evaluation of liver disease than nondrinkers. Such bias can be avoided only if the likelihood of identifying persons with significant liver disease is similar for drinkers and nondrinkers. The easiest way to do so is from a population-based study that includes persons with mild or minimal liver disease. However, because of the requirement of liver biopsy to ascertain the presence of cirrhosis, such studies are difficult to perform. Other potentially unbiased sources of patients could come from transfusion studies, blood donor studies, and hospital admissions or clinic patients screened for anti-HCV regardless of the presence of liver disease.

A question critical to both clinical practice and public health is whether the effect of alcohol consumption insufficient to cause liver disease by itself increases the risk of liver disease in patients with HCV infection. Another way to frame the issue is to ask: what is the safe limit of alcohol consumption in HCV infection? (7) This question is of central importance because the large majority of drinkers are light to moderate consumers. In the general U.S. population, 85% of drinkers reported consuming fewer than three drinks per day (10) and about 65% of drinkers with antibody to HCV consumed fewer than three drinks per day (Table I). Because the risk of liver disease is low in persons who consume this level of alcohol and do not have other causes of liver disease, an additive interaction would be shown if light or moderate alcohol consumers with HCV infection had higher rates of liver disease than nondrinkers infected with hepatitis C [Eq. (7)].

Interactions between HCV Infection and Moderate Alcohol Use

Two reports provided information relevant to the issue of cirrhosis and moderate alcohol consumption in persons infected with HCV. (57,58) Although neither found a greater risk of cirrhosis with moderate drinking relative to non or minimal drinking, the precision of the risk estimates was poor due to the small sample size of either exposed or unexposed groups (Table III). Another study found moderate to heavy consumption of 30–80 g per day to be associated with cirrhosis, but not higher levels. (59) Although no odds ratios were provided for this matched analysis, an unmatched analysis from data in the paper gives these odds ratios and 95% confidence intervals: 2.3 (1.0–5.8) for 30–80 g per day versus <30 g per day and 2.1 (0.74–6.4) for >80 g per day versus <30 g per day. A study of a small sample from a well-characterized cohort of Irish women who received immunoglobulin contaminated with HCV found a nonstatistically significant higher degree of fibrosis in women who drank, even though consumption averaged only 8 g per day. (60) Two other studies found an increasing fibrosis score associated with an increasing level of lifetime alcohol consumption, but it is impossible to interpret these results in terms of risk with moderate consumption. (45,61) In one of these studies, persons who were either moderate consumers (30–60 g/day) or heavy consumers (>60 g/day) were not more likely to have cirrhosis than nondrinkers and lighter drinkers. (61) In the other study, only 3 of 233 patients were not drinking at the time of diagnosis of HCV, too few for a meaningful comparison to drinkers. (45) A large French study suggested that fibrosis would progress more quickly among consumers of 1–49 g per day than among nondrinkers; however, the difference between these two groups was not statistically significant. (62) If these "rates" (which were actually the mean fibrosis score divided by an estimated duration of infection) were extrapolated to 20 years from time of infection, then the mean fibrosis score on a scale of 0 to 4 would be 2.5 in nondrinkers and 2.9 in moderate drinkers, a rather modest difference. One study examined the association of moderate consumption with the elevation of serum alanine aminotransferase activity (ALT), an imprecise surrogate for chronic liver disease. Japanese patients with HCV infection who consumed less than 46 g/day had higher mean ALT activity than nondrinkers. (63)

   To summarize, neither of the two studies that directly addressed the issue of cirrhosis with moderate alcohol consumption among patients with HCV found an increased risk. (57,58) Other studies examined different consumption levels or outcome measures other than cirrhosis. Thus an increased risk of cirrhosis with moderate alcohol consumption among patients with HCV has not been established, but the evidence in either direction is slim because of both small samples and flawed designs.

TABLE III Severity of Liver Disease According to Alcohol Consumption in Persons Infected with Hepatitis C Virus[a]

Reference	Study design	Ascertainment	N	Alcohol use	Outcome
Corrao et al. (57)	Case control of decompensated cirrhosis and hospitalized controls	Three Italian hospitals		Alcohol by nearest 25 g	Cirrhosis odds ratio and 95% CI
			18	0 g/day	1
			91	<50 g/day	1.01 (0.17–4.3)
			48	50–99 g/day	1.7 (0.24–10.0)
			79	≥ 100 g/day	3.8 (0.49–24.3)
Khan et al. (58)	Cross-sectional	Patients with HCV at Australian referral center		Past alcohol intake	Cirrhosis (%)
			186	<10 g/day	23
			78	10–40 g/day	15
			43	41–80 g/day	11
			69	81–120 g/day	16+
			35	>120 g/day	23+
					+p NS, but <0.001 for degree of fibrosis on multivariate analysis
Serfaty et al. (58)	Matched case control	French referral center of patients with HCV	84	Cirrhotics	Matched odds ratio of cirrhosis for alcohol intake (relative to <30 g/day)
			84	Non-cirrhotics matched for age, sex, mode of infection, HCV duration	30–80 g/day: $p < 0.05$
					>80 g/day: $p > 0.05$
Sachithanandan et al. (60)	Cross-sectional, cohort derived	Irish women Immune globulin recipients with liver disease			Inflammation (0–18)
			16	Non/minimal drinkers (8 g/day)	3
			12		5.5 ($p = 0.07$)
					Fibrosis (0–4)
			16	Non/minimal drinkers (8 g/day)	0.3
			12		1.5 ($p = 0.08$)
Ostapowicz et al. (61)	Cross-sectional	Australian referral center		Mean lifetime total alcohol consumption (kg)	Fibrosis score
			15	101	0
			119	200	1
			35	185	2
			11	243	3
			50	289 ($p = 0.02$ vs other groups)	Cirrhosis
Pessione et al. (45)	Cross-sectional	French referral center of patients with HCV		Mean alcohol consumption prior to diagnosis	Fibrosis score
			94	16 g/day	0
			100	22.1 g/day	1
			28	27.0 g/day	3
			9	34.8 g/day	Cirrhosis
				$p < 0.001$ trend in mean consumption	

(continued)

TABLE III—_Continued_

Reference	Study design	Ascertainment	N	Alcohol use	Outcome
Poynard et al. (62)	Cross-sectional	Referred for biopsy, France	598	0	Fibrosis progression/ year 0.12 (0.11–0.14)
			330	1–49 g/day	0.14 (0.12–0.16)
			111	≥50 g/day	0.17 (0.13–0.17)
Katakami et al. (63)	Cross-sectional	Screening study in high-risk area for HCC Kobe, Japan	90	Nondrinker	Mean ALT (U/liter) 44.4
			63	<46 g/day	72.6 ($p < 0.0001$)
			10	≥46 g/day	59.2 ($p = 0.91$)
Shen et al. (65)	Cross-sectional	Natives of Taiwan	10	Nonalcoholic	Elevated ALT or AST 10.0%
			16	Alcoholic	37.5%
Wiley et al. (67)	Cross-sectional	Patients under-going liver biopsy	45	>5 years <40–60 g/day[b]	Cirrhosis after ≥ 20 years of HCV 33%
			40	≥40–60 g/day	70% ($p < 0.01$)
Mathurin et al. (68)	Case Control	Two French re-ferral centers of patients with HCV	1	Cases <50 g/day	Odds ratio for severe fibrosis
			3	>50 g/day	27.5 (1.7–1468),
			55	Controls <50 g/day	$p = 0.007$
			6	>50 g/day	
Frieden et al. (69)	Case control	Hospitalized patients in inner city New York	6	Cases with HCV[c] <80 g/day	Odds ratio for chronic liver disease
			24	≥80 g/day	2.5 (0.75–9.5)
			15	Controls <80 g/day	
			24	≥80 g/day	
Strasser (31)	Cross-sectional	Biopsied pa-tients at Australian referral center	<180[d]	<60 g/day	Percentage with cirrhosis 55%
			<162	≥60 g/day	39% ($p = 0.08$)
Hourigan et al. (71)	Cross-sectional	Referral for biopsy and treatment in Brisbane, Australia		Past alcohol consumption Cases	Prevalence ratio for severe fibrosis 1.25 (0.71–2.21)
			20	≤50 g/day	
			16	>50 g/day	
			52	Controls ≤50 g/day	
			56	>50 g/day	
Pol et al. (72)	Cross-sectional	Anti-HCV-positive in-jection drug users in Paris, France	97	Anti-HIV negative ≤80 g/day	Prevalence of cirrhosis 11.3%
			53	>80 g/day	24.5% ($p = 0.04$)
			37	Anti-HIV positive ≤80 g/day	29.7%
			23	>80 g/day	30.4% ($p = 0.95$)

(_continued_)

■ **TABLE III—Continued**

Reference	Study design	Ascertainment	N	Alcohol use	Outcome
Shiomi et al. (73)	Nonconcurrent prospective	Laparascopic diagnosis of cirrhosis at Japanese hospital[c]	87 46	<80 g/day ≥80 g/day	5-year mortality 22% 55% ($p < 0.01$)
Smith et al. (64)	Nonconcurrent prospective	"Look back" of blood donors and recipients Newcastle, UK	19 5 19 5	≤28 units/week >28 units/week ≤28 units/week >28 units/week	Inflammation (0–18) 3.2 6.4 ($p = 0.002$) Fibrosis (0–6) 0.9 4.2 ($p = 0.001$)
Healey et al. (74)	Cross-sectional	Patients with HCV at English referral center	19 23	Average units of alcohol per week 6.4 17.8 ($p = 0.01$)	AST activity Persistently normal Elevated
Shev et al. (75)	Nonconcurrent prospective	Patients with HCV at Swedish referral center	14 6	Nondrinkers Occasional heavy drinkers (≥70 g/day)	Mean HAI score change in 9–16 years 1.3 4.6 ($p < 0.05$)
Cromie et al. (44)	Cross-sectional and prospective (4.4 months)	Referral for interferon treatment in Melbourne, Australia	22 23 23	Baseline ≤10 g/day 71 g/day (range = 30–100 g/day) Follow-up 71 g/day → 13 g/day (range = 0–50 g/day)	Mean ALT activity (U/liter) 150 269 ($p = 0.008$) 269 → 144 ($p = 0.002$)

[a] HAI, hepatitis activity index; AST, aspartate aminotransferase; ALT, alanine aminotransferase.
[b] 40 g/day in women, 60 g/day in men
[c] Diagnosis of HCV based on first-generation EIA.
[d] There were 342 in the total study of whom 152 were biopsied, but breakdown was not given by alcohol consumption.

Studies Needed to Demonstrate Effects of Moderate Alcohol Intake on HCV Infection

What sort of study would best address this critical issue of the effects of moderate alcohol use in hepatitis C? Optimal would be a cross-sectional study in a sample of patients with HCV infection that is chosen without respect to the presence of liver disease for the reasons described earlier. The population could be truly population based, but could also be participants of a defined health program, such as a health maintenance organization or the U.S. Veterans Affairs outpatient clinics. Best would be a population in whom the duration of infection can be ascertained, such as patients who were diagnosed with HCV after exposure to infective blood products. (60,64) The prevalence of cirrhosis or other defined severe liver injury would be compared across alcohol consumption levels, obtained though a carefully performed, standardized interview performed without regard to the presence of liver disease. A second approach to this issue would be a cohort study such as in patients with mild liver disease who are followed for a number of years for worsening of fibrosis. An example would be blood donors determined to be infected with HCV who are followed with periodic liver biopsy. Such a study is now difficult to conduct because alcohol consumption would likely decline markedly after diagnosis and many patients, particularly those with more severe liver disease, would be treated for hepatitis C. A third approach would be a case-control study of persons with HCV infection that would compare alcohol consumption between cases with cirrhosis to controls without significant liver disease. Simple in concept, such a study is difficult to design and execute because the controls should be chosen from the same reference population as the cases and a large number of controls would need to be screened to identify enough with HCV. This is roughly the approach taken by Corrao and colleagues, (57) in which a total of 462 hospitalized cases with decompensated cirrhosis and 651 hospitalized controls were evaluated for HCV and alcohol consumption at three centers. Only 27 controls were positive for HCV and only 3 of these were nondrinkers. Although it will be difficult to establish a precise relationship between moderate consumption and cirrhosis in HCV-infected persons, there is considerable current and ongoing interest in the issue of interaction of alcohol and HCV. For example, all but one of the studies cited in Table III have been published since 1995.

A second issue involving interaction is whether the presence of heavy alcohol consumption in patients with HCV increases the risk of cirrhosis more than would be expected from the presence of either alone. This issue is of less clinical and public health importance than moderate consumption and HCV infection. Consumption of alcohol in a quantity sufficient to increase the risk of serious liver disease substantially should be discouraged vigorously regardless of the presence of HCV or other risk factors for liver disease. It is also more difficult to determine the presence of additive interaction of HCV with heavy alcohol consumption than with moderate consumption. With moderate consumption, the risk in uninfected individuals can be assumed to be near 0, which means the risks in infected individuals only need to be known [Eqs. (7) and (8)]. However, the precision of estimating the interaction of HCV and heavy alcohol depends on the measurement of at least three risks: the risk in persons exposed to HCV alone, to alcohol alone, and to both together. A fourth measurement of cirrhosis risk in nondrinkers without HCV would also be needed if this risk was found to be nonnegligible. Bias and imprecision in measurement in one or more of these statistics weaken any judgment regarding interaction, even in large data sets. (56) Because all studies suffer from inaccuracies in measuring aspects of exposure to HCV and alcohol, claims of interaction should be greeted skeptically. Nevertheless, several studies have suggested either the presence (57,65) or the absence (66) of interaction

Effects of High Alcohol Consumption on HCV Infection

Many studies have addressed the issue of high alcohol consumption, HCV, and increased risk of liver disease (Table III). The same studies that found no association of cirrhosis with moderate consumption found a high risk of cirrhosis with greater consumption, although the estimates of the increased risk were not precise. (57,58) Studies that did not establish an upper limit of consumption generally found an increased risk of cirrhosis or chronic liver disease relative to lower consumption. (67–69) Oddly, one study from Australia found a nonsignificantly *lower* prevalence of cirrhosis in persons who drank at least 60 g/day than persons who drank less. (70) Another Australian study found no association with consumption of at least 50 g/day. (71) A study of anti-HCV-positive injection drug users found that drinking more than 80 g/day increased the risk of cirrhosis in patients not infected with human immunodeficiency virus, but had no effect on cirrhosis risk in coinfected patients. (72) A prospective study of patients with cirrhosis found that mortality was much worse in patients infected with HCV who drank more than 80 g/day than in infected patients who drank less. (73)

Studies of hepatic fibrosis, similar to the studies of cirrhosis, have also found more severe degrees of fibrosis correlated with greater alcohol consumption in HCV-infected patients. (45,61,62,64) Similarly, inflammation and serum aminotransferase activities were usually higher among infected individuals who drank the most, (64,74,75) although this was not always the case. (63) One study found that ALT activities fell by nearly half after patients reduced their alcohol consumption from a mean of 70 to 13 g/day. (44) Additional reports of a relationship of HCV, alcohol, and liver disease that did not provide enough information to quantify an effect were not included in Table III. (66,76–80) A study of individual histological features found that patients with HCV infection and alcoholic liver disease had more pericellular fibrosis and a somewhat greater fatty change, but few other differences, when compared with persons with HCV alone. (81) In contrast, several features of liver injury have appeared more pronounced in persons with HCV infection and alcoholic liver disease than in persons with alcoholic liver disease alone. (32,81,82)

The issue of liver injury and HCV could be addressed indirectly in the third National Health and Nutrition Examination Survey, which, as noted earlier, determined HCV status using a second-generation EIA with confirmatory testing, alcohol consumption history, and serum ALT activity. The prevalence of elevated ALT did vary with alcohol consumption, but not in a clearly explicable pattern. The lightest drinkers had the highest prevalence of abnormal ALT, whereas there was little difference in the prevalence between nondrinkers and the heaviest drinkers (Table IV). Factors that appeared to be related to a higher prevalence of ALT were younger age, non-Hispanic black and Mexican American ethnicity, not smoking, higher body mass index, and past hepatitis B infection (presence of antibody to hepatitis B core antigen in the absence of hepatitis B surface antigen). On multivariate logistic regression analysis, no clear association was seen with alcohol consumption (Table V). The only features that were associated significantly with elevated ALT ($p < 0.05$) were increasing overweight and never having smoked. Thus we are reminded that not only has moderate alcohol consumption not been shown unequivocally to increase the risk of liver injury in HCV infection, but that we should not neglect to look for other factors that may influence disease progression, including common conditions such as obesity. (71,83)

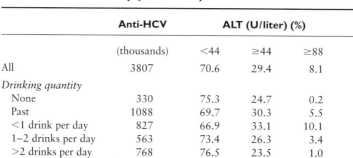

TABLE IV   Alanine Aminotransferase Activity (ALT) among Anti-HCV-Positive Participants in the Third U.S. National Health and Examination Survey (1988–1994)

	Anti-HCV	ALT (U/liter) (%)		
	(thousands)	<44	≥44	≥88
All	3807	70.6	29.4	8.1
Drinking quantity				
None	330	75.3	24.7	0.2
Past	1088	69.7	30.3	5.5
<1 drink per day	827	66.9	33.1	10.1
1–2 drinks per day	563	73.4	26.3	3.4
>2 drinks per day	768	76.5	23.5	1.0
Unknown	113	82.4	17.6	3.5

Basis of Advice Regarding Moderate Alcohol Use in Patients with Hepatitis C

Some physicians might argue that it is prudent for patients with HCV infection to remain abstinent from alcohol, even in the absence of evidence that moderate consumption increases injury. (84) Implicit in this view is that alcohol can only be harmful to infected patients. However, ample evidence indicates that moderate alcohol consumption can have beneficial health effects. Numerous studies have shown that moderate consumption is associated with a reduction of both overall morbidity and mortality. (85–87) The reduction in mortality results from decreased deaths from coronary heart disease, which has been estimated to be at about 25% with consumption of one to two drinks per day. (88,89) Because coronary heart disease is the leading cause of death in Western countries (about 30% of deaths in the United States), (90) the potential public health benefit of moderate alcohol consumption is not trivial. If such cardiovascular disease benefits of drinking were also found to apply to patients with HCV infection, then it would become imperative to determine whether drinking at a level that is beneficial to the heart also increases the risk of cirrhosis.

TABLE V   Odds Ratios for Abnormal Alanine Aminotransferase Activity (≥44 U/liter) among Anti-HCV-Positive Participants in the Third U.S. National Health and Examination Survey (1988–1994)[a]

Drinking quantity	Odds ratio	95% confidence interval	p value
None/past	1	—	—
<1 drink per day	1.95	0.57–6.71	0.28
1–2 drinks per day	1.55	0.40–6.06	0.52
>2 drinks per day	0.93	0.32–2.74	0.90

[a] Controlled for age, sex, ethnicity, smoking, body mass index, and past evidence of hepatitis B infection by antibody to hepatitis B core antigen by multivariate logistic regression.

ALCOHOL CONSUMPTION AND HEPATOCELLULAR CARCINOMA IN HCV-INFECTED PERSONS

HCV infection and alcoholic liver disease are both risk factors for HCC, although the risk is considerably higher and more consistent with hepatitis C. (79, 91–95) With the exception of areas of the world in which hepatitis B is endemic, it is uncommon to find HCC in the absence of cirrhosis. (96,97) For example, a case-control study from Greece found that cases with HCC were more likely than controls without liver disease to be positive for hepatitis B surface antigen (HBsAg) and anti-HCV positive and heavy alcohol users, but when compared with controls with liver cirrhosis, HBsAg was the only factor associated with HCC. (98) Similarly, an Italian multicenter study found that relative to patients without hepatic disease, alcohol abuse was found more commonly in patients with HCC and cirrhosis but not in patients with HCC without cirrhosis. (99) Thus a combined effect of HCV and alcohol might act largely through an increased risk of cirrhosis. Among cirrhotic patients who are heavy consumers of alcohol, the presence of HCV infection appears to increase the risk of HCC. (1,100–102) However, it is uncertain whether alcohol consumption may increase the risk of HCC further in HCV-related cirrhosis. Of the studies that have examined the joint relationship of alcohol consumption and HCV for risk of HCC among persons with cirrhosis, two found a statistically significant positive association, (1,103) two a statistically nonsignificant positive association, (100, 104) and one a nonsignificant protective effect (101) (Table VI). None of these studies examined the risk of HCC with moderate consumption . Other studies that compared HCC with noncirrhotic liver disease or to controls without liver disease also found a modest effect of alcohol. (79,94,105) One additional study of this type found independent associations for HCV and alcohol abuse without interaction. (98)

JOINT EFFECTS OF HCV INFECTION AND ALCOHOL ON THE PATHOGENESIS OF FIBROSIS

For a biologically significant interaction to occur, alcohol and HCV would need to harm the liver through a common pathway. In animal models of alcohol-related fibrosis, numerous factors, including cytokines, such as TNF-α, and long chain fatty acid imbalances (106–108) and cellular responses, such as Kupffer cells to endotoxin, (109) are thought to play important roles. It is unknown whether these factors may exacerbate HCV-related fibrosis in which the immune response is thought to play a primary role.

While a host of immune changes (lymphocyte subpopulations, cytokines, immune responses, etc.) may be seen in heavy drinkers once liver disease is established, there are relatively few, major changes seen in either nonproblematic drinkers or heavy drinkers without liver disease. Perhaps one relevant issue for an interaction between alcohol and HCV may be whether Th1/Th2 lymphocyte differentiation is altered in the HCV-directed immune response in alcohol drinkers (heavy or otherwise). There are rationales for this idea. In experimental animals treated chronically with alcohol, lymphocyte (thymocyte and B cell)

TABLE VI   Hepatocellular Carcinoma (HCC) in Persons Infected with Hepatitis C Virus (HCV) According to Alcohol Consumption

Reference	Study design	Ascertainment	N	Alcohol Use	Outcome
De Bac et al. (1)	Cross-sectional	Cirrhotic patients at 21 Italian centers		With HCC	HCC prevalence ratio (95% CI)
			90	<60–80 g/day[a]	1.55 (1.15–2.10),
			62	>60–80 g/day	$p = 0.005$
				Without HCC	
			783	<60–80 g/day	
			325	>60–80 g/day	
Chiba et al. (103)	Cross-sectional	Hospitalized Japanese patients with HCV and cirrhosis		With HCC	HCC odds ratio (95% CI)
			58	<80 g/day	3.3 (1.5–7.3)
			70	>80 g/day	
				Without HCC	
			63	<80 g/day	
			13	>80 g/day	
Miyakawa et al. (100)	3-year prospective	Japanese patients with HCV and cirrhosis			Cumulative incidence of HCC
			176	≤72 g/day	23%
			81	>72 g/day	28% ($p > 0.05$)
Suzuki et al. (104)	Cross-sectional	Hospitalized Japanese patients with HCV and cirrhosis		With HCC	HCC odds ratio (95% CI)
			16	>130 g/day	2.0 (0.82–4.9)
			20	Nondrinkers	
				without HCC	
			23	>130 g/day	
			58	Nondrinkers	
Simonetti et al. (101)	Matched case-control	Hospitalized cases with HCC and cirrhosis controls without HCC		Cases HCV positive[b]	HCC odds ratio (95% CI) 0.55 (0.28–1.08)
			96	≤80 g/day	
			38	>80 g/day	
				Controls HCV positive	
			36	≤80 g/day	
			26	>80 g/day	
Donato et al. (94)	Case-control	Two Italian hospitals		Cases HCV positive	HCC odds ratio (95% CI) 1.8 (0.46–8.3), $p = 0.37$
			41	≤80 g/day	
			24	>80 g/day	
				Controls HCV positive	
			12	≤80 g/day	
			4	>80 g/day	
Ikeda et al. (79)	Nonconcurrent prospective cohort	1500 Japanese patients with chronic hepatitis		Lifetime alcohol	Multivariate hazard rate ratio
			1228	<500 kg	1.96 (1.06–3.62),
			272	≥500 kg	$p = 0.03$
Noda et al. (105)	Cross-sectional	Transfused patients with HCV			Mean years to cancer occurrence
			67	<46 g/day	31 ± 9 years
			18	≥46 g/day	26 ± 6 years ($p < 0.05$)

[a] 60 g/day for women; 80 g/day for men.
[b] Diagnosis of HCV based on first-generation EIA.

populations are depleted and T-cell population distributions are also abnormal, suggesting impaired lymphocyte maturation and compartmentalization. (110, 111) Furthermore, alcohol-fed mice have an impaired ability to generate cellular immune and cytokine responses after DNA vaccination with HCV core- and NS5A-expressing plasmids, with restoration of immunity when coimmunized with IL-2 or GM/CSF expressing DNA plasmids. (112) In humans, lymphocyte populations appear to be reduced in alcoholic liver disease, but less marked changes are seen in alcohol abusers without liver disease. However, the latter group may still have abnormalities of lymphocyte cell populations, and cell surface marker studies indicate that circulating lymphocytes, particularly $CD8^+$ cells, are in a state of persistent activation. (36) The significance of these studies, especially the specificity of this activation, remains to be determined. Cytokine profiles in alcoholics and alcohol-fed animals indicate a shift toward a Th2 response, which may be influenced by abnormalities of the innate immune system. (113) In this regard, glutathione depletion in lymphocytes has been demonstrated to affect the balance of Th1 vs Th2 responses. (114) Interestingly, glutathione depletion has been demonstrated in several models of alcohol consumption, (115,116) and its reduction in lymphocytes has been correlated with thymocyte apoptosis, (117) but whether such a mechanism may account for immune dysfunction in humans is speculative. Finally, abnormalities of cytokine production, particularly IFN-γ production, can also be seen after brief acute exposures to moderate doses of ethanol in healthy subjects. (118,119)

Although the preceding paragraph points to theoretical mechanisms of interaction, it is difficult to meaningfully ascribe a mechanism of worsened fibrosis in HCV to contributory factors related to alcohol consumption. Regardless of any interaction that may occur between HCV and alcohol, the final common pathway to hepatic fibrosis of most causes is thought to ultimately depend on stellate cell activation. (120) How this cell may integrate and respond to the two fibrogenic risk factors remains to be elucidated.

EFFECT OF ALCOHOL ON HCV INFECTION TREATMENT OUTCOME

Patients with HCV infection who drink heavily have largely been excluded from clinical trials, so there is limited evidence as to how alcohol affects the response to treatment. Several reports from Japan have suggested that alcohol consumption worsens the response to treatment with interferon-α. (42,46,121–123) Reasons for this low response rate are not clear. High levels of virus are associated with a low response rate, but reports are inconsistent regarding the association of alcohol consumption on HCV levels and how this might affect response. (42, 43,46) Heavy drinkers with HCV infection tend to have high levels of hepatic iron, and hepatic iron is associated with a poorer response to therapy. (124, 125) The immunosuppressive effects of alcohol noted earlier may diminish the effectiveness of interferons, which are themselves immune modulators. Thus alcoholics have been reported to have a diminished physiological response to administered interferon. (126) Heavy alcohol consumers may not be as compliant with treatment or may have more side effects, resulting in curtailed treatment, but these possibilities have not been fully examined. There is also concern—

based on reasonable caution but little evidence—that heavy drinkers may have an increased risk of psychiatric side effects from interferon treatment, particularly anxiety and mood disorders. Much more information is needed on the effect of drinking on treatment outcome if only because a disproportionate number of infected persons drink.

HCV and alcohol-related end-stage liver disease are the two leading indications for liver transplantation, accounting for nearly half of all liver transplantations. (127) More than 7% of these patients carry both diagnoses. Nearly all programs require that alcoholics abstain from drinking for at least several months prior to transplantation. (128) For this and other reasons, perhaps related to the transplant experience itself, a relapse to heavy drinking after transplantation occurs in fewer than 20% of patients. (129) It is not known if the rate of drinking relapse differs in patients who are also infected with HCV. In the United States, 3-year graft survival is similar for patients with alcoholic liver disease and HCV (63.2%) and patients with HCV alone (65.4%) and patient survival is also similar. (127) Because greater graft loss and mortality would be expected later, studies with longer follow-up are needed. When cirrhosis does recur in patients with pretransplant alcoholic liver disease and HCV, it is generally more characteristic of HCV than alcohol. (130)

There is no evidence that alcohol increases the risk of acute liver failure in HCV, but case reports do suggest a risk of analgesic-induced hepatic failure in persons with HCV who drink heavily. (131)

CONCLUSION

Because alcohol and hepatitis C virus infection are the leading causes of chronic liver disease in most of the developed world, much interest has focused on the relationship of these two factors. Although alcohol use can be expressed in a number of ways, it is average daily consumption that has been applied most often to studies of liver disease. Persons who drink, particularly who drink excessively, are more likely to be infected with HCV, probably because of increased exposure to the virus rather than increased susceptibility. A substantial proportion of cirrhosis among alcoholics can actually be attributed to HCV infection. Alcohol consumption at a level that can cause cirrhosis also increases the risk of cirrhosis in persons infected with HCV. It is unclear whether there is an interaction between these two factors such that the risk of cirrhosis is increased disproportional to the amount of alcohol consumed in patients with chronic hepatitis C. In addition, it is unknown whether there is a safe level of drinking in persons with hepatitis C. Heavy alcohol consumption may increase the risk of hepatocellular carcinoma, but much of this risk can be attributed to an increased risk of cirrhosis. Plausible pathophysiological interactions, mostly of an immunological basis, have been proposed for alcohol and HCV infection, although they are inadequate for ascribing a common pathway in fibrogenesis. There is limited evidence that heavy alcohol consumption increases the level of HCV RNA in the blood and decreases the probability of response to interferon-α therapy. At present, most patients with hepatitis C are advised to cease alcohol consumption completely, yet there is little evidence that modest or moderate alcohol intake affects the natural history of chronic hepatitis C adversely.

REFERENCES

1. De Bac C, Stroffolini T, Gaeta G B, Taliani G, Giusti G. Pathogenic factors in cirrhosis with and without hepatocellular carcinoma: a multicenter Italian study. Hepatology 1994;20:1225–30.
2. Corrao G, Zambon A, Torchio P, Arico S, La Vecchia C, di Orio F. Attributable risk for symptomatic liver cirrhosis in Italy. Collaborative Groups for the Study of Liver Diseases in Italy. J Hepatol 1998;28:608–14.
3. Bellentani S, Tiribelli C, Saccoccio G, et al. Prevalence of chronic liver disease in the general population of northern Italy: the Dionysos Study. Hepatology 1994;20:1442–9.
4. Stroffolini T. Alcohol, HCV infection, and liver cirrhosis: is the cup half full or half empty? J Hepatol 1998;28:728–30.
5. Arico S, Corrao G, D'Amicis A, Klatsky A L. Alcoholic liver cirrhosis after the advent of hepatitis C virus: some reflections on its epidemiology and on the concept of attributable risk. Collaborative GESIA and AISF Groups. Gruppo Epidemiologico della Societa Italiana di Alcologia and Associazione Italiana per lo Studio del Fegato. Ital J Gastroenterol Hepatol 1997;29:75–80.
6. Schiff E R. Hepatitis C and alcohol. Hepatology 1997;26(Suppl 1):39S–42S.
7. Grellier L F, Dusheiko G M. The role of hepatitis C virus in alcoholic liver disease. Alcohol Alcohol 1997;32:103–11.
8. Seeff L B. Chronic hepatitis C: beware the older drinking male: fibrosis progression beckons! Hepatology 1997;26(4):1074–6.
9. American Psychiatric Association. Diagnostic and statistical manual of mental disorders, 4th ed. Washington, DC: Ameican Psychiatric Association; 1994.
10. Caetano R, Tam T, Greenfield T, Cherpitel C, Midanik L. DSM-IV alcohol dependence and drinking in the U.S. population: a risk analysis. Ann Epidemiol 1997;7(8):542–9.
11. Midanik L T, Clark W B. Drinking-related problems in the United States: description and trends, 1984–1990. J Stud Alcohol 1995;56(4):395–402.
12. Arico S, Galatola G, Tabone M, et al. The measure of life-time alcohol consumption in patients with cirrhosis: reproducibility and clinical relevance. Liver 1995;15(4):202–8.
13. Morabia A, Moore M, Wynder E L. Reproducibility of food frequency measurements and inferences from a case-control study. Epidemiology 1990;1(4):305–10.
14. Skinner H A, Sheu W J. Reliability of alcohol use indices. The Lifetime Drinking History and the MAST. J Stud Alcohol 1982;43(11):1157–70.
15. Lemmens P H. Measuring lifetime drinking histories. Alcohol: Clin Exp Res 1998;22(2 Suppl):29S–36S.
16. Poikolainen K. Underestimation of recalled alcohol intake in relation to actual consumption. Br J Addict 1985;80(2):215–6.
17. Uchalik D C. A comparison of questionnaire and self-monitored reports of alcohol intake in a nonalcoholic population. Addict Behav 1979;4(4):409–13.
18. Verbaan H, Hoffmann G, Lindgren S, Nilsson S, Widell A, Eriksson S. Long-term outcome of chronic hepatitis C infection in a low-prevalence area. Scand J Gastroenterol 1998;33(6):650–5.
19. Corrao G, Bagnardi V, Zambon A, Torchio P. Meta-analysis of alcohol intake in relation to risk of liver cirrhosis. Alcohol Alcohol 1998;33(4):381–92.
20. Corrao G, Arico S, Zambon A, et al. Is alcohol a risk factor for liver cirrhosis in HBsAg and anti-HCV negative subjects? Collaborative Groups for the Study of Liver Diseases in Italy. J Hepatol 1997;27(3):470–6.
21. Becker U, Deis A, Sorensen T I, et al. Prediction of risk of liver disease by alcohol intake, sex, and age: a prospective population study. Hepatology 1996;23(5):1025–9.
22. Bellentani S, Saccoccio G, Costa G, et al. Drinking habits as cofactors of risk for alcohol induced liver damage. The Dionysos Study Group. Gut 1997;41(6):845–50.

23. Prieto D J, Carrion B J, Bandres M F. [Prevalence of hepatitis C virus and excessive consumption of alcohol in a nonhospital worker population]. Gastroenterol Hepatol 1997;20(10):479–83.

24. Ezzati T M, Massey J T, Waksberg J, Chu A, Maurer K R. Sample design: Third National Health and Nutrition Examination Survey. Hyattsville, MD: U.S. Department of Health and Human Services, 1992: DHHS Publ. No. (PHS) 92–1387, 1–113.

25. Anonymous. Plan and operation of the Third National Health and Nutrition Examination Survey, 1988–94. Washington, DC: 1994;1(32).

26. Befrits R, Hedman M, Blomquist L, et al. Chronic hepatitis C in alcoholic patients: prevalence, genotypes, and correlation to liver disease. Scand J Gastroenterol 1995;30(11):1113–8.

27. Coelho-Little M E, Jeffers L J, Bernstein D E, et al. Hepatitis C virus in alcoholic patients with and without clinically apparent liver disease. Alcohol: Clin Exp Res 1995;19(5):1173–6.

28. Rosman A S, Waraich A, Galvin K, Casiano J, Paronetto F, Lieber C S. Alcoholism is associated with hepatitis C but not hepatitis B in an urban population. Am J Gastroenterol 1996;91(3):498–505.

29. Mendenhall C L, Moritz T, Rouster S, et al. Epidemiology of hepatitis C among veterans with alcoholic liver disease. The VA Cooperative Study Group 275. Am J Gastroenterol 1993;88(7):1022–6.

30. Verbaan H, Andersson K, Eriksson S. Intravenous drug abuse—the major route of hepatitis C virus transmission among alcohol-dependent individuals? Scand J Gastroenterol 1993;28(8):714–8.

31. Strasser S I. Hepatitis C: questions to be answered. Questions remain about virus transmission, the natural history of infection and the role of interferon in management. Med J Aust 1996;164(3):132–3.

32. Fong T L, Kanel G C, Conrad A, Valinluck B, Charboneau F, Adkins R H. Clinical significance of concomitant hepatitis C infection in patients with alcoholic liver disease. Hepatology 1994;19(3):554–7.

33. Smith F E, Palmer D L. Alcoholism, infection and altered host defenses: a review of clinical and experimental observations. J Chronic Dis 1976;29(1):35–49.

34. Adams H G, Jordan C. Infections in the alcoholic. Med Clin North Am 1984;68(1):179–200.

35. MacGregor R R. Alcohol and immune defense. JAMA 1986;256(11):1474–9.

36. Cook R T. Alcohol abuse, alcoholism, and damage to the immune system—a review. Alcohol: Clin Exp Res 1998;22(9):1927–42.

37. MacGregor R R, Louria D B. Alcohol and infection. Curr Clin Top Infect Dis 1997;17:291–315.

38. Mendenhall C L, Theus S A, Roselle G A, Grossman C J, Rouster S D. Biphasic in vivo immune function after low- versus high-dose alcohol consumption. Alcohol 1997;14(3):255–60.

39. Zignego A L, Foschi M, Laffi G, et al. "Inapparent" hepatitis B virus infection and hepatitis C virus replication in alcoholic subjects with and without liver disease. Hepatology 1994;19(3):577–82.

40. Nalpas B, Thiers V, Pol S, et al. Hepatitis C viremia and anti-HCV antibodies in alcoholics. J Hepatol 1992;14(2–3):381–4.

41. Sata M, Fukuizumi K, Uchimura Y, et al. Hepatitis C virus infection in patients with clinically diagnosed alcoholic liver diseases. J Viral Hepatitis 1996;3(3):143–8.

42. Oshita M, Hayashi N, Kasahara A, et al. Increased serum hepatitis C virus RNA levels among alcoholic patients with chronic hepatitis C. Hepatology 1994;20(5):1115–20.

43. Sawada M, Takada A, Takase S, Takada N. Effects of alcohol on the replication of hepatitis C virus. Alcohol Alcohol Suppl 1993;1B:85–90.

44. Cromie S L, Jenkins P J, Bowden D S, Dudley F J. Chronic hepatitis C: effect of alcohol on hepatitic activity and viral titre. J Hepatol 1996;25(6):821–6.

45. Pessione F, Degos F, Marcellin P, et al. Effect of alcohol consumption on serum hepatitis C virus RNA and histological lesions in chronic hepatitis C. Hepatology 1998;27(6):1717–22.

46. Mochida S, Ohnishi K, Matsuo S, Kakihara K, Fujiwara K. Effect of alcohol intake on the efficacy of interferon therapy in patients with chronic hepatitis C as evaluated by multivariate logistic regression analysis. Alcohol: Clin Exp Res 1996;20(9 Suppl):371A–7A.

47. Sherman K E, Mendenhall C, Thee D L, O'Brien J, Rouster S D. Hepatitis C serotypes in non-alcoholic and alcoholic patients. Dig Dis Sci 1997;42(11):2285–91.

48. Sherman K E, Rouster S D, Mendenhall C, Thee D. Hepatitis cRNA quasispecies complexity in patients with alcoholic liver disease. Hepatology 1999;30(1):265–70.

49. Brillanti S, Masci C, Siringo S, Di Febo G, Miglioli M, Barbara L. Serological and histological aspects of hepatitis C virus infection in alcoholic patients. J Hepatol 1991;13(3):347–50.

50. Rothman K J. Modern epidemiology. Boston, MA: Little, Brown, 1986.

51. Parés A, Barrera J M, Caballeria J, et al. Hepatitis C virus antibodies in chronic alcoholic patients: association with severity of liver injury. Hepatology 1990;12(6):1295–9.

52. Quintela A G, Alende R, Aguilera A, et al. Hepatitis-C virus-antibodies in alcoholic patients. Revi Clin Espan 1995;195(6):367–72.

53. Mendenhall C L, Seeff L, Diehl A M, et al. Antibodies to hepatitis B virus and hepatitis C virus in alcoholic hepatitis and cirrhosis: their prevalence and clinical relevance. The VA Cooperative Study Group (No. 119). Hepatology 1991;14(4 pt 1):581–9.

54. Shimizu S, Kiyosawa K, Sodeyama T, Tanaka E, Nakano M. High prevalence of antibody to hepatitis C virus in heavy drinkers with chronic liver diseases in Japan. J Gastroenterol Hepatol 1992;7(1):30–5.

55. Cooksley W. Chronic liver disease: do alcohol and hepatitis C virus interact. J Gastroenterol Hepatol 1996;11(2):187–92.

56. Rothman K J, Greenland S. Modern epidemiology, 2nd ed. Philadelphia, PA: Lippincott-Raven, 1998:1.

57. Corrao G, Torchio P, Zambon A, Ferrari P, Arico S, di Orio F. Exploring the combined action of lifetime alcohol intake and chronic hepatotropic virus infections on the risk of symptomatic liver cirrhosis. Eur J Epidemiol 1998;14(5):447–56.

58. Khan M H, Thomas L, Byth K, et al. How much does alcohol contribute to the variability of hepatic fibrosis in chronic hepatitis C? J Gastroenterol Hepatol 1998;13(4):419–26.

59. Serfaty L, Chazouilleres O, Poujol-Robert A, et al. Risk factors for cirrhosis in patients with chronic hepatitis C virus infection: results of a case-control study. Hepatology 1997;26(3):776–9.

60. Sachithanandan S, Kay E, Leader M, Fielding J F. The effect of light drinking on HCV liver disease: the jury is still out. Biomed Pharmacother 1997;51(6–7):295–7.

61. Ostapowicz G, Watson K J, Locarnini S A, Desmond P V. Role of alcohol in the progression of liver disease caused by hepatitis C virus infection. Hepatology 1998;27(6):1730–5.

62. Poynard T, Bedossa P, Opolon P. Natural history of liver fibrosis progression in patients with chronic hepatitis C. The OBSVIRC, METAVIR, CLINIVIR, and DOSVIRC groups. Lancet 1997;349:825–32.

63. Katakami Y, Ohishi H, Komatsu H, Kirizuka K. Alcohol intake increases hepatitis C virus-induced hepatocellular injury. Intern Med 1995;34(12):1153–7.

64. Smith B C, Chapman C E, Burt A D, Toms G L, Bassendine M F. Outcome of post-transfusion hepatitis C: disease severity in blood-component recipients and their implicated donors. QJM 1997;90(9):587–92.

65. Shen C Y, Lee H S, Huang L C, Tsai K S, Chen D S, Cheng A T. Alcoholism, hepatitis B and C viral infections, and impaired liver function among Taiwanese aboriginal groups. Am J Epidemiol 1996;143(9):936–42.

66. Alemy-Carreau M, Durbec J P, Giordanella J, et al. Lack of interaction between hepatitis C virus and alcohol in the pathogenesis of cirrhosis. A statistical study. J Hepatol 1996;25(5):627–32.

67. Wiley T E, McCarthy M, Breidi L, Layden T J. Impact of alcohol on the histological and clinical progression of hepatitis C infection. Hepatology 1998;28(3):805–9.

68. Mathurin P, Moussalli J, Cadranel J F, et al. Slow progression rate of fibrosis in hepatitis C virus patients with persistently normal alanine transaminase activity. Hepatology 1998;27(3):868–72.

69. Frieden T R, Ozick L, McCord C, et al. Chronic liver disease in central harlem: the role of alcohol and viral hepatitis. Hepatology 1999;29(3):883–8.

70. Strasser S I, Watson K J, Lee C S, Coghlan P J, Desmond P V. Risk factors and predictors of outcome in an Australian cohort with hepatitis C virus infection. Med J Aust 1995;162(7):355–8.

71. Hourigan L F, Macdonald G A, Purdie D, et al. Fibrosis in chronic hepatitis C correlates significantly with body mass index and steatosis. Hepatology 1999;29(4):1215–9.

72. Pol S, Lamorthe B, Thi N T, et al. Retrospective analysis of the impact of HIV infection and alcohol use on chronic hepatitis C in a large cohort of drug users. J Hepatol 1998;28(6):945–50.

73. Shiomi S, Kuroki T, Minamitani S, et al. Effect of drinking on the outcome of cirrhosis in patients with hepatitis B or C. J Gastroenterol Hepatol 1992;7(3):274–6.

74. Healey C J, Chapman R W, Fleming K A. Liver histology in hepatitis C infection: a comparison between patients with persistently normal or abnormal transaminases. Gut 1995;37(2):
274–8.

75. Shev S, Dhillon A P, Lindh M, et al. The importance of cofactors in the histologic progression
of minimal and mild chronic hepatitis C. Liver 1997;17(5):215–23.

76. Ohta S, Watanabe Y, Nakajima T. Consumption of alcohol in the presence of hepatitis C virus
is an additive risk for liver damage. Prev Med 1998;27(3):461–9.

77. Kondili L A, Tosti M E, Szklo M, et al. The relationships of chronic hepatitis and cirrhosis to
alcohol intake, hepatitis B and C, and delta virus infection: a case-control study in Albania.
Epidemiol Infect 1998;121(2):391–5.

78. Verbaan H, Widell A, Bondeson L, Andersson K, Eriksson S. Factors associated with cirrhosis
development in chronic hepatitis C patients from an area of low prevalence. J Viral Hepatitis
1998;5(1):43–51.

79. Ikeda K, Saitoh S, Suzuki Y, et al. Disease progression and hepatocellular carcinogenesis in patients with chronic viral hepatitis: a prospective observation of 2215 patients. J Hepatol 1998;
28(6):930–8.

80. Seeff L B, Buskell-Bales Z, Wright E C, et al. Long-term mortality after transfusion-associated
non-A, non-B hepatitis. The National Heart, Lung, and Blood Institute Study Group. N Engl J
Med 1992;327(27):1906–11.

81. Uchimura Y, Sata M, Kage M, Abe H, Tanikawa K. A histopathological study of alcoholics
with chronic HCV infection: comparison with chronic hepatitis C and alcoholic liver disease.
Liver 1995;15(6):300–6.

82. Rosman A S, Paronetto F, Galvin K, Williams R J, Lieber C S. Hepatitis C virus antibody in alcoholic patients. Association with the presence of portal and/or lobular hepatitis. Arch Intern
Med 1993;153(8):965–9.

83. Corrao G, Ferrari P A, Galatola G. Exploring the role of diet in modifying the effect of known
disease determinants: application to risk factors of liver cirrhosis. Am J Epidemiol 1995;
142(11):1136–46.

84. Marsano L S, Pena L R. The interaction of alcoholic liver disease and hepatitis C. Hepatogastroenterology 1998;45(20):331–9.

85. Poikolainen K. Alcohol and overall health outcomes. Ann Med 1996;28(5):381–4.

86. Poikolainen K. Alcohol and mortality: a review. J Clin Epidemiol 1995;48(4):455–65. [Er-
ratum, J Clin Epidemiol 1995;48(9):i]

87. Rehm J, Bondy S. Alcohol and all-cause mortality: an overview. Novartis Found Symp 1998;
216:223–32.

88. Makela P, Valkonen T, Poikolainen K. Estimated numbers of deaths from coronary heart disease "caused" and "prevented" by alcohol: an example from Finland. J Stud Alcohol 1997;
58(5):455–63.

89. Rehm J T, Bondy S J, Sempos C T, Vuong C V. Alcohol consumption and coronary heart disease morbidity and mortality. Am J Epidemiol 1997;146(6):495–501.

90. Peters K D, Kochanek K D, Murphy S L. Deaths: final data for 1996. Hyattsville, MD: National
Center for Health Statistics, 1998:19.

91. Nalpas B, Pol S, Thepot V, Berthelot P, Brechot C. Hepatocellular carcinoma in alcoholics. Alcohol 1995;12(2):117–20.

92. Di Bisceglie A M. Hepatitis C and hepatocellular carcinoma. Hepatology 1997;26(3 Suppl 1):
34S–8S.

93. Ikeda K, Saitoh S, Koida I, et al. A multivariate analysis of risk factors for hepatocellular carcinogenesis: a prospective observation of 795 patients with viral and alcoholic cirrhosis. Hepatology 1993;18(1):47–53.

94. Donato F, Tagger A, Chiesa R, et al. Hepatitis B and C virus infection, alcohol drinking, and
hepatocellular carcinoma: a case-control study in Italy. Brescia HCC Study. Hepatology 1997;
26(3):579–84.

95. Chang C C, Yu M W, Lu C F, Yang C S, Chen C J. A nested case-control study on association between hepatitis C virus antibodies and primary liver cancer in a cohort of 9,775 men in Taiwan. J Med Virol 1994;43(3):276–80.

96. Fattovich G. Progression of hepatitis B and C to hepatocellular carcinoma in Western countries. Hepatogastroenterology 1998;45(Suppl 3):1206–13.

97. Donato F, Boffetta P, Puoti M. A meta-analysis of epidemiological studies on the combined effect of hepatitis B and C virus infections in causing hepatocellular carcinoma. Int J Cancer 1998;75(3):347–54.

98. Goritsas C P, Athanasiadou A, Arvaniti A, Lampropoulou-Karatza C. The leading role of hepatitis B and C viruses as risk factors for the development of hepatocellular carcinoma. A case control study. J Clin Gastroenterol 1995;20(3):220–4.

99. Pagliaro L, Simonetti R G, Craxi A, Spano C, Ligippazzo M G, Palazzo V. Alcohol and HBV infection as risk factors for hepatocellular carcinoma in Italy: a multicentric, controlled study. Hepatogastroenterology 1983;30:48–50.

100. Miyakawa H, Izumi N, Marumo F, Sato C. Roles of alcohol, hepatitis virus infection, and gender in the development of hepatocellular carcinoma in patients with liver cirrhosis. Alcohol: Clin Exp Res 1996;20(1 Suppl):91A–4A.

101. Simonetti R G, Camma C, Fiorello F, et al. Hepatitis C virus infection as a risk factor for hepatocellular carcinoma in patients with cirrhosis. A case-control study. Ann Intern Med 1992;116(2):97–102.

102. Takase S, Tsutsumi M, Kawahara H, Takada N, Takada A. The alcohol-altered liver membrane antibody and hepatitis C virus infection in the progression of alcoholic liver disease. Hepatology 1993;17(1):9–13.

103. Chiba T, Matsuzaki Y, Abei M, et al. Multivariate analysis of risk factors for hepatocellular carcinoma in patients with hepatitis C virus-related liver cirrhosis. J Gastroenterol 1996;31(4):552–8.

104. Suzuki M, Suzuki H, Mizuno H, et al. Studies on the incidence of hepatocellular carcinoma in heavy drinkers with liver cirrhosis. Alcohol Alcohol, Suppl 1993;1B:109–14.

105. Noda K, Yoshihara H, Suzuki K, et al. Progression of type C chronic hepatitis to liver cirrhosis and hepatocellular carcinoma—its relationship to alcohol drinking and the age of transfusion. Alcohol: Clin Exp Res 1996;20(1 Suppl):95A–100A.

106. Pawlosky R J, Flynn B M, Salem N J. The effects of low dietary levels of polyunsaturates on alcohol-induced liver disease in rhesus monkeys. Hepatology 1997;26(6):1386–92.

107. Pawlosky R J, Salem N J. Alcohol consumption in rhesus monkeys depletes tissues of polyunsaturated fatty acids and alters essential fatty acid metabolism. Alcohol: Clin Exp Res 1999;23(2):311–7.

108. Mezey E. Dietary fat and alcoholic liver disease. Hepatology 1998;28(4):901–5.

109. Thurman R G. II. Alcoholic liver injury involves activation of Kupffer cells by endotoxin. Am J Physiol 1998;275(4 pt 1):G605–11.

110. Saad A J, Jerrells T R. Flow cytometric and immunohistochemical evaluation of ethanol-induced changes in splenic and thymic lymphoid cell populations. Alcohol: Clin Exp Res 1991;15(5):796–803.

111. Kruger T E, Jerrells T R. Effects of ethanol consumption and withdrawal on B cell subpopulations in murine bone marrow. Clin Exp Immunol 1994;96(3):521–7.

112. Geissler M, Gesien A, Wands J R. Inhibitory effects of chronic ethanol consumption on cellular immune responses to hepatitis C virus core protein are reversed by genetic immunizations augmented with cytokine-expressing plasmids. J Immunol 1997;159(10):5107–13.

113. Waltenbaugh C, Vasquez K, Peterson J D. Alcohol consumption alters antigen-specific Th1 responses: mechanisms of deficit and repair. Alcohol Clin Exp Res 1998;22(5 Suppl):220S–3S.

114. Peterson J D, Herzenberg L A, Vasquez K, Waltenbaugh C. Glutathione levels in antigen-presenting cells modulate Th1 versus Th2 response patterns. Proc Natl Acad Sci U S A 1998;95(6):3071–6.

115. Colell A, Garcia-Ruiz C, Miranda M, et al. Selective glutathione depletion of mitochondria by ethanol sensitizes hepatocytes to tumor necrosis factor. Gastroenterology 1998;115(6):1541–51.

116. Calabrese V, Randazzo G, Ragusa N, Rizza V. Long-term ethanol administration enhances

age-dependent modulation of redox state in central and peripheral organs of rat: protection by metadoxine. Drugs Exp Clin Res 1998;24(2):85–91.

117. Wang J F, Spitzer J J. Alcohol-induced thymocyte apoptosis is accompanied by impaired mito-chondrial function. Alcohol 1997;14(1):99–105.

118. Szabo G. Monocytes, alcohol use, and altered immunity. Alcohol: Clin Exp Res 1998;22 (5 Suppl):216S–9S.

119. Szabo G, Chavan S, Mandrekar P, Catalano D. Acute alcohol consumption attenuates inter-leukin-8 (IL-8) and monocyte chemoattractant peptide-1 (MCP-1) induction in response to ex vivo stimulation. J Clin Immunol 1999;19(1):67–76.

120. Bissell D M, Maher J J. Zakim D, Boyer T D, eds. Hepatology: a textbook of liver disease, 3rd ed. Philadelphia, PA: Saunders, 1996:506–25.

121. Okada S, Ishii H, Nose H, et al. Effect of heavy alcohol intake on long-term results after cura-tive resection of hepatitis C virus-related hepatocellular carcinoma. Jpn J Cancer Res 1996; 87(8):867–73.

122. Okazaki T, Yoshihara H, Suzuki K, et al. Efficacy of interferon therapy in patients with chronic hepatitis C. Comparison between non-drinkers and drinkers. Scand J Gastroenterol 1994; 29(11):1039–43.

123. Ohnishi K, Matsuo S, Matsutani K, et al. Interferon therapy for chronic hepatitis C in habit-ual drinkers: comparison with chronic hepatitis C in infrequent drinkers. Am J Gastroenterol 1996;91(7):1374–9.

124. Olynyk J K, Reddy K R, Di Bisceglie A M, et al. Hepatic iron concentration as a predictor of response to interferon alfa therapy in chronic hepatitis C. Gastroenterology 1995;108(4): 1104–9.

125. Izumi N, Enomoto N, Uchihara M, et al. Hepatic iron contents and response to interferon-alpha in patients with chronic hepatitis C. Relationship to genotypes of hepatitis C virus. Dig Dis Sci 1996;41(5):989–94.

126. Ono K, Sata M, Murashima S, Fukuizumi K, Suzuki H, Tanikawa K. Biological responses to administered interferon in alcoholics. Alcohol Clin Exp Res 1996;20(9):1560–3.

127. Belle S H, Beringer K C, Detre K M. Liver transplantation for alcoholic liver disease in the United States: 1988 to 1995. Liver Transplant Surg 1997;3(3):212–9.

128. Everhart J E, Beresford T P. Liver transplantation for alcoholic liver disease: a survey of trans-plantation programs in the United States. Liver Transplant Surg 1997;3(3):220–6.

129. Everson G, Bharadhwaj G, House R, et al. Long-term follow-up of patients with alcoholic liver disease who underwent hepatic transplantation. Liver Transplant Surg 1997;3(3):263–74.

130. Lee R G. Recurrence of alcoholic liver disease after liver transplantation. Liver Transplant Surg 1997;3(3):292–5.

131. Leach M, Makris M, Gleeson D C, Preston F E. Acute liver failure induced by alcohol and paracetamol in an HCV-infected haemophiliac. Br J Haematol 1998;103(3):891–3.

20
HEPATITIS C IN CHILDREN

MAUREEN M. JONAS

Division of Gastroenterology
Children's Hospital
and Harvard Medical School
Boston, Massachusetts

INTRODUCTION

Since the original descriptions of the hepatitis C virus (HCV) in 1989 and its elucidation as the cause of most cases of non-A, non-B hepatitis, a great deal has been learned about the virus itself and the clinical diseases it causes. However, knowledge about HCV infection in children has accrued at a much slower rate. This is due to the small proportion of HCV-infected individuals that are children and the lack of clinical manifestations of this infection during childhood. Nonetheless, children may acquire HCV infection and develop chronic hepatitis in most cases. Although rare, cirrhosis and end-stage liver disease have been associated with childhood HCV infection. There may be important differences in modes of acquisition, natural history, complications, and treatment between pediatric and adult HCV infection. Elucidation of these features will enhance not only management of children exposed to or infected with HCV, but also understanding of the pathogenesis of this disease and the interactions of this virus with physiologically different hosts.

INCIDENCE AND PREVALENCE IN CHILDREN

Infection with HCV occurs throughout the world, and this is true for children as well as adults. The highest risk group by age for acquisition of HCV infection is young adults. An estimated 28,000 new infections occur each year in the United States (1); the proportion of these cases in children less than 18 years of age is not clearly defined. Prior to 1990, the predominant risk for acquisition of HCV infection by children was via blood or blood product transfusion. Although this mode of transmission is responsible for many current cases of pediatric HCV infection, new infections in children are primarily due to perinatal (vertical) transmission, as has been demonstrated in Italy. (2) The incidence of new infections in children through this mechanism is not known, but could be estimated from the prevalence of HCV infection in women of childbearing age and the risk of transmission with each pregnancy (see later).

The prevalence of HCV infection in the United States is 1.8%; this was determined by the seroprevalence of antibody to HCV (anti-HCV) in the *Third National Health and Nutrition Examination* conducted from 1988 to 1994 (1) and represents approximately 3.9 million people. However, there is great variation in prevalence among subgroups, with up to 60 to 90% in those with repeated percutaneous exposures and 1% in health care workers. Volunteer blood donors, who represent the lowest risk group, have a seroprevalence of <0.5%. For children, the seroprevalence is 0.2% for those less than 12 years of age and 0.4% for those 12 to 19 years of age. (3)

EPIDEMIOLOGY AND MODES OF TRANSMISSION IN CHILDREN

The epidemiology of HCV infection has been examined in some pediatric groups. Children at risk for HCV infection are listed in Table I. The prevalence varies both by risk factors and by geographical location. Children from all parts of the world who have been multiply transfused with either blood or blood products, such as those with thalassemia (4,5) or hemophilia, (6) have infection rates from 50 to 95%. Children with moderate but not ongoing transfusion exposure, such as those who had been treated for childhood malignancies, (7,8) those who had been treated with hemodialysis (9,10) or extracorporeal membrane oxygenation, (11) or those who had undergone surgery for congenital heart disease, (12) have intermediate seroprevalence rates of 10 to 20%. Studies in general pediatric populations, without identifiable risk factors, have reported seroprevalence rates from 0% in Japan (13) and Taiwan, (14) 0% in Egypt, (15) 0.4% in Italy, (16) 0.9% in Saudi Arabia, (17) and up to 14.5% in Cameroon. (18) For the United States, unpublished CDC data indicate a childhood prevalence of HCV infection of 0.2–0.4%. (3) In a large urban adolescent population in Boston, a 0.1% seroprevalence for anti-HCV was detected. (19) Socioeconomic differences have been postulated but not proven to explain these geographic differences.

TABLE I   Children at Risk for HCV Infection

Children transfused repeatedly with blood or blood products for
  Thalassemia
  Sickle cell anemia
  Other congenital anemias
  Hemophilia
  Hemodialysis
  Hypogammaglobulinemia or other immunodeficiency (IVIG)
Children with a history of transfusion prior to 1992 for
  Childhood malignancy, especially leukemia
  Major surgery—cardiac, orthopedic
  Prematurity, neonatal intensive care
  Conditions requiring extracorporeal membrane oxygenation
Adolescents with high risk behaviors
  Intravenous drug use
  Intranasal drug use
  Body piercing and/or tattooing
Infants of HCV-infected mothers

Transfusion-Associated HCV in Children

Until recently, receipt of blood or blood products has been the major mode of transmission of HCV to children. (12,20) In addition to erythrocyte and platelet transfusions, implicated products have included clotting factors, (6,21) plasma, and intravenous immunoglobulin. (22) Transmission to children has also been demonstrated by transplanted organs or tissues. (10,23) In general, as has been described for adults, the risk of HCV acquisition increases with the number or units of blood or blood products received. (9,11,15) Screening of donated blood for anti-HCV, the use of recombinant and heat-inactivated clotting factors, and the addition of virus-inactivating physicochemical processes in the production of immunoglobulin have drastically reduced the incidence of HCV transmission by these means. However, these are relatively recent advances, instituted in the early to mid-1990s. While many children infected with HCV via these products are being followed in clinical practices, many others are probably yet to be identified.

Perinatal Transmission of HCV

The frequency of anti-HCV seropositivity in newborns of HCV-infected women was shown to be 14 to 100% using first- and second-generation ELISA testing. In most instances, this antibody was present only transiently, indicating that it had been acquired passively through placental transfer. (24–27) The true delineation of the frequency of perinatal transmission required use of the polymerase chain reaction (PCR) technique to detect viral genome in the serum of exposed infants. It then became clear that vertical transmission of the virus does occur, albeit at a low rate. (25,28–31) Various studies have confirmed that the rate of transmission from anti-HCV seropositive women is 5 to 6%; this increases to 10 to 11% in most reports and up to 33% in one Italian study (32) for women who have HCV RNA in serum at the time of delivery. This compares to a frequency of 40 to 90% for the perinatal transmission of hepatitis B virus. Maternal coinfection with the human immunodeficiency virus (HIV) increases the rate of perinatal HCV transmission, (33–38) even without concomitant HIV transmission.

In the absence of HIV coinfection, the likelihood of HCV transmission increases with higher levels of maternal HCV viremia. In several studies, no women with less than 10^6 copies/ml of serum HCV RNA transmitted the infection to their newborns, (27,39–41) although this was not the case in one report from Italy. (42) Some studies have raised the question of whether vaginal delivery is a risk factor versus cesarean delivery, (41) but sporadic cases of HCV transmission after cesarean births have been reported. (36) In one report, transmission frequency after vaginal delivery was 4% and after cesarean delivery was 6%. (42) The possibility of *in utero* transmission in at least some cases was suggested by the detection of viremia in six infants on the day of birth. (42) HCV transmission has been documented in women who have acute infection during the last trimester of pregnancy. (43) In some instances, viremia in the neonates is transient and is not associated with the development of liver disease. (27)

One report indicates a correlation between the duration of breast feeding and HCV infection, (39) but, in others, breast feeding did not increase the frequency of infection in neonates. (42,44,45) Whether factors such as maternal viremia levels or duration of breast feeding will turn out to be significant remains to be determined.

Because the rate of perinatal transmission of HCV is low, the risk factors that increase this rate are not fully defined, and there is no intervention for the neonate at this time, routine screening of all pregnant women is not warranted. Pregnant women, or those considering pregnancy, with risk factors such as intravenous drug use (IVDU), blood transfusions prior to 1992, or unexplained alanine aminotransferase (ALT) elevations should be offered screening for anti-HCV. Those found to be anti-HCV seropositive should undergo testing with PCR to confirm active infection. At the present time, no specific recommendations are made to physicians caring for HCV-infected pregnant women in an attempt to reduce the frequency of perinatal transmission. (46) Postexposure prophylaxis with immune globulin does not appear to be effective in preventing HCV infection and is not recommended for infants born to HCV-infected women. Infants born to mothers infected with HCV during pregnancy or at delivery should be tested after 1 year of age for anti-HCV. A positive test at that time is likely to correlate with true infection, as maternal antibody will have disappeared by that age.

Intrafamilial and Other Horizontal Transmission of HCV

There are two pediatric issues to be addressed regarding horizontal HCV transmission: how often children are infected from other family members and how often HCV-infected children transmit infection to others in the home or at school.

Studies of household transmission have been done in Europe, South America, and Asia. In general, they entail screening of household contacts of index cases (known HCV-infected individuals) for anti-HCV; in some, further testing of seropositive contacts with PCR for HCV RNA and even comparative genotype analysis (47) was done. The prevalence of anti-HCV seropositivity in household contacts varied from 0 to 14.8%. (48–55) Nonsexual (nonspouse) seroprevalence rates were 0 to 6.5%. Higher rates were seen in the households of HCV-infected individuals with liver disease compared to those who were asymptomatic carriers, (51) and in the households of those with risk factors as opposed to those without. (52) The risk of anti-HCV positivity increased with age and/or duration of exposure for sexual and nonsexual contacts. (50,52) Rates were particularly low in households of HCV-infected hemophiliacs. (56) In these studies, it is difficult to distinguish the risk to children in the households of chronically HCV-infected individuals from perinatal risk. This risk can be inferred to be quite low, as prevalence rates were very low (approaching zero) in the youngest children and increased steadily with increasing age. (49,53,57) Because the mechanism of nonsexual, nonperinatal infection of children in these families is not known, counseling to prevent this transmission is limited to avoidance of sharing household items such as razors, toothbrushes, and fingernail clippers. There is no justification at this time to have family members avoid sharing of eating utensils or bathrooms. HCV-infected adults should be educated about the extremely low likelihood of spreading HCV to their children by routine family contact, including kissing and day-to-day care.

There are few data regarding the transmission of HCV from infected children to others. In a Spanish study, 80 household contacts (without independent risk factors for infection) of 27 HCV-infected children were tested. None of the parents was found to be infected, but one infected sibling (1/32) was identified. (58) The proband had HCV infection presumed secondary to transfusion. In an Italian study of 44 index children with various sources of infection, one parent was infected through an accidental needle stick, and no transmission to other children was demonstrated. (59) Thus, it appears that horizontal transmission of HCV between children is quite rare. There is no need to restrict school or day-care attendance or participation in any routine activity, including contact sports, for HCV-infected children. (60) Although school nurses and other administrative personnel may be told of a child's HCV infection, this information should be kept confidential. They should also be assured that the routine universal precautions they are already utilizing for all children are adequate for children with HCV.

Other Modes of Transmission of HCV in Children

The most frequent mode of HCV transmission in adults is needle sharing for the purpose of intravenous illicit drug injection. To the extent that older children and teenagers participate in this activity, they are at risk for infection. In fact, it has been demonstrated that HCV infection occurs within 6 to 12 months after beginning injection in the majority of individuals. (61) Other percutaneous exposures, which may be more common than IVDU in children and adolescents, such as body piercing and tattooing, have been implicated as a risk in Italy, (62) but not in the United States. (63) Sexual transmission of HCV is thought to occur by both homosexual and heterosexual activity, (64,65) but its importance to the overall prevalence of HCV infection is controversial, (66) especially in the pediatric age group. The prevalence of HCV infection in children not currently explained by risk factors, i.e., sporadic or community-acquired HCV, is not known.

CLINICAL FEATURES OF HCV INFECTION IN CHILDREN

In adults, acute HCV infection has been described as mild and usually subclinical. There are no reports of clinical manifestations of acute HCV infection in children infected perinatally or via blood transfusion. Some of the children who were infected during the outbreak associated with intravenous immunoglobulin had acute, severe hepatitis with atypically high ALT values, jaundice, malaise, anorexia, and hepatomegaly. (67) The reasons for this unusually severe presentation are not clear, but may involve greater amounts of virus inoculated, repeated inoculations, or underlying immunodeficiency in the hosts. Anecdotally, when chronically infected children are identified, although biochemical evidence for "non-A, non-B hepatitis" may have been gathered in some transfused children, there is usually no history of recognized acute hepatitis. Fulminant hepatitis due to HCV has not been described in children.

There are no reports specifically describing clinical features of chronic HCV infection in children. Studies of epidemiology, natural history, and treatment in children often describe the patients as being asymptomatic or having nonspecific fatigue and/or abdominal pain, with normal or mildly abnormal ALT levels. (7, 12,20,68–72) Nonorgan-specific autoantibodies are commonly found: antinuclear antibodies have been described in 7.5–11%, smooth muscle antibodies in 9–17.5%, and type 1 liver–kidney microsomal antibodies in 10–13%. (73, 74) However, clinically apparent autoimmune manifestations are rare. The author has cared for a 13-year-old girl with cirrhosis due to chronic HCV infection, who also had nephrotic syndrome secondary to membranoproliferative glomerulonephritis, and a 6-year-old boy with chronic HCV infection and lichen planus (unpublished data). HCV-associated cryoglobulinemia, vasculitis, and porphyria cutanea tarda have not been reported in children. This lack of clinical signs or symptoms and the fact that "routine" serum ALT determinations are not done as part of pediatric medical care indicate that chronic HCV infection in children is probably underrecognized.

NATURAL HISTORY OF HCV INFECTION IN CHILDREN

Factors that have been implicated in the natural history of HCV infection in adults include age at acquisition, gender, mode of acquisition, concomitant infections, ethanol ingestion, comorbid disease, and viral genotype and level. Some of these factors have been examined in children as well, but the studies are small and less definitive. Age at acquisition and mode of acquisition are difficult to separate, as most reports of transfusion-associated infection include children older than those of perinatally infected children. The natural history of transfusion-associated HCV infection may differ according to the underlying disease for which transfusion is required. In a Japanese study, 45 to 50% of children who were transfused at the time of surgery for congenital heart disease developed chronic infection. (75) When 29 children infected in this manner were followed for a minimum of 4 years, only 50% of the children had persistent viremia. Although all who underwent biopsy had histologic chronic hepatitis, none had cirrhosis within this time period. (76) Very similar findings were reported in a study from Germany. (77) These authors studied 67 individuals who were infected with HCV in the first years of life, at the time of cardiac surgery. At an average follow-up of 17 years (range 12 to 27 years), only 55% of the anti-HCV-seropositive subjects were viremic. All but one of the infected patients had normal ALT values. Seventeen underwent liver biopsy: 14 had minimal changes, 2 had mild fibrosis, and 1, who had a history of prior HBV infection, had cirrhosis. Children treated for leukemia prior to 1990 had a very high rate of HCV infection. (78) Many of these children had an abnormal serologic response, with a delay in the development of anti-HCV for several years. However, extended follow-up (13–27 years) of these patients did not reveal serious liver disease. (79) The authors hypothesized that the acquisition of HCV during a period of immunosuppression induced by chemotherapeutic agents may have prevented the development of an immune response that plays a patho-genetic role in this disease. However, in a small series of American children, one child treated for leukemia developed cirrhosis within 2 years. (80) Children with thalassemia requiring chronic transfusion have a very high prevalence of HCV infection. (5) Secondary hemochromatosis contributes to the hepatic injury demonstrated frequently in this patient group, and the response to therapy may be affected by the degree of hepatic iron overload. (81) Although end-stage liver disease is not common in HCV-infected children with hemophilia, it has been demonstrated that HCV infection, which may have been acquired during childhood before recombinant clotting factor preparations were available, contributes to early mortality in these individuals. (82)

The role of the host immune response has been studied by describing the course of HCV infection in patients infected via intravenous immunoglobulin (IVIG). The chronicity rate for HCV infection in individuals with a variety of immune disorders is higher than that of the general transfused population (67, 83) and with a faster rate of progression to end stage liver disease. (84) Three children who acquired HCV infection from IVIG in our series had bridging fibrosis with architectural distortion when liver biopsies were examined from 1 to 3 years after infection. (84) Although some reports have suggested that boys with X-linked agammaglobulinemia (XLA) have a milder course than patients with other immune deficiencies, (85) perhaps because there is less immune pressure for the generation of mutant strains, (86) the author has cared for two boys with XLA infected by contaminated IVIG and both developed chronic hepatitis with fibrosis.

The natural history of perinatally acquired HCV infection will be particularly important to understand as it becomes the major route of infection for the pediatric population. Several small studies have addressed this issue. When 7 vertically infected infants were followed prospectively for 26 to 90 months, all had initial ALT abnormalities, but in 4 of the 7 ALT subsequently became normal. (87) However, all children remained viremic during follow-up, and all of the 5 who underwent liver biopsy had histologic chronic hepatitis. In contrast, a Japanese study in which 3 infants were followed from birth demonstrated transient viremia in 2 of the 3. (88) In addition, only 6 of 8 vertically infected children discovered retrospectively remained viremic when followed for 1.4 to 5 years. In the same study, transfusion-associated HCV infection persisted for the duration of follow-up (2.6 to 6.1 years) in 14 children (63.6% for perinatal vs 100% transfusion associated). Another Italian report describes 14 infected infants followed from birth; all had abnormal ALT for the first year, some remained viremic but with normal ALT in the long-term follow-up, and 2 resolved the infection. (72) When a cohort of older children with perinatally acquired HCV was followed, fluctuating or persistent viremia was the rule, all biopsies demonstrated chronic hepatitis, but most had normal or near-normal ALT values. (72) In general, it appears that HCV infection acquired vertically is frequently associated with biochemical evidence of hepatic injury early in life, persists for many years in most cases, and causes only mild liver disease in the first one or two decades.

The role of viral genotype has been reported in only one small study. In 36 Italian children, the genotype distribution closely resembled that of the general

HCV-infected Italian population and demonstrated the same geographic variation. There was no correlation of genotype with severity of liver disease in these
children. (89)

In summary, the natural history of HCV infection in childhood can be considered relatively benign, as it is rarely associated with severe or decompensated
liver disease during the childhood years. However, HCV acquired during childhood most often persists for many years, causes chronic hepatic damage, and
may, at least in some instances, be responsible for significant morbidity and mortality later in life.

HISTOPATHOLOGIC FEATURES OF THE LIVER IN HCV INFECTION IN CHILDREN

Histologic features of the liver associated with HCV infection in adults have
been described in several series and include portal inflammation with lymphoid
aggregates, varying degrees of steatosis, and bile duct injury. In HCV-infected
adults, the severity of histologic abnormalities does not correlate with biochemical parameters of hepatic dysfunction, such as ALT levels. The implication is
that patients may have progressive liver disease in the absence of clinical signs.
Thus, histopathologic examination of the liver is an important tool in the understanding of childhood HCV infection.

Several reports have described histologic features in small numbers of HCV-
infected children, but most were not systematically examined and scored or described in detail. (5,20,76,90) In these reports, varying degrees of necroinflammatory activity were noted, and fibrosis was not uniformly described; cirrhosis
was reported in 0 to 11% of cases.

Three papers have focused primarily on histologic findings, with results of
scoring, in large series of children. In all series, the characteristic histopathologic lesions of HCV infection, including portal lymphoid aggregates or follicles,
steatosis, sinusoidal lymphocytes, and steatosis, were seen with approximately
the same frequency as in adults (84,91,92) (Table II). (93–96) Kage et al., (91)
who described the findings in 109 Japanese children infected primarily via transfusion, reported an average histologic activity (Scheuer system) of 3.8. No cases

**TABLE II   Comparison of Histopathologic Features
of the Liver in Children and Adults with HCV Infection**

Feature	Adult (%) (93–96)	Pediatric (%) (84)
Sinusoidal lymphocytosis	26–78	74
Lymphoid aggregates	49–78	48
Steatosis	54–72	50
Bile duct damage	22–90	28
Bridging fibrosis	9.3	36
Cirrhosis	1–58	8
Centrilobular pericentral fibrosis	NR[a]	52

[a] Not reported.

of cirrhosis were encountered, and only 3.6% of the children had bridging fibrosis with architectural distortion (stage 3). Viral genotypes were not reported, and the mean duration of infection was only 2.6 years. In contrast, although histologic activity (Scheuer and METAVIR schemes) was generally mild in a series of children in the United States, portal fibrosis was much more frequent, described in 78% of specimens from 40 children. (84) Fibrosis was mild in 26%, moderate in 22%, severe in 22%, and cirrhosis was found in 8%. Two of the children with cirrhosis were young adolescents who had acquired HCV infection perinatally. A newly described finding was pericellular fibrosis, typically around the central veins, in 52% of specimens; whether this abnormality is unique to pediatric HCV infection has yet to be determined, and this fibrosis was not included in the histologic grading. In this series, 60% of children had HCV of genotype 1a and 32% had genotype 1b. The mean duration of infection, in those children in whom it could be determined accurately, was 6.8 ± 5.3 years. In a series of 80 children from Italy and Spain, (92) most of whom were infected with HCV genotype 1a and 1b and with a mean duration of infection of 3.5 ± 4.3 years, inflammatory scores were generally quite low (grade 1 or 2). The frequency and severity of the bile duct damage and lymphoid follicles increased with patient age. Like the American series, fibrosis was present in 72.5% of cases and increased with duration of disease and patient age. Only 1 (1.25%) child had cirrhosis.

Histologic features of chronic HCV infection in childhood are quite similar to those reported in adults. However, although necrosis and inflammation are usually mild, fibrosis is commonly seen and progresses with increasing age and duration of infection. Thus, the natural history of HCV infection acquired in childhood may, in some instances, be associated with significant morbidity as the children progress into young adulthood.

TREATMENT OF HCV INFECTION IN CHILDREN

There have not been any large, multicenter, randomized, controlled therapeutic trials in children with HCV infection. Reports of treatment in children are limited in number and scope, most often uncontrolled, and sometimes refer only to selected patient groups, such as hemophiliacs or thalassemics. (71,97–105) The NIH Consensus Statement on the Management of Hepatitis C (106) indicates that "firm recommendations . . . cannot be made for patients younger than age 18 . . . because of incomplete data." Nonetheless, studies that have been reported demonstrate that treatment with interferon-α (IFN-α) may eradicate HCV infection in a minority of chronically infected children (Table III). Sustained virologic response has been achieved in 30 to 45% of children treated with various preparations of IFN-α, in dosages of 3 to 10 MU/m² body area or 0.1 MU/kg body weight, for 6 to 12 months. This is significantly higher than the response rate reported in adults who received IFN monotherapy. Factors that might be expected to correlate with response, such as viral load and/or genotype, duration of infection, and route of infection, although determined in some of these trials, could not be evaluated systematically due to small patient numbers. In general, children tolerated IFN-α well and were able to complete the

TABLE III Reported Trials of Interferon (IFN) Treatment of Chronic Hepatitis C in Children[a]

Refer-ence	No. Patients		Type IFN	Dose (MU/m² TIW)	Rx duration (months)	% SBR		% SVR	
	Rx	Cont				Rx	Cont	Rx	Cont
3	12	0	α2b	3	6	45	ND	NA	NA
98[b]	5	0	α2b	1.75, 3	6	0	ND	0	ND
6	11	10	LB	3	12	45	10	45	10
97[c]	13	0	Natural	0.1 MU/kg[d]	6	46	ND	38	ND
94	18[b]	0	Natural	0.1 MU/kg[d]	6	61	ND	56	ND
95	14	13	α2b	5	12 (4 in 4 pts)	43	7.5	43	0
99	22	0	α2b	0.1 MU/kg[d]	6			36	ND
100[e]	14 (8 ped)	0	Natural	10	6	73	ND	35	ND
101[e]	67 (? ped)	0	α2b	5 (for 2 m), then 3	12	40	ND	40	ND
71	21	0	α2a	3	6–12	38	ND	33	ND

[a] LB, lymphoblastoid; MU, million units; SBR, sustained biochemical response; SVR, sustained virologic response; ND, not done; NA, not available.
[b] All subjects had hemophilia.
[c] All subjects were leukemia survivors.
[d] Dosed by body weight rather than surface area.
[e] Adults were included.

courses of treatment. No long-term sequelae of IFN-α therapy have been reported, but whether they were systematically sought is not clear. Several infants treated with IFN-α for life-threatening hemangiomas developed spastic diplegia, (107) and one young child with HCV infection had seizures, (108) so toxicity to the central nervous system may be a concern in very young children. Criteria for patient selection, optimal dose, schedule, and duration of IFN-α treatment of children with chronic HCV infection have not been defined.

Combination therapy with IFN-α and ribavirin has been proven superior to IFN monotherapy in adults. There are no data regarding the use of ribavirin for chronic HCV in children. Because this drug has significant teratogenic and mutagenic potential, its use in young children may require careful monitoring and adaptation. Scant pharmacokinetic data in children have been derived in the HIV-infected population (109) and may not be applicable to those with HCV or in the setting of combination therapy.

CONCLUSION

Although the incidence of new HCV infections in the United States is decreasing, the 4 million estimated existing cases are expected to cause an increase in the number of people with end-stage liver disease in the next decade or two. The contribution of pediatric cases to this health care burden is difficult to quantify because the majority of HCV-infected children have probably not yet been identified. In addition, new pediatric infections will primarily be caused by perinatal transmission. Because most HCV-infected women of childbearing potential have probably not yet been recognized or treated and there is as yet no way to prevent perinatal transmission, new childhood infections will continue to occur. For these reasons, elucidation of the mechanisms of perinatal infection, factors affecting progression of disease, and optimal therapies of childhood HCV infection warrant further study.

REFERENCES

1. Alter M J. Epidemiology of hepatitis C. Hepatology 1997;26:62S–5S.
2. Bortolotti F, Resti M, Giacchino R, et al. Changing epidemiologic pattern of chronic hepatitis C virus infection in Italian children. J Pediatr 1998;133:378–81.
3. Committee on Infectious Diseases, American Academy of Pediatrics. Hepatitis C virus infection. Pediatrics 1998;101:481–5.
4. Resti M, Azzari C, Rossi M E, et al. Hepatitis C virus antibodies in a long-term follow-up of beta-thalassaemic children with acute and chronic non-A, non-B hepatitis. Eur J Pediatr 1992;151:573–6.
5. Lai M E, DeVirgilis S, Argiolu F, et al. Evaluation of antibodies to hepatitis C virus in a long-term prospective study of posttransfusion hepatitis among thalassemic children: comparison between first- and second-generation assay. J Pediatr Gastroenterol Nutr 1993;16:458–64.
6. Blanchette V S, Vorstmann E, Shore A, et al. Hepatitis C infection in children with hemophilia A and B. Blood 1991;78:285–9.
7. Locasciulli A, Gornati G, Tagger A, et al. Hepatitis C virus infection and chronic liver disease in children with leukemia in long-term remission. Blood 1991;78:1619–22.
8. Rossetti F, Cesaro S, Pizzocchero P, et al. Chronic hepatitis B surface antigen-negative hepatitis after treatment of malignancy. J Pediatr 1992;121:39–43.
9. Jonas M M, Zilleruelo G E, LaRue S I, Abitbol C, Strauss J, Lu Y. Hepatitis C in a pediatric dialysis population. Pediatrics 1992;89:707–9.
10. Greco M, Cristiano K, Leozappa G, et al. Hepatitis C infection in children and adolescents on haemodialysis and after renal transplant. Pediatr Nephrol 1993;7:424–7.
11. Nelson S P, Jonas M M. Hepatitis C infection in children who received extracorporeal membrane oxygenation. J Pediatr Surg 1996;31:644–8.
12. Ni Y-H, Chang M-H, Lue H-C, et al. Posttransfusion hepatitis C virus infection in children. J Pediatr 1994;124:709–13.
13. Tanaka E, Kiyosawa K, Soeyama T, et al. Prevalence of antibody to hepatitis C virus in Japanese schoolchildren: comparison with adult blood donors. Am J Trop Med Hyg 1992;46:460–4.
14. Lee S-D, Chan C-Y, Wang Y-J, et al. Seroepidemiology of hepatitis C virus infection in Taiwan. Hepatology 1991;13:830–3.
15. Khalifa A S, Mitchell B S, Watts D M, et al. Prevalence of hepatitis C viral antibody in transfused and nontransfused Egyptian children. Am J Trop Med Hyg 1993;49:316–21.
16. Gessoni G, Manoni F. Prevaence of anti-hepatitis C virus antibodies among teenagers in the Venetian area: a seroepidemiological study. Eur J Med 1993;2:79–82.
17. al-Faleh F Z, Ayoola E A, al-Jeffry M, et al. Prevalence of antibody to hepatitis C virus among Saudi Arabian children: a community-based study. Hepatology 1991;14:215–8.
18. Ngatchu T, Stroffolini T, Rapicetta M, et al. Seroprevalence of anti-HCV in an urban child population: a pilot survey in a developing area, Cameroon. J Trop Med Hyg 1992;95:57–61.
19. Jonas M M, Robertson L M, Middleman A B. Low prevalence of antibody to hepatitis C virus in an urban adolescent population. J Pediatr 1997;131:314–6.
20. Bortolotti F, Jara P, Diaz C, et al. Posttransfusion and community-acquired hepatitis C in childhood. J Pediatr Gastroenterol Nutr 1994;18:279–83.
21. Kanesaki T, Kinoshita S, Tsujino G, et al. Hepatitis C virus infection in children with hemophilia: characterization of antibody response to four different antigens and relationship of antibody response, viremia, and hepatic dysfunction. J Pediatr 1993;123:381–7.
22. Bresee J S, Mast E E, Coleman P J, et al. Hepatitis C virus infection associated with administration of intravenous immunoglobulin. JAMA 1996;276:1563–7.

23. Pastore M, Willems M, Cornu C, et al. Role of hepatitis C virus in chronic liver disease occurring after orthotopic liver transplantation. Arch Dis Child 1995;75:363–5.

24. Fortuny C, Ercilla M G, Barrera J M, et al. HCV vertical transmission: prospective study in infants born to HCV seropositive mothers. In: Hollinger F B, Lemon S M, Margolis H S, eds. Viral hepatitis and liver disease. Baltimore, MD: Williams & Wilkins, 1991:418–9.

25. Thaler M M, Park C K, Landers D V, et al. Vertical transmission of hepatitis C virus. Lancet 1991;338:17–8.

26. Reinus J F, Leikin E L, Alter H J, et al. Failure to detect vertical transmission of hepatitis C virus. Ann Intern Med 1992;117:881–6.

27. Giacchino R, Tasso L, Timitilli A, et al. Vertical transmission of hepatitis C virus infection: Usefulness of viremia detection in HIV-seronegative hepatitis C virus-seropositive mothers. J Pediatr 1998;132:167–9.

28. Wejstal R, Widell A, Mansson A-S, et al. Mother to infant transmission of hepatitis C virus. Ann Intern Med 1992;117:887–90.

29. Lam J P H, McOmish F, Burns S M, et al. Infrequent vertical transmission of hepatitis C virus. J Infect Dis 1993;167:572–6.

30. Roudot-Thoraval F, Pawlotsky J-M, Thiers V, et al. Lack of mother-to-infant transmission of hepatitis C virus in human immunodeficiency virus-seronegative women: a prospective study with hepatitis C virus RNA testing. Hepatology 1993;17:772–7.

31. Marcellin P, Bernuau J, Martinot-Peignoux M, et al. Prevalence of hepatitis C virus infection in asymptomatic anti-HIV1 negative pregnant women and their children. Dig Dis Sci 1993;38:2151–5.

32. Sabatino G, Ramenghi L A, di Marzio M, Pizzigallo E. Vertical transmission of hepatitis C virus: an epidemiological study on 2,980 pregnant women in Italy. Eur J Epidemiol 1996;12:443–7.

33. Giovanninni M, Tagger A, Ribero M L, et al. Maternal-infant transmission of hepatitis C virus and HIV infections: a possible interaction. Lancet 1990;335:1166.

34. Novati R, Theirs V, Monforte AA, et al. Mother-to-child transmission of hepatitis C virus detected by nested polymerase chain reaction. J Infect Dis 1992;165:720–3.

35. Zanetti A R, Tanzi E, Paccagnini S, et al. Mother-to-infant transmission of hepatitis C virus. Lombardy Study Group on Vertical HCV Transmission. Lancet 1995;345:289–91.

36. Paccagnini S, Principi N, Massironi E, et al. Perinatal transmission and manifestation of hepatitis C virus infection in a high risk population. Pediatr Infect Dis J 1995;14:195–9.

37. Zuccotti G V, Ribero M L, Giovannini M, et al. Effect of hepatitis C genotype on mother-to-infant transmission of virus. J Pediatr 1995;127:278–80.

38. Tovo P A, Palomba E, Ferraris G, et al. Increased risk of maternal-infant hepatitis C virus transmission for women coinfected with human immunodeficiency virus type 1. Italian Study Group for HCV Infection in Children. Clin Infect Dis 1997;25:1121–4.

39. Ohto H, Terazawa S, Sasaki N, et al. Transmission of hepatitis C virus from mothers to infants. N Engl J Med 1994;330:744–50.

40. Lin H H, Kao J H, Hsu H Y, et al. Possible role of high-titer maternal verimia in perinatal transmission of hepatitis C virus. J Infect Dis 1994;169:638–41.

41. Granovsky M O, Minkoff H L, Tess B H, et al. Hepatitis C virus infection in the mothers and infants cohort study. Pediatrics 1998;102:355–9.

42. Resti M, Azzari C, Mannelli F, et al. Mother to child transmission of hepatitis C virus: prospective study of risk factors and timing of infection in children born to women seronegative for HIV-1. Br Med J 1998;317:437–41.

43. Maggiore G, Ventura A, De Giacomo C C, Silini E, Cerino A, Mondelli M U. Vertical transmission of hepatitis C. Lancet 1995;345:1122–3.

44. Lin H-H, Kao J-H, Hsu H-Y, et al. Absence of infection in breast-fed infants born to hepatitis C virus-infected mothers. J Pediatr 1995;126:589–91.

45. Manzini P, Saracco G, Cerchier A, et al. Human immunodeficiency virus infection as a risk factor for mother-to-child hepatitis C virus transmission; persistence of anti-hepatitis C virus in children is associated with the mother's anti-hepatitis C virus immunoblotting pattern. Hepatology 1995;21:328–32.

46. Hunt C M, Carson K L, Sharara A I. Hepatitis C in pregnancy. Obstet Gynecol 1997;89:883–90.

47. Honda M, Kaneko S, Unoura M, Kobayashi K, Murakami S. Risk of hepatitis C virus infection

through household contact with chronic carriers: analysis of nucleotide sequences. Hepatology 1993;17:971–6.

48. Takahashi M, Yamada G, Tsuji T. Intrafamilial transmission of hepatitis C. Gastroenterol Jpn 1991;26:483–8.

49. Al Nasser M N. Intrafamilial transmission of hepatitis C virus (HCV): a major mode of spread in the Saudi Arabia population. Ann Trop Pediatr 1992;12:211–5.

50. Pramoolsinsap C, Kurathong S, Lerdverasirikul P. Prevalence of anti-HCV antibody in family members of anti-HCV-positive patients with acute and chronic liver disease. Southeast Asian J Trop Med Public Health 1992;23:12–6.

51. Buscarini E, Tanzi E, Zanetti AR, et al. High prevalence of antibodies to hepatitis C virus among family members of patients with anti-HCV-positive chronic liver disease. Scand J Gastroenterol 1993;28:343–6.

52. Chang T T, Liou T C, Young K C, et al. Intrafamilial transmission of hepatitis C virus: the important role of inapparent transmission. J Med Virol 1994;42:91–6.

53. Nakashima K, Ikematsu H, Hayashi J, Kishihara Y, Mutsutake A, Kashiwagi S. Intrafamilial transmission of hepatitis C virus among the population of an endemic area of Japan. JAMA 1995;274:1459–61.

54. Demelia L, Vallebona E, Poma R, Sanna G, Masia G, Coppola RC. HCV transmission in family members of subjects with HCV related chronic liver disease. Eur J Epidemiol 1996;12:45–50.

55. Arif M, al-Swayeh M, al-Faleh F Z, Ramia S. Risk of hepatitis C virus infection among household contacts of Saudi patients with chronic liver disease. J Viral Hepatitis 1996;3:97–101.

56. Brackmann S A, Gerritzen A, Oldenburg J, Brackmann H H, Schneweis K E. Search for intrafamilial transmission of hepatitis C virus in hemophilia patients. Blood 1993;81:1077–82.

57. Diago M, Zapater R, Tuset C, et al. Intrafamily transmission of hepatitis C virus: sexual and non-sexual contacts. J Hepatol 1996;25:125–8.

58. Camarero C, Martos I, Delgado R, Suarez L, Escobar H, Mateos M. Horizontal transmission of hepatitis C virus in households of infected children. J Pediatr 1993;123:98–9.

59. Vegnente A, Iorio R, Saviano A, et al. Lack of intrafamilial transmission of hepatitis C virus in family members of children with chronic hepatitis C infection. Pediatr Infect Dis J 1994;13:886–9.

60. American Academy of Pediatrics. Hepatitis C. In: Peter G, ed. 1997 Red Book: Report of the Committee on Infectious Diseases. Elk Grove Village, IL: American Academy of Pediatrics, 1997:99,260–4.

61. Garfein R S, Vlahov D, Galai N, Doherty M C, Nelson K E. Viral infections in short-term injection drug users: the prevalence of the hepatitis C, hepatitis B, human immunodeficiency, and human T-lymphotropic viruses. Am J Public Health 1996;86:655–61.

62. Mele A, Corona R, Tosti M E, et al. Beauty treatments and risk of parenterally transmitted hepatitis: results from the hepatitis surveillance system in Italy. Scand J Infect Dis 1995;27:441–4.

63. Conroy-Cantilena C, VanRaden M, Gibble J, et al. Routes of infection, viremia, and liver disease in blood donors found to have hepatitis C virus infection. N Engl J Med 1996;334:1691–6.

64. Alter M J, Coleman P J, Alexander J, et al. Importance of heterosexual activity in the transmission of hepatitis B and non-A, non-B hepatitis. JAMA 1989;262:1201–5.

65. Tedder R S, Gilson R J C, Briggs M, et al. Hepatitis C virus: evidence for sexual transmission. BMJ 1991;302:1299–302.

66. Osmond D H, Padian N S, Sheppard H W, et al. Risk factors for hepatitis C virus seropositivity in heterosexual couples. JAMA 1993;269:361–5.

67. Jonas M M, Baron M J, Bresee J S, Schneider L C. Clinical and virologic features of hepatitis C virus infection associated with intravenous immunoglobulin. Pediatrics 1996;98:211–5.

68. Hsu S-C, Chang M-H, Chen D-S, et al. Non-A,non-B hepatitis in children: a clinical, histologic, and serologic study. J Med Virol 1991;35:1–6.

69. Bortolotti F, Vajro P, Cadrobbi P, et al. Cryptogenic chronic liver disease and hepatitis C virus infection in children. J Hepatol 1992;15:73–6.

70. Bortolotti F, Vajro P, Barbera C, et al. Hepatitis C in childhood: epidemiological and clinical aspects. Bone Marrow Transplant 1993;12 (Suppl):s21–3.

71. Jonas M M, Ott M J, Nelson S P, Badizadegan K, Perez-Atayde A R. Interferon-alpha treatment of chronic hepatitis C virus infection in children. Pediatr Infect Dis J 1998;17:241–6.

72. Bortolotti F, Resti M, Giacchino R, et al. Hepatitis C virus infection and related liver disease in children of mothers with antibodies to the virus. J Pediatr 1997;130:990–3.

73. Bortolotti F, Vajro P, Balli F, et al. Non-organ specific autoantibodies in children with chronic hepatitis C. J Hepatol 1996;25:614–20.

74. Lang T, Vogt M, Schön C, et al. Prevalence, autoimmune phenomena, and clinical outcome of posttransfusion HCV infection after cardiac surgery in pediatric patients: a study on 45 patients. Hepatology 1997;26:463A.

75. Matsuoka S, Tatara K, Hayabuchi Y, Nii M, Mori K, Kuroda Y. Post-transfusion chronic hepatitis C in children. J Paediatr Child Health 1994;30:544–6.

76. Matsuoka S, Tatara K, Hayabuchi Y, et al. Serologic, virologic, and histologic characteristics of chronic phase hepatitis C virus disease in children infected by transfusion. Pediatrics 1994;94:919–22.

77. Vogt M, Lang T, Hess J, et al. Prevalence and clinical outcome of hepatitis C infection in children undergoing cardiac surgery before blood donor screening. N Engl J Med 1999;341:866–70.

78. Aricò M, Maggiore G, Silini E, et al. Hepatitis C virus infection in children treated for acute lymphoblastic leukemia. Blood 1994;84:2919–21.

79. Locasciulli A, Testa M, Pontisso P, et al. Prevalence and natural history of hepatitis C infection in patients cured of childhood leukemia. Blood 1997;90:4628–33.

80. Monteleone P M, Andrzejewski C, Kelleher J F. Prevalence of antibodies to hepatitis C virus in transfused children with cancer. Am J Pediatr Hematol/Oncol 1994;16:309–13.

81. Clemente M G, Congia M, Lai M E, et al. Effect of iron overload on the response to recombinant interferon alpha treatment in transfusion-dependent patients with thalassemia major and chronic hepatitis C. J Pediatr 1994;125:123–8.

82. Makris M, Preston F E, Rosendaal F R. The natural history of chronic hepatitis C in haemophiliacs. Br J Haematol 1996;94:746–52.

83. Bjøro K, Frøland S S, Yun Z, Samdal H H, Haaland T. Hepatitis C infection in patients with primary hypogammaglobulinemia after treatment with contaminated immune globulin. N Engl J Med 1994;331:1607–11.

84. Badizadegan K, Jonas M M, Ott M J, Nelson S P, Perez-Atayde A R. Histopathology of the liver in children with chronic hepatitis C viral infection. Hepatology 1998;28:1416–23.

85. Adams G, Kuntz S, Rabalais G, Bratcher D, Tamburro CH, Kotwal GJ. Natural recovery from acute hepatitis C virus infection by agammaglobulinemic twin children. Pediatr Infect Dis J 1997;16:533–4.

86. Kumar U, Monjardino J, Thomas H C. Hypervariable region of hepatitis C virus envelope glycoprotein (E2/NS1) in an agammaglobulinemic patient. Gastroenterology 1994;106:1072–5.

87. Palomba E, Manzini P, Fiammengo P, Maderni P, Saracco G, Tovo P-A. Natural history of perinatal hepatitis C virus infection. Clin Infect Dis 1996;23:47–50.

88. Sasaki N, Matsui A, Momoi M, Tsuda F, Okamoto H. Loss of circulating hepatitis C virus in children who developed a persistent carrier state after mother-to-baby transmission. Pediatr Res 1997;42:263–7.

89. Bortolotti F, Vajro P, Balli F, et al. Hepatitis C virus genotypes in chronic hepatitis C of children. J Viral Hepatitis 1996;3:323–7.

90. Inui A, Fujisawa T, Miyagawa Y, et al. Histologic activity of the liver in children with transfusion-associated chronic hepatitis C. J Hepatol 1994;21:748–53.

91. Kage M, Fujisawa T, Shiraki K, et al. Pathology of chronic hepatitis C in children. Hepatology 1997;26:771–5.

92. Guido M, Rugge M, Jara P, et al. Chronic hepatitis C in children: the pathological and clinical spectrum. Gastroenterology 1998;115:1525–9.

93. Bach N, Thung S N, Schaffner F. The histological features of chronic hepatitis C and autoimmune chronic hepatitis: a comparative analysis. Hepatology 1992;15:572–7.

94. Lefkowitch J H, Schiff E R, Davis G L, et al. Pathological diagnosis of chronic hepatitis C: a multicenter comparative study with chronic hepatitis B. Gastroenterology 1993;104:595–603.

95. Scheuer PJ, Ashrafzadeh P, Sherlock S, et al. The pathology of hepatitis C. Hepatology 1992;15:567–71.

96. Shakil A O, Conry-Cantilena C, Alter H J, et al. Volunteer blood donors with antibody to hepatitis C virus: clinical, biochemical, virologic, and histologic features. The Hepatitis C Study Group. Ann Intern Med 1995;123:330–7.

97. Ruíz-Moreno M, Rua M J, Castillo I, et al. Treatment of children with chronic hepatitis C with recombinant interferon-alfa: a pilot study. Hepatology 1992;16:882–5.
98. Fujisawa T, Inui A, Ohkawa T, Komatsu H, Miyakawa Y, Onoue M. Response to interferon therapy in children with chronic hepatitis C. J Pediatr 1995;127:660–2.
99. Bortolotti F, Giacchino R, Vajro P, et al. Recombinant interferon-alfa therapy in children with chronic hepatitis C. Hepatology 1995;22:1623–7.
100. Iorio R, Pensati P, Porzio S, Fariello I, Guida S, Vegnente A. Lymphoblastoid interferon alfa treatment in chronic hepatitis C. Arch Dis Child 1996;74:152–6.
101. Komatsu H, Fujisawa T, Inui A, et al. Efficacy of interferon in treating chronic hepatitis C in children with a history of acute leukemia. Blood 1996;87:4072–5.
102. Zwiener R J, Fielman B A, Cochran C, et al. Interferon-alpha-2b treatment of chronic hepatitis C in children with hemophilia. Pediatr Infect Dis J 1996;15:906–8.
103. Matsuoka S, Mori K, Nakano O, et al. Efficacy of interferons in treating children with chronic hepatitis C. Eur J Pediatr 1997;156:704–8.
104. Marcellini M, Kondili L A, Comparcola D, et al. High dosage alpha-interferon for treatment of children and young adults with chronic hepatitis C disease. Pediatr Infect Dis J 1997;16:1049–53.
105. Di Marco V, Lo Iacono O, Almasio P, et al. Long-term efficacy of alpha-interferon in beta-thalassemics with chronic hepatitis C. Blood 1997;90:2207–12.
106. National Institutes of Health. Management of hepatitis C. NIH Consensus Statement, Management of Hepatitis C, Bethesda, MD: U.S. Department of Health and Human Services, 1997.
107. Barlow C F, Priebe C J, Mulliken J B, et al. Spastic diplegia as a complication of interferon alfa-2a treatment of hemangiomas of infancy. J Pediatr 1998;132:527–30.
108. Miller V S, Zwiener R J, Fielman B A. Interferon-associated refractory status epilepticus. Pediatrics 1994;93:511–2.
109. Connor E, Morrison S, Lane J, Oleske J, Sonke R L, Connor J. Safety, tolerance, and pharmacokinetics of systemic ribavirin in children with human immunodeficiency virus infection. Antimicrob Agents Chemother 1993;37:532–9.

21
HEPATITIS C AND PREGNANCY

AUGUSTO E. SEMPRINI* AND ALESSANDRO R. ZANETTI†
Department of Obstetrics and Gynecology* and Institute of Virology†
University of Milan Medical School
Italy

INTRODUCTION

Hepatitis C during pregnancy offers several challenges in management and therapy. Chronic hepatitis C does not appear to adversely affect pregnancy, delivery, or perinatal health of the mother or newborn. Thus, a woman known to have hepatitis C virus (HCV) infection should not be counseled against becoming pregnant unless she has advanced hepatic disease. (1–3) Rather, the major issues in management should be to ensure the safety of the pregnancy for mother and child and to reduce the risk of transmission of the virus to the newborn. Counseling before pregnancy and attentive obstetric care can affect both factors favorably. Transmission of hepatitis C can occur during pregnancy, at the time of delivery, or postnatally. The relative roles of each of these times of transmission remain unclear, but most evidence indicates that the peripartum period is most important. Maternal characteristics, such as high levels of HCV RNA in serum or presence of human immunodeficiency virus (HIV) infection, may increase the likelihood of transmission. The role of obstetric factors such as cesarean versus vaginal delivery and the use of monitoring devices and different instruments are still under investigation. Most studies indicate that breast feeding and the usual maternal–infant postnatal contacts are not risk factors for transmission. The importance of maternal–infant transmission of HCV is underscored by the finding that this mode of spread is now the major cause of HCV infection among children. This chapter focuses on the prevalence of HCV infection among pregnant women in different populations, factors that influence the risk of transmission, reproductive counseling, obstetric care of women infected with HCV, and future perspectives for improved management and control of hepatitis C during pregnancy.

PREVALENCE OF HCV INFECTION AMONG PREGNANT WOMEN

Between 1 and 2% of women in childbearing age groups in western Europe, the United States, Japan, Taiwan, and Australia are reactive for antibody to HCV (anti-HCV). (1,4–15) Higher rates of anti-HCV, ranging from 2 to 5%, have been reported from eastern Europe, the Middle East, and north Africa (16, 17) and rates above 5% from some sub-Saharan populations. (18,19) The geographical variability of rates of anti-HCV among young women no doubt mirrors the differences in hepatitis C prevalence found in the general population of these countries.

In Western countries, injection drug use is the most common risk factor for hepatitis C reported among anti-HCV-positive women. Other important risk factors include previous blood transfusion and possible parenteral exposures occurring during surgery or dental care or with body piercing and tattooing. Importantly, in most studies, as many as 50% of anti-HCV-positive women had no identifiable risk factors. Because of this, half of HCV-infected women would be missed by selective antenatal screening based on reported high-risk behaviors. (9) Because hepatitis C is relatively uncommon among women of childbearing age and means of prevention of transmission are not available, public health agencies have not recommended routine screening of all pregnant women for anti-HCV.

Among pregnant women found to be anti-HCV positive, 55 to 80% have HCV RNA detectable in blood reflecting ongoing infection. (5–7,9,13,15,20) The variability in the prevalence of viremia in different studies may reflect differences in the characteristics of maternal populations (socioeconomic status, presence of coinfection with HIV, serum aminotransferase elevations, history of chronic liver disease, and injection drug use) as well as different sensitivities of the methods used to detect HCV RNA.

RISK FACTORS FOR MOTHER-TO-CHILD TRANSMISSION OF HCV

The reported rate of mother-to-infant transmission of HCV has varied widely, probably due partially to methodological differences in the various studies. (4–9,13,20–32) Thus, reported rates of transmission have ranged from 0 to 100%, based on sample sizes ranging from 4 to more than 100 mother–infant pairs. Use of standardized diagnostic criteria along with application of sensitive virological testing and frequent but set intervals need to be applied to lessen differences across studies. In a systemic review, (8) a total of 976 eligible infants from 28 studies were identified who were followed for a sufficient time with adequate serological and virological testing to calculate reliable transmission rates. Overall, maternal–infant transmission rates were less than 10% in most populations and averaged 6%.

Transmission of hepatitis C is largely restricted to infants whose mothers are viremic and the risk increases with increasing levels of HCV RNA in maternal blood. However, a specific level of HCV RNA that reliably predicts transmission cannot be defined. (4,6–9,29–32) In many studies, different methods for quantitation of HCV RNA were used, which makes comparisons difficult, but transmission was rarely reported from mothers with serum HCV RNA levels less than 10^6 copies/ml. The genotype of HCV RNA appears to have no effect on the rate of transmission. (4,6,7,9,13,33) A maternal history of chronic liver disease or elevated serum alanine aminotransferase (ALT) also does not appear to increase the likelihood of perinatal spread of hepatitis C. Studies that included women coinfected with HIV have reported higher rates of HCV transmission among coinfected maternal–infant pairs. (7–9,28,30) The increase in transmission associated with HIV coinfection is likely due to the effects of immune suppression on HCV replication and the higher levels of HCV RNA among coinfected mothers. However, in these studies, most HIV-infected women were injection drug users, and the practice of injecting drugs during and after pregnancy might also have been a risk factor for transmission. (8,9,32) Others factors, such as the quasispecies diversity of HCV and the titers of anti-HCV in maternal serum, may also influence the rate of transmission, but have not been evaluated adequately. (34) These factors may also be affected by HIV coinfection.

Current evidence indicates that rates of maternal–infant transmission of HCV infection are similar after vaginal delivery as after cesarean section. (1–3, 8,9,30,32) However, studies of the mode of delivery have not controlled adequately for other important cofactors, and definitive conclusions about the relative risks and safety of vaginal or cesarean delivery cannot be made. The role of obstetric variables such as invasive procedures (prenatal amniocentesis, fetal scalp monitoring), gestational age at birth, type of vaginal delivery (spontaneous, induced, operative), duration of rupture of membranes, and timing of cesarean section (before or during labour) remains largely unexplored. The presence of HCV infection should encourage caution in using any invasive procedure that might expose the fetus or neonate to maternal blood.

HCV can be found in low levels in breast milk, but many studies have found no association of breast feeding with maternal–infant transmission. (1–9,13, 27,30,32,35–39) Factors that might modify the risk of transmission by breast feeding, such as duration of practice, levels of HCV RNA in colostrum and milk, and exposure to chapped nipples, have not yet been sufficiently addressed.

REPRODUCTIVE COUNSELING OF WOMEN INFECTED WITH HCV

Women infected with HCV may desire to have a child and ask whether the pregnancy will affect the course of their hepatitis adversely, whether the hepatitis C will affect the course of pregnancy adversely or interfere with fertility, whether they can infect their sexual partner, whether the child will become infected with hepatitis C, and how the risk of transmission can be reduced. None of these questions are easily answered, and what answers can be given are limited by the lack of information and the lack of effective means of intervention to prevent transmission and limit the course of liver disease.

Effect of Pregnancy on Hepatitis C

Preliminary studies have indicated that pregnancy does not affect the course of chronic hepatitis C adversely; indeed serum aminotransferases often improve during pregnancy, although titers of HCV RNA can increase slightly during gestation. (40) Flares of hepatitis C following delivery are also uncommon. Women infected with HCV should, therefore, be counseled that pregnancy is unlikely to affect the underlying liver disease and their long-term prognosis negatively. (2,3) An important exception to this is the prospective mother with advanced liver disease, significant coagulopathy, thrombocytopenia, or portal hypertension. (41–43) These complications are associated with an increased risk of esophageal hemorrhage during pregnancy and obstetric hemorrhagic problems.

Prophylactic use of β blockers to prevent esophageal variceal hemorrhage may be helpful and can be given safely during pregnancy. (44) Women with chronic hepatitis C may also have an increased risk of cholestasis of pregnancy. (45) This complication is usually benign and disappears spontaneously shortly after delivery. Itching is usually limited to arms and legs and is worse at night. If severe, itching can be treated safely with ursodiol, cholestyramine, or, in countries where it is available, S-adenosylmethionine. (46,47)

Effect of Hepatitis C on Pregnancy

Chronic hepatitis C does not appear to affect the normal course of pregnancy adversely. The rates of spontaneous abortion and prematurity, as well as congenital anomalies, are similar among anti-HCV-positive as -negative mothers. Infection with HCV is not associated with decreased fertility. Use of fertility drugs and sex hormones need not be avoided in women with mild to moderate chronic hepatitis C, but these should be avoided in women with advanced disease or decompensated cirrhosis.

Sexual Transmission of Hepatitis C to Partner

Sexual transmission of hepatitis C is uncommon, particularly between monogamous sexual partners. Although HCV RNA has been reported to be detectable in female genital fluids, (48) instances of female-to-male sexual transmission of HCV are quite rare. (49) Currently, the use of condoms or other safe sex techniques is not recommended for monogamous couples and no precautions are advised in couples interested in having children. (2,3)

Infertile couples in whom either partner is infected with HCV may require assisted reproductive techniques in order to have a child. There are insufficient data on the interaction between HCV infection and assisted reproductive techniques to make recommendations. However, if the woman is infected, the couple should receive specific counseling on the potential risk of mother-to-child transmission of HCV as conception, in this setting, involves medical intervention. Obviously, both insemination attempts or *in vitro* fertilization procedures carry no risk of infection for the uninfected male. However, when the man is infected there is a potential risk of HCV transmission to the female if semen contains HCV. However, a specific study on semen of males infected with HCV has failed to detect HCV RNA in seminal fractions. (50) Furthermore, in the author's practice, over 1400 intrauterine inseminations attempts with processed semen of males infected with HCV have been performed without a case of transmission to the uninfected female partner.

Heterologous gamete donation can be required for assisted reproductive techniques. There is no report of HCV transmission through heterologous gametes donated by individuals infected with HCV, but is advisable to select uninfected donors.

Maternal–Infant Transmission of Hepatitis C

The risks of maternal–infant transmission of hepatitis C should be discussed thoroughly with prospective parents. As summarized earlier, the overall risk of transmission of hepatitis C from mother to newborn is approximately 6% and may be higher for mothers with high levels of circulating HCV RNA or with HIV coinfection. While transmission is uncommon, when it occurs, it usually results in chronic infection in the infant and the ultimate prognosis of hepatitis C in children is unsettled.

There are no known effective means of prevention of transmission of hepatitis C. Use of interferon-α and particularly ribavirin should be avoided during pregnancy as both have adverse effects on fetal development. The effects of obstetric variables on the risk of vertical transmission have yet to be evaluated adequately. Attempts should be made to avoid or reduce exposure of the fetus or newborn to maternal blood and serum. However, because cesarean delivery is not associated with either a decrease or an increase in maternal–infant transmission, the presence of HCV should not affect the decision for the type of delivery. Breast feeding is also not associated with HCV transmission and should not be discouraged. However, mothers with HCV–HIV coinfection probably should be delivered by cesarean section and should not breast feed.

Apart from the possibility of maternal–infant transmission of hepatitis C, there is little to suggest that hepatitis C in the mother affects the newborn adversely during the perinatal period. Women who develop cholestasis in pregnancy appear to be at increased risk of premature delivery and fetal distress. (51) Furthermore, women with hepatitis C may have additional risk factors for complications of pregnancy, such as drug addiction or coinfection with HIV, requiring specific reproductive counseling.

OBSTETRIC CARE OF HCV-INFECTED WOMEN

The obstetric care of women with hepatitis C should include attempts to limit further liver damage, to control the consequences of the established liver disease on the course of pregnancy, and to reduce the likelihood of maternal–infant transmission. Most women with chronic hepatitis C are asymptomatic of liver disease, have mild-to-moderate degrees of liver injury, and may expect an uneventful course of pregnancy. Nevertheless, the obstetric care of HCV-positive women should focus on avoiding or limiting the use of medications to a minimum, particularly those that require extensive hepatic metabolism. (52) When surgery is needed, preference should be given to spinal peripheral anesthesia or anesthetic agents that are not hepatotoxic.

Management of Woman with HCV-Related Cirrhosis

In women with cirrhosis, particularly those with decompensation, special attention must be paid to the management of pregnancy. The coagulopathy of liver disease can be exacerbated during pregnancy because of an increased need and monitoring of prothrombin time and administration of vitamin K may be necessary. The increased risk of hemorrhage at the time of delivery should be anticipated. Some degree of portal hypertension is present in patients with cirrhosis due to hepatitis C, and the expansion of plasma volume with pregnancy can increase the risk of esophageal or gastric variceal bleeding. (53) In instances of severe hemorrhage, delivery of the fetus may be necessary. (41,42) Variceal hemorrhage that does not respond to medical therapy, sclerotherapy, or esophageal banding may require emergency portacaval shunting, which can be carried out during pregnancy, although with a significant risk of fetal death. (54) In general, cirrhosis from hepatitis C with decompensation is an indication for liver transplantation. While liver transplantation should not be performed during pregnancy, normal pregnancies and deliveries have been reported in women after a successful liver transplant. (55–57) Risks of the immunosuppressive regimen are limited, and the increased risk of premature delivery in liver transplant patients is often acceptable to the prospective mother with a transplant. (58) Pregnancy itself does not cause a deterioration in graft function or increase the risk of rejection.

Special Obstetric Procedures in HCV-Infected Women

The safety of special obstetric procedures during pregnancy in mothers with hepatitis C is not well documented. Most evidence suggests that the transmission of hepatitis C occurs at or around the time of delivery. HCV RNA has not been found in the amniotic fluid at midgestation or at term. (59) Thus, the placenta may be an effective barrier against the transmission of HCV. Because the integrity of the placenta can be compromised by invasive prenatal procedures, such as chorionic villous sampling, amniocentesis, or cord blood sampling, these should be avoided in women infected with HCV. The vascular integrity of the placenta may also break during the contractions of labor. In women with HIV infection, a blood-borne virus that can be transmitted perinatally, a cesarean section performed before labor has been associated with a reduction in the rate of transmission of HIV. (60,61) However, in the case of hepatitis C, there is no evidence of a lesser risk of transmission with cesarean delivery compared to vaginal delivery.

CONCLUSION

Women with hepatitis C usually experience a normal and uneventful pregnancy and delivery. Maternal infection does not appear to affect pregnancy aversely nor does pregnancy have adverse effects on the course of the liver disease. The major issue raised by HCV infection during pregnancy is how to decrease the risk of transmission of the virus to the newborn. Although the rate of transmission is low, the consequences of transmission to the child may be significant. Because the level of viremia in the mother has been found to be a major risk factor for transmission, future attempts to reduce the rate of maternal–infant transmission might focus on lowering the level of viremia in the mother. In this regard, antiviral therapy of hepatitis C would seem to be a reasonable approach to control of transmission. At present, however, the antiviral agents available are tezatogenic (ribavirin) or have adverse effects on fetal growth (interferon) and should be avoided. Transmission might also be prevented by postexposure prophylaxis as is practiced for hepatitis B. However, vaccines against hepatitis C have yet to be developed and immune globulin appears to be ineffective in the prevention or spread of hepatitis C. Other approaches to reducing the rate of vertical transmission will await better studies of associated risk factors. Furthermore, antiviral treatment of women in childbearing ages before planned pregnancy may be a more rational approach to reducing the risk. At present, screening for hepatitis C during pregnancy should be limited to women who are to undergo a prenatal invasive procedure. Routine screening of all pregnant women for hepatitis C is not currently recommended, but the future availability of effective drugs to treat established infections in women and children and interventions to prevent mother-to-child infections may change this strategy.

REFERENCES

1. American Academy of Pediatrics. Hepatitis C. In: Peter G, ed. Redbook: Report of the Committee on Infectious Diseases, 24th ed. Elk Grove Village, IL: American Acadamy of Pediatrics, 1997:260–5.
2. National Institutes of Health. Consensus Development Conference, Panel Statment: Management of Hepatitis C. Hepatology 1997;26(Suppl 1):2S–10S.
3. EASL. International Consensus Conference on Hepatitis C. Consensus Statement. J Hepatol 1999;30:956–61.
4. Ohto H, Terazawa S, Sasaki N, et al. Transmission of hepatitis C virus from mothers to infants. N Engl J Med 1994;330:744–50.
5. Manzini P, Saracco G, Cerchier A, et al. Human immunodeficiency virus infection as risk factor for mother-to-child hepatitis C virus transmission: persistence of anti-hepatitis C virus in children is associated with the mother's anti-hepatitis C virus immunoblotting pattern. Hepatology 1995;21:328–32.
6. Matsubara T, Sumazaki R, Takita H. Mother-to-infant transmission of hepatitis C virus: a prospective study. Eur J Pediatr 1995;154:973–8.
7. Zanetti A R, Tanzi E, Paccagnini S, et al. Mother-to-infant transmission of hepatitis C virus. Lancet 1995;345:289–90.
8. Thomas S L, Newell M L, Peckham C S, Ades A E, Hall A J. A review of hepatitic C virus (HCV) vertical transmission: risks of transmission to infants born to mothers with and without HCV viraemia or human immunodeficiency virus infection. Int J Epidemiol 1998;27:108–17.
9. Zanetti A R, Tanzi E, Newell M L. EASL International Consensus Conference on Hepatitis C. Risk factors for mother-to-infant transmission of hepatitis C virus (HCV). J Hepatol 1999;31 (Suppl 1):96–100.
10. Roudot-Thoraval F, Pawlotsky J, Deforges L, Girollet P, Dhumeaux D. Anti-HCV seroprevalence in pregnant women in France. Gut, 1993 (Suppl 2):S55–6.
11. Wahl M, Hermonsson S, Leman J, Lindholm A, Wejstal R, Norkrans G. Prevalence of antibodies against hepatitis B and C virus among pregnant women and female blood donors in Sweden. Serodiagn Immunother Infect Dis 1994;6:127–9.
12. Lin H, Kao J, Huang S, Lee T, Chen P, Chen D. Prevalence, genotypes and antibody titer of hepatitis C virus in pregnant women in Taiwan. J Obstet Gynaecol 1995;21:557–62.
13. Moriya T, Sasaki F, Mizui M, et al. Transmission of hepatitis C virus from mothers to infants: its frequency and risk factors revisited. Biomed Pharmacother 1995;49:59–64.
14. Garner J J, Gaughwin M, Dodding J, Wilson K. Prevalence of hepatitis C infection in pregnant women in South Australia. Med J Australia 1997;167(9):470–2.
15. Chang M-H. Mother-to-infant transmission of hepatitis C virus. Clin Invest Med 1996;19: 368–72.
16. El Guneid A M, Gunaid A A, O'Neil A M, Zureikat N I, Coleman J C, Murray-Lyon I M. Prevalence of hepatitis B, C and D virus markers in Yemeni patients with chronic liver disease. J Med Virol 1993;40:330–3.
17. Hassan N F, Kotkat A. Prevalence of antibodies to hepatitis C virus in pregnant women in Egypt. J Infect Dis 1993;168:248.
18. François-Gerard C, Nkurunziza J, De Clerq C, Stouffs L, Sondag D. Seroprevalence of HIV, HBV and HCV in Rwanda. 7th Int Conf AIDS, Amsterdam, 1992;C249 [abstract].

19. Ndumbe P M, Skalsky J. Hepatitis C virus infection in different populations in Cameroon. Scand J Infect Dis 1993;25:689–92.

20. Reinus J F, Leikin E L, Alter Hj, et al. Failure to detect vertical transmission of hepatitis C virus. Ann Intern Med 1992;117:881–6.

21. Thaler M M, Park C K, Landers D V, et al. Vertical transmission of hepatitis C virus. Lancet 1991;338:17–8.

22. Weintrub P S, Veereman-Wauters G, Cowan M J, Thaler M M. Hepatitis C virus infection in infants whose mothers took street drug intravenously. J Pediatr 1991;119:869–74.

23. Novati R, Thiers V, D'Arminio Monforte A, et al. Mother-to-child transmission of hepatitis C virus detected by nested polymerase chain reaction. J Infect Dis 1992;165:720–3.

24. Wejstal R, Widell A, Mansson A-S, Hermodsson S, Norkrans G. Mother-to-infant transmission of hepatitis C virus. Ann Intern Med 1992;117:887–90.

25. Lam J P H, McOmish F, Burns S M, Yap P L, Mok J Y Q, Simmonds P. Infrequent vertical transmission of hepatitis C virus. J Infect Dis 1993;167:572–6.

26. Roudot-Thorval F, Pawlotsky J-M, Thiers V, et al. Lack of mother-to-infant transmission of hepatitis C virus in human immunodeficiency virus-seronegative women: a prospective study with hepatitis C virus RNA testing. Hepatology 1993;17:772–7.

27. Fischler B, Lindh G, Lindgren S, et al. Vertical transmission of hepatitis C virus infection. Scand J Infect Dis 1996;28:353–6.

28. Dienstag J L. Sexual and perinatal transmission of hepatitis C. Hepatology 1997;26(Suppl 1):66S–70S.

29. Mazza C, Ravaggi A, Rodella A, et al. Prospective study of mother-to-infant transmission of HCV infection. J Med Virol 1998;54:12–9.

30. Terrault N A. Epidemiological evidence for perinatal transmission of hepatitis C virus. Viral Hepatitis 1998;4:245–58.

31. Thomas D L, Villano S A, Riester K A, et al. Perinatal transmission of hepatitis C virus from human immunodeficiency virus type1-infected mothers. J Infect Dis 1998;177:1480–88.

32. Resti M, Azzari C, Mannelli F, Motino M, Vierucci A, Tuscany Study Group on HCV Infection in Children. Mother to child transmission of HCV: prospective study of risk factors and timing of infection in children born to women seronegative for HIV-1. BMJ 1998;317:437–41.

33. Zuccotti G V, Ribero M L, Giovannini M, et al. Effect of hepatitis C genotype on mother-to-infant transmission of virus. J Pediatr 1995;127:278–80.

34. Kudo T, Yanase Y, Ohshiro M, et al. Analysis of mother-to-infant transmission of hepatitis C Virus: Quasispecies nature and buoyant densities of maternal virus populations. J Med Virol 1997;51:225–30.

35. Centers for Disease Control and Prevention. Recommendations for prevention and control of hepatitis C virus (HCV) infection and HCV-related chronic disease. MMWR 1998;47 (Suppl RR-19):9.

36. Gurakan B, Oran O, Ygit, S. Vertical transmission of hepatitis C virus. N Engl J Med 1994;331:399.

37. Lin H H, Kao J H, Hsu H Y, et al. Absence of infection in breast-fed infants born to hepatitis C virus-infected mothers. J Pediatr 1995;126:589–91.

38. Ruiz-Extremera A, Gimenez-Sanchez F, Perez-Ruiz M, Torres C, Ros R, Salmeron, J. Can breastmilk contribute to perinatal transmission of hepatitis C virus (HCV)? J Hepatol 1995;23(Suppl 1):191.

39. Zimmermann R, Perucchini D, Fauchere J C, et al. Hepatitis C virus in breast milk. Lancet 1995;345:928.

40. Wejstal R, Widell A, Norkrans G. HCV-RNA levels increase during pregnancy in women with chronic hepatitis C. Scand. J Infect Dis 1998;30(2):111–3.

41. Borhanmanesh F, Haghighi P. Pregnancy in patients with cirrhosis of the liver. Obstet Gynecol 1970;36:315–8.

42. Cheng Y S. Pregnancy in liver cirrhosis and/or portal hypertension. Am J Obstet Gynecol 1977;128:812.

43. Schreyer P, Caspi E, El-Hindi J M, et al. Cirrhosis, pregnancy and delivery: a review. Obstet Gynecol Surv 1982;37:304–10.

44. Briggs G G, Freeman R K, Jaffe S J. Drugs in pregnancy and lactation, 5th ed. Baltimore, MD: Williams & Wilkins, 1998.

45. Riely C A. Hepatic disease in pregnancy. Am J Med 1994;96(1A):18S–22S.
46. Laatikainen T J. Effect of cholestiramine and phenobarbital on pruritus and serum bile acid levels in cholestasis of pregnancy. Am J Obstet Gynecol 1978;132:501–6.
47. Nicastri P L, Diaferia A, Tartagni M, Loizzi P, Fanelli M. A randomised placebo-controlled trial of ursodeoxycolic acid and S-adenosylmethionine in the treatment of intrahepatic cholestasis of pregnancy. Br J Obstet Gynaecol 1998;105(11):1205–7.
48. Tang Z, Yang D, Hao L, Tang Z, Huang Y, Wang S. Detection and significance of HCV RNA in saliva, seminal fluid and vaginal discharge in patients with hepatitis C. J Tongji Med Univ 1996;16(1):11–3,24.
49. Brettler D B, Mannucci P M, Gringeri A, et al. The low risk of hepatitis C virus transmission among sexual partner of hepatitis C-infected hemophilic males: an international, multicenter study. Blood 1992;80(2):540–3.
50. Semprini A E, Persico T, Thiers V, et al. Absence of hepatitis C virus and detection of hepatitis G virus/GB virus C RNA sequences in the semen of infected men. J Infect Dis 1998;177:848–54.
51. Reid R, Ivey K J, Rencozet R H, Storej B. Fetal complications of obstetric cholestasis. BMJ 1976;1:870–2.
52. McCormack W M, George H, Donner A, et al. Hepatotoxicity of erythromycin estolate during pregnancy. Antimicrob Agents Chemother 1997;12:630.
53. Britton R C. Pregnancy and esophageal varices. Am J Surg 1982;143(4):412–5.
54. Krol-Van Straaten J, De Maat C E. Successful pregnancies in cirrhosis of the liver before and after portocaval anastomosis. Neth J Med 1984;27(1):14–5.
55. Radomski J S, Moritz M J, Munoz S J, Cater J R, Jarrell B E, Armenti VT. National transplantation pregnancy registry: analysis of pregnancy outcomes in female liver transplant recipients. Liver Transplant Surg 1995;1(5):281–4.
56. Jain A, Venkataramanan R, Fung J J, et al. Pregnancy after liver transplantation under tacrolimus. Transplantation 1997;64(4):559–65.
57. Wu A, Nashan B, Messner U, et al. Outcome of 22 successful pregnancies after liver transplantation. Clin Transplant 1998;12(5):454–64.
58. Casele H L, Laifer S A. Association of pregnancy complications and choice of immunosuppressant in liver transplant patients. Transplantation 1998;65(4):581–3.
59. Semprini A E, Persico T, Morsica G, et al. Amniocentesis at mid-gestation in women infected with hepatitis C and GBV/C virus. Submitted for publication.
60. European Mode of Delivery Collaboration. Elective caesarean section versus vaginal delivery in prevention of transmission of vertical HIV-1 transmission: a randomized clinical trial. Lancet 1999;353:1035–9.
61. International Perinatal HIV Group. The mode of delivery and the risk of vertical transmission of human immunodeficiency virus type 1—A meta-analysis of 15 Prospective Cohort Studies. N Engl J Med 1999;340:977–87.

22

HEPATITIS C AND IRON

JOHN K. OLYNYK AND BRUCE R. BACON
Division of Gastroenterology and Hepatology
Department of Internal Medicine
Saint Louis University School of Medicine
St. Louis, Missouri

INTRODUCTION

Hepatitis C is the most common form of chronic viral hepatitis in western countries. Of individuals exposed to the hepatitis C virus, approximately 70 to 85% develop chronic hepatitis and of those, approximately 20 to 30% develop cirrhosis usually over a 20- to 30-year period of time. Of those with cirrhosis, a small subset will develop hepatic failure and/or hepatocellular carcinoma. Results of controlled trials have shown that interferon-α and, more recently, the combination of interferon-α and ribavirin are effective treatments for patients who have chronic hepatitis C. With interferon-α, approximately 10 to 15% of patients develop a sustained response, whereas with the combination of interferon and ribavirin, approximately 35 to 40% of patients can achieve a sustained response [normalization of serum alanine aminotransferase (ALT) levels and loss of hepatitis C virus (HCV) RNA at 6 months off treatment]. (1–3) Unfortunately, the use of interferon or interferon plus ribavirin is expensive and has well-documented side effects. Accordingly, there is a need to identify alternative or complementary therapies that can increase the proportion of patients who experience a sustained response. Pretreatment characteristics of a successful response include age, sex, duration of infection, mode of acquisition, liver histology, HCV RNA levels, and HCV genotype. (4–11) More recently, there has been considerable interest in the role of iron in the pathogenesis of chronic hepatitis C and also in the role of iron depletion therapy as an adjunctive measure for the treatment of liver disease due to chronic hepatitis C infection. While iron is an essential element for the survival of all cells, excess amounts of iron can result in tissue injury. (12) It is now apparent that iron can also modulate disease states and cellular function at levels much below those observed in classical iron overload, such as that seen in hereditary hemochromatosis. This chapter reviews the current state of knowledge pertaining to the role of iron in chronic hepatitis C.

SERUM AND HEPATIC IRON STUDIES IN HEPATITIS C

The study of serum and hepatic iron parameters in chronic liver disease has been achieved readily through the use of several standard methods. Serum transferrin saturation and ferritin levels, while useful in the assessment of iron overload in conditions such as hereditary hemochromatosis, are not as useful in the determination of iron status in chronic inflammatory liver diseases. These inaccuracies are due to the effect of inflammation and proinflammatory mediators on serum iron levels and hepatic transferrin and ferritin protein synthesis. (13) The "gold standard" for defining hepatic iron content is the biochemical measurement of the hepatic iron concentration. (14) The hepatic iron concentration can be determined from fresh or paraffin-embedded tissue (15) using colorimetric, (16) or atomic absorption spectrophotometry-based (17) methods. Additionally, a semiquantitative grading of iron deposition and cellular distribution can be accomplished using a histological assessment of sections stained for iron using the Perls' Prussian blue method. (18)

It has long been known that serum and hepatic iron parameters can be increased in chronic liver diseases of diverse etiologies, including hereditary hemochromatosis and other secondary iron overload disorders. (19) As early as 1974, Blumberg and colleagues described abnormal iron studies in patients with hepatitis B. (20,21) Interest in the role of iron in chronic hepatitis became rekindled in 1992 when Di Bisceglie et al. (22) noted that up to 36% of patients with chronic hepatitis C had elevated serum iron parameters, but only 5% had elevated hepatic iron concentrations to the degree generally seen in hemochromatosis. Similar observations have been reported subsequently by other groups. (23, 24) Following these observations, Van Thiel et al. (25) reported in a group of patients with chronic viral hepatitis of varying etiologies that the hepatic iron concentration of interferon responders was lower than that of interferon nonresponders and that the hepatic iron concentration could perhaps "predict" the response to interferon. Olynyk et al. (26) studied the effect of hepatic iron concentration on the response to interferon therapy in patients with chronic hepatitis C. This study demonstrated that the hepatic iron concentration was higher in nonresponders to interferon therapy compared with responders. More specifically, a hepatic iron concentration >1100 µg/g predicted a nonresponse to interferon in nearly 90% of patients. In contrast, hepatic iron concentrations ranging up to 700 µg/g were frequently seen in patients who responded to interferon. In keeping with the biochemical measurement of hepatic iron concentration, more patients demonstrated low-grade stainable hepatic iron in the nonresponder group. Additionally, the hepatic iron concentration was similar in cirrhotic patients as in noncirrhotic patients, suggesting that increased hepatic iron was not related to the histological severity of the underlying liver disease. Serum ferritin concentrations were significantly higher in the "high" iron nonresponder group than in the "low" iron nonresponder groups. However, the marked overlap of ferritin concentration between these groups precluded using an increased serum ferritin concentration to predict response. The overlap in ferritin concentrations may be due to the acute-phase reactant properties of ferritin in the setting of chronic inflammatory liver disease. Finally, responders and nonresponders had similar HCV RNA levels and there were no significant relationships among HCV RNA levels and the hepatic iron concentration, the presence of an elevated serum ferritin level, or the level of ALT. Many additional studies have been published regarding the role of iron in chronic hepatitis C. (27–41) Most have confirmed the findings that increased serum and/or hepatic iron parameters are associated with a lower likelihood of response to interferon therapy in patients with chronic hepatitis C.

Several studies have indicated that the distribution of iron within the hepatic lobule and the cell type affected by the iron may be important in determining the effect that iron has on chronic hepatitis C. It appears that the iron deposition within zone 1, portal tracts, and sinusoidal lining cells is associated with a higher likelihood of nonresponse to interferon therapy (Fig. 1). (27–34) In our study, (26) we noted that 18 of 24 responders had no stainable iron in hepatocytes or Kupffer cells. The remaining 6 responders had grade 1 stainable iron distributed equally between hepatocytes and Kupffer cells. However, 19 of 34 nonresponders showed grade 1 stainable iron distributed equally between hepatocytes and Kuppfer cells. Banner and colleagues (32) conducted a careful, morphological study of the frequency with which stainable iron occurred in sections of liver biopsies taken from patients with chronic hepatitis C. These investigators noted that interferon nonresponders had a greater accumulation of iron in sinusoidal lining cells and in portal tracts. Ikura et al. (31) found that the presence and degree of portal iron deposition had an inverse correlation with response to treatment with interferon. The presence of stainable iron has been shown to correlate with inflammation and fibrosis in patients with chronic hepatitis C, suggesting that the increased iron may have arisen from damaged hepatocytes. (41,42) In contrast, the absence of stainable iron is associated with a higher likelihood of response to interferon. (43,44) Other groups have suggested that iron may be a more significant factor in certain hepatitis C genotypes, in particular genotype lb. In a preliminary study by D'Alba et al., (45) patients with chronic hepatitis C and genotype lb had higher hepatic iron concentrations compared to patients with other hepatitis C genotypes. Genotype and hepatic iron concentration remained predictive factors of nonresponse to interferon on multivariate analysis.

HFE MUTATIONS AND HEPATITIS C

The discovery of the *HFE* gene containing two missense mutations (C282Y and H63D), of which the C282Y mutation is strongly associated with disordered iron metabolism, raises the possibility that abnormal *HFE* genotypes could contribute to iron-related cell injury in chronic hepatitis C. (46) Studies have analyzed the relationship of *HFE* mutations and iron overload in chronic hepatitis C. (46–49) Patients with chronic hepatitis C have frequencies of *HFE* mutations that are no different from the general population. However, heterozygosity for the C282Y mutation (C282Y/wt) is often associated with increased iron stores and with more advanced liver fibrosis. (50) There is a much stronger association among *HFE* gene mutations, abnormal iron status, and HCV infection in patients with porphyria cutanea tarda. (47,51,52) Thus, in this group of patients, it is possible that iron could play a more significant role in the pathogenesis of hepatitis C-related liver injury, but this remains to be confirmed in additional prospective studies.

PATHOPHYSIOLOGY OF IRON TOXICITY IN CHRONIC HEPATITIS C

The mechanisms by which iron may cause liver disease have been recently reviewed. (12) The concept that iron can act in a synergistic fashion with other hepatotoxins has been described previously. Iron has been shown to be a synergistic factor in the pathogenesis of alcohol and carbon tetrachloride-induced liver diseases. (53–55) It is generally accepted that iron increases the formation of reactive oxygen intermediates, which can result in lipid peroxidation and then lead to oxidative damage to proteins, membrane phospholipids, and nucleic acids. Subsequently, this can result in organelle dysfunction, fibrosis, and eventually hepatocellular carcinoma. Although these findings were initially based on studies in experimental iron overload, lipid peroxidation products have been shown in the plasma (56) and in liver biopsies (57,58) from patients with chronic hepatitis C. Farinati et al. (57) studied whether HCV could have a direct cytopathic effect on hepatocytes through the occurrence of iron-dependent lipid peroxidation. Patients with chronic hepatitis C had significantly greater lobular inflammation, more steatosis, higher serum ferritin levels, transferrin saturation levels, tissue iron levels, glutathione levels, and malondialdehyde levels compared with patients with other forms of chronic hepatitis not related to HCV infection. These results suggested that altered iron metabolism and iron accumulation in chronic hepatitis C could be related to a specific effect of the virus on parenchymal or nonparenchymal cell function. In liver tissue, lipid peroxidation products are mainly observed in portal tract macrophages. (58) Lipid peroxidation products have been shown to stimulate collagen production in activated hepatic stellate cells and in cultured human fibroblasts. (59,60) Alternatively, lipid peroxidation products may increase the production of transforming growth factor-β (TGF-β) or other profibrogenic substances produced by Kupffer cells, which may then activate hepatic stellate cells. (61,62)

It is well known that the risk for development of hepatocellular carcinoma is increased substantially in both hereditary hemochromatosis and in patients with long-standing chronic hepatitis C with cirrhosis. (63) Mechanisms responsible for the development of hepatocellular carcinoma in chronic liver disease are not clear, but several potential mechanisms exist. Chronic infection with HCV may be directly oncogenic. (64) Alternatively, HCV-induced chronic liver injury may culminate in cirrhosis with an increased risk for the development of hepatocellular carcinoma. (65) As cirrhosis develops, hepatocellular necrosis is followed by an attempted secondary proliferative response of mature hepatocytes. (66–69) However, this proliferative response is often impaired in patients with chronic liver disease. An alternative mechanism for hepatocyte regeneration in chronic liver disease involves stem cell proliferation and differentiation into hepatocytes. In humans, oval cells have been reported in hepatitis B-associated hepatocellular carcinoma and chronic liver disease associated with ductular proliferation. (70,71) We have shown that oval cells are present in patients with hereditary hemochromatosis and chronic hepatitis C. (72) Further-

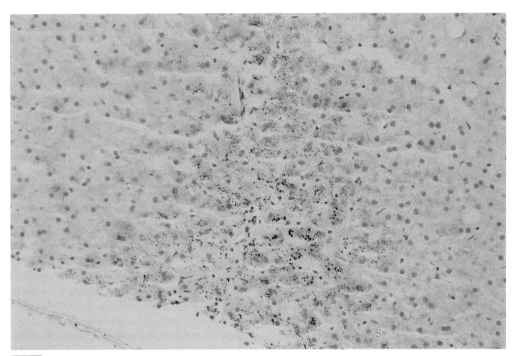

FIGURE 1 Hepatic iron deposition in chronic hepatitis C. This photomicrograph shows 1+ deposition of iron, which is found in sinusoidal lining cells (Kupffer cells) and in hepatocytes; 20×, Perls' Prussian blue (photographs courtesy of Dr. Elizabeth M. Brunt).

A

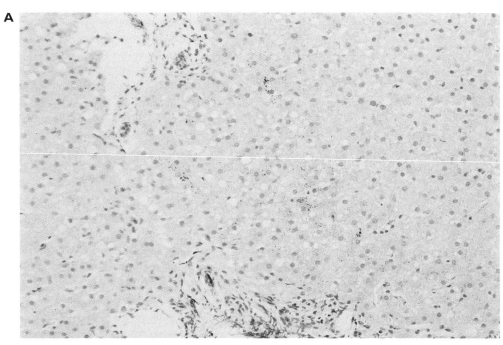

B

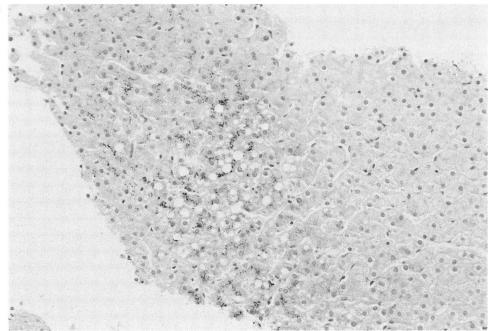

FIGURE 3   Hepatic iron deposition in chronic hepatitis C following treatment with interferon and ribavirin. Ribavirin-induced hemolysis results in increased iron deposition predominantly in Kupffer cells. (A) Before treatment, 20×, Perls' Prussian blue; and (B) after treatment, 20×, Perls' Prussian blue (photographs courtesy of Dr. Elizabeth M. Brunt).

more, oval cell numbers increase significantly with the progression of disease severity in each of the groups studied, suggesting that oval cell proliferation is not disease specific, but rather occurs in response to progressive liver injury and fibrosis. The association between severity of liver disease and increasing number of oval cells is consistent with the hypothesis that oval cell proliferation is associated with the increased risk for development of hepatocellular carcinoma, particularly when cirrhosis is present. Finally, iron could contribute to the increased risk of hepatocellular carcinoma in chronic hepatitis C through DNA damage from iron-induced adduct formation and chromosomal damage. (73,74)

   The pathophysiological mechanisms whereby iron exerts its effects in chronic hepatitis C are unknown. Much evidence has accumulated supporting an immunopathological mechanism that underlies liver injury in chronic hepatitis C. (75–77) Virus-specific T cells are present in the liver tissue and peripheral blood of patients with chronic hepatitis C infection and are able to contribute to hepatocellular injury, but are not able to eliminate the viral infection. (78,79) Previous studies have shown that persistent hepatitis B virus infection is associated with iron overload. (20,21,80) It is also known that patients with iron overload are more susceptible to bacterial infections. (81) Iron has been shown to impair antigen-specific immune responses and generation of cytotoxic T cells, decrease functional T helper precursor cells, and enhance T suppressor activity. (82,83) Natural killer cell activity has also been reported to be decreased in conditions of iron overload. (84–86) Lymphocyte proliferation is inhibited by ferritin. (87,88) Ferritin molecules, particularly those rich in heavy (H) subunits, bind to activated T cells (89) and H-ferritin receptors are expressed by T cell lines. (90,91) These data suggest that iron could impair the host lymphocyte-dependent clearance of HCV virus. Interferon-α possesses multiple actions, including direct antiviral effects and enzyme modulation. (92) The actions of interferon are not known to be dependent on intracellular iron, although it is possible that iron may also interfere in some way with these actions, resulting in reduced antiviral activity. It has been suggested that transferrin and nontransferrin-bound iron-uptake pathways may be affected by necroinflammatory conditions. (93) As a result, patients with chronic hepatitis C who fail to respond to interferon may have increased iron uptake and hepatic iron deposition when compared with those who respond. Increased hepatic iron deposition in hepatitis C may then result in increased oxidative stress in the liver, decreased glutathione levels, and increased lipid peroxidation and formation of malondialdehyde adducts. (29,32,39,40,56–58) The type of storage molecule from which iron is released could modulate these effects further. It is well known that ferritin and hemosiderin release iron to different degrees, a property that may influence the ability of iron to participate in biological actions. (94)

   It is possible that iron deposition in sinusoidal lining cells, especially Kupffer cells, could alter the immune responsiveness of macrophages. This hypothesis is supported by observations that iron deposition within zone 1, portal tracts, and sinusoidal lining cells is associated with a higher likelihood of nonresponsiveness to interferon therapy. (27–34) There are reports of impaired phagocytic function by monocytes taken from patients with hereditary hemochromatosis. (95,96) Intracellular killing of microorganisms may also be impaired by iron overload. (96,97) Interleukin-2 production by cytotoxic T cells is reduced in the presence of iron overload. (83) We have studied the effect of chronic iron overload on Kupffer cell cytokine production. (98) Kupffer cells from iron-loaded animals exhibit reduced proinflammatory cytokine production compared with Kupffer cells from control animals. Thus, iron loading could impair immune clearance mechanisms via impaired macrophage function or interfere with the actions of interferon-α on macrophage function.

IRON STATUS AND LIKELIHOOD OF RESPONSE TO INTERFERON THERAPY

Following reports of the relationship between iron status and likelihood of response to interferon, investigators began evaluating the possibility that patients might benefit by being depleted of iron by repeated therapeutic phlebotomy before treatment with interferon in naïve patients or to improve response rates in previous interferon nonresponders. Hayashi et al. (34) reported that iron reduction alone led to the normalization of serum ALT levels in 5 of 10 patients with chronic hepatitis C. Four to 13 phlebotomies, with removal of 1 to 3 g of iron, over 2 to 9 months were required to achieve iron removal as judged by serum ferritin levels dropping to <10 ng/ml. Seven patients underwent repeat biopsy within 2 months of iron depletion with no apparent change in the severity of portal fibrosis or inflammation. In another study of 8 patients with chronic hepatitis C who had previously failed to respond to treatment with interferon-α, serum ALT levels fell in 7 of 8 following iron reduction. (38) Van Thiel et al. (99) randomized 30 interferon nonresponders to either iron depletion followed by an increased dose of interferon-α or to an increased dose of interferon alone. Twelve of 15 (80%) patients treated with iron depletion and interferon-α had a virological response at 6 months compared with 6 of 15 (40%) in the interferon alone group. Significantly higher sustained virological response rates were seen in the iron-depleted group (60%) compared with the interferon alone group (13%) ($p < 0.05$). Iron chelation with desferrioxamine has also been shown to improve the response to interferon therapy. (100) However, there have been no clear effects of iron reduction on levels of HCV RNA in serum. (100–102)

Fong et al. (43) conducted a randomized study that evaluated the effect of iron depletion on aminotransferase activity, HCV RNA levels, and response to interferon-α therapy in patients with chronic hepatitis C. Serum ALT levels decreased in 15 of 17 patients following phlebotomy. Changes in iron indices and in ALT levels were not accompanied by changes in HCV RNA levels. At the end of 24 weeks of interferon therapy, similar numbers of patients who had undergone phlebotomy (7 of 17) had a biochemical response compared to control patients (6 of 21). However, after 6 months of follow-up, 5 of 17 patients who had undergone phlebotomy remained HCV RNA negative compared with only 1 of 21 control patients ($p = 0.07$). Tsai et al. (103) have also shown that phlebotomy therapy may result in a sustained response in up to 15% of patients who have not responded previously to treatment with interferon but who are retreated following phlebotomy therapy.

Boucher et al. (27) have provided additional information on the possible relationships between hepatic iron metabolism and chronic hepatitis C. In their study, 55 patients were treated with interferon-α for 6 months and the hepatic iron concentration and distribution of iron were evaluated before and after therapy. They found no difference in hepatic iron concentration between patients who responded to interferon and those who did not respond. However, they did identify a relation between hepatic iron concentration and inflammatory activity, such that the iron load was higher in those patients with the greatest degree of histological inflammatory activity. Interestingly, the hepatic iron concentration decreased following treatment with interferon. This was related to iron that was apparently depleted from sinusoidal lining cells and appeared regardless of whether patients responded to interferon therapy or not. These findings suggest that increased iron stores may be present in patients with chronic hepatitis C predominantly as a result of the degree of inflammatory activity, presumably correlating with cell injury or necrosis, with subsequent phagocytosis by Kupffer cells resulting in progressive increases in Kupffer cell iron loading.

We have completed a multicenter study wherein 97 patients who had failed previously to respond to interferon-α were randomly divided to receive either phlebotomy alone or phlebotomy with interferon-α retreatment for 6 months. Phlebotomy therapy was well tolerated and resulted in a significant reduction in serum ALT levels, a significant reduction in inflammatory activity on serial liver biopsy, but no change in HCV RNA levels (see Fig. 2). (104,105) These results suggest a histological and biochemical benefit by iron reduction therapy for patients who are unable to achieve a sustained virologic response with antiviral therapy.

Combination therapy with interferon-α and ribavirin is increasingly being used to treat patients with chronic hepatitis C who are either naïve to therapy or who have relapsed. (3,106) Interestingly, despite an increase in sustained response rates, there is an increase in hepatic iron concentration due to the effects

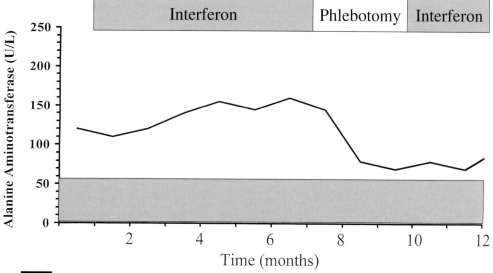

FIGURE 2 Typical ALT response to iron reduction therapy in patients with chronic hepatitis C. During an initial 6-month course of interferon, there is no reduction in serum ALT levels in a patient who fails to respond. Weekly phlebotomy renders the patient iron deficient and the ALT level is reduced by about 40%. Retreatment with interferon fails to lower ALT into the normal range.

of ribavirin-induced hemolysis with a subsequent stimulus to increased iron absorption (see Fig. 3). (107) This would suggest that the synergistic antiviral effect of ribavirin, when added to interferon-α, is of greater importance than the negative effects from the increase in iron deposition. Studies examining the efficacy and safety of iron reduction therapy prior to and/or during treatment with interferon and ribavirin have not been completed.

CONCLUSION

In summary, iron clearly influences the response of chronic hepatitis C to treatment and perhaps to the natural history of chronic hepatitis C. Mechanisms responsible for the effects of iron are not clear, but emerging data would suggest that the cellular location of iron within the hepatic lobule and the subsequent effects on immune function may well be critical determinants for these effects. Continued evaluation of therapies for chronic hepatitis C that either remove iron or interfere with the action of iron at the cellular level may prove useful clinically and may provide some insights into the mechanisms of cellular injury in this disease.

REFERENCES

1. Davis G L, Balart L, Schiff E R, et al. Treatment of chronic hepatitis C with recombinant interferon alfa. A multicenter randomized, controlled trial. N Engl J Med 1989;321:501–6.
2. Saracco G, Rizzetto M. The long-term efficacy of interferon alfa in chronic hepatitis C patients: A critical review. J Gastroenterol Hepatol 1995;10:668–73.
3. McHutchison J G, Gordon S C, Schiff E R, et al. Interferon alfa-2b alone or in combination with ribavirin as initial treatment for chronic hepatitis C. N Engl J Med 1998;339:1485–92.
4. Caussse X, Godinot H, Chevallier M, et al. Comparison of 1 or 3 MU of interferon alfa-2b and placebo in patients with chronic non-A, non-B hepatitis. Gastroenterology 1991;101:497–502.
5. Lin R, Grierson J, Schoeman M N, et al. Can the response to interferon treatment be predicted in patients with chronic active hepatitis C? Aust N Z J Med 1991;21:387–92.
6. Perez P, Pravia R, Linares A, et al. Response related factors in recombinant interferon alfa-2b treatment of chronic hepatitis C. Gut, Suppl 1993;S139–40.
7. Lau J Y N, Davis G L, Kniffen J, Qian K P. Significance of serum hepatitis C virus RNA levels in chronic hepatitis C. Lancet 1993;341:1501–4.
8. Tsubota A, Chayama K, Arase Y, et al. Factors useful in predicting the response to interferon therapy in chronic hepatitis C. J Gastroenterol Hepatol 1993;8:535–9.
9. Mita E, Hayashi N, Hagiwara H, et al. Predicting interferon therapy efficacy from hepatitis C virus genotype and RNA titer. Dig Dis Sci 1994;39: 977–82.
10. Pagliarc L, Craxi A, Cammaa C, et al. Interferon-α for chronic hepatitis C: An analysis of pretreatment clinical predictors of response. Hepatology 1994;19:820–8.
11. Davis G L. Prediction of response to interferon treatment of chronic hepatitis C. J Hepatol 1994; 21:1–3.
12. Britton R S, Ramm G A, Olynyk J, Singh R, O'Neill R, Bacon B R. Pathophysiology of iron toxicity. Adv Exp Med Biol 1994;356:239–53.
13. Worwood M. Serum ferritin. Clin Sci 1986;70:215–20.
14. Powell L W, Jazwinska E, Halliday J W. Primary iron overload. In: Brock J H, Halliday J W, Pippard M J, Powell L W, eds. Iron metabolism in health and disease. London: Saunders 1994; 227–70.
15. Olynyk J K, O'Neill R, Britton R S, Bacon B R. Determination of hepatic iron concentration in fresh and paraffin-embedded tissue: diagnostic implications. Gastroenterology 1994;106: 674–7.

16. Torrance J D, Bothwell T H. Tissue iron stores. In: Cook J D, ed. Iron. Methods in hematology, Vol. 1. New York: Churchill-Livingstone, 1980:90–115.

17. Olynyk J, Hall P, Sallie R, Reed W, Shilkin K, Mackinnon M. Computerized measurement of iron in liver biopsies: comparison with biochemical iron measurement. Hepatology 1990;12: 26–30.

18. Searle J W, Kerr J F R, Halliday J W, Powell L W. Iron storage disease. In: MacSween R N M, Anthony P P, Scheuer P J, eds. Pathology of the liver, 2nd ed. New York: Churchill-Livingstone, 1987;181–201.

19. Prieto J, Barry M, Sherlock S. Serum ferritin in patients with iron overload and with acute and chronic liver diseases. Gastroenterology 1975;68:525–33.

20. Sutnik A L, Blumberg B S, Lustbader E D. Elevated serum iron levels and persistent Australian antigen (HBsAg). Ann Intern Med 1974;81:855–6.

21. Lustbader E D, Hann H W L, Blumberg B S. Serum ferritin as a predictor of host response to hepatitis B virus infection. Science 1983;220:423–5.

22. Di Bisceglie A M, Axiotis C A, Hoofnagle J H, Bacon B R. Measurement of iron status in patients with chronic hepatitis. Gastroenterology 1992;102:2108–13.

23. Riggio O, Montagnese F, Fiore P, et al. Iron overload in patients with chronic viral hepatitis: how common is it? Am J Gastroenterol 1997;92:1298–301.

24. Arber N, Konikoff F M, Moshkowitz M, et al. Increased serum iron and iron saturation without iron accumulation distinguish chronic hepatitis C from other chronic liver diseases. Dig Dis Sci 1994;39:2656–9.

25. Van Thiel D H, Friedlander L, Faginoli S, Wright H I, Irish W, Gavaler J S. Response to interferon-α therapy is influenced by the iron content of the liver. J Hepatol 1994;20:410–5.

26. Olynyk J K, Reddy K R, Di Bisceglie A M, et al. Hepatic iron concentration as a predictor of response to interferon alfa therapy in chronic hepatitis C. Gastroenterology 1995;108:1104–9.

27. Boucher E, Bourienne A, Adams P, Turlin B, Brissot P, Deugnier Y. Liver iron concentration and distribution in chronic hepatitis C before and after interferon treatment. Gut 1997;41: 115–20.

28. Fargion S, Fracanzani A L, Sampietro M, et al. Liver iron influences the response to interferon alpha therapy in chronic hepatitis C. Eur J Gastroenterol Hepatol 1997;9:497–503.

29. Paradis V, Mathurin P, Kollinger M, et al. In situ detection of lipid peroxidation in chronic hepatitis C: correlation with pathological features. J Clin Pathol 1997;50:401–6.

30. Izumi N, Enomoto N, Uchihara M, et al. Hepatic iron contents and response to interferon-alpha in patients with chronic hepatitis C. Relationship to genotypes of hepatitis C. Dig Dis Sci 1996;41:989–94.

31. Ikura Y, Morimot H, Johmura H, Fukui M, Sakurai M. Relationship between hepatic iron deposits and response to interferon in chronic hepatitis C. Am J Gastroenterol 1996;91:1367–73.

32. Banner B F, Barton A L, Cable E E, Smith L, Bonkovsky H L. A detailed analysis of the Knodell score and other histologic parameters as predictors of response to interferon therapy in chronic hepatitis C. Mod Pathol 1995;8:232–8.

33. Barton A L, Banner B F, Cable E E, Bonkovsky H L. Distribution of iron in the liver predicts response of chronic hepatitis C infection to interferon therapy. Am J Clin Pathol 1995;103: 419–24.

34. Hayashi H, Takikawa T, Nishimura N, Yano M. Improvement of serum aminotransferase levels after phlebotomy in patients with chronic active hepatitis C and excess hepatic iron. Am J Gastroenterol 1994;89:986–8.

35. Piperno A, D'Alba R, Fargion S, et al. Liver iron concentration in chronic viral hepatitis: a study of 98 patients. J Gastroenterol Hepatol 1995;7:1203–308.

36. Di Marco V, Iacono O L, Almasio P, et al. Long-term efficacy of α-interferon in β-thalassemics with chronic hepatitis C. Blood 1997;90:2207–12.

37. Hayashi H, Takikawa T, Nishimura N, Yano M. Serum aminotransferase levels as an indicator of the effectiveness of venesection for chronic hepatitis C. J Hepatol 1995;22:268–71.

38. Bacon B R, Rebholz A E, Fried M, Di Bisceglie A M. Beneficial effect of iron reduction therapy in patients with chronic hepatitis C who failed to respond to interferon-α. Hepatology 1993; 18:90A.

39. Piperno A, Sampietro M, D'Alba R, et al. Iron stores, response to α-interferon therapy, and effects of iron depletion in chronic hepatitis C. Liver 1996;16:248–54.

40. Clemente M G, Congia M, Lai M E, et al. Effect of iron overload on the response to recombinant interferon-alfa treatment in transfusion-dependent patients with thalassemia major and chronic hepatitis C. J Pediatr 1994;125:123–8.

41. Beinker N K, Voigt M D, Arendse M, Smit J, Stander I A, Kirsch R E. Threshold effect of liver iron content on hepatic inflammation and fibrosis in hepatitis B and C. J Hepatol 1996;25: 633–8.

42. Kaji K, Nakanuma Y, Sasaki M, Unoura M, Kobayashi K, Nonomura A. Hemosiderin deposition in portal endothelial cells: a novel hepatic hemosiderosis frequent in viral hepatitis B and C. Hum Pathol 1995:26:1080–5.

43. Fong T, Han S, Tsai N, et al. A pilot randomized, controlled trial of the effect of iron depletion on long-term response to α-interferon in patients with chronic hepatitis C. J Hepatol 1998;28: 369–74.

44. Kaserer K, Fiedler R, Steindl P, Muller C H, Wrba F, Ferenci P. Liver biopsy is a useful predictor of response to interferon therapy in chronic hepatitis C. Histopathology 1998;32:454–61.

45. D'Alba R, Sampietro M, Fargion S, et al. Iron stores and virus genotypes in chronic hepatitis C: relation with α-interferon response. Hepatology 1995;22:180A.

46. Bacon B R, Powell L W, Adams P C, Kresina T F, Hoofnagle J H. Molecular medicine and hemochromatosis: at the crossroads. Gastroenterology 1999;116:193–207.

47. Stuart K A, Busfield F, Jazwinska E C, et al. The C282Y mutation in the haemochromatosis gene (HFE) and hepatitis C virus infection are independent cofactors for porphyria cutanea tarda in Australian patients. J Hepatol 1998;28:404–9.

48. Kazemi-Shirazi L, Datz C, Maier-Dobersberger T, et al. The relation of iron status and hemochromatosis gene mutations in patients with chronic hepatitis C. Gastroenterology 1999;116: 127–34.

49. Bacon B R, Olynyk J K, Brunt E M, Britton R S, Wolff R K. *HFE* genotype in patients with hemochromatosis and other liver diseases. Ann Intern Med 1999;130:953–62.

50. Smith B C, Gorve J, Guzail M A, et al. Heterozygosity for hereditary hemochromatosis is associated with fibrosis in chronic hepatitis C. Hepatology 1998;27:1695–9.

51. Bonkovsky H, Poh-Fitzpatrick M, Pimstone N, et al. Porphyria cutanea tarda, hepatitis C and *HFE* gene mutations in North America. Hepatology 1998;27:1661–9.

52. Roberts A G, Whatley S D, Morgan R R, Worwood M, Elder G H. Increased frequency of the haemochromatosis Cys282Tyr mutation in sporadic porphyria cutanea tarda. Lancet 1997; 349:321–3.

53. Stal P, Hultcranz R. Iron increases ethanol toxicity in rat liver. J Hepatol 1993;17:108–15.

54. Olynyk J, Mackinnon M, Reed W, Williams P, Kerr R, Mackinnon M. A long-term study of the interaction between iron and alcohol in an animal model of iron overload. J Hepatol 1995;22: 671–6.

55. Mackinnon M, Clayton C, Plummer J, et al. Iron overload facilitates hepatic fibrosis in the rat alcohol/low-dose carbon tetrachloride model. Hepatology 1995;21:1083–8.

56. Higueras V, Raya A, Rodrigo J M, Serra M A, Roma J, Romero F J. Interferon decreases serum lipid peroxidation products of hepatitis C patients. Free Radical Biol Med 1994;16:131–3.

57. Farinati R F, Cardin R, DeMaria N, et al. Iron storage, lipid peroxidation and glutathione turnover in chronic anti-HCV positive hepatitis. J Hepatol 1995;22:449–56.

58. Kikuyama M, Kobayashi Y, Kawasaki T, Yoshimi T. Hepatic lipid peroxidation in chronic hepatitis C. Hepatology 1995;22:276A.

59. Maher J J, Zia S, Tzagarakis C. Acetaldehyde-induced stimulation of collagen synthesis and gene expression is dependent on conditions of cell culture: studies with rat lipocytes and fibroblasts. Alcohol: Clin Exp Res 1994;18:403–9.

60. Maher J J, Tzagarakis C, Gimenez A. Malondialdehyde stimulates collagen production by hepatic lipocytes only upon activation in primary culture. Alcohol Alcohol 1994;29:605–10.

61. Leonarduzzi G, Scavazza A, Biasi F, et al. The lipid peroxidation end product 4-hydroxy-2, 3-nonenal up-regulates transforming growth factor beta-1 expression in the macrophage lineage: a link between oxidative injury and fibrosclerosis. FASEB J 1997;11:851–7.

62. Parola M, Muraca R, Dianzani I, et al. Vitamin E dietary supplementation inhibits transforming growth factor beta-1 gene expression in the rat liver. FEBS Lett 1992;308:267–70.

63. Roudot-Thoraval F, Bastie A, Pawlotsky J M, Dhumeaux D. Epidemiological factors affecting the severity of hepatitis C virus-related liver disease: a French survey of 6,664 patients. The

Study Group for the Prevalence and the Epidemiology of Hepatitis C Virus. Hepatology 1997; 26:485–90.

64. Ikeda K, Saitoh S, Koida Y, et al. A multivariate analysis of risk factors for hepatocellular carcinogenesis: a prospective observation of 795 patients with viral and alcoholic cirrhosis. Hepatology 1993;18:47–53.

65. Kew M C. Hepatic tumors and cysts. In: Feldman M, Scharschmidt B F, Sleisenger M H, eds. Sleisenger and Fordtran's gastrointestinal and liver diseases: Pathophysiology/diagnosis/management. Philadelphia, PA: Saunders, 1998;1364–87.

66. Sell S, Dunsford H A. Evidence for the stem cell origin of hepatocellular carcinoma and cholangiocarcinoma. Am J Pathol 1989;134:1347–63.

67. Lemire J M, Shiojiri N, Fausto N. Oval cell proliferation and the origin of small hepatocytes in liver injury induced by D-galactosamine. Am J Pathol 1991;139:535–52.

68. Evarts R P, Nagy P, Marsden E, Thorgeirsson S S. A precursor-product relationship exists between oval cells and hepatocytes in rat liver. Carcinogenesis 1987;8:1737–40.

69. Hixson D C, Fowler L C. Development and phenotypic heterogeneity of intrahepatic biliary epithelial cells. In: Sirica A E, Longnecker D S, eds. Biliary and pancreatic ductal epithelia: pathobiology and pathophysiology. New York: Dekker, 1997:1–40.

70. Ray M B, Mendenhall C L, French S W, Gartside P S. Bile duct changes in alcoholic liver disease. The Veterans Administration Cooperative Study Group. Liver 1993;13:36–45.

71. Hsia C C, Evarts R P, Nakatsukasa H, Marsden E R, Thorgeirsson S S. Occurrence of oval-type cells in hepatitis B virus-associated human hepatocarcinogenesis. Hepatology 1992;16:1327–33.

72. Lowes K N, Brennan B A, Yeoh G C, Olynyk J K. Oval cell numbers in human chronic liver diseases are directly related to disease severity. Am J Pathol 1999;154:537–41.

73. Edling J E, Britton R S, Grisham M B, Bacon B R. Increased unwinding of hepatic double-stranded DNA (dsDNA) in rats with chronic dietary iron overload. Gastroenterology 1990;98:A585.

74. Nordenson I, Ritter B, Beckman A, Beckman L. Idiopathic haemochromatosis and chromosomal damage. Hum Hered 1992;42:143–5.

75. Gonzalez-Peralta R P, Davis G L, Lau J Y N. Pathogenetic mechanisms of hepatocellular damage in chronic hepatitis C virus infection. J Hepatol 1994;21:255–9.

76. Mondelli M U, Cerino A, Bellotti V, de Koning A. Immunobiology and pathogenesis of hepatitis C virus infection. Res Virol 1993;144:269–74.

77. Cerny A, Chisari F V. Immunological aspects of HCV infection. Intervirology 1994;37:119–25.

78. Sherman K E, O'Brien J, Gutierrez A G, et al. Quantitative evaluation of hepatitis C virus RNA in patients with concurrent human immunodeficiency virus and the hepatotropic viruses. J Clin Microbiol 1993;31:2679–82.

79. Horvath J, Raffanti S P. Clinical aspects of the interactions between human immunodeficiency virus and the hepatotropic viruses. Clin Infect Dis 1994;18:339–47.

80. Senba M, Nakamura T, Itakura H. Statistical analysis of relationship between iron accumulation and hepatitis B surface antigen. Am J Clin Pathol 1985;84:340–2.

81. Bullen J J, Spalding P B, Ward C G, Guttenridge J M. Hemochromatosis, iron and septicemia caused by *Vibrio vulnificus*. Arch Intern Med 1991;151:1606–9.

82. Good M F, Powell L W, Halliday J W. Iron status and cellular immune competence. Blood Rev 1988;2:43–9.

83. Good M F, Chapman D E, Powell L W, Halliday J W. The effect of experimental ironoverload on splenic T cell function: analysis using clonal techniques. Clin Exp Immunol 1987;68:375–83.

84. Gascon P, Zoumbos N C, Young N S. Immunological abnormalities in patients receiving multiple blood transfusions. Ann Intern Med 1984;100:173–7.

85. Kaplan J, Sarnaik S, Gitlin J, Lusher J. Diminished helper/suppressor lymphocyte ratios and natural killer activity in recipients of repeated blood transfusions. Blood 1984;64:308–10.

86. Akbar A N, Fitzgerald-Bocarsly P A, De Sousa M, Giardina P J, Hilgartner M W, Grady R W. Decreased natural killer activity in thalassemia major: a possible consequence of iron overload. J Immunol 1986;136:1635–40.

87. Matzner Y, Hershko C, Polliack A, Konijn A M, Izak G. Suppressive effect of ferritin on in vitro lymphocyte function. Br J Haematol 1979;42:345–53.

88. Harada T, Bab M, Torii I, Morikawa S. Ferritin selectively suppresses delayed-type hypersensitivity responses at induction and effector phase. Cell Immunol 1987;109:75–88.

89. Pattananpanyasat K, Hoy T G, Jacobs A. The response of intracellular and surface ferritin after T-cell stimulation in vitro. Clin Sci 1987;73:605–11.

90. Konijn A M, Meyron-Holtz E G, Levy R, Ben-Bassat H, Matzner Y. Specific binding of placental acidic isoferritin to cells of the T-cell line HD-MDR. FEBS Lett 1990;263:229–32.

91. Moss D, Powell L W, Arosio P, Halliday J W. Characterization of the ferritin receptors of human T-lymphoid (MOLT-4) cells. J Lab Clin Med 1992;119:273–9.

92. Chelbi-Alix MK, Thang MN. Multiple molecular forms of interferon display different specific activities in the induction of the antiviral state and $2'5'$ oligoadenylate synthetase. Biochem Biophys Res Commun 1986;141:1042–50.

93. Bacon B R, Fried M W, Di Bisceglie A M. A 39-year-old man with chronic hepatitis, elevated serum ferritin values, and a family history of hemochromatosis. Semin Liver Dis 1993;13:101–5.

94. Ward R J, O'Connell M J, Dickinson D P E, et al. Biochemical studies of the iron cores and polypeptide shells of haemosiderin isolated from patients with primary or secondary haemochromatosis. Biochim Biophys Acta 1989;993:131–3.

95. Van Asbeck B S, Verbrugh H A, van Oost B A, Marx J J, Imhof H W, Verhoef J. Listeria monocytogenes meningitis and decreased phagocytosis associated with iron overload. BMJ 1982;284:542–4.

96. Van Asbeck B S, Marx J J M, Struyvenberg J, Verhoef J. Functional defects in phagocytic cells from patients with iron overload. J Infect Dis 1984;8:232–40.

97. Ballart I J, Estevez M E, Sen L, et al. Progressive dysfunction of monocytes associated with iron overload and age in patients with thallasemia major. Blood 1986;67:105–9.

98. Olynyk J, Clarke S L. Functional heterogeneity of Kupffer cells in iron overload. Hepatology 1998;28:1115A.

99. Van Thiel D H, Friedlander L, Malloy P, et al. Retreatment of hepatitis C interferon nonresponders with larger doses of interferon with and without phlebotomy. Hepatogastroenterology 1996;43:1557–61.

100. Bayraktar Y, Koseoglu T, Kayhan B, Uzunalimoglu B, Gurakar A, Van Thiel D H. The use of desferrioxamine infusion to enhance the response rate to interferon-α treatment of chronic viral hepatitis. Gastroenterology 1995;108:1031A.

101. Kugelmas M, Liebennan B Y, Carey W D. Deironization in chronic hepatitis C patients previously nonresponsive to interferon improves transaminases but not viral activity. Gastroenterology 1995;108:1104A.

102. Yano M, Kakumu S, Hayashi H, Takikawa T, Nishimura N. Phlebotomy followed by α-interferon therapy in patients with chronic hepatitis C. Hepatology 1995;22:119A.

103. Tsai N C, Zuckerman E, Han S, Goad K, Redeker A G, Fong T L. Effect of iron depletion on long-term response to interferon-α in patients with chronic hepatitis C who previously did not respond to interferon therapy. Am J Gastroenterol 1997;92:1831–4.

104. Di Bisceglie AM, Bonkovsky H, Krawitt E, et al. Iron reduction therapy in chronic hepatitis C. Hepatology 1997;26:214A.

105. Di Bisceglie A M, Bassett S E, Bacon B R, Lanford R E. Effect of dietary iron loading in chimpanzees with chronic hepatitis C virus infection. Gastroenterology 1998;114:A1234.

106. Davis G L, Esteban-Mur R, Rustigi V, et al. Interferon alfa-2b alone or in combination with ribavirin for the treatment of relapse of chronic hepatitis C. N Engl J Med 1998;339:1549–50.

107. Di Bisceglie A M, Bacon B R, Kleiner D E, Hoofnagle J H. Increase in iron stores following prolonged therapy with ribavirin in patients with chronic hepatitis C. J Hepatol 1994;21:1109–12.

23
COMPLEMENTARY AND ALTERNATIVE MEDICINE IN HEPATITIS C

DORIS B. STRADER AND HYMAN J. ZIMMERMAN[1]
Veterans Affairs Medical Center and Georgetown University School of Medicine
Washington, DC

INTRODUCTION

For centuries, the use of herbal or botanical agents, acupuncture, and massage has been the cornerstone of medical treatment in east Asia, on the Indian subcontinent, and in some remote parts of South America. Increasingly, the Western world is turning to the use of these "alternative" medical therapies; in most cases to supplement, but in a few cases to completely replace conventional medical treatments. A study on trends in the use of alternative medicine in the United States (1) reported that the use of at least one alternative therapy within the previous year increased from 34% in 1990 to 42% in 1997. There was no medical insurance coverage for 60% of alternative therapies and only partial coverage for another 23%. As a result, approximately two-thirds of alternative therapy users pay entirely out of pocket, spending $12.2 billion of the estimated $21.1 billion spent on alternative medical therapies in 1997. (1)

The rationale for the increased use of traditional, or complementary and alternative, medicine (CAM) in the United States is complex and involves a number of factors. First, CAM users report an increased sense of control, as well as a disillusionment with current physician-prescribed medications. Often conventional medicine is perceived as impersonal and technical, with patients expected to play only a passive role. Studies suggest that many CAM users have chronic or incurable diseases such as diabetes, AIDS, arthritis, and cancer and often feel that conventional medicine has failed them. (2,3) CAM therapy reportedly provides patients with the opportunity to participate actively in their own health care and use products with centuries of experience behind them. Second, the impression that CAM, particularly herbs and botanicals, is more natural and therefore more healthful than conventional therapies appeals to Americans recent desire to return to a more holistic, nature-oriented lifestyle. Third, many patients have shown an increasing reluctance to have invasive conventional medical/surgical procedures, but rather have embraced noninvasive CAM

---

[1]Deceased. Formerly of the Armed Forces Institute of Pathology, WRAMC, Washington, DC and Professor of Medicine, Emeritus, George Washington University, Washington, DC

therapies, including massage, acupuncture, biofeedback, and imagery. Fourth, the assumption that all medicines packaged in pill form are approved by the Food and Drug Administration, as well as the relative lack of information regarding the adverse effects of alternative medical therapies in the lay literature, has led to the impression that CAM therapies are safe. (2) Finally, most medical professionals have a limited knowledge of possible the risks and benefits of CAM. As a result, many patients seek out herbalists, faith healers, and other alternative health providers to discuss therapies they feel may provide them with more options.

COMPARISON OF WESTERN MEDICINE AND TRADITIONAL MEDICINE

Paramount to understanding the use of CAM is the recognition that practitioners of traditional medicine have a different concept of the human body than practitioners of Western medicine. Traditional medicine teaches that energy flows through the body along energy paths, or meridians, and that this energy flows within, around, and through all things in the universe. (4) Energy cannot be destroyed, but can be affected negatively, leading to flow imbalance or disease. Traditional medicine does not view disease as an invasion or poisoning of the body by foreign organisms, but instead sees disease as the human body being out of balance. (4) Healing, therefore, is the art of manipulating the flow of energy to reestablish balance in the whole person rather than just the area of complaint. Spirituality is an integral part of traditional medicine and, as a result, traditional medical therapy can be very individualized, with no two persons receiving the same treatment, despite similar complaints. When used properly, herbs are considered benign, albeit essential for restoring the flow of energy in the acutely ill. In addition, traditional medicine considers itself a preventive rather than curative discipline, (4) as practitioners will often give advice on diet, environment, and lifestyle to guard against further imbalances. Finally, traditional medicine involves the use of information from many sources, including classic texts, but just as often incorporates popular belief and folk medicine.

In contrast, Western medicine tends to divide the body into compartments and measures function by evaluating tissues and examining body fluids. Although there is a great deal of knowledge regarding the body's complex interactions, abnormalities are often diagnosed and treated as individual entities. Western physicians frequently subspecialize and view disease as an invasion of the body by foreign organisms or a proliferation of individual cells out of proportion to their surrounding environment. The focus of Western medicine is to provide a cure for specific ailments. To that end, the scientific method is applied rigorously and claims of efficacy must be documented and proved by repeated independent study. Therapies and products are standardized and patients are treated according to standard of care. Like traditional medicine, however, Western medicine also advocates some changes in diet, environment, and lifestyle to promote health.

In recent years, there has been a move toward integrating traditional and Western medicine. Approximately 60% of medical schools in the United States have created alternative medicine programs and teach alternative medicine practices to their students. (5) Physicians are being encouraged to treat the whole patient—with equal emphasis on the physical as well as spiritual health. Similarly, there is an attempt to subject many traditional therapies to controlled, scientific study and to set standards for practice and products. (5) These developments signal a new attitude of cooperation and an attempt to access the best of both disciplines in providing patient care.

Alternative therapy encompasses a wide variety of treatment modalities, including herbal medicines, folk remedies, hypnosis and imagery, and prayer and spiritual healing. This chapter is devoted to the discussion of the major herbal preparations used in the treatment of hepatitis, particularly hepatitis C. Other forms of alternative therapy will not be discussed.

TRADITIONAL MEDICINES AS HEPATOPROTECTANTS

The primary criticism of traditional medicine is that claims of efficacy are often based solely on anecdotal or personal experience. This has prompted a number of investigators to attempt to test the scientific validity of the proposed benefits of traditional products. Many initial studies were performed to test the "hepatoprotective" effects of traditional medicines, i.e., their ability to prevent injury in liver cells exposed to known toxic agents. It was felt that the claims of efficacy might be bolstered if it could be demonstrated that traditional products protect against acute, toxin-induced injury. What follows is a summary of several of those studies (Table I).

Milk Thistle

Much has been published about the hepatoprotective effects of the herb *Silybum marianum* (milk thistle) since it was first described by Dioscores almost 2000 years ago. The active flavinoid components, silybin, silydianin, and silychristine, collectively known as silymarin, have been studied extensively and reported in over 450 peer-reviewed research manuscripts. Silybin has the greatest degree of biologic activity, and standard silymarin extracts contain at least 70% silybin. (6,7) The reported mechanism of hepatoprotection by silymarin includes antioxidant effects, (8–11) inhibition of lipid peroxidation, (11–15) and protection

TABLE I   Herbal Medications Reported to Have Hepatoprotective Properties[a]

Aloe vera
Gallic acid
Shi-Quan-Da-Bu-Tang (TJ-48)
Silymarin (milk thistle)
Sho-saiko-to (TJ-9)
Solanum alatum
Syh-Mo-Yiin, Guishi-Fuling-Wan, Shieh-Qing-Wan, Syh-Nih-Saan
Vitamin C

[a] Each herb is given shortly before or after administration of an hepatotoxic agent.

against glutathione depletion. (10,16,17) A study by Dehmlow and co-workers (18) published in 1996 evaluated the effects of silybin on rat Kupffer cell functions, specifically the formation of superoxide anions, nitric oxide, tumor necrosis factor-α (TNF-α), prostaglandin E_2 (PGE$_2$), and leukotriene B4. Silybin had a dose-dependent inhibitory effect on superoxide and nitric oxide production, but did not affect TNF-α formation. There was no inhibition of PGE$_2$ formation, but there was a strong inhibitory effect of leukotriene B4 production, suggesting that silybin-induced effects on the cyclooxygenase and 5-lipooxygenase pathways of arachadonic acid metabolism are opposite. The concentration of silybin needed to decrease the production of free radicals by activated Kupffer cells was quite high (>80 μmol/liter). In contrast, inhibition of the lipooxygenase pathway occurred at concentrations achieved *in vivo*, leading investigators to propose that the inhibition of leukotriene production by Kupffer cells was partly responsible for the hepatoprotective effects of silybin.

Other *in vivo* and *in vitro* experiments using silymarin in partially hepatectomized rats have demonstrated significant increases in DNA and protein synthesis in the remaining liver, consistent with the stimulation of hepatic regeneration. (19) The increases in protein synthesis were noted only in hepatectomized animals and did not occur in either control animals or cultured malignant cell lines. Silymarin has also been demonstrated to have significant anti-inflammatory effects characterized by mast cell stabilization (20,21) and inhibition of neutophil migration. (22) In addition, another report has shown a 75% decrease in the toxin-induced proliferation of rat hepatic stellate cells after exposure to silymarin. Finally, other hypothesized hepatoprotective effects of silymarin include an inhibitory effect on selected cytochrome P450 enzymes (24–26) and improvement in immunomodulatory markers such as T-cell and CD8$^+$ cell percentages in patients with cirrhosis. (27,28) These studies have resulted in the general acceptance of the potential hepatoprotective effects of silymarin and have led to its use as the standard agent to which other proposed hepatoprotective agents are compared.

Syh-Mo-Yiin, Guizhi-Fuling-Wan, Sheih-Qing-Wan, Syh-Nih-Sann

Tsai and co-workers (29) tested the ability of aqueous extracts of four traditional medicines to protect against acute liver injury induced by carbon tetrachloride (CCl$_4$) and D-galactosamine (D-GalN). The four agents, Syh-Mo-Yiin (prescribed for regulation of the flow of Qi), Guizhi-Fuling-Wan (for treating blood disorders), Sheih-Qing-Wan (for heat clearing), and Syh-Nih-Sann (for mediation), were compared simultaneously with silymarin in two groups of 11 rats. The first group was injected with saline alone (control), CCl$_4$ alone, or aqueous extracts of the other five agents concomitantly with CCl$_4$. Two additional injections of the aqueous extracts were given 24 and 48 hr later. The second group received injections of saline alone (control), D-GalN alone, or aqueous extracts of the other five agents 2 hr after D-GalN. The rats were sacrificed 24 and 72 hr after D-GalN and CCl$_4$ injection, respectively. Blood was sampled for aspartate aminotransferase (AST) and alanine aminotransferase (ALT) activity, and liver tissue was examined histologically for evidence of necrosis, steatosis, and inflammatory infiltrate.

Serum AST and ALT levels were markedly elevated in rats injected with

CCl_4 alone and D-GalN alone when compared to control animals. Rats injected with aqueous extracts of the five traditional agents had significantly lower AST and ALT levels when compared to animals injected with the toxin alone ($p < 0.01$). Histological evaluation of the liver tissue of rats injected with either CCl_4 alone or D-GalN alone revealed varying degrees of focal necrosis and inflammatory infiltrates, mitoses, steatosis, sinusoidal dilatation, and Kupffer cell injury. Animals injected with traditional agents or silymarin had only mild histological changes. (29)

This simple but elegant experiment suggests that the four traditional agents provide some protection against toxin-induced liver injury. Serologic markers of inflammation, as well as histological evidence of toxic liver injury, were minimal in groups pretreated with traditional agents. It should be stressed that this study provided information about the protective effects of these agents in the immediate posttoxin exposure period. It is unclear whether these agents provide any prophylactic benefit or could minimize liver injury if given more than 2 hr after the hepatotoxic agent. Further experiments to identify the active ingredients and to elucidate the mechanisms of action should be undertaken.

Gallic Acid

Similar protective effects against CCl_4 hepatic injury in the rat model have been described for 3,4,5-trihydroxy benzoic acid or gallic acid, (30) the recently isolated active ingredient in the herbal agent *Terminalia belerica*. (31) Hexobarbitone-induced sleep and zoxazolamine-induced paralysis, as well as serum aminotransferase and bilirubin levels, were measured as parameters of liver function. Eight groups of rats and eight groups of mice received CCl_4 alone, a control vehicle alone, one of four doses of gallic acid 1 hr before CCl_4, or one of two doses of silymarin 1 hr before CCl_4. The normal hexabarbitone-induced "sleep time" and zoxazolamine-induced "paralysis time" were increased significantly in animals receiving CCl_4 alone ($p < 0.01$). Each pretreatment dose of gallic acid and silymarin reduced the sleep time and paralysis time significantly in all animals ($p < 0.03$). Pre- and post-CCl_4 studies of the four doses of gallic acid and the two doses of silymarin were then performed to assess prophylactic and curative effects. Gallic acid and silymarin (pre- and post- CCl_4) resulted in dose-related decreases in AST, ALT, and bilirubin that achieved statistical significance ($p < 0.03$). Finally, the livers of rats who received either CCl_4 alone or a single dose of gallic acid (200 mg/kg orally) or silymarin (50 mg/kg orally) were excised, homogenized, and evaluated for lipid peroxidation, hepatic triglyceride level, microsomal drug metabolizing enzymes, specifically aminopyrine N-demethylase, and membrane-bound glucose-6-phosphatase. Significant increases were noted in lipid peroxidation and hepatic triglyceride levels (both $p < 0.01$) after CCl_4 alone, which were reversed significantly in rats treated with either traditional agent ($p < 0.05$). (30) The content of microsomal drug-metabolizing enzymes and membrane-bound glucose-6-phosphatase was increased, suggesting that the structural and functional integrity of hepatocytes was restored.

In the same paper, the authors were able to fractionate the bioactive component of the herb *T. belerica*, gallic acid, and perform rather sophisticated bioassays of antioxidant activity. They demonstrated a reversal of the increases in CCl$_4$-induced serum and hepatic parameters of injury in the animals pre-treated with gallic acid. In addition, *in vivo* functional studies showed that gallic acid decreased the prolonged CCl$_4$-induced "sleep and paralysis" times, which reportedly reflects a restoration of impaired hepatic monooxygenase activity. (32) In these clever experiments, the authors not only identified the active agent in *T. belerica*, but suggested that the mechanism of action involves antioxidant and free radical-scavenging activities.

Sho-Saiko-To (TJ-9)

Several Japanese investigators have used rat models of hepatic injury to demonstrate that traditional products can inhibit liver fibrosis and prevent cirrhosis. Most reports focused on the Chinese herb, Sho-saiko-to (TJ-9), a traditional medicine made from seven herbs. Two published studies from Yamaguchi University deserve mention. The aim of the first study was to determine whether Sho-saiko-to had an inhibitory effect on the development of liver fibrosis and premalignant lesions in rats. Liver fibrosis was induced by administering a choline-deficient L-amino acid-defined diet. (33) Treated rats received Sho-saiko-to in the diet, and all animals had serum and liver specimens evaluated for the presence of markers of fibrosis and malignancy. Sho-saiko-to-treated rats showed an "inhibition of the increase" of hyaluronic acid, a serum marker of fibrosis, when compared to untreated rats. These levels remained decreased despite an increase in aminotransferases. Examination of liver tissue revealed reduced hydroxyproline content, decreased expression of type III procollagen α 1 mRNA, and decreased proliferation of activated stellate cells when compared to controls. (33) Further examination of liver tissue for enzyme-altered, premalignant lesions, specifically cells that stained positively for the placental form of glutathione *S*-transferase, revealed a decrease in development of these lesions in the Sho-saiko-to-treated rats. The authors concluded that Sho-saiko-to prevents fibrosis and the development of preneoplastic lesions, not by inhibiting hepatic cell death, but by inhibiting the activation of hepatic stellate cells.

To further elucidate the effects of Sho-saiko-to on hepatic stellate cells, the same group performed a second study using stellate cells isolated from rats. (34) The stellate cells were exposed to varying concentrations of aqueous extracts of Sho-saiko-to and were observed for morphologic changes by phase-contrast microscopy. Flow cytometric analysis was performed to determine the potential for proliferation, and Northern blot analysis was carried out to determine the expression of types I and III procollagen mRNA. The two highest concentrations of Sho-saiko-to (500 and 1000 μg/ml) inhibited the morphologic transformation of stellate cells to myofibroblast cells, accumulated cells in the G$_0$/G$_1$ phase significantly ($p < 0.0001$), and decreased the number of cells in the G$_2$/M phase significantly ($p < 0.0001$). Expression of types I and III procollagen mRNA was suppressed significantly by the 500- and 1000-μg/ml concentrations of Sho-saiko-to when compared to controls ($p < 0.05$ and $p < 0.0001$, respectively). The lower concentrations of Sho-saiko-to (10,100, and 250 μg/ml) had no statistically significant effects on any of the parameters studied. The authors concluded that Sho-saiko-to has inhibitory effects on stellate cell activation, thereby inhibiting hepatic fibrosis.

Another group of investigators showed similar inhibitory effects of Sho-saiko-to on rat hepatic stellate cells. (35) In addition, this group demonstrated that the interaction of each of the individual components of Sho-saiko-to was necessary for its activity. When the active constituents were administered alone, the suppression of hepatic stellate cells was diminished. Finally, Sho-saiko-to was administered to 70% hepatectomized normal and liver-injured rats and resulted in an increase in liver weight and number of cells in S phase over time. However, observed histologic changes suggested that the site of action of Sho-saiko-to was different in the regenerating normal liver than in the regenerating injured liver.

These studies appear to have been well thought out and executed elegantly. Data suggest that Sho-saiko-to prevents the development of fibrosis and pre-neoplastic lesions by inhibiting the activation of hepatic stellate cells, primarily by increasing the number of cells in the S phase. Of interest is the fact that Sho-saiko-to leads to hepatic regeneration in both 70% hepatectomized normal and liver-injured rats, but that the site of action of regeneration appears to be different in each group. Although no explanation was given for this difference, further study should shed light on this phenomenon.

Summary of Animal Studies

Accumulated data suggest that a number of traditional agents may lead to a short-term decrease in biochemical and histologic markers of liver inflammation in experimental animals. As with most initial studies attempting to show the protective effects of an agent, the environment created in the laboratory does not usually mimic that found in human disease. The agents used in these studies were often given immediately before or soon after administration of the offending toxin. The microenvironment of the organism was then tested and changes in biochemical or biological markers were considered protective if they differed significantly from controls. Unfortunately, diseases in clinical practice tend to be chronic, with months to years passing before patients seek medical attention. Protective effects noted experimentally do not necessarily translate into a reversal of chronic injury or prevention of further injury in a patient with chronic disease. Whether the improvements in biochemical and histological markers noted in the rat would also occur in humans and, more importantly, whether they would lead to a loss of viremia or a decrease in hepatocellular injury in patients with viral hepatitis is unclear and has been the focus of a few studies. The reader is referred to several other reports (36–40) suggesting the hepatoprotective effects of other traditional medicines.

TRADITIONAL MEDICINES FOR TREATMENT OF HEPATITIS C

It is important to understand that practitioners of traditional medicine rarely separate diseases into discrete categories. A naturopath in Washington, DC explained traditional medicine's view of hepatitis this way, "because Chinese doctors mainly deal with symptomatic patients and because testing of these patients is also limited, the analysis of symptoms and the alleviation of these symptoms are a primary concern. For traditional doctors, the fact that the virus now involved is 'C' rather than 'B' has little significance in relation to treatment. Rather, the important factors are the symptom manifestation and the fact, known from modern science, that a virus is involved." In other words, the choice of herbal treatment in hepatitis is based primarily on symptoms and, to a lesser extent, on the broad category of disease encountered (e.g., viral or toxic). Consequently, data on herbs used to specifically treat hepatitis C are sparse. In addition, many studies evaluating the use of traditional medicine in the treatment of hepatitis were published before serologic testing for hepatitis C became available. As a result, patients with hepatitis B and non-A, non-B hepatitis were included in the same study. In addition, there have been no publications of "look-back" studies aimed at determining the number of non-A, non-B hepatitis cases that were actually due to hepatitis C. Investigators have attempted to study the responses to traditional medicines in the different types of viral hepatitis separately.

Because the processes used by naturopaths, or practitioners of traditional medicine, are unfamiliar to most physicians, a summary of traditional Chinese medical analysis of hepatitis C is necessary as a background to explain the basic concepts and to describe methods of diagnosis and treatment. The second portion of this section focuses on herbs used for the treatment of viral hepatitis, particularly hepatitis C. One should keep in mind that there are many herbs or possible combinations thereof (Table II). This text is not a comprehensive ac-

TABLE II   Some Commonly Used Herbs for the Treatment of Hepatitis

Allium sativa (garlic)[a]
Bupleurum falcatumz
Camellia[a]
Catechin
Chelidonium majus[a]
CH100[b]
Curcuma longa (tumeric)[a]
Dictamnus
Duchesnia
Glycyrrhiza glabra (licorice)[b]
Goou plus Yutan[b]
Hu-chang
Lithospermum
Lonicera
Oldenlandia
Phyllanthus
Picrorhiza kurroa (kutkin)[a]
Sho-saiko-to (TJ-9)[b]
Silymarin (milk thistle)[b]
Solanum alatum[a]
Sophora (oxymatrine)[b]
Thymus extracts[b]
9–11 granules[b]

[a] Studied in uncontrolled trials.
[b] Studied in controlled trials.

count of all traditional medical therapies used to treat hepatitis, but rather a summary of the controlled trials of the most commonly used herbs.

Traditional Concepts of Hepatitis C

Several texts and articles have attempted to explain the traditional concepts of diagnosis and treatment of hepatitis. (41,42) The major points about disease characteristics and treatment are summarized.

Toxic Pathogens in Nutritive (Ying) and Blood (Xue) Levels

Most people are infected via blood or plasma transfusion, and the respective pathogen therefore immediately enters the nutritive layer (rather than making its way slowly through the outer defensive layers of the body). Hepatitis C is an example of a toxic pathogen. In response, one should "vitalize" the blood (increase the circulation) and resolve toxin via the use of herbs that can both move blood and resolve toxin such as lithospermum, hu-chang, moutan, red peony, rhubarb, curcuma, and oldenlandia.

Accummulation of Toxic Stasis Leads to Disease

Hepatitis C is different from other types of liver disease in that it does not present as a "warm" disease. Although the pathogen enters the blood directly, there are usually no symptoms of a warm disease, such as a high fever, skin inflammation, boils, a cough with thick, yellow phlegm, dry tongue, unusual thirst, dry stools, scanty urination, delirium, red tongue, bleeding, and loss of consciousness. Rather, hepatitis C is classified as a yin-type disease, a "damp toxin," which causes indigestion, loss of appetite, nausea, diarrhea, cloudy urine, fatigue, and heavy and sore limbs. These characteristics are consistent with a chronic disease that does not respond well to treatment. As a result, one should attempt to disperse the liver qi (that level responsible for fever, jaundice, and digestive symptoms) with herbs such as bupleurum, blue citrus, cyperus, and magnolia bark.

Age-Dependent Susceptibility to Disease

As one ages, declining kidney function may increase the likelihood of development or worsening of hepatitis. Because many patients diagnosed with hepatitis C are over 40, it is recommended that herbs that "tonify" the liver and kidney be used in moderate amounts. These herbs include morinda, epimedium, curculigo, cuscuta, and fenugreek.

Treatment to Clear Pathogens, Remove Toxins, and Prevent Stasis

Protocols for hepatitis C should focus on treatments that (a) clear pathogens and resolve toxins, (b) remove toxins by strengthening the qi level, and (c) transform stasis to prevent cancer formation. These concepts suggest that the mode of infection and the clinical symptom complex dictate therapy. In the diagnosis of hepatitis C, the symptoms indicate "chronicity" and the herbs chosen for treatment would "regulate" or augment the functioning of a chronically infected liver. This gross oversimplification of Chinese medical principles is a little difficult to understand, but it is clear that there is the potential for overlap in clinical symptoms. This may result in a great deal of variability in treatment recommendations. In fact, several articles agree with the diagnostic classification of hepatitis C mentioned previously, but recommend a different group of herbs for therapy. (43–45) The reader is referred to texts of traditional Chinese medicine for detailed explanations of diagnosis and treatment.

COMMONLY USED HERBS FOR HEPATITIS C (TABLE III)

Silymarin (Milk Thistle)

Despite the fact that silymarin has been used for centuries to treat various liver diseases, there have been no published randomized, double-blind, placebo-controlled trials using silymarin in the treatment of hepatitis C (HCV). Several studies have documented the effectiveness of silymarin in the treatment of Amanita mushroom poisoning in both humans and animals, (46–51) as well as its effectiveness in treating toxic exposures to organophosphates (52,53) and psychotropic medications. (54) A number of double-blind studies using silymarin to treat acute hepatitis A and B have been reported. In one study, 57 patients with acute hepatitis A or B were randomized to receive either silymarin in a dose of 140 mg orally three times a day or a placebo for at least 3 weeks. (6,55) Mean levels of ALT, AST, and bilirubin were significantly lower in the treated group when compared to the placebo group 5 days after beginning therapy. There was no difference in the number of patients who went on to develop immunity in either group. A second study of inpatients with acute hepatitis A or B demonstrated a significantly shorter length of hospital stay (23.3 days vs 30.4 days) in patients receiving silymarin. In addition, there was a shorter length of time (30.4 vs 41.2 days) for the appearance of antibody to HBsAg (anti-HBs) in patients with hepatitis B treated with silymarin. (56) In neither study was the presence of underlying liver disease, use of alcohol, or viral levels and viral markers discussed.

Double-blind studies of silymarin therapy in patients with chronic alcoholic liver disease have shown significant decreases in aminotransferase levels, (57,58) bilirubin, (57) and histological improvement on liver biopsy when compared to

TABLE III   Herbal Medicines Used in the Treatment of Hepatitis C[a]

CH100
Glycyrrhiza glabra (licorice)
Goou plus Yutan
Sho-saiko-to (TJ-9)
Silymarin (milk thistle)
Sophora (oxymatrine)
Thymus extracts
9–11 granules

[a] Represents those discussed in detail in this chapter; not an exhaustive list.

placebo therapy. (57) Conflicting results have been reported in controlled trials of patients with acute alcoholic hepatitis treated with silymarin. (59,60)

Several trials using silymarin to treat chronic liver disease have been reported. Unfortunately, it is unclear whether viral hepatitis, particularly hepatitis C, was the primary disease being treated. In one study, 170 patients with cirrhosis (92 alcoholic, 78 nonalcoholic) were asked to abstain from alcohol and were then randomized to receive either silymarin 140 mg three times a day or placebo for 2–6 years. (6,61) Survival improved in the treated group (77% vs 67% overall, 82% vs 68% at 2 years) and was highest among alcoholic patients. There was no change in biochemical markers in either group. Another study reported no difference in biochemical markers, with a trend toward improvement in histological activity in patients treated for 12 months with silymarin. (62) Unfortunately, this study was hampered by incomplete follow-up in approximately one-half of its patients. Finally, a large study of over 2500 patients with chronic liver disease treated with high-dose silymarin (560 mg/day) for 8 weeks reported a decrease in symptoms in two-thirds of enrolled patients, a fall in aminotransferase levels by approximately 35%, and a decrease in physical findings, specifically hepatomegaly. (63) However, as mentioned previously, neither study reported the viral hepatitis status of patients with chronic liver disease or cirrhosis, thereby making it difficult to ascertain the effect of silymarin on the treatment of chronic viral hepatitis. It has been reported that silybin bound to phosphatidylcholine lowered aminotransferase levels significantly in patients with chronic hepatitis B and C. (64) In addition, there are ongoing, long-term studies of high-dose silymarin in patients with hepatitis C who had not responded to a course of interferon-α.

Discussion

The studies on silymarin have suffered from two major flaws. First, the studies in hepatitis C were not randomized, double blind, nor placebo controlled. Patients with hepatitis B and C were often included in the same study under the broad heading of chronic viral hepatitis. Similarly, responses to treatment were usually undifferentiated, making it difficult to determine whether the subtypes of viral hepatitis had varying susceptibilities to silymarin therapy. Although practitioners of traditional medicine tend not to separate the types of viral hepatitis in terms of treatment, Western physicians view the types of viral hepatitis as quite different entities. Second, the accepted definition of response to treatment in Western medicine involves the return of serum aminotransferase levels to normal *and* a loss of HCV RNA from serum, indicative of resolution of viremia. In no study of silymarin were either of these criteria met. Rather, there were trends toward improvement as evidenced by decreases in aminotransferase levels, improvements in liver histology, decreases in hospital stay, or subjective reports of resolution of symptoms. It is possible that these findings may have been the consequence of lifestyle changes and not related directly to treatment with silymarin. At present, accumulated data do not indicate that silymarin is effective in treating patients with hepatitis C. To address the possible role of silymarin as therapy of hepatitis C adequately, prospective randomized, controlled trials with a careful documentation of changes in serum aminotransferase levels, liver histology, and HCV RNA levels both during and after therapy need to be performed.

Glycyrrhizin (Licorice)

Glycyrrhizin is a major component of the licorice root, *Glycyrrhiza glabra* or *Glycyrrhiza uralensis*. It has been used for the treatment of peptic ulcer disease, aphthous stomatitis, and eczema in many different countries. (64) In addition, it has been reported to have a number of beneficial effects on liver tissue, including stabilization of hepatic cellular membranes, (65) inhibition of the production of prostaglandin E_2, (66) and augmentation of the effects of interferon. (67) In Japan, glycyrrhizin is used to treat both acute and chronic viral hepatitis and is administered as a product called Stronger Neominophagen C (SNMC), which contains 200 mg of glycyhrrizin, 100 mg of cysteine, and 2000 mg of glycine in 100 ml of saline. The cysteine component is felt to be an antiallergin, whereas the glycine component prevents the aldosterone-like action of glycyrrhizin. (68,69) Most studies have used daily intravenous injections of SNMC, but more recent studies suggest that an oral form may have equivalent efficacy.

Yamamoto (70) was the first to report the use of SNMC as treatment of chronic hepatitis and noted an improvement in serum aminotransferase levels. His data soon led to the widespread use of SNMC for the treatment of chronic liver disease in Japan. Suzuki et al. (71) later attempted to confirm the beneficial effects of SNMC on serum aminotransferase levels in a randomized, controlled, double-blind trial. In this study, 133 patients with chronic hepatitis were randomized to receive daily intravenous doses of either 40 ml of SNMC or a placebo for 4 weeks. (71) Forty-three patients were HBsAg positive (no further data were given regarding the type of hepatitis). There were no differences between control and treatment groups with respect to age, sex, history of blood transfusion, alcohol consumption, use of concomitant medicines, or histological classification of liver disease. Serum aminotransferase levels were evaluated at regular intervals during and for 2 months after completion of the trial. Mean aminotransferase levels showed a statistically significant decrease from baseline in both placebo and SNMC-treated groups and remained decreased during the 2-month follow-up period. Importantly, both AST and ALT levels were lower in the SNMC-treated group when compared to the placebo group ($p = 0.001$) throughout the treatment period, the greatest difference being at week 2. However, within 2 weeks of follow-up there was no longer a statistical difference in AST and ALT levels between the two groups. Nevertheless, the authors concluded that there was a significant difference in the "general improvement rating of liver function" in the SNMC-treated group when compared to placebo and that "SNMC was shown to be clearly useful for the treatment of chronic active liver disease." In view of the short-term nature of the study, they noted that no conclusions could be made regarding the long-term effectiveness of SNMC. (71)

Although there were statistically significant differences in AST and ALT levels between SNMC-treated and placebo groups throughout the treatment period, it should be noted that HCV RNA remained present, that differences in AST and ALT levels disappeared within 2 weeks after completion of the trial, and that aminotransferase levels decreased in both treatment and placebo groups.

These findings suggest that SNMC results in a greater decline in aminotransferase levels in patients with chronic liver disease, but that it has no lasting benefit once therapy is stopped.

Another study of SNMC evaluated its combination with interferon-α in patients with hepatitis C who had not responded to a course of interferon alone. (72) Twenty-eight patients with chronic hepatitis C who had no response (defined as persistently abnormal enzymes) to 12 weeks of therapy with interferon-α were randomized to either continued interferon-α alone or receive both interferon and SNMC for 12 more weeks. Subsequently, ALT levels became normal in 33% of patients on interferon alone and 64% of patients treated with the combination, and HCV RNA became undetectable in 13% of interferon alone and 38.5% of combination recipients. Finally, liver biopsies revealed a trend toward a greater reversal of histological grade in combination-treated patients. However, none of these differences were statistically significant, perhaps because of the small sample size. The authors recommend further studies to resolve these issues.

More recently, investigators in Toranomon Hospital, Tokyo, assessed whether long-term treatment with SNMC prevents the development of hepatocellular carcinoma (HCC) in patients with chronic hepatitis C. (73) This retrospective study evaluated 453 patients diagnosed with hepatitis C between January 1979 and April 1984. Of the 453 patients, 84 (group A) had been treated with SNMC at a dose of 100 ml daily for 8 weeks and then two to seven times weekly for 2–16 years (median, 10.1 years). Group B consisted of 109 control, untreated patients who did not receive either interferon-α or SNMC during the period of observation (because of the lack of home health professionals to give intravenous injections). These patients frequently received "other" herbal therapy, which was not defined, and were followed for 1–16 years (median, 9.2 years). The remaining 210 patients received a small amount of SNMC (not defined), corticosteroids, or immunosuppressive agents. Only groups A and B were compared with respect to the development of HCC, and they were similar with respect to age, gender, transfusion history, HCV genotype (most 1b), histological grade, and aminotransferase levels at the time of first liver biopsy. Average ALT levels declined toward normal (<50 IU/ml) in 36% of patients in group A and in 6% of patients in group B, but this difference did not achieve statistical significance. No mention was made of HCV RNA levels. The cumulative 10-year incidence of HCC incidence was 7% for the 83 patients in group A and 12% for the 93 patients in group B who completed the study. The 15-year rates were 12 and 25%, respectively, with a relative risk of HCC incidence of 2.5 in patients not treated with SNMC. In addition, 71 patients in group A and 81 patients in group B had repeat liver biopsies (interval not defined). Cumulative 10- and 15-year incidence rates for cirrhosis were 12 and 21% in group A and 20 and 37% in group B. (73) Univariate analysis showed liver histology stage ($p = 0.0000$), age ($p = 0.0052$), SNMC therapy ($p = 0.0319$), and ALT level ($p = 0.0437$) to be significant factors associated with the development of HCC. The authors concluded that improvements in ALT levels by long-term therapy with SNMC in chronic hepatitis C may be associated with protection against HCC.

Although several of the studies of glycyrrhizin and SNMC were randomized, double-blind controlled trials, they suffered several shortcomings. As with other trials of traditional medicine in the treatment of viral hepatitis, the study by Suzuki et al. failed to differentiate between patients with hepatitis B and hepatitis C. The authors interpreted the decreases in aminotransferase levels and mild improvements in liver histology as a trend toward benefit, but virological responses were not documented and the treatment and follow-up times were too short to demonstrate a lasting benefit. A randomized, controlled trial of SNMC in patients with hepatitis C lasting at least 6 months with at least 6 months of follow up is required to answer whether SNMC has any role in the therapy of hepatitis C. The study comparing SNMC plus interferon with interferon alone in patients with chronic hepatitis C who previously failed interferon therapy provided interesting results, but the differences, although large (64% vs 33%), did not achieve statistical significance due to the small numbers of patients in the study. A further study of the combination of SNMC and interferon is warranted. Finally, the study done on the use of SNMC to prevent cirrhosis and HCC was a nonrandomized, retrospective analysis of patients who were either treated or not treated. Unfortunately, as with most retrospective studies, it is difficult to control for factors that introduce bias. The authors claimed there were no differences between patients treated with SNMC and those who were not aside from the availability of health personnel to deliver treatment. However, there was no mention of the use of alcohol, the presence of comorbid conditions, or the subsequent use of other therapies for hepatitis C that might have had an impact on the incidence of HCC. In addition, patients in group B received other unidentified herbal medicines. Finally, if the reason for the lack of health personnel to deliver treatment to patients in group B was financial, then it is possible that these patients may not have been able to afford regular clinic visits or other lifestyle changes, which could decrease the likelihood of development of HCC. More careful studies are needed before a conclusion can be made about the impact of SNMC on the development of HCC in hepatitis C. Thus, data do not support the use of SNMC alone for the treatment of hepatitis C. Preliminary data on the combination of SNMC plus interferon, although not statistically significant, warrant further study. Similarly, the impact of SNMC treatment on the development of HCC requires further study.

CH100

CH100 is the code name for an herbal tablet developed by Cathay Herbal in conjunction with hepatologists in China and is composed of 19 different herbs. (74) These herbs are often used in traditional Chinese medicine to treat chronic liver diseases, but are not used in a standardized tablet formulation. It is unclear how the choice of herb, and its subsequent concentration in the formula, was determined for this study.

The effects of CH100 treatment in patients with chronic hepatitis C were reported by Batey and co-workers (75) from Australia. Forty-four patients were randomized to receive either CH100 tablets or placebo, and 40 completed the study (20 in each group). Patient demographics were similar in the two groups. Eight patients in the treatment group and six patients in the placebo group had relapsed after previous interferon therapy. Mean ALT levels decreased significantly ($p = 0.03$) in the treatment group as compared with the placebo group, and four patients, all in the treatment group, had normalization of ALT levels throughout the 6-month study period. Only one of these patients had persistently normal ALT levels 18 months after stopping CH100. All patients continued to have HCV RNA detectable in serum. Significant side effects were experienced by four patients receiving CH100: one patient with palpitations (in whom the drug was stopped), one with abdominal pain, and two with diarrhea. The authors concluded that CH100 led to statistically significant decreases in ALT levels in patients with chronic hepatitis C. They further state that the use of herbs in a standardized tablet form as opposed to traditional individualized non-tablet formulation was "likely to reduce the efficacy of Chinese herbal treatment."

Discussion

Although the number of patients studied was small, these findings suggest that CH100 treatment leads to a 20% end of treatment response (ETR) and a 5% sustained biochemical response without a virological response. The clinical significance of the changes in ALT levels was unclear. It is possible that if more patients were studied over a longer period of time, a role of CH100 in the suppression of disease activity in hepatitis C might be identified. At present, CH100 cannot be considered to be clinically effective in the treatment of hepatitis C.

Thymus Extracts

A number of oral thymus preparations are available over the counter. The components include bovine glandular extracts of thymus, thymopoeitin, thymic humoral factor, herbs, vitamins, and enzymes. (76) Two double-blind studies of thymus extracts in the treatment of hepatitis B have suggested that the immunological properties of thymus preparations result in a therapeutic effect in both acute and chronic disease. (77,78) The immunological properties include stimulation of interferon production, enhanced T-cell-dependent antibody production, enhanced helper T-cell activity, and increased production of suppressor cells and natural killer cell activity. (79–81)

There have been four published studies on the efficacy of thymus extract in hepatitis C. A preliminary study of a 6-month course of injectable thymosin-α1 extract in 10 patients with hepatitis C reported no effect. (82) However, in an open-label study, Rasi et al. (83) reported a sustained loss of HCV RNA in 5 of 11 interferon naïve and 1 of 4 interferon nonresponders treated with the combination of interferon and thymosin-α1. Similarly, a randomized, controlled trial of thymosin-α1 plus interferon suggested that the combination resulted in a greater biochemical response than interferon alone. (84) More recently, a randomized controlled trial of oral thymus extract for patients who had previously failed to respond to a course of interferon was reported from the University of Alabama. (85) Thirty-eight patients (36 patients who did not respond and 2 who were intolerant to interferon) were randomized to receive either six tablets of thymus extract twice daily (20 patients) or a placebo (18 patients) for 12 weeks. The code was broken at 12 weeks, and all patients receiving placebo were offered thymus extract. All patients could receive 6 months of thymus extract if they wished. Baseline clinical and demographic characteristics were similar in each group. No patient became HCV RNA negative by the end of the initial 12-week period and average HCV RNA and aminotransferase levels did not differ between treatment and placebo groups during therapy. Results for patients who completed 6 months of thymus extract treatment were similar. HCV viremia persisted and there were no significant changes in aminotransferase levels from baseline. One patient taking thymus extract developed thrombocytopenia during the fifth month of treatment. No other adverse events were reported.

Few conclusions can be drawn from the published studies of thymus extract therapy of hepatitis C. All were hampered by a small sample size, use of differing forms of thymus extract (including oral versus parenteral preparations), and different doses and regimens. Two studies suggested that thymus extract in combination with interferon-α was more effective than interferon alone; two studies showed no benefit of thymus extract monotherapy. Some authors have suggested that the thymus extract has a beneficial effect in interferon-naïve patients but no efficacy in patients who are intolerant or fail to respond to interferon. This conclusion is somewhat contradictory. If a standardized formulation of thymus extract could be developed and shown to have some effect in chronic hepatitis C, further investigation in large controlled trials would be warranted.

Sho-saiko-to (TJ-9)

Sho-saiko-to is a Japanese Kampo formula consisting of seven herbs: *Bupleurum falcatum* (Chinese thoroughwax), *G. glabra* (licorice root), *Panax ginseng* root, *Scutellaria baicalensis* (Chinese skullcap root), *Zizyphus jujuba* (jujube fruit), *Zingiber officinale* (ginger root), and *Pinella ternata* (half summer root). It is widely prescribed in Asia as a treatment of chronic viral liver disease. As mentioned earlier, it has been suggested that Sho-saiko-to enhances the immune system, decreases the progression of hepatic fibrosis, and suppresses the development of HCC.

A study from Osaka University Hospital Department of Pediatrics suggested that Sho-saiko-to was efficacious in hepatitis B. (86) Fourteen children with chronic hepatitis B were treated with Sho-saiko-to at dosages equivalent to the adult dose of 7.5 g daily. (86) Fifty-percent of treated children became HBeAg negative over an average follow-up period of 6 months compared with the natural yearly conversion rate of 23% observed in 22 untreated control children. Four of the 7 HBeAg-negative children also developed anti-HBe. In addition, ALT levels normalized in 6 children after 12 months of therapy. Other uncontrolled studies have shown that Sho-saiko-to results in moderate biochemical improvement in patients with undifferentiated chronic viral hepatitis. (87–89)

There have been few controlled trials of Sho-saiko-to in chronic hepatitis C. The most often sited study was a prospective, randomized, but nonblinded controlled trial from Osaka City Hospital that analyzed the effects of long-term Sho-saiko-to therapy on the development of HCC in patients with either hepatitis B or non-B-related cirrhosis. (86) Two-hundred-sixty patients were randomized to receive either Sho-saiko-to or placebo, of whom 37 were HBsAg positive. There was some overlap among the 54 patients who had a history of blood transfusions and 57 patients who were heavy drinkers. Seventy-six of the 94 patients without hepatitis B who had pretreatment serum tested were positive for anti-HCV. Patients were monitored prospectively for 5 years and both survival and rates of HCC were calculated. The cumulative 5-year incidence of HCC was lower in the treated group than controls ($p = 0.071$), and differences reached statistical significance for treated patients with non-hepatitis B-related cirrhosis ($p = 0.024$). Similarly, survival was improved in the treated group, but treated patients with non-hepatitis B-related cirrhosis had a statistically significant increase in survival compared with treated patients with hepatitis B-related cirrhosis ($p = 0.043$). Unfortunately, no mention was made of the status of biochemical markers or the level of viremia, and the relationship of therapy to viral clearance and outcome could not be determined.

The Osaka City Hospital study suggested that Sho-saiko-to may have more efficacy against cirrhosis due to hepatitis C than hepatitis B. Subsequently, a number of investigators have measured the *in vitro* effects of Sho-saiko-to on the production of cytokines by peripheral blood mononuclear cells (PBMC) from patients with hepatitis C. Resultant data suggest that Sho-saiko-to induces the production of granulocyte/colony-stimulating factor, (90) returns decreased IL-10 production and excessive IL-4 and IL-5 levels toward normal, (91) and induces tumor necrosis factor-α (92) in patients infected with HCV. An additional reports states that Sho-saiko-to induces apoptosis in cultured HCC cell lines. (93)

Sho-saiko-to (TJ-9) has shown some success in the treatment of hepatitis B and is often used for the treatment of viral hepatitis in Japan. Reliable data on the effects of Sho-saiko-to in hepatitis C are sparse. The study done at Osaka City Hospital demonstrated a decreased incidence of HCC and increased survival rates in treated patients, but statistical significance was not achieved. The authors were able to show a statistically significant decrease in HCC incidence and increase in survival in the subgroup of patients with non-hepatitis B-related cirrhosis. The assumption is made that most of these patients had hepatitis C. Unfortunately, it is unclear which patients were anti-HCV positive, and of those, which had improved survival. In addition, a first-generation enzyme immunoassay (EIA), not confirmed with recombinant immunoblot assay (RIBA), was used to identify anti-HCV in these stored samples, increasing the likelihood of false-positive results. Based on these data, one must conclude that treatment with Sho-saiko-to has yet to be shown to decrease the incidence of HCC or to improve survival in patients with chronic viral hepatitis.

Of concern is the side effect profile of Sho-saiko-to. Between 1995 and 1997, 66 patients treated with Sho-saiko-to have been reported to develop drug-induced interstitial pneumonitis and 55% of cases occurred in anti-HCV-positive patients. (90,94) Nine patients died, of whom 8 had hepatitis C. It is unclear whether this pneumonitis represented an allergic or autoimmune phenomenon and why patients with hepatitis C had increased mortality. A study from Tokyo General Hospital reported a 0.7% incidence of drug-induced pneumonitis among patients with chronic hepatitis or cirrhosis given Sho-saiko-to only, a 0.5% incidence in those treated with interferon-α alone, and a 4% incidence in those given both Sho-saiko-to and interferon-α. (95) In most patients, the pneumonitis responded to corticosteroid therapy. Given this side effect profile and the lack of convincing evidence that Sho-saiko-to is effective in hepatitis C, it is prudent to recommend that this agent not be used in patients with hepatitis C until there is further documentation of its efficacy and safety.

Goou (Bovine Gallstone) and Yutan (Bear Gall) Powders

Goou and Yutan are crude animal products used for the treatment of liver disease throughout Asia. Goou consists of bile acids, particularly cholic acid, bilirubin, and taurine. It is believed to promote bile acid secretion and suppress leucocyte aggregation. (96) Yutan contains ursodeoxycholic acid (UDCA) and its taurine-conjugated derivatives. It also promotes bile acid secretion as well as dissolution of gallstones and reduction of cholesterol. (97) A preliminary report discusses the effectiveness of these two agents in the treatment of patients with chronic liver disease.

Twenty-three patients (13 with hepatitis B and 10 with hepatitis C) were given either 200 mg of Goou per day alone (6 patients, all with cirrhosis) or 200 mg of Goou plus 60 mg Yutan per day (17 patients, 11 with chronic hepatitis, 6 with cirrhosis). (98) The 11 patients with chronic hepatitis treated with Goou plus Yutan, regardless of type of viral hepatitis, showed statistically significant improvements in AST and ALT levels 1 month after treatment. Similar results were noted in the 6 cases of cirrhosis given both drugs. No patient receiving Goou alone had a statistically significant decline in aminotransferase levels. In addition, no patient in either group had normalization of AST or ALT; however, all patients, regardless of biochemical response, had symptomatic improvement. Viral loads and hepatitis genotypes were not measured in this study.

The combination of Goou and Yutan may lower serum aminotransferase levels slightly, but the clinical significance of such changes is unclear. It is safe to conclude that neither Goou alone nor Goou plus Yutan appears to be effective in the treatment of hepatitis B or C.

Oxymatrine (Sophora)

Oxymatrine is one of several alkaloids isolated from sophora root, either *Sophora flavescens* or *S. subprostrata*. Oxymatrine has been reported to inhibit viral infections (particularly hepatitis B), enhance cellular immune functions, and reduce liver fibrosis. In China, *S. subprostata* has been an ingredient in many hepatitis B decoctions, and sophora root extract injections have been used experimentally and clinically for a variety of disorders since 1976. (99) More recently, (100) 40 patients with hepatitis C were randomized to receive either oxymatrine 600 mg/day by intramuscular injection or liver-protecting herbs and vitamins given orally. The treatment duration was 3 months. Of the 20 patients receiving oxymatrine injections, 17 completed the trial, and HCV RNA fell below the level of detection in 8 (47%) patients. In the control group, 18 of 23 patients completed the study and only 1 (5%) had undetectable HCV RNA by the end of the study. Aminotransferase levels decreased in both groups, but it was not stated whether levels returned to normal. Nearly all patients experienced pain at the injection site, and 1 patient had an allergic reaction (pruritis), which did not require an adjustment in dose.

This small trial had several flaws. Importantly, it was neither placebo controlled nor double blind. The study subjects received intramuscular injections, whereas the controls were given oral herbs and vitamins. The authors explained that placebo controls are not accepted in China, hence the use of the unspecified liver-protecting herbs. Unfortunately, this introduces bias caused by the patient's awareness that they are not receiving the potentially beneficial medication. A second shortcoming of the study was that the purity of the oxymatrine was not described and the identity of the liver-protecting herbs and vitamins was unknown. This lack of standardization makes it difficult to interpret results as each patient may have received a different combination of herbs. Finally, the 47% potential cure rate reported was an ETR, not a sustained response; no information was given on HCV RNA or aminotransferase levels 6 months after treatment. Although it is compelling that the ETR achieved by intramuscular oxymatrine was similar to that of the combination of interferon-α and ribavirin, further study is needed to document that this response rate is reproducible and that responses are maintained.

911-GRANULES

911-granules is an herbal remedy consisting of Minor Bupleurum combination, Cinnamon and Hoelen formula, and capillaris; agents previously reported to be effective against liver disease. Accordingly, the formula may include any of the following ingredients: bupleurum, scute, pinellia, ginger, licorice, jujube, ginseng, cinnamon twig, moutan, hoelen, persica, peony, capillaris, and tang-kuei. Three hundred thirty patients with hepatitis C were enrolled in a randomized study; 170 patients were treated with the 911-granules and 160 served as controls. (101) Study patients received two packets of 911-granules daily for 200 days, whereas controls received vitamins and standard liver-protecting herbs. Effectiveness was determined by testing for HBV and HCV antibodies with EIA before and 3–6 months after treatment. Anti-HCV became undetectable in 29% of patients receiving 911-granules but in only 8% of controls. No information is given regarding aminotransferase or HCV RNA levels.

This single study of 911-granules suffered from a lack of placebo controls and a lack of standardization of the herbs used. In addition, loss of anti-HCV was used as the measure of treatment effect, an unusual outcome measure of uncertain clinical significance. HCV RNA levels and aminotransferase levels, the more reliable and traditional measures of outcome, were not reported, making it impossible to conclude that 911-granules have any effect in hepatitis C.

HEPATOTOXICITY OF TRADITIONAL MEDICINES

The hepatotoxic effects of conventional medicines are well recognized and described. Until recently, little was known about the potentially harmful effects of traditional medicines. This is due to the misconception that herbs are natural and, therefore, safer than conventional drugs. The lack of FDA regulation of traditional medicines has fueled unchecked claims of the purity and harmlessness of herbal constituents. Over the past few years, however, the hepatotoxic effects of a number of traditional medicines have been reported. The most common class of hepatotoxic herbs are the pyrrolizidine alkaloids, including *Symphytkum officinale* (comfrey), *Ilex* (Mate tea), *Teucrium chamaedrys* (germander), *Larrea tridentata* (chapparal), *Valeriana offinalis* (valerian), *Viscum album* (mistletoe), and *Labiatae* sp. (pennyroyal oil). Some Chinese herbal preparations, including teas, have also been noted to have hepatotoxic potential (Table IV).

TABLE IV   **Herbal Products That Can Lead to Hepatic Injury**

Herb	Type of hepatic injury
Comfrey	VOD[a]
Gordolobo herbal tea	VOD
Mate tea	VOD
Chinese herb preparations	
Medicinal tea	VOD
"Chinese herbs"	Hepatitis
Jin Bu huan	Hepatitis, microvesicular steatosis
Germander	Necrosis (zone 3), chronic hepatitis, cirrhosis
Chaparral leaf	Necrosis (zone 3)
Chapparal, valerian root, skullcap	Hepatitis
Mistletoe	Chronic hepatitis
Margosa oil	Microvesicular steatosis
Pennyroyal oil	Necrosis (zone 3), microvesicular steatosis

[a] Venoocclusive disease.

In addition to the adverse effects on the liver, it has been noted that some traditional medicines used to treat liver disease have extrahepatic side effects. For example, glycyrrhizin at doses of greater than 100 mg per day, or the crude root preparation of more than 3 g per day for 6 months, led to symptoms of hyperaldosteronism. (64) CH100 has been associated with mild gastrointestinal side effects and to one case of cardiac arrhythmias, necessitating discontinuation of the drug. Mild allergic reactions have been reported with silymarin and thymus extracts. Of greatest concern are the reports of interstitial pneumonitis associated with the use of Sho-saiko-to (TJ-9) with or without interferon for the treatment of chronic hepatitis C. A detailed listing of all reported hepatotoxic effects of traditional medicines is beyond the scope of this chapter. The reader is referred to excellent review articles (102) and textbooks on hepatotoxicity. (103)

CONCLUSION

Anecdotal evidence and several small and inadequately controlled studies of herbal preparations as therapy of hepatitis C have suggested that these agents may be effective either in promoting recovery or in ameliorating the ongoing liver injury. None of these reports document the efficacy of these preparations in hepatitis C adequately and most provide insufficient evidence for safety. The few controlled trials of these agents were often limited by small size, lack of placebo control, high rate of drop out, and use of indefinite end points and outcome measures. The rigorous definitions of response to treatment that have been developed during the evaluation of interferon-α and ribavirin for hepatitis C should provide a framework with which to develop controlled trials that will define the possible role of these agents as therapy of this disease. The need for such studies is obvious. The promise of herbal preparations as a treatment of hepatitis C needs to be either confirmed or withdrawn.

ACKNOWLEDGMENTS

The authors thank K. K. Nazirahk and N. D. Amen, L.Ac, Naturopathic Physicians and Acupuncturists in Washington, DC, for advice and literature on herbal preparations used in the treatment of hepatitis.

REFERENCES

1. Eisenberg D M, Davis R B, Ettner S L, et al. Trends in alternative medicine use in the United States, 1990–1997. JAMA 1998;280:1569–75.
2. Winslow L C, Droll D J. Herbs as medicines. Arch Intern Med 1998;158:2192–9.
3. Brown J S, Marcy S A. The use of botanicals of heal purposes by members of prepaid health plans. Res Nurs Health 1991;14:339–50.
4. Craze R. Traditional Chinese medicine. Lincolnwood, IL: NTC Publishing Group, 1998.
5. Jonas W B. Alternative medicine—learning from the past, examining the present, advancing to the future. JAMA 1998;280:1616–7.
6. Flora K, Hahn M, Rosen H, Benner K. Milk Thistle (*Silybum marianum*) for the therapy of liver disease. Am J Gerontol 1998;93:139–43.
7. Luper S. A review of plants used in the treatment of liver disease: Part I. Alternative Med Rev 1998;3:410–21.
8. Mira L, Silva M, Mansco C F. Scavenging of reactive oxygen species by silibinin dihemisuccinate. Biochem Pharmacol 1994;48:753–9.
9. Halim A B, el-Ahmady O, Hassab-Allah S, Abdel-Galil F, Hafez Y, Darwish A. Biochemical effect of antioxidants on lipids and liver function in experimentally induced liver damage. Ann Clin Biochem 1997;34:656–63.
10. Pietroangelo A, Borella F, Casalgrandi G, et al. Antioxidant activity of silybin in vivo during long-term iron overload in rats. Gastroenterology 1995;109:1941–9.
11. Basaga H, Poli G, Tekkaya C, Aras I. Free radical scavenging and antioxidative properties of 'silibin' complexes on microsomal lipid peroxidation. Cell Biochem Funct 1997;15:27–33.
12. Bosisio E, Benelli C, Pirola O. Effect of flavanoligans of *Silybum marianum L.* on lipid peroxidation in rat liver microsomes and freshly isolated hepatocytes. Pharmacol Res 1992;25:147–54.
13. Rui Y C. Advances in pharmacological studies of silymarin. Mem Inst Oswaldo Cruz 1991;S2:79–85.
14. Carini R, Comoglio A, Albano E, Poli G. Lipid peroxidation and irreversible damage in the rat hepatocyte model: protection by the silybin-phospholipid complex IdB 1016. Biochem Pharmacol 1992;43:2111–5.
15. Valenzuela A, Barria T, Guerra R, Garrido A. Inhibitory effect of the flavinoid silymarin on the erythrocyte hemolysis induced by phenylhydrazine. Biochem Biophys Res Commun 1985;126:712–8.
16. Cabrera C. Milk Thistle: A clinician's report. Med Herbalism 1996;6:1–5.
17. Campos R, Garrido A, Guerra R, Valenzuela A. Silybin dihemisuccinate protects against glutathione depletion and lipid peroxidation induced by acetaminophen on rat liver. Planta Med 1989;55:417–9.
18. Dehmlow C, Erhard J, de Groot H. Inhibition of Kupffer Cell functions as an explanation for the hepatoprotective properties of silibin. Hepatology 1996;23:749–54.
19. Sonnenbichler J, Goldberg M, Hane L, Madubuny I, Vogel S, Zefl I. Stimulatory effect of silibinin on the DNA synthesis in partially hepatectomized rat livers: non-response in hepatoma and other malignant cell lines. Biochem Pharmacol 1986;35:538–41.
20. Fantozzi R, Brunelleschi S, Rubino A, Tarli S, Masini E, Mannaioni PF. FMLP-activated neutophils evoke histamine release from mast cells. Agents Actions 1986;18:155–8.
21. Lecomte J. Propriétés pharmacologiques générales de la silybine et de la silymarine chez la rat. Arch Int Pharmacody Ther 1975;214:165–76.
22. De la Puerta R, Martinez E, Bravo L. Effect of silymarin on different acute inflammation models and on leukocyte migration. J Pharm Pharmacol 1996;48:968–70.

23. Fuchs E C, Weyhenmeyer R, Weiner O H. Effects of silibinin and of a synthetic analogue on isolated rat hepatic stellate cells and myofibroblasts. Arzneim-Forsch 1997;47:1383–7.

24. Baer-Dubowska W, Szaefer H, Krajka-Kuzniak V. Inhibition of murine hepatic cytochrome P450 activities by natural and synthetic phenolic compounds. Xenobiotica 1998;28:735–43.

25. Miguez M P, Anundi I, Sainz-Pardo L A. Hepatoprotective mechanism of silymarin: no evidence for involvement of cytochrome P450-2E1. Chem-Biol Interact 1994;91:51–63.

26. Amdur M O, Doull J, Klaassen C D. Casarett and Doull's toxicology: the basic science of poisons, 4th ed. New York: McGraw-Hill, 1991.

27. Deak G, Muzes G, Lang I. Immunomodulator effect of silymarin therapy in chronic alcoholic liver diseases. Orv Hetil 1990;131:1291–6.

28. Lang I, Nekam K, Gonzalez-Cabello R. Hepatoprotective and immunological effects of antioxidant drugs. Tokai J Exp Clin Med 1990;15:123–7.

29. Tsai C-C, Kao C-T, Hsu C-T, Lin C-C, Lin J-G. Evaluation of four prescriptions of traditional Chinese medicine: Syh-Mo-Yiin, Guizhi-Fuling-Wan, Shieh-Qing-Wan and Syh-Nih-Sann on experimental acute liver damage in rats. J Ethnopharmacol 1997;55:213–22.

30. Anand K K, Singh B, Saxena A K, Chandan V N, Gupta V N, Bhardwaj V. 3,4,5-Trihydroxy benzoic acid (Gallic acid), the hepatoprotective principle in the fruits of *Terminalia belerica*— bioassay guided activity. Pharmacol Res 1997;36:315–21.

31. Anand K K, Singh B, Saxena A K, Chandan K, Gupta V N. Hepatoprotective studies of fraction from the fruits of *Terminalia belerica* Roxb. on experimental liver injury in rodents. Phytother Res 1994;8:287–92.

32. Dreyfuss J, Peffer D A, Schreiber E C. The effect of analgesics on the hexobarbital sleeping times of rats, dogs and rhesus monkeys: a species difference. Toxicol Appl Pharmacol 1970;16:597–605.

33. Sakaida I, Matsumura Y, Akiyama S, Hayashi K, Ishige A, Okita K. Herbal medicine Sho-saiko-to (TJ-9) prevents liver fibrosis and enzyme-altered lesions in rat liver cirrhosis induced by a choline-deficient L-amino acid-defined diet. J Hepatol 1998;28:298–306.

34. Kayano K, Sakaida I, Uchida K, Okita K. Inhibitory effects of the herbal medicine Sho-saiko-to (TJ-9) on cell proliferation and procollagen gene expressions in cultured rat hepatic stellate cells. J Hepatol 1998;29:642–9.

35. Miyamura M, Masahide O, Shojiro K, Nishioka Y. Effects of Sho-saiko-to extract on fibrosis and regeneration of the liver in rats. J Pharm Pharmacol 1998;50:97–105.

36. Shamaan N A, Kadir K A, Rahmat A, Wan-Ngah W Z. Vitamin C and Aloe Vera supplementation protects from chemical hepatocarcinogenesis in the rat. Nutrition 1998;14:846–52.

37. Pines M, Knopov V, Genina O, Lavelin I, Nagler A. Halofuginone, a specific inhibitor of collagen type I synthesis, prevents dimethylnitrosamine-induced liver cirrhosis. J Hepatol 1997;27:391–8.

38. Torres M I, Fernandez M I, Gil A, Rios A. Dietary nucleotides have cytoprotective properties in rat liver damaged by thioacetamide. Life Sci 1998;62:13–22.

39. Tatsuta M, Iishi H, Miyako B, Nakaizumi A, Uehara H. Inhibition by Shi-Quan-Da-Bu-Tang (TJ-48) of experimental hepatocarcinogenesis Induced by N-nitrosomorpholine in Sprague-Dawley rats. Eur J Cancer 1994;30A:74–8.

40. Lin C-C, Lin W-C, Yang S-R, Shieh D-E. Anti-inflammatory and hepatoprotective effects of *Solanum alatum*. Am J Chin Med 1995;23:65–9.

41. Lihau C. Hepatitis C: Characteristics and TCM treatment methods. J Traditional Chin Med 1994;10.

42. Shi J, Quanliang C. Clinical manifestations of hepatitis C and hepatitis B: A comparative approach utilizing TCM differential diagnosis. J Traditional Chin Med 1994;9.

43. Huiwen H. Analysis of clinical and therapeutic specificity in treating chronic hepatitis B and C. J Traditional Chin Med 1997;38:732–4.

44. Hougen L. Qingtui Fang applied in treating 128 cases of chronic hepatitis C. Chin J Integr Traditional West Med Liver Dis 1994;4:40.

45. Songxin Y et al. Clinical research on hepatitis C treating with oral liquid. J Traditional Chin Med 1996;37:673–5.

46. Desplaces A, Choppin J, Vogel G. The effects of silymarin on experimental phalloidine poisoning. Arzneim-Forsch 1975;25:89–96.

47. Vogel G, Tuchweber B, Trost W. Protection by silibinin against *Amanita phalloides* intoxication in beagles. Toxicol Appl Pharmacol 1984;73:355–62.

48. Hruby K, Csomos G, Fuhrmann M, Thaler H. Chemotherapy of *Amanita phalloides* poisoning with intravenous silibinin. Hum Toxicol 1983;2:183–95.

49. Sabeel A I, Kkurkkus J, Lindholm T. Intensive hemodialysis and hemoperfusion treatment of Amanita mushroom poisoning. Mycopathologia 1995;131:107–14.

50. Carducci R, Armellino N I, Volpe C, et al. Silibinin and acute poisoning with *Amanita phalloides*. Minerva Anestesiol 1996;62:187–93.

51. Rambousek V, Janda I, Sikut M. Severe Amanita phalloides poisoning in a 7-year-old girl. Cesk Pediatr 1993;48:332–3.

52. Boari C, Montanuri F, Galletti G, et al. Silymarin in the protection against exogenous noxae. Drugs Exp Clin Res 1981;7:115–20.

53. Szilard S, Szentgyorgyi D, Demeter I. Protective effect of Legalon in workers exposed to organic solvents. Acta Med Hung 1988;45:249–56.

54. Saba P, Galeone F, Salvadorini F, et al. Effetti terapeutica della silimarina nelle epatopatie croniche indotte da psicofarmaci. Gazz Med Ital 1976;135:236–51.

55. Magliulo E, Gagliardi B, Fiori G P. Zur Wirkung von Silymarin bei der Behandlung der akuten Virushipatitis. Med Klin 1978;73:1060–5.

56. Cavalieri S. Kontrollierte klinische Pruefung von Legalon. Gazz Med Ital 1974;133:628.

57. Feher J, Deak G, Muzes G, et al. Hepatoprotective activity of silymarin (Legalon) therapy in patients with chronic liver disease. Orv Hetil 1989;130:2723–7.

58. Salmi H A, Sarna S. Effect of Silymarin on chemical, functional, and morphological alternations of the liver: a double-blind controlled study. Scand J Gastroenterol 1982;17:517–21.

59. Fintelmann V, Albert A. Nachweis der therapeutischen Wirksamkeit von Legalon bei toxishenc Lebererkrankungen im Doppelblindversuch. Therapiewoche 1980;30:5589–94.

60. Trinchet I C, Coste T, Levy V G. Treatment of alcoholic hepatitis with silymarin. A double-blind comparative study in 116 patients. Gastroenterol Clin Biol 1989;13:120–4.

61. Ferenci P, Dragosics B, Dittrich H, et al. Randomized controlled trial of silymarin treatment in patients with cirrhosis of the liver. J Hepatol 1989;9:105–13.

62. Kiesewetter E, Leodolter I, Thaler H. Ergebnisse zweier Doppelblindstudien zur Wirksamkeit von Silymarin bie chronischer Hepatitis. Leber Magen Darm 1977;7:318–23.

63. Albrecht M, Frerick H, et al. Therapy of toxic liver pathologies with Legalon. Z Klin Med 1992;47:87–92.

64. Reichert R. Phytotherapeutic alternatives for chronic active hepatitis. Q Rev Nat Med 1997;Summer:103–8.

65. Watari N. An electronmicroscopic study of the effects of glycyrrhizin on experimentally injured liver. Mini Med Rev 1973;11:12–7.

66. Ohuchi K, Tsurufuji A. A study of the anti-inflammatory mechanism of glycyrrhizin. Mino Med Rev 1982;27:188–93.

67. Acharya S K, Dasarathy S, Tandon A, Jushi Y, Tandon B. A preliminary open trial on interferon stimulator (SNMC) derived from *Glycyrrhiza glabra* in the treatment of subacute hepatic failure. Indian J Med Res 1993;98:75–8.

68. Hikino H, Kiso Y. Natural products for liver diseases. In: Wagner H, Hikino H, Farnsworth N R, eds. Economic and medicinal plant research, Vol. 2. New York: Academic Press, 1988:49.

69. Werbach M R, Murray M T. Botanical influences on illness. Tarzana, CA: Third Line Press, 1994:178–9.

70. Yamamoto S, Maekawa Y, Imamura M, Hisajima T. Treatment of hepatitis with the anti-allergic drug, Stronger Neo-Minophagen C. Clin Med Pediatr 1958;13:73.

71. Suzuki H, Ohta T, Takino T, Fujisawa K, Hirayama C. Effects of glycyrrhizin on biochemical tests in patients with chronic hepatitis: double-blind trial. Asian Med J 1983;26:423–38.

72. Abe Y, Ueda T, Kato T, Kohli Y. Effectiveness of interferon, glycyrrhizin combination therapy in patients with chronic hepatitis C. Nippon Rinsho 1994;52:1817–22.

73. Arase Y, Ikeda K, Murashima N, et al. The long term efficacy of glycyrrhizin in chronic hepatitis C patients. Cancer 1997;79:1494–500.

74. Salmond S. Herbs and hepatitis C. Int J Alternative Comp Med 1997;15:24–7.

75. Batey R G, Bensoussan A, Fan Y, Ballipo S, Hossain M A. Preliminary report of a randomized, double-blind placebo-controlled trial of a Chinese herbal medicine preparation CH-100 in the treatment of chronic hepatitis C. J Gastroenterol Hepatol 1998;13:244–7.

76. Burgstiner C B. Complete thymic formula [label]. Duluth, GA: Preventive Therapeutic, Inc.

77. Galli M, Crocchiola P, Negri C, Caredda F, Lazzarin A, Moroni M. Attempt to treat acute type

B hepatitis with an orally administered thymic extract (thymomodulin): preliminary results. Drugs Exp Clin Res 1985;11:665–9.

78. Dworniak D, Tchorzewski H, Pokoca L, et al. Treatment with thymic extract TFX for chronic active hepatitis B. Arch Immunol Ther Exp 1991;39:537–47.

79. Serrate S A, Schulof R S, Leondaridis L, Goldsterin A L, Sztein M B. Modulation of human natural killer cell activity, lymphokine production, and interleukin 2 receptor expression by thymic hormones. J Immunol 1987;139:2338–43.

80. Low T L, Goldstein A L. Thymosins: structure, function and therapeutic applications. Thymus 1984;6:27–42.

81. Sztein M B, Goldstein A L. Thymic hormones—a clinical update. Springer Semin Immunopathol 1986;9:1–18.

82. Rezakovic I, Zavaglia C, Botelli R, Ideo G. A pilot study of thymosin-alpha 1 therapy in chronic active hepatitis C. Hepatology 1993;252A.

83. Rasi G, DiVirgilio D, Mutchnick M G, et al. Combination thymosin-alpha 1 an lymphoblastoid interferon treatment in chronic hepatitis C. Gut 1996;39:679–83.

84. Sherman K E, Sjögren M H, Creager R L, et al. Thymosin-alpha 1 plus interferon combination therapy for chronic hepatitis C: results of a randomized controlled trial. Hepatology 1993; 402A.

85. Raymond R S, Fallon M B, Abrams G A. Oral thymic extract for chronic hepatitis C in patients previously treated with interferon: a randomized, double-blind, placebo-controlled trial. Ann Intern Med 1998;129:797–800.

86. Oka H, Yamamoto S, Kuroki T, et al. Prospective study of chemoprevention of hepatocellular carcinoma with Sho-saiko-to (TJ-9). Cancer 1995;76:743–9.

87. Oka H, Fujiwara K, Oda T. Ziao-chai-hu-tang and Gui-zhi-fu-ling-wan for treatment of chronic hepatitis. In: Oda T, Needham J, Otsuka Y, Gur-bin L, eds. Recent advances in traditional medicine in the East Asia. Amsterdam: Excerpta Medica, 1984;232–7.

88. Fujiwara K, Ohta Y, Ogata I, et al. Treatment trial of traditional Oriental medicine in chronic viral hepatitis. In: Ota Y, ed. New trends in peptic ulcer and chronic hepatitis: Part II. Chronic hepatitis. Tokyo: Excerpta Medica, 1987:141–6.

89. Yamamoto M, Uemura T, Nakama S, et al. A fundamental study of chronic hepatitis treated with saiko agents. Proc Symp Wakan-Yaku 1983;16:245–8.

90. Yamashiki M, Nishimura A, Nobori T, et al. *In vitro* effects of Sho-saiko-to on production of granulocyte colony-stimulating factor by mononuclear cells from patients with chronic hepatitis C. Int J Immunopharmacol 1997;19:381–5.

91. Yamashiki M, Nishimura A, Suzuki H, Sakaguchi S, Kosaka Y. Effects of the Japanese herbal Medicine Sho-saiko-to (TJ-9) on *in vitro* interleukin-10 production by peripheral blood mononuclear cells of patients with chronic hepatitis C. Hepatology 1997;25:1390–7.

92. Yamashiki M, Nishimura A, Nomoto M, Suzuki H, Kosaka Y. Herbal medicine Sho-saiko-to induces tumour necrosis factor-alpha and granulocyte colony-stimulating factor *in vitro* in peripheral blood mononuclear cells of patients with hepatocellular carcinoma. J Gastroenterol Hepatol 1996;11:137–42.

93. Yano H, Mizoguchi A, Fukuda K, et al. The herbal medicine Sho-saiko-to inhibits proliferation of cancer cell lines by inducing apoptosis and arrest at the G_0/G_1 phase. Cancer Res 1994;54: 448–54.

94. Ishizaki T, Sasaki F, Ameshima S, et al. Pneumonitis during interferon and/or herbal drug therapy in patients with chronic active hepatitis. Eur Respir J 1996;9:2691–6.

95. Nakagawa A, Yamaguchi T, Takoa T, Amano H. Five cases of drug-induced pneumonitis due to Sho-saiko-to or interferon-alpha or both. Nippon Kyobu Shikkan Gakkai Zasshi 1995;33: 1361–6.

96. Takagi K, Kimura M, Harada M, Ootsuka H. Goou. Pharmacology of medicinal herbs in East Asia. Nanzando, Tokyo, 1982.

97. Takagi K, Kimura M, Harada M, Ootsuka H. Yutan. Pharmacology of medicinal herbs in East Asia. Nanzando, Tokyo, 1982.

98. Matsumoto N, Nakashima T, Kashima K. Effectiveness of bovine gallstone (Goou) and bear gall (Yutan) on chronic liver diseases: a preliminary report. Tokai J Exp Clin Med 1995;20: 9–16.

99. Yeung, H. Handbook of Chinese herbal formulas, 2nd ed. Institute of Chinese Medicine, 1995.

100. Jiqiang L, Chao-qun L, Mingde Z, et al. A preliminary study on therapeutic effect of Oxymatrine in treating patients with chronic hepatitis C. Chin J Integr Traditional West Med 1998; 18:227–9.
101. Zhen Y, Maocai L, Chaolian W. A preliminary report on the effect of 911 Granules on chronic viral hepatitis of the B and C types. Chin J Integr Traditional West Med 1995;15(3).
102. Schiano T D. Liver injury from herbs and other botanicals. In: Cullen J H, Schmidt R, Gitlin N, Black M, eds. Clinics in liver disease: Drug-induced liver disease. Philadelphia, PA: Saunders, 1998:607–30.
103. Zimmerman H J. Hepatotoxicity: the adverse effects of drugs and other chemicals on the liver. Philadelphia, PA: Lippincott-Williams-Wilkins, 1999.

24
DEVELOPMENT OF NOVEL THERAPIES FOR HEPATITIS C

JOHNSON Y. N. LAU * **AND DAVID N. STANDRING**†

*Department of Research and Development
ICN Pharmaceuticals
Costa Mesa, California

†Department of Antiviral Therapy
Schering-Plough Research Institute
Kenilworth, New Jersey

"If I have seen further it is by standing on the shoulders of giants."

Sir Isaac Newton 1642–1727
In *Correspondence* Vol. 1:
Letter to Robert Hooke, 1676

INTRODUCTION

With the discovery of the hepatitis C virus (HCV) by Dr. Choo and colleagues (1) and the development of assays by Dr. Kuo and colleagues, (2) a large body of knowledge on the natural history, clinical features, disease pathogenesis, and virology has been generated. These rapid advancements were achieved through the collective efforts of the many clinicians and scientists. Therapies have already been developed and are beneficial to a proportion of patients infected with this viral infection. It is and will continue to be the knowledge generated by the scientific community that forms the basis for the development of future therapeutic strategies.

Up until May 1998, interferon-α was the only approved therapy for treating patients with chronic HCV infection. (3) Unfortunately, only a small proportion of patients (<10%) responded virologically to interferon-α monotherapy in a completed and sustained fashion. In June and December 1998, interferon-α-2b/ribavirin combination therapy (Rebetron, Schering-Plough, Kenilworth, NJ) was approved by the Food and Drug Administration of the United States for the treatment of patients with chronic HCV infection who relapsed after previous interferon-α treatment and who have never been treated (naïve patients), respectively. This combination therapy was also approved by the European Union Health Authority in February 1999. This combination therapy improves the complete and sustained virological response rate to 49% for patients who relapsed after a previous course of interferon-α therapy and 41% for treatment of naïve patients. (4–6)

TABLE I Potential Antiviral Targets Present in the HCV Genome

Target	Biological role	Other properties	Enzymatic or functional activity	*In vitro* assay	Interest level in antiviral development
5′ UTR	Translational control	Unique RNA structure	IRES	Yes	Moderate high
Core (C)	Capsid protein	Membrane association	Homotypic multimerization		Moderate
E1	Envelope protein	Membrane association	Homo- and hetero-typic interactions	No	Low
E2	Envelope protein	Membrane association	Homo- and hetero-typic interactions	No	Low
p7	Unknown	Unknown	Unknown	No	None
NS2/3	Metalloprotease	Unknown	NS2/3 cleavage	Yes	Low
NS3	Protease	Structure known	Releases NS proteins	Yes	High
NS3	Helicase	Structure known	Unwinds viral nucleic acid	Yes	High
NS4A	Cofactor for NS3 protease	Membrane association	Essential for cleavage at 4A/4B and 4B/5A sites		
NS4B	Unknown	Membrane association	Unknown	No	None
NS5A	Viral replication?	Confers resistance to interferon?	Unknown	Yes (for ISDR)	Low
NS5B	Polymerase	Membrane association	Replicates RNA	Yes	High
3′ UTR	Regulates replication	Unique RNA structure		No	Further information needed

Despite the improved efficacy of the combination therapy, 50–60% of the patients failed to respond in a sustained fashion. The current combination therapy also requires a treatment period of 6–12 months. Hence, newer and better anti-HCV therapies are still needed.

It is important to know and understand the strength and weakness of our enemy (i.e., HCV, the target). The molecular virology of HCV has been summarized in another chapter. As detailed later, knowledge of the function of the viral genome and its encoded viral proteins is essential in determining the validity of these targets for anti-HCV drug discovery and development (Table I). Equally important is the understanding of the role of the host immune system in the pathogenesis of chronic hepatitis C. In chronic HCV infection, the current understanding is that the host immune response is ineffective in controlling and eliminating HCV infection. Hence, it is possible that augmentation of the HCV-specific immune response may assist the host in clearing the viral infection.

ISSUES AND APPROACHES TO ANTIVIRAL THERAPY FOR HCV

HCV poses some major challenges in antiviral discovery and immunotherapy development. One key issue is the lack of a reproducible infectious tissue culture system, which has precluded the detection of antiviral compounds through conventional cell-based virological screening. This also limits our understanding of HCV biology. For example, we still do not know the nature of the genetic elements that control HCV replication or the functions of all the HCV proteins. The availability of full-length infectious HCV clones promises to shed some light on these important questions. (7–9) However, because there is no HCV small animal model, the only way to investigate HCV biology *in vivo* is by infecting chimpanzees with mutated HCV genomes. Thus, we can anticipate that the progress will be limited and slow.

Given this scenario, the drug discovery process to date has had to rely on the following types of strategy: (i) generate and characterize recombinant HCV proteins, (ii) use these recombinant proteins for *in vitro* screening of anti-HCV compounds, and (iii) aid the optimization of anti-HCV drugs through structure–function studies. While such an approach can lead to the identification of promising inhibitors, the assessment of their biological activity against HCV remains a challenge. As noted earlier, no HCV tissue culture or small animal model is available at present. In lieu of these systems, there has been considerable interest in surrogate viruses such as BVDV or GBV-B, which are most closely related to HCV and hence offer the hope of providing surrogate models capable of predicting the activity of antiviral compounds against HCV. Although these models are important for drug development at present, it should be cautioned that activity against these viruses *in vivo* may not translate into anti-HCV activity in patients. Needless to say, the activity against HCV will ultimately have to be evaluated in HCV-infected chimpanzees or in the clinic.

Another issue concerns the genetic heterogeneous nature of HCV. There are six HCV clades. (10) Further genotyping revealed more genotypes and subtypes. This raises two concerns. First, it is important to develop an anti-HCV drug with a broad spectrum of activity against different HCV isolates/subtype/genotype/clade. Second, rapid resistance may develop against drugs that target HCV genome/protein, based on our knowledge of antivirals against other chronic viral infections, including human immunodeficiency virus (HIV) and hepatitis B virus (HBV) infection. Hence, it is likely that combination therapy will be required for effective treatment of chronic HCV infection.

Before we proceed to discuss the various approaches, let us consider the ideal and acceptable anti-HCV therapy profile, which will guide us in evaluating the potential of the possible therapeutic strategies. The ideal profile should be an oral drug, taken for a short period of time, potent, with minimal side effects (i.e., with good specificity and therapeutic ratio), and clear the infection in a sustained fashion. What we want may not be what we can develop. Given the public health implications of this viral infection, a parenteral adminstration (e.g., subcutaneous injection), taken for a longer period of time (e.g., 1 year) and with some side effects (e.g., side effects similar to that with interferon-α and ribavirin), should be acceptable.

As discussed previously, antivirals and immunotherapy represent two of the most attractive approaches for the development of anti-HCV therapies. Other approaches aim at targeting the virus through antisense, ribozyme, single chain anti-HCV, or through viral interference, either through dominant negative mutants or defective interfering viruses.

DEVELOPMENT OF SMALL MOLECULE ANTI-HCV DRUGS

The potential antiviral targets for HCV are summarized in Table I along with their known or putative properties. Altogether 10 distinct HCV proteins have been shown to be processed from the polyprotein. (11) Added to these 10 potential antiviral targets are discrete viral genetic elements located within the 5'- and 3'-untranslated regions (UTR) of the genomic RNA that are responsible for the translation and replication of viral RNA. The possibility that further critical genetic elements exist in other regions of the viral RNA has not been ruled out at the present time.

Perusal of Table I shows that only a few of the potential HCV antiviral targets are being pursued seriously by various investigators and pharmaceutical companies. These targets were favored because (1) this class of viral proteins are known to be good targets for drug development (e.g., protease), (2) soluble recombinant viral proteins that are active can be generated, (3) a robust assay can be developed for some targets, and (4) crystal structures are available for rational drug design.

To date, most of the effort to develop inhibitors has centered on key viral-specific enzymatic targets, including HCV protease, helicase, and polymerase. Viral protease and polymerase have been shown to be good targets for drug development for other viruses. Soluble protease and helicase, and recently polymerase, have been generated. These activities are well characterized from an enzymatic standpoint. Robust assays can be developed for these targets. In the case of HCV protease and helicase, X-ray crystallographic structures have been determined. Among nonprotein targets, the relatively well-characterized internal ribosomal entry site (IRES) translational control element poses an interesting discovery target. The 3'X end, which is likely to be involved in viral replication, is also an attractive target but assay development is challenging.

The 5' UTR

The translation of most cellular mRNAs involves a scanning mechanism in which the 43S initiation complex binds to the m7Gppp cap structure at the 5' terminus of the mRNA. The complex scans along the mRNA 5' leader sequence, which is typically short (50–70 nucleotides in length) and relatively unstructured, until it finds the first AUG codon which is then used as the initiation site. In contrast, certain viruses, including picornaviruses and HCV, (12) as well as a few cellular genes encoding regulatory proteins (e.g., the PDGF-2 mRNA), use a very different mechanism to translate their RNAs. A number of these highly structured elements have been characterized and are collectively known as IRES, which is a class of cis-acting genetic elements that regulate translation in a m7G cap- and end-independent manner. The highly conserved nature of HCV sequence in this region is another attractive feature for antiviral development.

Although the mechanism by which HCV IRES element functions is largely unknown, it presumably depends on specific interactions with unidentified host proteins (and perhaps also viral proteins) that result in enhancement of translation. Given that each IRES element has a distinctive structure, the interaction with other functional proteins may also be IRES specific. It is important to note that the HCV IRES is a type 3 IRES, which is structurally distinct from cellular and picornavirus IRESs, suggesting that specific inhibitors against this viral target can be developed based on either (i) their precise structural differences per se or (ii) the different binding proteins.

There is precedence for the feasibility of developing small molecule antiviral drugs for the selective inhibition of RNA–protein interactions. Neomycin B, an aminoglycoside antibiotic, specifically blocks the binding of the HIV Rev protein to its viral RNA recognition element, RRE. This binding specifically antagonizes Rev function and inhibits HIV production *in vitro*. (13)

Several pharmaceutical companies have small molecule-based HCV IRES drug discovery programs. The challenges for developing this type of inhibitor are to determine the precise mechanism of inhibition and to build specificity into this inhibition. The highly conserved nature of the HCV IRES sequence also make this target attractive for the development of HCV nucleotide sequence-specific targeting approaches, including the use of antisense and ribozyme molecules.

HCV Structural Proteins

Structural proteins, comprising the core protein (C), the two envelope proteins (E1 and E2), and possibly the p7 peptide (the nature and functional role are unknown), are processed cotranslationally from the HCV polyprotein by host signal peptidase. By mechanisms that remain to be elucidated, HCV core proteins assemble, through an array of homotypic and heterotypic interactions, into subviral capsid structures, including specifically packed viral RNA. These capsids then acquire an envelope coat and become infectious virions. The viral envelope proteins, E1 and E2, are also involved in homotypic and heterotypic interactions. Thus, small molecules that interfere with capsid assembly and envelope/core protein interactions will inhibit HCV viral particle assembly and hence the viral life cycle. HCV core antigen has also been shown to exhibit other functions, including binding to RNA, modulation of transcription, interacting with host proteins, including tumor necrosis factor (TNF) receptor, and regulating host immune response. (14–16) Hence, inhibitors that bind to HCV core may also interfere with other important functions of core in addition to viral assembly.

This approach has a number of hurdles. First, the nature of the interactions between monomeric core proteins has not been defined. The capsid assembly pathway, as well as the nature of capsid assembly intermediates, also remains unknown. Second, the exact mechanism responsible for viral RNA capsid assembly has not been defined. These factors, in conjunction with the lack of a reliable cell culture model, limit the scope of a detailed structure–activity relationship analysis and drug development. Similar issues exist for the development of inhibitors that interfere with core/envelope or envelope E1/E2 protein assembly.

HCV E2 has been shown to bind to CD81 on the cell surface. (17) Although there is no evidence that this binding is sufficient to support viral entry and replication, data suggest that CD81 may be a coreceptor for HCV, similar to the chemokine receptors for HIV. Although the biologic relevance of this interaction remains to be determined, blockade of this type of interaction has been shown to be successful in disrupting the viral life cycle of HIV. Thus, inhibitors that block CXCR4 usage or HIV gp41 inhibit viral entry or fusion in both *in vitro* (for CXCR4 blockade) and *in vivo* studies (for interfering HIV gp41 cell fusion). (18,19) This inhibition was evident through a reduction in HIV viremia. Whether a similar approach is useful for treating HCV infection remains to be evaluated.

HCV NS2 Metalloprotease

Isolates known to have defective cleavage at the NS2/NS3 site by the NS2 metalloprotease were identified in a small number of patients with chronic HCV infection. Although these data need confirmation and the biologic significance of these variants is not known, the possible existence of these variants challenges the validity of HCV NS2 metalloprotease as a good anti-HCV drug target. The difficulty encountered in the generation of soluble recombinant HCV NS2 protein for the screening assay further reduces the enthusiasm of developing inhibitors against this viral target.

HCV NS3 Protease

Serine protease activity encoded by amino (N)-terminal 181 amino acids of NS3 is responsible for the proteolytic processing of four downstream sites in the viral polyprotein (NS3/NS4A, NS4A/4B, NS4B/5A, and NS5A/5B). (20) The enzymatic activity of the HCV NS3 protease is well characterized. (21) The NS3 protein contains three highly conserved residues, His[57], Asp[81], and Ser[139], which represent the catalytic triad of the serine proteinase family. Substitutions of any of these residues abolish proteolytic processing. Studies in a related flavivirus (yellow fever virus) and pestivirus (BVDV) have shown that the NS3 protease is indispensable for virus growth. Hence, HCV protease is an attractive target for anti-HCV drug development.

The 54 amino acid NS4A protein functions as a cofactor for NS3 protease activity. NS4A is essential for cleavages at NS3/4A, NS4A/4B, and NS4B/5A junctions and enhances cleavage at the NS5A/5B site. Mutagenesis experiments have shown that the N-terminal region of NS3 between amino acids 15–22 interacts with amino acids 21–34 of NS4A. (22) Structural studies of the NS3/4A complex have confirmed these observations, indicating that the NS4A polypeptide is intercalated into the NS3 structure in the active complex. (23) The X-ray crystal structure of the HCV NS3 serine protease domain revealed that it is structurally similar to previously characterized proteases. The molecular fold consists of two β barrels and resembles that of the chymotrypsin class of serine proteases. The catalytic residues, His[57], Asp[81], and Ser[139], participate in a hydrogen-bond network, which is a signature of serine proteases. The catalytic triad spans the β barrels, as does the proposed substrate-binding site. There is a structural zinc atom in the enzyme complex. The substrate binding site is a shallow, hydrophobic cleft rather than the deeper pocket lined with some charged residues that characterize elastase.

Our understanding of the biochemical behavior and crystal structure shed light on the anti-HCV protease drug design. The substrate-binding site, the zinc atom site, and the interaction between NS3 and NSS4A are possible targets for anti-HCV protease drug development. However, the shallow substrate-binding site suggests that targeting this pocket is inherently difficult. Inhibitors that eject the zinc atom are likely to be reactive and nonspecific. The tight binding between NS3 and NS4A also casts doubt on the potential of developing inhibitors to interfere with this interaction.

Many pharmaceutical and biotechnology companies have anti-HCV NS3 programs. Most effort has centered on peptidic molecules (peptidomimetics) based on the natural substrate.

HCV Helicase

Viral replication, like cellular DNA replication and mRNA transcription and translation, typically requires a separation of duplex nucleic acids. This reaction is mediated by a class of unwinding enzymes called helicases, which use energy derived from coupled NTP hydrolysis. The exact mechanism of unwinding is not clear, but it is believed to involve recognition of an unpaired nucleic acid followed by a processive energy-dependent translocation of the helicase along the nucleic acid or a cooperative binding of the protein–nucleic acid complex.

Positive-stranded RNA viruses with a genome size greater than 5.8 kb generally encode a helicase. (24) The requirement for the helicase function has been demonstrated for the plum pox potyvirus RNA helicase and the bovine viral diarrhea virus NS3 protein. (25,26) Mutation of the helicase moiety in these viruses rendered them noninfectious. Virus-encoded helicases can be divided into three superfamilies based on characteristic amino acid motifs. The HCV helicase, located in the carboxyl-terminal two-thirds of NS3 protein, belongs to the superfamily II, the same family for virus-like plum pox potyvirus and bovine viral diarrheal virus helicases. Hence, specific inhibitors against HCV helicase are likely to be effective in interrupting the HCV replication cycle.

The biochemical characteristics of HCV NS3-4A helicase activity have been determined. The enzyme can utilize all four ribonucleotides (NTPs) as the energy source for nucleic acid unwinding. (27) This hydrolysis is stimulated in the presence of nucleic acid polymers. The enzyme unwinds all homo- and heteroduplexes of DNA and RNA, provided that a 3' overhang is present in one of the strands. This information will certainly assist the development of anti-HCV drugs directed toward this target.

The crystal structure of HCV helicase has been resolved. (28) The structure reveals an HCV helicase divided into three domains. Domain I contains NTP- and Mg^{2+}-binding sites, whereas domain II is speculated to contain a nucleic acid-binding domain in the form of a interdomain grove, with many of the conserved sequences clustered near this interdomain channel. These features indicate the mechanistic importance of this cleft, making it an attractive target for anti-HCV drug design. The structure suggests that domain II can pivot relative to the other domains. A specific hinge or "switch" region has been proposed to control this conformational change, which is thought to accompany NTP hydrolysis. In principle, the NTPase site, the nucleic acid-binding region, and the switch region can all serve as targets for helicase inhibitors. Our understanding of the crystal structure of this enzyme provides us an excellent opportunity for structure-based drug design.

Many pharmaceutical and biotechnology companies have anti-HCV helicase programs. A number of inhibitors with low potency have been reported. The major challenges are to identify the best chemical structure and to optimize the potency and selectivity of the compound through a combination of structural activity analyses and fine structural studies.

NS5A

The function of HCV NS5A in HCV viral cycle and pathogenesis is not known. NS5A can be inferred to be part of the replication process by analogy with Dengue fever virus where NS5A and NS5B are included in a single protein. Reports suggest that HCV NS5A contains an interferon sensitivity determinant region (ISDR), which may be an important factor in determining the patient's response to interferon-α therapy. (29) Based on a two-hybrid system, this ISDR region was found to interact with PKR, a kinase induced by interferon-α. (30) However, there is also a large body of literature that fail to confirm the clinical significance of ISDR in response to interferon-α therapy. Whether this is a good target for anti-HCV drug development remains to be established.

NS5B RNA-Dependent RNA Polymerase (RdRp)

HCV NS5B RdRp is the key enzyme that drives the HCV genome replication and thus is essential for viral growth. HCV replication can be divided into two steps: (1) synthesis of the (−)-stranded RNA replication intermediate from the 3′ end of the input (+)-stranded RNA genome and (2) synthesis of progeny (+)-stranded RNA genome from the (−)-stranded RNA replication intermediate. As HCV RdRp is likely to be the viral enzyme that drives both steps of replication, HCV RdRp is an attractive therapeutic target. It should be noted that viral polymerases have proved to be good targets for drug discovery and development.

Biochemical characterization of this viral enzyme revealed that its polymerization activity requires an RNA template and primer. (31,32) The processivity of NS5B is rather low, estimated to be around 100–200 nucleotides per minute. By analogy with other polymerases that lack a proofreading capability, the misincorporation rate of the NS5B is presumed to be high, which contributes to the genetic heterogeneous nature of HCV. NS5B can utilize a DNA primer, although less efficiently than an RNA primer, and does not have any preference for viral RNA as a specific template. (33) This lack of specificity may reflect the notion that additional viral or cellular factors are required for specific recognition of the replication signal, most likely present at the 3′UTR. Indeed, a host protein known as polypyrimidine tract-binding protein (PTB) has been shown to bind specifically to the highly structured 3′X tail at the end of the HCV genome. (34) This information will certainly aid in the development of anti-HCV drugs.

NS5B is a virus-specific enzyme with no functional homologues in the host, and therefore, inhibitors may have the advantage of less toxicity/side effects. Sequence analysis has demonstrated that NS5B is highly conserved among all six clades of HCV. Thus, it is possible to develop anti-HCV polymerase inhibitors with broad-spectrum antiviral activities. These features provide additional enthusiasm for developing inhibitors against this viral target.

A number of pharmaceutical and biotechnology companies have anti-HCV polymerase program. The challenges are conventional. With nucleoside analogue-based inhibitors, attention to nonspecific activity against host polymerases should be evaluated carefully. As for HIV and HBV, drug resistance may develop against both nucleoside- and nonnucleoside-based inhibitors.

3'X End

The HCV genome contains a highly conserved, highly structured domain of 98 nucleotides at the 3' end, which is believed to be important for HCV replication. (35,36) Because the biology of this element has not been worked out, it is difficult to address the validity of this target or to develop a useful assay.

ANTI-HCV IMMUNOTHERAPY

The host immune response is important in controlling HCV infection. The failure to eliminate HCV infection leads to a continual host immune response against infected cells, which results in chronic inflammation and liver damage. (37) It is important to note that patients with acute HCV infection who mount a vigorous CD4$^+$ immune response against HCV NS3 are more likely to clear HCV infection. (38) In patients with chronic HCV infection, the presence of a cytotoxic T lymphocyte response against HCV in liver was shown to be associated with a better subsequent response to interferon-α therapy. (39) In addition, an induction of a CD4$^+$ T-cell response against HCV NS3 and NS4 during interferon-α therapy was associated with a sustained virologic response. (40) These data suggest that host immune responses play an important role in determining the clinical outcome and response to interferon-α therapy.

With this background, it is logical to consider immunotherapy as a possible therapeutic strategy against HCV infection. Immunotherapy against HCV can be classified into two categories: HCV specific and HCV nonspecific. These two approaches have different clinical and pathobiological implications. HCV-specific immunotherapy is expected to be more specific (targeting at HCV-infected cells), with less nonspecific side effects (e.g., systemic side effects), and development is driven by a rationale approach based on our knowledge of HCV-specific immune response. However, HCV-nonspecific immunotherapy (e.g., a cytokine with antiviral activities) is likely to be associated with systemic side effects (which may limit the therapeutic index) and therapeutic development is based mainly on trial and error in clinics.

HCV-Specific Immunotherapy

Obviously, HCV-specific immunotherapy requires HCV-specific stimulation. This is usually accomplished through the use of HCV-specific proteins (i.e., antigens), HCV-specific peptides, or a DNA-based, HCV-specific vaccine. Most investigators/pharmaceutical and biotechnology companies that are working on an HCV vaccine are focused on developing preventive vaccines. Hence, their current focus is on HCV envelope antigens, with the aim of triggering a vigorous B-cell response and the development of neutralization antibodies.

Chiron has reported the B-cell response of their gpE1/gpE2 and gpE2 vaccine. A proportion of chimpanzees immunized with a good B-cell response developed a high anti-HCV antibody titer and did not develop HCV infection on homologous viral challenge. (41) However, they also reported that chimpanzees immunized with their vaccine were not protected from heterologous HCV challenge. It is interesting to note that although the vaccine is not very protective against HCV challenge, a much smaller proportion of chimpanzees developed chronic HCV infection. Whether this protected effect against chronic HCV infection is associated with a B-cell or a T-cell response is not clear.

Similarly, Innogenetics reported that two chimpanzees immunized with their HCV gpE1 vaccine had a significant induction of anti-E1 titer, an improvement in liver histology, and a reduction of HCV core antigen expression in the chimpanzees' liver. (42) However, the effect of their immunotherapeutic approach on HCV viremia in these two chimpanzees was minimal. HCV-specific, T-cell response in these chimpanzees were not reported.

A number of HCV-specific, CD4$^+$ and CD8$^+$ T-cell epitopes have been reported. The lack of a small animal model hinders testing of the therapeutic potential of these epitopes in conjunction with other immunomodulating strategies. We have not yet seen any reports on the use of these epitope peptides as immunotherapy in clinics. It is interesting to note that the research group at the National Cancer Institute reported the engineering of an epitope in HCV core region with better *in vitro* and *in vivo* activity. (43) This type of epitope enhancement strategy may be useful in optimizing HCV-specific immunotherapy.

DNA-based, HCV-specific immunization approaches have also been tested. Based on this approach, a T-cell response to both structural and nonstructural proteins has been demonstrated in a murine model. (44,45) Whether these interesting results can be translated into a therapeutic strategy in patients with chronic HCV infection remains to be determined.

HCV-Nonspecific Immunotherapy

A nonspecific immune response includes complement, interferons and other cytokines, and natural killer cells. There is no report that indicates the involvement of complement in the host defense against HCV infection. Interferons are induced by most acute viral infections. However, interferons are rarely detectable in serum/plasma in patients with chronic diseases/infection. It is important to note that interferon-α is effective in controlling HCV replication (as reflected by a reduction of HCV viremia during therapy) and is able to clear HCV infection in a small proportion of patients with chronic HCV infection. As discussed earlier, patients with a detectable HCV-specific, CD8$^+$ response respond more favorably to interferon-α therapy. (39) Whether interferon-α works through its immunomodulatory or antiviral activities, or a combination of both, remains to be established.

Other cytokines, including interleukin 2 (IL-2), IL-12, and granulocyte/ macrophage colony-stimulating factor (GM/CSF), have also been tested in patients with chronic HCV infection. As we do not have a good cell culture or animal model for HCV infection, testing the efficacy of cytokines in chronic HCV infection is mostly by trial and error in clinics. The general principles guiding the use of cytokines are still based on a combination of its direct antiviral effects and their capabilities to induce a good CD4$^+$ (in particular, Th1 response), CD8$^+$ response.

Dendritic cells have been shown to play an important role in the induction of a host immune response. Cytokines, including FLT-3 ligand and a combination of IL-4 and GM/CSF, have been shown to increase the number of dendritic cells as well as augmenting its response. Whether augmenting the dendritic cell response (with or without HCV-specific stimulation) represents a good therapeutic strategy against HCV remains to be tested.

Our understanding of the paradigm of the Th1 and Th2 response can guide the development of HCV-nonspecific immunotherapy (Fig. 1). It is now known

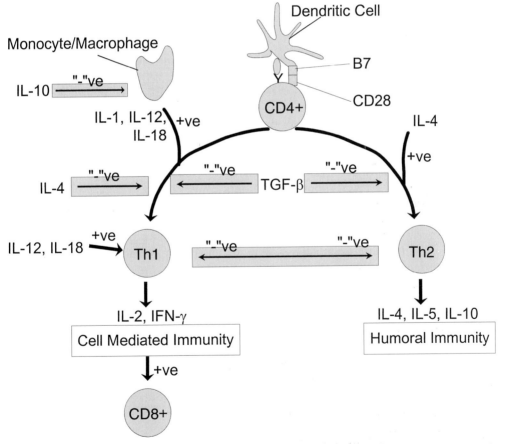

FIGURE 1   Host T-cell response and cytokines that drive the Th1/Th2 response. Cytokines with a positive effect are shown with a solid arrow with a +vs sign. Cytokines with a negative effect are shown with an arrow with a shaded box and are indicated with "−"ve.

that the CD4$^+$ Th1 response is an important component of the cell-mediated immunity by secreting Th1 cytokines and activating CD8$^+$ cells. Hence, the Th1 response is likely to be important in the host defense against HCV infection. In contrast, the Th2 response is more involved in the humoral response and, hence, is more important in the recovery process. It is important to note that the Th1 and Th2 response regulate each other negatively. It is believed that the balance between the Th1 and the Th2 response directs the host immune system to control and clear a viral infection (through a Th1 response) followed by a humoral response for long-term immune protection (mediated by the Th2 response). Cytokines are involved in the regulation of the Th1/Th2 balance as well as serving as effectors of the response. Therefore, it is not surprising that a number of investigators and pharmaceutical/biotechnology companies are trying various cytokines in an attempt to induce a Th1 response in order to control/clear HCV infection.

Stimulation of the CD8$^+$ response is also an attractive strategy. However, our understanding of the mechanisms involved in directing the CD8$^+$ response is rather poor. Cytokines that are known to activate CD8$^+$ cells, including IL-2, remain the focus of HCV-nonspecific, CD8$^+$ stimulation immunotherapy.

Combination Therapy

It is possible that a combination of HCV-specific and HCV-nonspecific immunotherapies may be more effective than either one of them alone. Of particular interest is the combination of the dendritic cell approach combined with HCV-specific immunotherapy. Although this sounds promising, the use of a combination of different biologics for therapeutic usage is still not well established. The side effects/toxicity profile resulting from the combined use of different biologics is also of concern.

As HCV persists in most patients in the presence of a host immune response, it is possible that a robust host immune response may prime the patients to respond better to anti-HCV therapy. Conversely, immunomonotherapy may not be sufficient. The demonstration that patients with an intrahepatic CD8$^+$ response respond better to interferon-α therapy is in keeping with this hypothesis. (39) Therefore, it is possible that combination therapy of anti-HCV drugs and immunotherapy represents the best therapeutic approach for chronic HCV infection.

OTHER APPROACHES

The antisense approach is being developed for HCV infection. The main obstacle to developing an antisense approach is the delivery of the antisense molecules to the circulation (i.e., route of administration), to the liver cells, and to the specific compartment where HCV replicates. At body temperature, the antisense molecule may also bind nonspecifically to host RNA/DNA, and therapeutic specificity is another hurdle to overcome. In a study based on antisense olignonucleotide therapy in chimpanzees, a minimal effect on serum and liver HCV RNA was seen in three chimpanzees and a moderate effect was seen in one chimpanzee. (46)

Ribozyme, an RNA molecule with catalytic efficiency to cleave a targeted sequence, is also being developed for HCV. (47) As with the antisense approach, delivery and specificity represent hurdles for development.

Gene therapy may also be adopted for HCV infection. Molecules including antisense RNA, ribozyme, anti-HCV single chain molecule, and cytokine genes may be delivered through gene therapy. Again, the route of administration and the duration of therapy remain as major challenges for this form of therapy. Dominant-negative HCV mutant and viral interfering particles are also possible strategies from a scientific standpoint. Much more work is needed before the potential of these therapeutic strategies is realized.

CONCLUSION

HCV is an elusive pathogen. Given the flexibility of HCV to adapt through its genetic evolution, the development of resistance to therapies targeted at HCV enzymes is a given. Combination therapies attacking various steps of the viral life cycle and boostering the host immune response represent the most attractive approach at present. HCV will remain a scientific challenge for the development of novel therapies in the many years to come.

"When we do the best that we can, we never know what miracle is wrought in our life, or in the life of another"

Helen Keller
In: *Out of the Dark,* 1913

ACKNOWLEDGMENTS

Our knowledge on HCV disease/virology/pathogenesis was secured by many scientists and clinicians. Neither space nor time allowed us to be comprehensive. For those contributions that we failed to mention, we apologize. This review was written based on the information available in the literature and the authors have attempted to be as objective as possible. JYNL was the Senior Director and DNS is an Associate Director in the Department of Antiviral Therapy, Schering-Plough Research Institute, Kenilworth, New Jersey. JYNL is currently senior Vice President, Research and Development, ICN Pharmaceuticals, Costa Mesa, CA 92626.

REFERENCES

1. Choo Q L, Kuo G, Weiner A J, Overby L R, Bradley D W, Houghton M. Isolation of a cDNA clone derived from a blood-borne non-A, non-B viral hepatitis genome. Science 1989;244:59–362.
2. Kuo G, Choo Q L, Alter H, et al. An assay for circulating antibodies to a major etiologic virus of human non-A, non-B-hepatitis. Science 1989;244:362–4.
3. Davis G L, Balart L A, Schiff E R, et al. Treatment of chronic hepatitis C with recombinant interferon alfa. A multicenter randomized, controlled trial. Hepatitis Interventional Therapy Group. N Engl J Med 1989;321:1501–6.
4. McHutchison J G, Gordon S C, Schiff E R, et al. Interferon alfa-2b alone or in combination

with ribavirin as initial treatment for chronic hepatitis C. Hepatitis Interventional Therapy Group. N Engl J Med 1998;339:1485–92.

5. Poynard T, Marcellin P, Lee S S, et al. Randomized trial of interferon alpha2b plus ribavirin for 48 weeks or for 24 weeks versus interferon alpha2b plus placebo for 48 weeks for treatment of chronic infection with hepatitis C virus. International Hepatitis Interventional Therapy Group (IHIT). Lancet 1998;352:1426–32.

6. Davis G L, Esteban-Mur R, Rustgi V, et al. Interferon alfa-2b alone or in combination with riba- virin for the treatment of relapse of chronic hepatitis C. International Hepatitis Interventional Therapy Group. N Engl J Med 1998;339:1493–9.

7. Kolykhalov A A, Agapov E V, Blight K J, Mihalik K, Feinstone S M, Rice C M. Transmission of hepatitis C by intrahepatic inoculation with transcribed RNA. Science 1997:25;277:570–4.

8. Yanagi M, St Claire M, Shapiro M, Emerson S U, Purcell R H, Bukh J. Transcripts of a chimeric cDNA clone of hepatitis C virus genotype 1b are infectious in vivo. Virology 1998;244:161–72.

9. Hong Z, Beaudet-Miller M, Lanford R E, et al. Generation of transmissible hepatitis C virions from a molecular clone in Chimpanzees. Virology 1999;256:36–44.

10. Robertson B, Myers G, Howard C, et al. Classification, nomenclature, and database devel- opment for hepatitis C virus (HCV) and related viruses: proposals for standardization. Inter- national Committee on Virus Taxonomy. Arch Virol 1998;143:2493–503.

11. Grakoui A, Wychowski C, Lin C, Feinstone S M, Rice C M. Expression and identification of hepatitis C virus polyprotein cleavage products. J Virol 1993;67:1385–95.

12. Brown E A, Zhang H, Ping L H, Lemon S M. Secondary structure of the 5′ nontranslated re- gions of hepatitis C virus and pestivirus genomic RNAs. Nucleic Acids Res 1992;20:5041–5.

13. Zapp M L, Stern S, Green M R. Small molecules that selectively block RNA binding of HIV-1 Rev protein inhibit Rev function and viral production. Cell 1993;74:969–78.

14. Hwang S B, Lo S Y, Ou J H, Lai M M C. Detection of cellular proteins and viral core protein in- teracting with the 5′ untranslated region of hepatitis C virus RNA. J Biomed Sci 1995;2:227–36.

15. Zhu N, Khoshnan A, Schneider R, et al. Hepatitis C virus core protein binds to the cytoplas- mic domain of tumor necrosis factor (TNF) receptor 1 and enhances TNF-induced apoptosis. J Virol 1998;72:3691–7.

16. Lo S Y, Masiarz F, Hwang S B, et al. Differential subcellular localization of hepatitis C virus core gene products. Virology 1995;213:455–61.

17. Pileri P, Uematsu Y, Campagnoli S, et al. Binding of hepatitis C virus to CD81. Science 1998; 282:938–41.

18. Labrosse B, Brelot A, Heveker N, et al. Determinants for sensitivity of human immunodeficiency virus coreceptor CXCR4 to the bicyclam AMD3100. J Virol 1998;72:6381–8.

19. Kilby J M, Hopkins S, Venetta T M, et al. Potent suppression of HIV-1 replication in humans by T-20, a peptide inhibitor of gp41-mediated virus entry. Nat Med 1998;4:1302–7.

20. Ggrakoui A, McCourt D W, Wychowski C, Feinstone S M, Rice C M. Characterization of the hepatitis C virus-encoded serine protease: determination of proteinase-dependent polyprotein cleavage. J Virol 1993;67:2832–43.

21. Bartenschlager R, Rhlborn-Laake L, Mous J, Jacobson H. Kinetics and structural analysis of hepatitis C virus polyprotein processing. J Virol 1994;68:5045–55.

22. Satoh S, Tanji Y, Hijikata M, Kimura K, Shimotohno K. The N-terminal region of hepatitis C virus non-structural protein (NS3) is essential for stable complex formation with NS4A. J Virol 1995;69:4255–60.

23. Kim J L, Morgenstern K A, Lin C, et al. Crystal structure of the hepatitis C virus NS3 protease domain complexed with a synthetic NS4A cofactor peptide. Cell 1996;87:343–55.

24. Kadare G, Haenni A L. Virus-encoded RNA helicases. J Virol 1997;71:2583–90.

25. Fernandez A, Guo H S, Saenz P, Simon-Buela L, Gomez de Cedron M, Garcia J A. The motif V of plum pox potyvirus CI RNA helicase is involved in NTP hydrolysis and is essential for virus RNA replication. Nucleic Acids Res 1997;25:4474–80.

26. Warrener P, Collett M S. Pestivirus NS3 (p80) protein possesses RNA helicase activity. J Virol 1995;69:1720–6.

27. Tai C L, Chi W K, Chen D S, Hwang L H. The helicase acctivity associated with hepatitis C vi- rus non-structural protein 3 (NS3). J Virol 1996;70:8477–84.

28. Yao N, Hesson T, Cable M, et al. Structure of the hepatitis C virus RNA helicase domain. Nat Struct Biol 1997;4:463–7.

29. Enomoto N, Sakuma I, Asahina Y, et al. Mutations in the nonstructural protein 5A gene and response to interferon in patients with chronic hepatitis C virus 1b infection. N Engl J Med 1996;334:77–81.
30. Gale M J Jr, Korth M J, Tang N M, et al. Evidence that hepatitis C virus resistance to interferon is mediated through repression of the PKR protein kinase by the nonstructural 5A protein. Virology 1997;230:217–27.
31. Behrens S E, Tomei L, De Francesco R. Identification and properties of the RNA-dependent RNA polymerase of hepatitis C virus. EMBO J 1996;15:12–22.
32. Lohmann V, Korner F, Herian U, Bartenschlager R. Biochemical properties of hepatitis C virus NS5B RNA-dependent RNA polymerase and identification of amino acid sequence motifs essential for enzymatic activity. J Virol 1997;71:8416–28.
33. Ferrari E, Wright-Minogue J, Fang J W, Baroudy B M, Lau J Y, Hong Z. Characterization of soluble hepatitis C virus RNA-dependent RNA polymerase expressed in *Escherichia coli.* J Virol 1999;73:1649–54.
34. Ito T, Lai M M. Determination of the secondary structure of and cellular protein binding to the 3'-untranslated region of the hepatitis C virus RNA genome. J Virol 1997;71:8698–706.
35. Takamizawa A, Mori C, Fuke I, et al. Structure and organization of the hepatitis C virus genome isolated from human carriers. J Virol 1991;65:1105–13.
36. Kolykhalov A A, Feinstone S M, Rice C M. Identification of a highly conserved sequence element at the 3'terminus of hepatitis C virus genome RNA. J Virol 1996;70:3363–71.
37. Nelson D R, Marousis C G, Davis G L, et al. The role of hepatitis C virus-specific cytotoxic T lymphocytes in chronic hepatitis C. J Immunol 1997;158:1473–81.
38. Diepolder H M, Zachoval R, Hoffmann R M, et al. Possible mechanism involving T-lymphocyte response to non-structural protein 3 in viral clearance in acute hepatitis C. Lancet 1995;346:1006–7.
39. Nelson D R, Marousis C G, Ohno T, Davis G L, Lau J Y N. Intrahepatic hepatitis C virus-specific cytotoxic T lymphocyte activity and response to interferon alfa therapy in chronic hepatitis C. Hepatology 1998;28:225–30.
40. Lohr H F, Gerken G, Roth M, et al. The cellular immune responses induced in the follow-up of interferon-alpha treated patients with chronic hepatitis C may determine the therapy outcome. J Hepatol 1998;29:524–32.
41. Houghton M, Choo Q L, Kuo G, et al. HCV Vaccine: interim report. 9th Trienn Int Symp Viral Hepatitis Liver Dis, Rome, April, 1996.
42. Maertens G, Ducatteeuw A, Priem S, et al. Therapeutic vaccination of chronically infected chimpanzees with the HCV E1 protein. Hepatology 1998;28:298A.
43. Sarobe P, Pendleton C D, Akatsuka T, et al. Enhanced in vitro potency and in vivo immunogenicity of a CTL epitope from hepatitis C virus core protein following amino acid replacement at secondary HLA-A2.1 binding positions. J Clin Invest 1998;15:1239–48.
44. Geissler M, Tokushige K, Wakita T, Zurawski V R Jr, Wands J R. Differential cellular and humoral immune responses to HCV core and HBV envelope proteins after genetic immunizations using chimeric constructs. Vaccine 1998;16:857–67.
45. Encke J, zu Putlitz J, Geissler M, Wands J R. Genetic immunization generates cellular and humoral immune responses against the nonstructural proteins of the hepatitis C virus in a murine model. J Immunol 1998;161:4917–23.
46. Dailey P J, Collins M L, Urdea M S, Wilber J C. Quantitation of HCV RNA in liver tissue by bDNA. Chapter 10 In: Lau J Y N, ed. Hepatitis C protocols. Clifton, NJ: Humana Press, 1998:119–29.
47. Roberts E C, Malmstrom T A, Pavco P A, et al. Synthesis and testing of nuclease resistant hammerhead ribozymes directed against hepatitis C virus RNA. Hepatology 1998;28:398A.

25
HEPATITIS C VACCINES

SARA GAGNETEN AND STEPHEN M. FEINSTONE
Laboratory of Hepatitis Viruses
Center for Biologics Evaluation and Research
Food and Drug Administration
Bethesda, Maryland

INTRODUCTION

Although the hepatitis C virus (HCV) presently causes an estimated 30,000 new cases of hepatitis each year in the United States, this rate has declined significantly from the 1980s when there were an estimated 180,000 infections each year. (1) The majority of these acute infections, however, progress to persistent, usually lifelong infections. This high rate of persistence has resulted in a large number of chronic carriers estimated to be as many as four million in the United States alone. These carriers form a continuing pool of HCV infection and maintain the virus in the population by serving as the source of new infections. How the virus is transmitted in the general population is not completely known. Parenteral transmission is clearly important. With the introduction of effective screening tests, the blood supply has been virtually eliminated as a source of new infections. At present, illicit use of intravenous drugs is probably the most common identifiable mode of transmission in the United States. (2) However, nonparenteral or apparently nonparenteral transmission must also be important. If these mechanisms of transmission were well understood, public health measures might be designed to interdict this transmission. HCV can be transmitted by sexual contact, but this type of transmission probably occurs at a much lower rate than is the case for hepatitis B transmission. Maternal–infant transmission may also occur but again at a relatively low rate. (3) Other forms of personal contact that might transmit HCV are largely unknown and may differ considerably in different populations that have different customs and behavior patterns. Without a clear understanding of how this virus is transmitted and maintained in the population, the best chance for breaking the chain of transmission would be the development and utilization of a prophylactic vaccine.

Viruses that produce chronic infections have become attractive targets for antiviral therapy. Most common viral infections produce acute, self-limited disease and do not require chemotherapeutic intervention. Hepatitis B virus, HCV, human immunodefficiency virus, and several herpes viruses have all been targeted for antiviral development with some degree of success. However, long-term antiviral therapy is generally costly, often requires continued oversight by health care professionals, and may be associated with significant side effects.

While HCV infections often become chronic, resulting in progressive liver disease, acute hepatitis C infections frequently go unnoticed as they are often subclinical. Acute infection may be far easier to eradicate than established chronic infection, but the opportunity for treatment during the acute stage of hepatitis C is rarely encountered. A vaccine to prevent infection would therefore be preferred over therapy of established chronic infection. In addition, the possibility for immunotherapy of chronic viral infections by means of therapeutic vaccines also has some attractive features, although to date, the practical application of this concept has met only limited success. Nevertheless, successful therapeutic vaccines may require only a few doses over a relatively short period of time, be much less expensive than the long-term administration of antiviral drugs and would generally be expected to have low rates of adverse events compared to many of the drugs in use today. Therefore, the vaccine approach has many advantages for both the prophylaxis and the therapy of HCV infection.

PROBLEMS OF HCV VACCINE DEVELOPMENT

The virology of hepatitis C has presented many obstacles to the successful development of vaccines. Although the hepatitis C virus has been known since the late 1980s, the virus has not yet been cultivated successfully *in vitro* at a level useful for viral production and for the performance of classical virologic studies. Due to the lack of a robust cell culture system, no *in vitro* assays are known to correlate with protection or neutralization. The genome of HCV is highly variable, resulting in at least six genotypes and multiple subtypes. In addition, there is a hypervariable region (HVR1) in the E2 glycoprotein that may be an important antigenic site. (4) Finally, HCV is highly host range restricted. The only established animal model for HCV infection is the chimpanzee, which cannot be used for routine experiments.

Genetic Variability of HCV

Like all RNA viruses, HCV has a relatively high rate of genetic variability. This is presumably due to the low fidelity of the viral-coded, RNA-dependent RNA polymerase (RDRP), which is responsible for the replication of the viral genome. (5) These viral RDRPs, which do not have a counterpart in mammalian cells, lack proofreading capability and are unable to correct misincorporated nucleotides. Although many such substitutions may be lethal, HCV seems to be relatively tolerant of mutations. High levels of sequence diversity between viral isolates have led to the concept of genotypes. The known viruses for which sequence data are available have been divided into six genotypes with a nucleotide sequence difference between genotypes of at least 30%. Each genotype has been further divided into subtypes. (6) There have been some correlation studies on phenotypic differences among these genotypes. For the purpose of vaccine development, it is important to know if these genotypes also constitute serotypes or even if the concept of serotype can be applied to HCV. Virus isolates that can be neutralized by the same antibody or antiserum define a serotype, whereas viruses that are not neutralized by the same antibody constitute distinct serotypes.

For example, polioviruses are divided into three serotypes. The antibody in a patient recovered from a polio type 1 infection will neutralize all polio type 1 viruses but not type 2 or 3 polio viruses.

Each HCV-infected patient carries a population of circulating viruses with different but closely related genomic sequences. These individual viruses have been termed quasispecies. Quasispecies would be found in any virus population, especially RNA viruses. However, for most viruses, the quasispecies that can be detected can still be neutralized by antibody for their serotype. In HCV infections, the quasispecies have most often been defined by the sequence in the HVR1 that codes for approximately the first 30 amino acids of the E2 glycoprotein. (4,7) In general, the greatest degree of genomic sequence diversity has been seen within this region, regardless of whether the comparison is made among viruses from different genotypes, isolates from the same genotype, or sequences of individual genomes isolated from an individual patient. There is a considerable amount of evidence that the HVR1 represents an important target for neutralizing antibodies. Immune pressure is responsible for the continual selection of variants in the HVR1, allowing viral escape from neutralization and possibly viral persistence. (8,9) If the HVR1 is the primary neutralization antigen in HCV and the HVR1 varies independently of genotype, there would be no recognizable correlation of serotype to genotype. In addition, if the HVR1 represents the neutralization epitope of HCV and HVR1 is broadly variable, then there may be an extremely large number of neutralization types and the concept of serotype cannot be applied to HCV. Therefore this issue has major implications for vaccine development.

Evidence that antibody to HVR1 can neutralize HCV was provided by an experiment in which antibody was raised to a synthetic oligopeptide representing the dominant HVR1 sequence of the HCV in patient H plasma. (9,10) A dilution of the patient H plasma that contained 64 chimpanzee infectious doses (CID50) of HCV was mixed and incubated with the hyperimmune rabbit anti-HVR1 peptide serum. This neutralization mixture was then inoculated into a chimpanzee. The animal became infected, but not with the virus that had the HVR1 sequence to which the rabbit antibody was raised, implying that this individual quasispecies had been neutralized. If the HVR1 indeed represents the only neutralization epitope of HCV, the approach to making a broadly reactive vaccine is not feasible. Chimpanzees that recovered from HCV infection could be reinfected with a virus of a different genotype, the same genotype, or even virus present within the same inoculum used in the initial inoculation. (11,12) Thus, infection and resolution do not produce an immune response that is broad or strong enough to protect against reinfection by all the quasispecies in the original inoculum. If antibody to the HVR1 is crucial for viral neutralization, it would present a great challenge to devise a technology to immunize against a broad array of antigens.

In Vitro Culture Systems for HCV

Numerous reports in the literature have shown that HCV replicates in a variety of cultured cells. (13–19) Cells of liver and lymphoid origin, both B cells and T cells, have served as substrates for HCV replication. In general, the systems used to measure HCV replication have relied on highly sensitive reverse tran-scriptase polymerase chain reaction (RT-PCR) technology. The viral yields of these cell culture systems have not been high enough to use standard virologic or immunologic detection methods, and this low yield has limited the utility of these *in vitro* culture systems. Nevertheless, the number of reports on success-ful *in vitro* cultivation of HCV gives credence to the concept that HCV does in-deed replicate at low level *in vitro* and provides hope that a useful cell culture system will be developed. Reports of successful *in vitro* culture systems need to be evaluated carefully as it is known that "sticking" of input virus to cultured cells can be detected by PCR for long periods of time without true replication. Studies in which strand-specific RT-PCR has been used to demonstrate the tran-scription of the positive-stranded viral RNA into a negative-stranded interme-diate suggest *de novo* viral replication; however, such evidence only supports RNA replication and not true viral production. Perhaps the most convincing evidence for *in vitro* replication of HCV has been provided by Shimizu and col-leagues in two experiments. In the first, HCV was grown in a B lymphocyte line termed HPBMa and was then passaged to a new drug-resistant cell line by co-cultivation in the presence of the drug, which was lethal for the HPBMa. Pas-sages between these cell lines therefore supported the replication of the virus-infected cells. (13) In the second experiment, HCV that had been cultured in Daudi cells for 58 days was harvested and inoculated into a chimpanzee, which then developed typical HCV infection. It seems unlikely but still possible that even after 58 days in culture, the infectious virus from the original inoculum persisted and infected the chimpanzee. (20) However, classical virology exper-iments in which virus can be serially diluted and amplified have not been done.

Whether HCV replicates in cell culture is less of an issue for vaccine devel-opment than the question of whether it replicates in a way that is useful for vi-rologic experiments. The level of virus production *in vitro* is far below what would be necessary for the production of a vaccine antigen or even for a live-attenuated viral vaccine. Although an *in vitro* neutralization has been described in HPBMa cells, (13) it is not clear that this assay represents a true infectivity neutralization or a blocking of HCV binding to the cells. In addition, the de-scribed system may not be readily applicable to classical viral titration and neu-tralization experiments. Therefore, the available cell culture systems to date have not been useful for the purpose of vaccine development.

In Vitro Correlates of Neutralization

Without a practical cell culture system, it would still be useful to find other *in vitro* correlates of virus neutralization. An assay in which recombinant E2 gly-coprotein expressed in mammalian cells was shown to bind specifically to cells susceptible to HCV infection has been developed. It has further been shown that this binding can be inhibited by certain antibodies to E2. (21) Inhibition of binding of E2 to this cell surface protein by antibody has been correlated with antibody-mediated protection against infection. This assay has been named neu-tralization of binding (NOB). A cell surface protein that binds E2 has been iden-tified as CD81, a member of the tetraspanin superfamily. (22) This molecule is expressed broadly in many tissues, including hepatocytes and lymphocytes. The extracellular domain of CD81 is not well conserved between species although it is nearly identical between humans and chimpanzees. (23) Although there is some evidence that supports the notion that the NOB assay correlates with the neutralization of infection, it is far from proven. While neutralization of infectivity could be achieved by blocking viral attachment to its cellular receptor, this mechanism of antibody-mediated viral neutralization is not the only way that viruses are neutralized. It could be argued that if the HCV genome can mutate with relative ease and escape antibody-mediated neutralization, those mutations would also likely affect the ability of the virus to infect cells if these mutations occurred in such a vital portion of the virion surface as the receptor-binding region. Because the CD81-binding region of E2 is not within HVR1, (24) there are probably other targets for antibody neutralization in addition to the putative neutralization epitope in the HVR1. At this time, the function of CD81 as the HCV receptor and the correlation with viral neutralization by blockage of this binding by antibody are still under investigation. If the NOB assay proves to be a good correlate of antibody-mediated neutralization, it will facilitate vaccine development and evaluation greatly.

Other systems that may correlate with HCV neutralization have been studied. The vesicular stomatitis virus (VSV) has been used to express either the HCV E1 or the E2 glycoprotein as pseudotype viral particles. The coding regions of the E1 and E2 ectodomains were appended to the transmembrane and cytoplasmic tail coding regions of the VSV G protein. These proteins could be expressed on the cell surface after transfection of the chimeric RNA transcript. In addition, if transfected cells expressing E1 or E2 were infected with a temperature-sensitive mutant of VSV at a nonpermissive temperature, a VSV/HCV pseudotyped virus was generated. It was shown that infection of new cells with this virus could be neutralized with serum from HCV-vaccinated chimpanzees. (25) Although this system is quite cumbersome, it does offer a possible direction for the development of an *in vitro* neutralization assay that could be correlated with *in vivo* protection.

Animal Models of HCV Infection

The only established animal model for HCV infections is the chimpanzee. Obviously this rare and very expensive animal model is not useful for routine experiments that require multiple data points. Many vaccine experiments have been performed in small animals, typically mice, and various types of immune responses induced. Because these animals cannot be infected with HCV and an acceptable *in vitro* neutralization assay has not been developed, mouse studies are of limited value. Mice have been used to mimic the human either as transgenic animals or by reconstituting immunodeficient mice with human tissue. This approach may have some utility for vaccine development.

IMMUNOPROTECTION AGAINST HCV

Vaccine development has not only been hampered by properties of the virus such as variability and antigenic diversity, but also by the nature of the virus–host interactions. HCV can persist in the host despite the presence of apparently adequate antibody and T-cell responses to the virus. Understanding of the immune mechanisms in patients who resolve HCV infection may allow determination of the type of immunity required for viral clearance as well as for vaccine development. The humoral and cellular immune responses during HCV infection are discussed extensively in other chapters. For illustration purposes, immunologic features important for vaccine development are highlighted here.

Humoral Immunity

Most HCV infections induce antibody responses to both structural and nonstructural proteins. Flaviviruses such as yellow fever virus and dengue can be neutralized by antibody to the major envelope glycoprotein. (26,27) However, it remains unclear whether effective neutralizing antibodies against either of the envelope glycoproteins develop following HCV infections. Examination of antibody responses in relation to outcome of infection reveals that the prevalence of specific antibodies to HVR1 of E2 appears early after infection in recovered patients. (10,28) However, antibodies to both structural and nonstructural proteins are detected less frequently in recovered patients as compared with patients with viral persistence. (29) In chimpanzees, there is little correlation between recovery and antibodies to the envelope glycoproteins. (30) In the course of natural infection, HCV appears to elicit a restricted neutralizing antibody response. HCV from a patient during the acute phase of a chronic infection could be neutralized *in vitro* by plasma obtained from the same patient 2 years later but not with plasma obtained 11 years later. (31) High-titer antibodies to HVR1 have been shown to prevent HCV infection after *in vitro* neutralization, but protection was incomplete, possibly due to a minor population of neutralization escape variants. (9) In a study of 34 patients with HCV infections, high levels of antibodies that block the binding of the E2 to human cells (NOB assay) were found in 7 patients who recovered from chronic hepatitis C but not in 5 patients who recovered naturally from acute hepatitis or in 22 patients who had unresolved chronic infection. (32) In multiply transfused humans and experimentally infected chimpanzees, acute self-limited infections did not confer protective immunity against reinfection by even the same inoculum used for the original infection, suggesting that antibody responses generated during the acute infection are not effective in neutralizing the virus. (11,12,33)

Cell-Mediated Immunity

Comparative studies of humoral and cellular immune responses in healthy individuals who are seropositive for HCV antibodies but negative for HCV RNA and individuals with chronic hepatitis C have been instrumental in defining the features of the immune response associated with disease resolution or chronic viral persistence. The CD4$^+$ T helper lymphocyte response to a range of HCV proteins is broader and stronger in patients who clear the virus than in patients with chronic hepatitis C. (29,34–38) In contrast, virus-specific antibody responses in patients who have cleared the virus in the past are both weaker and targeted at fewer antigens than in patients with continuing HCV replication.

T helper lymphocyte responses to HCV core, (29) NS3, (29,36) NS4, (29,35, 37) and NS5 (35,37) have all been found to correlate with a benign course of infection. Thus, control of HCV infection may be associated with effective activation of a vigorous T helper lymphocyte response to a broad range of HCV proteins. The dominant T helper lymphocyte response in patients who control viral replication is of the Th1 type, which promotes cellular effector mechanisms rather than humoral immune responses. There is growing evidence that resolution of HCV infection also correlates with a broad CD8$^+$ cytotoxic T lymphocyte (CTL) response directed against various regions of the HCV polyprotein and independently of the antibody response. (39,40) Although rare, spontaneous clearance of HCV in agammaglobulinemic patients who have been infected by therapy with contaminated immune globulin preparations provides additional evidence that resolution can occur independently of antibodies. (41–43) Strong cellular immune responses may not only contribute to the prevention of persistence, but may also be important for the control of established persistent viral infections. However, the presence of a strong and broad T helper cell response in individuals and chimpanzees who have undetectable viremia several years after exposure to HCV suggests that the liver or peripheral blood mononuclear cells (PBMC) may be a reservoir of infection and that the presence of these HCV-specific T lymphocytes may be responsible for suppressing viral replication. (44,45)

Similar immune response patterns have been observed in prospective studies in chimpanzees infected with HCV. Animals that terminated the infection generated a broad CD8$^+$ CTL response but poor antibody responses. Prospective studies in chimpanzees have shown that a critical factor for termination is the simultaneous emergence of multispecific CTLs early in the course of infection. (45) Persistently infected chimpanzees express a higher prevalence of antibody reactivity to structural and nonstructural proteins compared to chimpanzees that have cleared the virus. (46)

Host Genetic Factors

Cellular immune responses to infection are strongly dependent on genetic background, especially the major histocompatibility complex. Because HLA polymorphisms affect epitope presentation and recognition by T-cell receptors, some HLA alleles may be more effective presenters of viral neutralizing epitopes during the induction of T-cell responses. Studies designed to address the influence of HLA class II genotype on resolution of HCV infection have found that several class II alleles, DRB1*04, DQA1*03, DQB1*0301, and DRB1*0301, (47, 48) are associated with disease resolution. The association of specific alleles with viral clearance may reflect an optimal interaction of these particular alleles with both viral peptides and T-cell receptors. Nevertheless, many patients who express these class II alleles still develop chronic infections, suggesting a complex interplay of viral and host factors in determining the outcome. Correlation of outcomes of hepatitis C infection with different HLA haplotypes and HCV genotypes is likely to be very complex and would require extensive studies of a large number of patients and chimpanzees. (45,49)

The nature of the immune responses in patients who are able to control

HCV replication suggests that a successful vaccine will need to elicit powerful and multispecific T helper cell and CTL responses to a number of HCV proteins. The possibility that occult HCV infection persists in the liver of "recovered" patients suggests that therapeutic vaccines that could trigger a strong and broad cellular immune response could control virus replication in chronically infected patients.

PRECLINICAL STUDIES

Although the chimpanzee is the only established animal model for HCV infection and disease, much can be learned from experiments in small animals. Both the quality and the quantity of the immune response can be measured in animal models. Without an *in vivo* protection model or an *in vitro* correlate of neutralization, it is difficult to determine what the effect of the immune response would be on prevention or elimination of HCV infections in humans. Vaccines of several different types have been studied in mice, including recombinant proteins, vaccinia vectors expressing HCV antigens, synthetic peptides, naked DNA, and virus-like particles.

Small Animal Models and Chimpanzees

Evaluation of candidate HCV vaccines is particularly difficult due to the lack of suitable small animal models and efficient *in vitro* replication systems. Despite the inability for viral challenge, vaccination studies in mice are indispensable for preliminary evaluation of the potential of experimental HCV vaccines to induce either humoral or cellular immune responses.

The chimpanzee (*Pan troglodyte*) remains the only established animal model for HCV infection and disease in humans. The chimpanzee can be infected with HCV, resulting in disease similar to that of humans. In addition, the chimpanzee immune system resembles that of the human and many human-specific immunologic reagents work well in the chimpanzee. The chimpanzee offers the only opportunity to challenge vaccinated animals with live virus in order to actually test the efficacy of the vaccine. Although chimpanzees closely mimic the clinical response of humans, the fine details of the immune responses may be different. At this time, however, the sensitivity of chimpanzees to HCV infection relative to humans is not known. In addition, immune responses that are restricted by class I or class II MHC antigens in pathogenesis, recovery, or protection may differ from human. A considerable amount of information has become available on chimpanzee analogues of HLA antigens. In chimpanzees, these HLA analogues have been termed Patr antigens and some of them have been shown to be closely related to major HLA types and to even bind to the same peptides, implying that these animals could recognize the same epitopes as humans who express the analogous HLA.

Naked DNA Vaccines

Delivery of purified plasmid DNA-encoding antigens under the control of eukaryotic promoters can lead to expression of these antigens in the host cells, thereby triggering an immune response. Nucleic acid-based vaccines, which can be prepared with relative ease, allow the generation of constructs containing different HCV coding sequences, bicistronic messages, and messages coding for chimeric proteins or immune-enhancing elements. When administered to mice, these DNA vaccines can be tested using different combinations, delivery modes, or doses. Finally, DNA-based immunization, as with recombinant proteins, offers the advantage of inducing immune responses against both envelope proteins and internal proteins of the virus.

The HCV core protein is generally well conserved and, although not present on the virus surface, elicits an immune response that could contribute to a reduction in viral load in primary infections or in chronic carriers. Core-expressing plasmids have induced weak humoral and cellular responses in mice. (50,51) However, enhanced immunogenicity of the core protein was obtained when mice were coimmunized with DNA expression constructs encoding the HCV core protein, mouse interleukin (IL)-2, and mouse granulocyte macrophage colony-stimulating factor (GM/CSF). Coimmunization of core and IL-2 expressing plasmids produced the most significant increase in T-cell proliferative responses and CTL activity when compared with mice immunized with the core expressing plasmid alone. (52) Immunogenicity of the nonsecreted core protein was also enhanced using chimeric constructs expressing the core protein fused to various regions of the secreted hepatitis B envelope protein. (53, 54) CTL responses were investigated using contructs for HCV core, E1, and E2. Balb/C mice were immunized with vaccines expressing all three proteins, individual proteins, or various combinations of these proteins. All the plasmids elicited antibody responses to the specific immunogens. However, only plasmids that included the core antigen induced a CTL response in this mouse model. (55)

Recombinant E1 and E2 glycoproteins have been shown to induce protection against homologous challenge in the chimpanzee model. Several neutralizing determinants and CTL and T helper cell epitopes have been described within E2. Efficient induction of anti-E2 antibodies was obtained in mice following delivery of plasmids expressing the E2 glycoprotein alone (55–57) or expressing discrete domains of E2 fused to the hepatitis B surface antigen, which allowed the mapping of immunogenic domains on E2. (56,58) HCV envelope DNA vaccine vectors designed to enhance expression and secretion of the envelope glycoproteins were studied in buffalo rats. The signal sequence of E1 and E2 proteins was replaced with the signal sequence of the herpes simplex virus type 1 glycoprotein D, which has been shown to facilitate the secretion of HIV gp160. In addition, C-terminal hydrophobic regions of the envelope proteins were truncated. Both antibody and lymphocyte proliferative responses were induced against E1 and E2, but these responses were enhanced greatly by the simultaneous delivery of the GM-CSF. Various methods for codelivery of the GM-CSF and the envelope proteins were tested. The highest immune response was obtained with a bicistronic plasmid that expressed both the GM-CSF and the envelope proteins. The response was intermediate when the GM-CSF and the envelope proteins were codelivered in separate plasmids and was lowest for constructs expressing GM-CSF envelope fusion proteins. (59) A DNA vaccine that expressed a truncated form of the E2 glycoprotein that targeted the antigen to the cell surface was used to immunize both mice and macaques. The cell surface form induced an earlier and stronger antibody response in both mice and monkeys compared to the entire E2 glycoprotein. (60)

DNA vaccines expressing NS3, NS4, and NS5 nonstructural proteins were highly immunogenic in mice and buffalo rats. In mice, these nonstructural proteins induced strong immune responses, including specific antibody responses and CD4$^+$ T-cell responses with a predominant Th1 phenotype. Specific CD8$^+$ CTL responses were demonstrated for NS3 and NS5. (61) In buffalo rats the immune response to all three nonstructural proteins was increased when a bicistronic plasmid expressing nonstructural proteins and GM-CSF was used. (62)

In order to mimic the immune response in humans, a plasmid vaccine encoding the HCV core antigen (amino acids 1–191) was administered to transgenic mice that express HLA-A2.1. In this mouse model it was possible to induce CD8$^+$, HLA-A2.1-restricted CTLs specific for three epitopes within the core protein that had previously been shown to be presented by HLA-A2.1 to human CTLs with the A2.1 haplotype. In order to test the possible effectiveness of such a vaccine, vaccinated mice were challenged by an HCV surrogate, namely a recombinant vaccinia virus expressing the HCV core protein. Five days after inoculation, HCV vaccinia virus titers were measured in the ovaries. There was a greater than 10^6-fold reduction in virus titer in immunized mice compared with mock-immunized controls, and this protection was mediated by CD8$^+$ cells, in that it was completely abrogated by treating the mice with anti-CD8 antibodies. Similar results were obtained 2, 6, and 14 months after immunization. These results demonstrate that a vaccine designed to mainly induce a CTL response has potential to produce protective immunity. (63)

The delivery mode of DNA vaccines influences the induction of immune responses greatly. Intraepidermal delivery has been more effective than intramuscular delivery for most antigens, and vaccination schedules that include a booster with a different immunogen induce a stronger and longer-lasting response than a single primary DNA vaccination.

Synthetic Vaccines

Short peptides with amino acid sequences that mimic the antigenic sites of viruses have been used as immunogens in experimental vaccines. Due to the important role of T helper cells in the induction of CTL responses and in the maintenance of CTL memory, the role of T helper cell epitope peptides in the induction of HCV-specific CTLs was examined. Mice were immunized with peptides corresponding to CTL and helper T-cell epitopes of the HCV core. Cytotoxic T-cell activity against the HCV core was evaluated after immunization and after infecting the mice with a recombinant vaccinia virus expressing the HCV core. CTL responses induced by a conjugated CTL–T helper peptide were higher than those induced by a CTL epitope peptide alone or a mixture of T helper and CTL epitope peptides. (64)

Advances in epitope design are important in the development of synthetic vaccines or as components of other vaccines. Major histocompatibility complex (MHC)–peptide-binding assays have led to the characterization of many CTL epitopes in the HCV polyprotein. Immunogenicity of a peptide epitope may be enhanced by modifying the sequence of the peptide to increase the binding affinity for the MHC molecule without interfering with recognition by the T-cell receptor. A well-conserved HLA-A2.1-restricted CTL epitope in the HCV core antigen (amino acids 132–140) was studied by making a series of single amino acid-substituted nonapeptides at each amino acid position. Each of the modified peptides was tested for its ability to bind to HLA-A2.1 and for its ability to induce a CTL response in HLA-A2.1 transgenic mice. Peptides substituted at position 1 had a higher binding affinity, but paradoxically had poorer immunogenicity. One peptide termed 8A in which the leucine at position 8 was exchanged for an alanine exhibited both increased binding affinity and improved immunogenicity in HLA-A2.1 mice for the wild-type peptide. (65) This approach may be useful for enhancing the immune response to desired epitopes.

A novel approach for the development of epitope-based vaccines consists of using sera from HCV-infected patients to screen phage-displayed peptide libraries and select peptides that react specifically with sera from infected patients. (66) Sera from HCV infected individuals were used to screen a vast repertoire of HVR1 peptides expressed in a bacteriophage library to select peptides that are antigenic and immunogenic mimics of a large number of naturally occurring HVR1 variants. Mixtures of peptides with the highest cross-reactivity were injected into mice and shown to induce highly cross-reacting responses to 95% of a panel of 40 natural HVR1 peptides. (67)

Live Recombinant Viral Vectors

Live recombinant vaccines consist of live-attenuated viruses or bacteria that carry heterologous genes encoding the appropriate protective antigens. Replication-defective recombinant adenoviruses can express heterologous proteins efficiently and may induce specific immune responses against a diversity of epitopes from these foreign antigens. Recombinant adenovirus containing the core and E1 genes of HCV in place of the adenoviral E1 gene region have stimulated specific CTL responses in mice against HCV antigens effectively. The cytotoxic T-cell response was H-2^d restricted, lasted for at least 100 days, and was mediated by T cells with the classic CD4$^-$CD8$^+$ phenotype. (68) Interestingly, studies aimed at assessing host immune responses in mice inoculated with vaccinia/HCV recombinant viruses revealed that recombinants expressing the HCV core protein exhibited strong immunosuppressive effects. These results suggest that expression of the HCV core protein may affect the immunogenicity of a vaccine strongly and, in chronically infected patients, could contribute to the establishment of a persistent infection. (69)

Virus-like Particles

Virus-like genomeless particles may represent a potential HCV vaccine approach. HCV-like particles have been produced in insect cells using a recombinant baculovirus system expressing HCV structural proteins. (70) Mice immunized with partially purified HCV-like particles generated antibodies to the core and envelope proteins as well as T-cell proliferative responses and CTL responses. (71)

Recombinant Envelope Proteins

It has been shown for several flaviviruses that antibody to the envelope glycoprotein provided protection from infection. Therefore, either one or both of the envelope glycoproteins of HCV may be used as a vaccine. A series of vaccination experiments were performed by the Chiron group in chimpanzees. Both the E1 and the E2 glycoproteins were expressed originally in HeLa cells by a recombinant vaccinia virus. The glycoproteins were purified and mixed with an oil/water microemulsified adjuvant and inoculated intramuscularly into seven chimpanzees in varying doses and schedules. Two to 3 weeks after the final boost, the chimpanzees were challenged with 10 chimpanzee infectious doses (CID50) of HCV-1 (genotype 1a), which was the same virus from which the vaccine had been made. The five animals that had the highest anti-E1/E2 responses were completely protected from infection by the challenge virus. The two low responders became infected but both resolved their infections. In contrast, four unvaccinated but challenged chimpanzees all became chronically infected. (72) This result has to be viewed in light of the reported 30% rate of chronicity in HCV-infected chimpanzees. (46)

In later studies, an E1/E2 expression Chinese hamster ovary (CHO) cell line was used as the source of the antigen for further chimpanzee studies. Of 4 vaccinated and challenged chimpanzees, 3 developed mild, self-limited infections and 1 developed a persistent infection. The 5 protected animals from the original experiment were reboosted with the CHO cell-derived E1/E2 and rechallenged with 10 CID50 of a homotypic though heterologous strain of HCV (HCV-H, genotype 1a). In this case, all 5 animals were infected, although none developed persistent infections. Similar results were obtained in other vaccine experiments in chimpanzees. A total of 13 chimpanzees received the E1/E2 vaccine and were challenged. Ten of these chimpanzees resolved their infections and 3 became persistently infected. Among 13 unvaccinated chimpanzees that were challenged, 9 became chronically infected and 4 resolved their infections (Houghton M: personal communication). These experiments showed that antibodies to the envelope glycoproteins induced by a subunit vaccine could affect the outcome of a subsequent HCV infection by reducing the severity of the acute infection and the likelihood of chronicity. These experiments, however, did not address the issue of the antigenic diversity of HCV. It is not at all clear what effect a vaccine based on a single envelop sequence would have on infection by widely different viruses.

Therapeutic Vaccination

The chimpanzee has been used to study the potential for an immunotherapeutic approach to the treatment of chronic HCV infections. The vaccine consisted of a recombinant E1 glycoprotein of an HCV genotype 1b isolate expressed in mammalian cells. The E1 was purified to homodimers and left to associate into monodispersed spherical particles averaging 9 nm in diameter. Two long-term chronically infected chimpanzees, one with genotype 1a and the other with 1b, were inoculated with a total of nine doses of the E1 vaccine (50 µg). The animals were studied for HCV viremia by RT-PCR, HCV antigens on liver biopsies by immunostaining, liver disease by monitoring ALT levels, and liver histology in biopsies. During the period in which the vaccines were administered, ALT levels decreased, liver histology became normal, and HCV antigens virtually disappeared from the liver. However, there was no change in HCV RNA levels in the serum as measured by RT-PCR. After the vaccine was stopped, inflammatory changes and HCV antigens reappeared in the liver and serum ALT levels rose to pretreatment levels. Although the animals were not cured, there was a measurable improvement in the liver disease associated with this chronic infection. (71)

Passive Immunization

The question of the role of antibody in protection from infection remains unanswered. However, a partial answer was provided by a chimpanzee neutralization experiment. Intravenous immunoglobulin (IGIV) (5% IgG) was prepared from more than 1000 donors who all had antibodies to HCV. A second preparation was made from donors who were antibody negative. Both preparations were inactivated for any potential residual HCV by the solvent detergent method. (73) Approximately 64 CID50 of HCV-H was mixed with each IGIV preparation, incubated overnight, and inoculated intravenously into chimpanzees. A control of 5% human serum albumin mixed with the HCV was also included. Chimpanzees receiving either the albumin/HCV or the anti-HCV negative IGIV/HCV mixture developed typical HCV infection with HCV viremia, ALT elevation, and positive anti-HCV within 10 weeks after inoculation. However, the chimpanzee inoculated with the anti-HCV-positive IGIV/HCV mixture never developed any signs of infection over more than 1 year of observation. After the disappearance of the passively acquired antibody, no new anti-HCV antibody developed (Yu MY: personal communication), demonstrating clearly that the antibody to HCV alone can neutralize the virus.

CLINICAL STUDIES

A version of the envelope vaccine developed at Chiron is presently in a phase I clinical trial to study primarily the safety of the vaccine with the MF59 adjuvant as well as a preliminary investigation of dose. No results of this initial human trial are available at this time.

SAFETY CONCERNS

Safety of any vaccine is an issue of paramount importance. Vaccines are intended to interact with the host immune system and therefore have the potential to induce long-lasting effects, some of which may not be desirable. In the particular case of HCV, it must be appreciated that the virus is associated with hepatocellular carcinoma and possibly lymphoproliferative disorders. It has been well established that some viral proteins can exert important biologic effects *in vitro*, in cell culture, and in transgenic mouse systems. (74) It has been shown that the core protein can modulate gene transcription, cell proliferation, and apoptosis through interaction with a variety of cellular factors, including tumor necrosis factor-α, nuclear factor κB, extracellular signal-regulated kinases, and the TATA box-binding protein. (75–77) Certain transgenic mice expressing the

HCV core protein develop profound steatosis in their livers and primary hepatocellular carcinomas. (78,79) The NS3 protein has been reported to transform mouse 3T3 cells. (80,81) The NS5A protein has been implicated in mediating interferon resistance and in inhibiting the PKR protein kinase. (82) There may be other interactions with cellular factors yet to be reported. Therefore, vaccines that are based on the expression of HCV proteins within host cells need to be evaluated carefully for their potential to alter cell functions. Because DNA-based hepatitis C vaccines may lead to the integration of HCV genes into the cellular genome with potential profound effects on cells, these safety considerations are more than hypothetical.

POTENTIAL USE OF A HEPATITIS C VACCINE

Which populations should receive a hepatitis C vaccine cannot be determined at this time. Vaccine strategies that target high-risk groups have not in general been successful in reducing the incidence of infections. However, until the actual composition of an approved HCV vaccine is known, the safety profile is determined, the effectiveness of the vaccine evaluated, and the duration of the protection determined, it will not be possible to decide who should be vaccinated. If an ideal, safe, and effective vaccine were developed, universal vaccination should be considered in order to reduce the rate of hepatitis C significantly in this country. Finally, a successful immunotherapeutic vaccine could also have broad utility among HCV carriers.

CONCLUSION

Presently, numerous obstacles to hepatitis C vaccine development remain. The large degree of genetic and immunologic diversity of the virus may be the most difficult to overcome. However, in limited studies, it has been shown that HCV can be neutralized by antibody and that even with the lack of solid protection from infection, the vaccine-induced antibody can alter the natural history of infection toward a short-lasting, mild disease. The prevention of chronic infection in itself would be important as the most serious outcomes of HCV infections are the result of viral persistence. It is hoped that detailed studies of the immune response to HCV infections will provide insights to solving many of these problems. New technologies being applied to vaccine development may eventually lead to effective immunoprophylaxis and therapy.

REFERENCES

1. Alter M J. Epidemiology of hepatitis C. Hepatology 1997;26:62S–5S.
2. Alter M J, Moyer L A. The importance of preventing hepatitis C virus infection among injection drug users in the United States. J Acquired Immune Defic Syndr Hum Retrovirol 1998;18 (Suppl 1):S6–10.
3. Dienstag J L. Sexual and perinatal transmission of hepatitis C. Hepatology 1997;26:66S-70S.
4. Weiner A J, Brauer M J, Rosenblatt J, et al. Variable and hypervariable domains are found in

the regions of HCV corresponding to the flavivirus envelope and NS1 proteins and the pestivirus envelope glycoproteins. Virology 1991;180:842–8.

5. Duarte E A, Novella I S, Weaver S C, et al. RNA virus quasispecies: significance for viral disease and epidemiology. Infect Agents Dis 1994;3:201–14.

6. Simmonds P. Variability of the hepatitis C virus genome. Curr Stud Hematol Blood Transfus 1998;6238–63.

7. Kato N, Ootsuyama Y, Ohkoshi S, et al. Characterization of hypervariable regions in the putative envelope protein of hepatitis C virus. Biochem Biophys Res Commun 1992;189:119–27.

8. Weiner A J, Geysen H M, Christopherson C, et al. Evidence for immune selection of hepatitis C virus (HCV) putative envelope glycoprotein variants: potential role in chronic HCV infections. Proc Natl Acad Sci U S A 1992;89:3468–72.

9. Farci P, Shimoda A, Wong D, et al. Prevention of hepatitis C virus infection in chimpanzees by hyperimmune serum against the hypervariable region 1 of the envelope 2 protein. Proc Natl Acad Sci U S A 1996;93:15394–99.

10. Zibert A, Meisel H, Kraas W, Schulz A, Jung G, Roggendorf M. Early antibody response against hypervariable region 1 is associated with acute self-limiting infections of hepatitis C virus. Hepatology 1997;25:1245–9.

11. Prince A M, Brotman B, Huima T, Pascual D, Jaffery M, Inchauspe G. Immunity in hepatitis C infection. J Infect Dis 1992;165:438–43.

12. Farci P, Alter H J, Govindarajan S, et al. Lack of protective immunity against reinfection with hepatitis C virus. Science 1992;258:135–40.

13. Shimizu Y K, Yoshikura H. Multicycle infection of hepatitis C virus in cell culture and inhibition by alpha and beta interferons. J Virol 1994;68:8406–8.

14. Seipp S, Mueller H M, Pfaff E, Stremmel W, Theilmann L, Goeser T. Establishment of persistent hepatitis C virus infection and replication in vitro. J Gen Virol 1997;78:2467–76.

15. Ikeda M, Kato N, Mizutani T, Sugiyama K, Tanaka K, Shimotohno K. Analysis of the cell tropism of HCV by using in vitro HCV-infected human lymphocytes and hepatocytes. J Hepatol 1997;27:445–54.

16. Iacovacci S, Bertolini L, Manzin A, et al. Quantitation of hepatitis C virus RNA production in two human bone marrow-derived B-cell lines infected in vitro. Res Virol 1997;148:147–51.

17. Iacovacci S, Manzin A, Barca S, et al. Molecular characterization and dynamics of hepatitis C virus replication in human fetal hepatocytes infected in vitro. Hepatology 1997;26:1328–37.

18. Kato N, Ikeda M, Sugiyama K, Mizutani T, Tanaka T, Shimotohno K. Hepatitis C virus population dynamics in human lymphocytes and hepatocytes infected in vitro. J Gen Virol 1998;79:1859–69.

19. Serafino A, Valli M B, Andreola F, Carloni G, Bertolini L. Morphological modifications induced by HCV infection in the TOFE human lymphoblastoid cell line. Res Virol 1998;149:299–305.

20. Shimizu Y K, Igarashi H, Kiyohara T, et al. Infection of a chimpanzee with hepatitis C virus grown in cell culture. J Gen Virol 1998;79:1383–6.

21. Rosa D, Campagnoli S, Moretto C, et al. A quantitative test to estimate neutralizing antibodies to the hepatitis C virus: cytofluorimetric assessment of envelope glycoprotein 2 binding to target cells. Proc Natl Acad Sci U S A 1996;93:1759–63.

22. Levy S, Todd S C, Maecker H T. CD81 (TAPA-1): a molecule involved in signal transduction and cell adhesion in the immune system. Annu Rev Immunol 1998;16:89–109.

23. Pileri P, Uematsu Y, Campagnoli S, et al. Binding of hepatitis C virus to CD81. Science 1998;282:938–41.

24. Habersetzer F, Fournillier A, Dubuisson J, Rosa D, Abrignani S, Wychowski C, et al. Characterization of human monoclonal antibodies specific to the hepatitis C virus glycoprotein E2 with in vitro binding neutralization properties. Virology 1998;249:32–41.

25. Lagging L M, Meyer K, Owens R J, Ray R. Functional role of hepatitis C virus chimeric glycoproteins in the infectivity of pseudotyped virus. J Virol 1998;72:3539–46.

26. Bray M, Lai C J. Dengue virus premembrane and membrane proteins elicit a protective immune response. Virology 1991;185:505–8.

27. Konishi E, Pincus S, Paoletti E, Shope R E, Burrage T, Mason P W. Mice immunized with a subviral particle containing the Japanese encephalitis virus prM/M and E proteins are protected from lethal JEV infection. Virology 1992;188:714–20.

28. Kobayashi M, Tanaka E, Matsumoto A, Ichijo T, Kiyosawa K. Antibody response to E2/NS1 hepatitis C virus protein in patients with acute hepatitis C. J Gastroenterol Hepatol 1997;12: 73–6.

29. Cramp M E, Carucci P, Rossol S, et al. Hepatitis C virus (HCV) specific immune responses in anti-HCV positive patients without hepatitis C viraemia. Gut 1999;44:424–29.

30. Bassett S E, Thomas D L, Brasky K M, Lanford R E. Viral persistence, antibody to E1 and E2, and hypervariable region 1 sequence stability in hepatitis C virus-inoculated chimpanzees. J Virol 1999;73:1118–26.

31. Farci P, Alter H J, Wong D C, et al. Prevention of hepatitis C virus infection in chimpanzees after antibody- mediated in vitro neutralization. Proc Natl Acad Sci U S A 1994;91:7792–6.

32. Ishii K, Rosa D, et al. High titers of antibodies inhibiting the binding of envelope to human cells correlate with natural resolution of chronic hepatitis C. Hepatology 1998;28:1117–20.

33. Lai M E, Mazzoleni A P, Argiolu F, et al. Hepatitis C virus in multiple episodes of acute hepatitis in polytransfused thalassaemic children. Lancet 1994;343:388–90.

34. Botarelli P, Brunetto M R, Minutello M A, et al. T-lymphocyte response to hepatitis C virus in different clinical courses of infection. Gastroenterology 1993;104:580–7.

35. Ferrari C, Valli A, Galati L, et al. T-cell response to structural and nonstructural hepatitis C virus antigens in persistent and self-limited hepatitis C virus infections. Hepatology 1994;19: 286–95.

36. Diepolder H M, Zachoval R, Hoffmann R M, et al. Possible mechanism involving T-lymphocyte response to non-structural protein 3 in viral clearance in acute hepatitis C virus infection. Lancet 1995;346:1006–7.

37. Lechmann M, Ihlenfeldt H G, Braunschweiger I, et al. T- and B-cell responses to different hepatitis C virus antigens in patients with chronic hepatitis C infection and in healthy anti-hepatitis C virus—positive blood donors without viremia. Hepatology 1996;24:790–5.

38. Missale G, Bertoni R, Lamonaca V, et al. Different clinical behaviors of acute hepatitis C virus infection are associated with different vigor of the anti-viral cell-mediated immune response. J Clin Invest 1996;98:706–14.

39. Koziel M J, Wong D K, Dudley D, Houghton M, Walker B D. Hepatitis C virus-specific cytolytic T lymphocyte and T helper cell responses in seronegative persons. J Infect Dis 1997;176: 859–66.

40. Hiroishi K, Kita H, Kojima M, et al. Cytotoxic T lymphocyte response and viral load in hepatitis C virus infection. Hepatology 1997;25:705–12.

41. Christie J M, Healey C J, Watson J, et al. Clinical outcome of hypogammaglobulinaemic patients following outbreak of acute hepatitis C: 2 year follow up. Clin Exp Immunol 1997;110: 4–8.

42. Bjoro K, Froland S S, Yun Z, Samdal H H, Haaland T. Hepatitis C infection in patients with primary hypogammaglobulinemia after treatment with contaminated immune globulin. N Engl J Med 1994;331:1607–11.

43. Adams G, Kuntz S, Rabalais G, Bratcher D, Tamburro CH, Kotwal G J. Natural recovery from acute hepatitis C virus infection by agammaglobulinemic twin children. Pediatr Infect Dis J 1997;16:533–4.

44. Haydon G H, Jarvis L M, Blair C S, et al. Clinical significance of intrahepatic hepatitis C virus levels in patients with chronic HCV infection. Gut 1998;42:570–5.

45. Cooper S, Erickson A L, Adams E J, et al. Analysis of a successful immune response against hepatitis C virus. Immunity 1999;10:439–49.

46. Bassett S E, Brasky K M, Lanford R E. Analysis of hepatitis C virus-inoculated chimpanzees reveals unexpected clinical profiles. J Virol 1998;72:2589–99.

47. Alric L, Fort M, Izopet J, et al. Genes of the major histocompatibility complex class II influence the outcome of hepatitis C virus infection. Gastroenterology 1997;113:1675–81.

48. Cramp M E, Carucci P, Underhill J, Naoumov N V, Williams R, Donaldson P T. Association between HLA class II genotype and spontaneous clearance of hepatitis C viraemia. J Hepatol 1998;29:207–13.

49. Kuzushita N, Hayashi N, Moribe T, et al. Influence of HLA haplotypes on the clinical courses of individuals infected with hepatitis C virus. Hepatology 1998;27:240–4.

50. Lagging L M, Meyer K, Hoft D, Houghton M, Belshe R B, Ray R. Immune responses to plasmid DNA encoding the hepatitis C virus core protein. J Virol 1995;69:5859–63.

51. Tokushige K, Wakita T, Pachuk C, et al. Expression and immune response to hepatitis C virus core DNA-based vaccine constructs. Hepatology 1996;24:14–20.
52. Geissler M, Gesien A, Tokushige K, Wands J R. Enhancement of cellular and humoral immune responses to hepatitis C virus core protein using DNA-based vaccines augmented with cytokine-expressing plasmids. J Immunol 1997;158:1231–7.
53. Major M E, Vitvitski L, Mink M A, et al. DNA-based immunization with chimeric vectors for the induction of immune responses against the hepatitis C virus nucleocapsid. J Virol 1995;69:5798–805.
54. Geissler M, Tokushige K, Wakita T, Zurawski V R J, Wands J R. Differential cellular and humoral immune responses to HCV core and HBV envelope proteins after genetic immunizations using chimeric constructs. Vaccine 1998;16:857–67.
55. Saito T, Sherman G J, Kurokohchi K, et al. Plasmid DNA-based immunization for hepatitis C virus structural proteins: immune responses in mice. Gastroenterology 1997;112:1321–30.
56. Fournillier A, Nakano I, Vitvitski L, et al. Modulation of immune responses to hepatitis C virus envelope E2 protein following injection of plasmid DNA using single or combined delivery routes. Hepatology 1998;28:237–44.
57. Tedeschi V, Akatsuka T, Shih J W, Battegay M, Feinstone S M. A specific antibody response to HCV E2 elicited in mice by intramuscular inoculation of plasmid DNA containing coding sequences for E2. Hepatology 1997;25:459–62.
58. Nakano I, Maertens G, Major M E, et al. Immunization with plasmid DNA encoding hepatitis C virus envelope E2 antigenic domains induces antibodies whose immune reactivity is linked to the injection mode. J Virol 1997;71:7101–9.
59. Lee S W, Cho J H, Sung Y C. Optimal induction of hepatitis C virus envelope-specific immunity by bicistronic plasmid DNA inoculation with the granulocyte-macrophage colony-stimulating factor gene. J Virol 1998;72:8430–6.
60. Forns X, Emerson S U, Tobin G J, Mushahwar I K, Purcell R H, Bukh J. DNA immunization of mice and macaques with plasmids encoding hepatitis C virus envelope E2 protein expressed intracellularly and on the cell surface. Vaccine 1999;17:1992–2002.
61. Encke J, zu P J, Geissler M, Wands J R. Genetic immunization generates cellular and humoral immune responses against the nonstructural proteins of the hepatitis C virus in a murine model. J Immunol 1998;161:4917–23.
62. Cho J H, Lee S W, Sung Y C. Enhanced cellular immunity to hepatitis C virus nonstructural proteins by codelivery of granulocyte macrophage-colony stimulating factor gene in intramuscular DNA immunization. Vaccine 1999;17:1136–44.
63. Arichi T, Saito T, Major M E, Belyakov I M, Shirai M, Engelhard V H, Feinstone S M and Berzofsky J A. Prophylactic DNA vaccine for hepatitis C virus (HCV) infection: HCV-specific cytotoxic T lymphocyte induction and protection from HCV-recombinant vaccinia infection in an HLA-A2.1 transgenic mouse model. Proc Natl Acad Sci U S A. 2000;97:297–302.
64. Hiranuma K, Tamaki S, Nishimura Y, et al. Helper T cell determinant peptide contributes to induction of cellular immune responses by peptide vaccines against hepatitis C virus. J Gen Virol 1999;80:187–93.
65. Sarobe P, Pendleton C D, Akatsuka T, et al. Enhanced in vitro potency and in vivo immunogenicity of a CTL epitope from hepatitis C virus core protein following amino acid replacement at secondary HLA-A2.1 binding positions. J Clin Invest 1998;102:1239–48.
66. Prezzi C, Nuzzo M, Meola A, et al. Selection of antigenic and immunogenic mimics of hepatitis C virus using sera from patients. J Immunol 1996;156:4504–13.
67. Puntoriero G, Meola A, Lahm A, et al. Towards a solution for hepatitis C virus hypervariability: mimotopes of the hypervariable region 1 can induce antibodies cross-reacting with a large number of viral variants. EMBO J. 1998;17:3521–33.
68. Bruna-Romero O, Lasarte J J, Wilkinson G, et al. Induction of cytotoxic T-cell response against hepatitis C virus structural antigens using a defective recombinant adenovirus. Hepatology 1997;25:470–7.
69. Large M K, Kittlesen D J, Hahn Y S. Suppression of host immune response by the core protein of hepatitis C virus: possible implications for hepatitis C virus persistence. J Immunol 1999;162:931–8.
70. Baumert T F, Ito S, Wong D T, Liang T J. Hepatitis C virus structural proteins assemble into viruslike particles in insect cells. J Virol 1998;72:3827–36.

71. 6th Int Symp Hepatitis C Relat Viruses, Bethesda, MD 1999.
72. Choo Q L, Kuo G, Ralston R, et al. Vaccination of chimpanzees against infection by the hepatitis C virus. Proc Natl Acad Sci U S A 1994;91:1294–8.
73. Horowitz B, Prince A M, Horowitz M S, Watklevicz C. Viral safety of solvent-detergent treated blood products. Dev Biol Stand 1993;81:147–61.
74. Brechot C. Molecular mechanisms of hepatitis B and C viruses related to liver carcinogenesis. Hepatogastroenterology. 1998;45(Suppl 3):1189–96.
75. Ray R B, Meyer K, Steele R, Shrivastava A, Aggarwal B B, Ray R. Inhibition of tumor necrosis factor (TNF-alpha)-mediated apoptosis by hepatitis C virus core protein. J Biol Chem 1998;273:2256–9.
76. Zhu N, Khoshnan A, Schneider R, et al. Hepatitis C virus core protein binds to the cytoplasmic domain of tumor necrosis factor (TNF) receptor 1 and enhances TNF-induced apoptosis. J Virol 1998;72:3691–7.
77. Marusawa H, Hijikata M, Chiba T, Shimotohno K. Hepatitis C virus core protein inhibits Fas- and tumor necrosis factor alpha-mediated apoptosis via NF-kappaB activation. J Virol 1999;73:4713–20.
78. Moriya K, Yotsuyanagi H, Shintani Y, et al. Hepatitis C virus core protein induces hepatic steatosis in transgenic mice. J Gen Virol 1997;78:1527–31.
79. Moriya K, Fujie H, Shintani Y, et al. The core protein of hepatitis C virus induces hepatocellular carcinoma in transgenic mice. Nat Med 1998;4:1065–7.
80. Sakamuro D, Furukawa T, Takegami T. Hepatitis C virus nonstructural protein NS3 transforms NIH 3T3 cells. J Virol 1995;69:3893–6.
81. Fujita T, Ishido S, Muramatsu S, Itoh M, Hotta H. Suppression of actinomycin D-induced apoptosis by the NS3 protein of hepatitis C virus. Biochem Biophys Res Commun 1996;229:825–31.
82. Gale M J J, Korth M J, Katze M G. Repression of the PKR protein kinase by the hepatitis C virus NS5A protein: a potential mechanism of interferon resistance. Clin Diagn Virol 1998;10:157–62.

■ INDEX

A

Acute hepatitis C, 71–80
  antiviral therapy
    combination therapy, 80
    interferon monotherapy,
      77–80
  cellular immune response, 153–
    155
  clinical course, 72–75
  convalescence, 73
  diagnosis, 43, 75–77
  icteric phase, 73
  incubation period, 72
  pathology, 108
  preicteric phase, 72
  progression to chronic hepati-
    tis C, 74–75, 185
  prospective studies, 86–89
Alcohol consumption
  alcohol abuse, 364
  alcohol dependence, 363–364
  chronic hepatitis C, 115–116
  cirrhosis and, 365, 367–368
  hepatic fibrosis and, 377, 379,
    381
  hepatocellular carcinoma and,
    250, 379, 380
  liver injury and, 365, 369–
    378

  moderate alcohol use, 372,
    375–376
  quantification of intake, 364–
    365
  studies, 372–378
ALT values
  alcohol consumption and, 372
  perinatally acquired HCV infec-
    tion, 395
  treatment of patients with nor-
    mal values, 224–225
Animal models, hepatitis C, 5–6,
  475
Antibodies, neutralizing, 129
Antigen presenting cells (APCs),
  148
Antigens, immunogenicity, 132–
  134
Anti-HCV
  hepatocellular carcinoma, 265–
    267
  HIV-HCV coinfection, 326
Anti-HCV immunotherapy, 461–
  464
Antisense molecule, 464
Antiviral therapy, 44–45, 203–
  236, 453–456. *See also*
    Complementary and alterna-
    tive medicine

  acute hepatitis C, 77–80
  after renal transplantation,
    343–344
  alcohol use and, 381–382
  benefits and risks, 204
  in children, 397–398
  chronic hepatitis C, 208–210,
    272, 420–422
  for cirrhotic patients, 255, 258,
    259, 273, 278
  combination therapy. *See*
    Ribavirin-interferon com-
    bination therapy
  contraindication to, 206–207
  cost-effectiveness, 208
  future therapies, 234–235
  genotypes and, 63–64
  HIV-HCV coinfection, 323–325
  indications for, 204–206
  inexpensive medications, devel-
    opment, 196–197
  initial therapy, 208–219
  interferon monotherapy. *See*
    Interferon monotherapy
  iron status and, 420–422
  for mixed cryoglobulinemia,
    303–304
  for nonresponding patients,
    222–224

Antiviral therapy (*continued*)
  nonresponse to, 222
  for patients with normal ALT values, 224–225
  for patients with renal disease, 336–338
  for porphyria cutanea tarda patients with HCV, 357–359
  posttransplant HCV disease, 277, 278–279, 287–290
  predicting response to, 233–234
  for relapsed patients, 219–222
  resistance to, 34, 45–46
  responses to, 207–208
  ribavirin therapy. *See* Ribavirin-interferon combination therapy
  side effects, 206–207, 226–233
  small molecule anti-HCV drugs, 456–461
Assays
  accuracy, 36
  HCV genotyping, 59–60
  precision and reproducibility, 35
  predictive value, 35
  quantitative, 35–36
  sensitivity, 35
  specificity, 35
  standardization, 36
Autoantibodies, hepatitis C and, 308–309
Autoimmune hepatitis, histology, 113

B
Bear gall, 443–444
Blood and blood products, HCV transmission, 172–173, 189
Blood-borne pathogens, 194
Blood donations, screening, 42, 193
Botanical agents. *See* Complementary and alternative medicine
Bovine gallstone, 443–444
Bupleurum falcatum, 442

C
CAPD (continuous ambulatory peritoneal dialysis) patients, hepatitis C and, 330–338
Capillaris, 445
Cell-mediated immunity, 474–475
Cellular immune response, 147–161
  acute hepatitis C, 153–155
  chronic hepatitis C, 155–156

cytotoxic T cells, 151–152, 153–155
  escape from, 160
  induction, 147–148
  kinetics, 152–153
  T helper cells, 148–151, 152, 155
CH100 (Cathay Herbal), 440–441
Chapparal, 445, 446
Children
  hepatitis C, 389–399
    antiviral therapy, 397–398
    chronic, 115
    clinical features, 393–394
    epidemiology, 389–390
    histology, 396–397
    natural history, 394–396
    transfusion-associated, 391
    transmission, 390–393
Chinese skullcap root, 442
Chinese thoroughwax, 442
Chronic hepatitis B, histology, 109, 113
Chronic hepatitis C, 203
  alcohol consumption and, 115–116
  antiviral therapy, 203–236
    benefits and risks, 204
    contraindications to, 206–208
    indications for, 204–206
    initial therapy, 208–219
    interferon monotherapy, 208–210, 272
    iron status and, 420–422
    for nonresponding patients, 222–224
    for patients with normal ALT values, 224–225
    predicting response to, 233–234
    relapsed patients, 219–222
    responses to, 207–208, 233–234
    ribavirin-interferon combination therapy, 210–219
    side effects, 206–207, 226–233
  children, 115
  cirrhosis and, 267–268
  diagnosis, 43
  grading, 117
  hepatocellular carcinoma and, 185, 273
  histologic differential diagnosis, 112–115
  histologic scoring, 117–121

histology, 109
  HIV-positive individuals, 116
  humoral mechanisms, 135–137
  iron toxicity in, 418–420
  liver biopsy, 107–108
  outcome, 203–204
  pathology, 108–112
  porphyria cutanea tarda and, 351–359
  posttransplantation evaluation of, 116–117
  pregnancy and, 408
  progression to cirrhosis, 242–243
  progression to from acute hepatitis, 74–75, 185
  prospective studies, 89–93
  retrospective studies, 93–96
  scoring, 117–121
  staging, 117
Chronic hepatitis D, histology, 109, 113
Cinnamon and Hoelen formula, 445
Cinnamon twig, 445
Cirrhosis, 241–260
  alcohol use and, 365, 367–368
  antiviral therapy
    combination therapy, 278
    interferon monotherapy, 255, 258, 259, 273, 278
  chronic hepatitis C and, 267–268
  clinical presentation, 243–245
  compensated. *See* Compensated cirrhosis
  defined, 112
  diagnosis, 112
  EUROHEP cohort study, 246, 251, 252
  and hepatocellular carcinoma, 246
  histology, 113
  laboratory features, 244–245
  management, 254–259
  mortality, 251–254
  outcomes, 91–92, 245–254
  pathology, 112
  physical examination in, 244
  pregnancy and, 409–410
  progression to, 242–243
  symptoms, 243–244
  uncompensated. *See* Uncompensated cirrhosis
Cocaine use, 172
Comfrey, 445

Compensated cirrhosis
  management, 254–255
  outcome, 91–92
Complementary and alternative
    medicine, 427–446
  comparison with Western medi-
    cine, 428–429
  concepts of hepatitis C, 435–
    436
  traditional medicines
    as hepatoprotectants, 429–
      433
    hepatotoxicity, 445–446
    treatment of hepatitis C,
      433–445
Continuous ambulatory peritoneal
    dialysis (CAPD) patients,
    hepatitis C and, 330–338
Counseling
  HCV-positive persons, 179–
    180, 195
  for pregnancy, 407–409
Cryoglobulins
  characterization, 297–298
  classification, 296–297
  detection, 297
  history, 295–296
Cutaneous vasculitis, mixed cryo-
    globulinemia, 300–301
Cytotoxic T cells, 151–152,
    153–155

D

Decompensated cirrhosis
  antiviral therapy, 257–259, 278
  clinical features, 245
  development of, 251
Dendritic cells, 148, 463
Dialysis patients, hepatitis C and,
    330–338
Drug-induced chronic hepatitis,
    histology, 113
Drug use
  HCV transmission, 171–172,
    190, 194
  HIV-HCV coinfection transmis-
    sion, 317

E

Education. See also Counseling
  HCV prevention and, 194–195
Egypt, hepatitis C, 191
Envelope proteins, 11
Enzyme immunoassays (EIAs),
    36–37
Epidemiology
  hepatitis C, 169–180, 185–189

children, 389–390
chronic liver disease, 170–171
global genotype distribution,
    186, 188–189
HCV genotypes, 56–57
in kidney disease patients,
    329–335
pregnancy and, 405–406
renal transplant patients,
    338–340
viral markers and, 45
hepatocellular carcinoma, 245–
    247
HIV-HVC coinfection, 316–
    318, 328
mixed cryoglobulinemia, 298–
    299
Epitopes, virus-neutralizing, 134,
    135, 138
EUROHEP cohort study, 246,
    251, 252

F

Fibrosis
  alcohol consumption and, 377,
    379, 381
  development of cirrhosis and,
    102
  staging, 89–90, 117, 120

G

Gallic acid, 431–432
Gene therapy, as HCV treatment,
    465
Genotyping assays, 41–42
Germander, 445, 446
Ginger root, 442, 445
Ginseng, 442, 445
Glomerulonephritis
  after renal transplantation,
    342–343
  membranoproliferative, 301–
    302, 307–308
Glycyrrhizin, 438–440
Goou, 443–444
Grading, 117
Guizhi-fuling-wan, 430–431

H

Half summer root, 442
HCV (hepatitis C virus)
  3′-untranslated region, 8
  5′-untranslated region, 6–8
  antigenic variability, 61
  coinfection with HIV, 315–326
  diagnostic assays, 61
  humoral response to, 128–139

in vitro culture systems, 471–
    472
molecular biology, 1–18
neutralizing antibodies, 129
nucleotide sequence variation,
    53–56
particle structure, 2
persistence, 29, 32, 158–161
polyproptein translation and
    processing, 8–10
protein structure, 10–15
quasispecies, 27–29, 32–33
replication, 16–18, 29, 32
tissue culture systems, 4–5
virion assembly, 17–18
HCV antigens, detection in tis-
    sues, 38
HCV core antigen assay, 38
HCV genome, 2–4, 53
  quasispecies, 27–29
  small molecule anti-HCV drugs,
    454, 456–461
  translation, 6–8
HCV genotypes, 25–26, 53–65
  antiviral therapy and, 63–64
  assays, 41–42, 59–60
  classification system, 53–56
  differences between, 60–64
  disease progression and, 62–63
  geographical distribution, 56–
    57
  global distribution, 186, 188–
    189
  HCV in HIV-infected patients,
    322–323
  HCV vaccines, 61–62, 470–
    471
  hemodialysis patients with HCV,
    336
  hepatocellular carcinoma and,
    250
  origins of, 57–59
  serotyping, 38
HCV infection. See Hepatitis C
HCV-positive persons, counseling,
    179–180, 195
HCV-related disease, pathogene-
    sis, 45
HCV testing, routine testing,
    178–179
HCV vaccines
  clinical studies, 481
  development, 197, 470–473
  HCV genotypes, 61–62,
    470–471
  immunoprotection against
    HCV, 473–476

HCV vaccines (*continued*)
  live recombinant vaccines, 479
  naked DNA vaccines, 476–478
  preclinical studies, 476–481
  recombinant envelope proteins,
    479–480
  safety, 481–482
  synthetic, 478–479
  therapeutic vaccination, 480–
    481
  virus-like particles, 479
Health care workers
  occupational risk, 174–175
  screening, 194
Helicase, as target of anti-HCV
  drugs, 459–460
Hemochromatosis, 113, 418
Hemodialysis, hepatitis C and,
  332–335
Hemophilia, HIV-HCV coinfection and, 316–317
Hepatitis, routing testing, 178
Hepatitis B
  hepatocellular carcinoma and,
    270
  histology, 109, 113
Hepatitis C
  acute. *See* Acute hepatitis C
  alcohol use and, 115–116,
    363–383
  animal models, 5–6, 475
  antiviral therapy. *See* Antiviral
    therapy
  in children, 115, 389–399
  chronic. *See* Chronic hepatitis C
  cirrhosis and, 241–260
  complementary and alternative
    medicine, 427–446
  counseling patients, 179–180,
    195
  epidemiology. *See* Epidemiology
  extrahepatic manifestations,
    306–307
    autoantibodies, 308–309
    glomerulonephritis, 301–302,
      307–308
    mixed cryoglobulinemia,
      295–306
    sialadenitis, 307
  global genotype distribution,
    186, 188–189
  hepatocellular carcinoma and,
    265–274
  HFE mutations, 417–418
  histology, 112–115, 156–157
  humoral response to, 125–139
  immunoprotection against. *See*
    Immunology

immunosuppression and, 342
incidence of, 171, 186, 196, 331
iron and, 415–422
liver transplant and, 277–291
mortality, 91
natural history, 85–102, 203–
  204
    HIV infected patients, 319–
      320
    renal failure patients, 335–
      336
outcome, 33
outcome studies, 85–102
pathology, 107–122
posttransplantation recurrence,
  34–35
pregnancy and, 405–411
prevalence, 147, 186–189, 196,
  315–316, 329–330, 405–
  406
prevention and control, 177–
  180, 193
prognosis, 43–44
progression, 62–63
relapse, 219–220
renal disease patients and, 329–
  338
renal transplant patients, 338–
  344
risk factors, 189–192
schistosomiasis and, 191
screening blood donations for,
  42
severity, 33, 43–44
spontaneous recovery, 101–102
traditional medicine, concepts
  of, 435–436
transmission. *See* Transmission
treatment. *See* Antiviral therapy
X-linked agammaglobulinemia
  and, 394
Hepatitis C vaccines. *See* HCV
  vaccines
Hepatitis C virus. *See* HCV
Hepatitis D, histology, 109, 113
Hepatocarcinogenesis, mechanisms of, 268–271
Hepatocellular carcinoma (HCC)
  age of infection and, 249–250
  alcohol consumption and, 250,
    379, 480
  anti-HCV, 265–267
  chronic hepatitis C and, 185
  cirrhosis and, 246
  development, 268–271
  diagnosis, 271
  epidemiology, 245–247
  etiology, 192

HBV infection and, 250
HCV genotype and, 250
hepatitis B coinfection and, 270
hepatitis C and, 265–274
incidence, 245
natural history, 267–268
porphyria cutanea tarda and,
  270
prevention, 271–273
risk factors, 246–251
Hepatoprotectants, herbal, 429–
  433
Herbal agents. *See* Complementary
  and alternative medicine
HFE mutations, 417–418
Histologic scoring, 117–121
Histology
  autoimmune hepatitis, 113
  hepatitis B, 109, 113
  hepatitis C, 112–115, 156–157
    in children, 396–397
  HIV-HCV coinfection, 323
HIV-HCV coinfection
  antiviral therapy, 323–325
  diagnosis, 322–323
  epidemiology, 316–318, 326
  hemophilia and, 316–317
  histology, 323
  natural history, 319–320
  pathogenesis, 320–322
  prevalence, 316–317
  transmission, 317–318
HIV infection, prevalence, 316
HIV-positive individuals, chronic
  hepatitis C, 116
Homosexual activity, HCV transmission and, 176
Host genetic factors, 475–476
Host immune response, 395
Humoral immunity, 125–130,
  135–137, 474

I
IgM assays, 38, 87
Ilex, 445
Immune-mediated liver injury,
  157–158
Immunization. *See* HCV vaccines
Immunoblot assays, 37
Immunology, 473–476
  cell-mediated immunity, 474–
    475
  cellular immune response, 147–
    161
  host genetic factors, 475–476
  host immune response, 395
  humoral immunity, 125–130,
    474

Immunosuppression, liver transplantation, 289–290
Immunotherapy, 461–464
Injection
  education in safe techniques, 194
  transmission of HCV and, 173–174, 189–190
Interferon-α, 203
Interferon monotherapy, 453–454
  acute hepatitis C, 77–80
  alcohol use and, 381–382
  in children, 397–398
  chronic hepatitis C, 208–210, 272
  cirrhosis, 255, 258, 259, 273, 278
  exacerbation of liver disease by, 228
  genotypes and, 63
  history, 453
  iron status and, 420–422
  long-term benefits, 207
  mixed cryoglobulinemia, 303
  outcomes, 241
  patients with renal disease, 336–338
  posttransplant HCV disease, 277, 288
  prevention of hepatocellular carcinoma, 255–257
  retreatment
    after relapse, 220
    of nonresponders, 222–224
  serious adverse events, 228, 229
  side effects, 206, 207, 226–229, 230–233
  three-month stop rule, 233–234
Interferon-ribavirin combination therapy. *See* Ribavirin-interferon combination therapy
Intranasal cocaine use, 172
Iron, hepatitis C and, 415–422
Iron overload, 114
Iron toxicity, in chronic hepatitis C, 418–420
Italy, hepatitis C, 192

J
Japan
  glycyrrhizin, 438–440
  hepatitis C in, 192
Jujube fruit, 442, 445

K
Kidney. *See* Renal
Kinetics, antiviral T-cell response, 152–153

L
Labiatae spp., 445
Larrea tridentata, 445
Licorice root, 442, 445
Liver, hepatoprotectants, herbal, 429–433
Liver biopsy, 107–108
  before antiviral therapy begins, 205–206
  scoring of, 117–118
Liver cancer. *See* Hepatocellular carcinoma
Live recombinant vaccines, 479
Liver inflammation
  chronic hepatitis C, 111
  scoring systems, 120
Liver injury
  alcohol use and, 365, 369–378
  immune-mediated, 157–158
Liver transplantation
  for decompensated cirrhosis, 257
  HCV-positive organ donors, 279
  HCV recurrence following, 34–35
  hepatitis C and, 277–291
  immunosuppression, 289–290
  indicators for, 382
  posttransplantation infection, 277, 278–287, 290
    antiviral therapy, 277, 279–287, 290
    complications, 286–287
    natural history, 280–283
    pathology, 286
    severity, 283–286
    source of infection, 279–280
  retransplantation, 290
Lymphocytic infiltrate, 158

M
Maternal transmission
  hepatitis C, 175, 190–191, 318, 391–392, 408–409
  HIV-HCV coinfection, 318
Mate tea, 445, 446
Membranoproliferative glomerulonephritis, hepatitis C and, 301–302, 307–308
METAVIR scoring system, 89, 117, 119–120, 121
Milk thistle, 429–430, 436–438
Minor Bupleurum combination, 445
Mistletoe, 445, 446
Mixed cryoglobulinemia, 295–306
  antiviral therapy, 303–304

bone marrow involvement, 302
  clinical manifestations, 299–300
  cryoglobulins
    characterization, 297–298
    classification, 296–297
    detection, 297
  cutaneous vasculitis, 300–301
  history, 295–296
  lymphoid involvement, 302–303
  membranoproliferative glomerulonephritis, 301–302
  pathogenesis, 304–306
  peripheral neuropathy, 302
  prevalence, 298–299
Mother-to-infant transmission, hepatitis C, 175, 190–191, 318, 391–392, 406–408
Moutan, 445

N
Naked DNA vaccines, 476–478
911-granules, 445
NS2 protein, 11–12, 453, 457
NS3 protein, 12–13, 153, 453, 457–458
NS4 protein, 13–14
NS5A protein, 14, 460
NS5B protein, 14–15, 460–461

O
Octacarboxylic porphyrin, 353
Outcome studies, 85–102
Oxymatrine, 444–445

P
Panax ginseng root, 442
Parenchymal inflammation, chronic hepatitis C, 111
Pathogenesis
  fibrosis in alcohol users, 379
  HCV-related disease, 45
  HIV-HCV coinfection, 320–322
  mixed cryoglobulinemia, 304–306
Pathology
  acute hepatitis C, 108
  chronic hepatitis C, 108–112
  iron toxicity in chronic hepatitis C, 418–420
Pennyroyal oil, 445
Peony, 445
Percutaneous needle biopsy, 107
Perinatal transmission, hepatitis C, 175, 190–191, 318, 391

Peripheral neuropathy, mixed cryoglobulinemia, 302
Persica, 445
Persistence, 29, 32, 158–161
Pinella ternata, 442
Pinellia, 445
Porphyria cutanea tarda (PCT)
  antiviral therapy for HCV, 357–359
  biochemical features, 353–356
  chronic hepatitis C and, 351–359
  hepatocellular carcinoma and, 270
  liver disease in, 352–353
Posttransplantation HCV infection, 277, 278–287, 290
  antiviral therapy, 277, 278–279, 287–290
  complications, 286–287
  natural history, 280–283
  pathology, 286
  severity, 283–286
  source of infection, 279–280
Pregnancy
  cirrhosis and, 409–410
  counseling of HIV-infected women, 407–409
  hepatitis C and, 405–411
  transmission, 406–409
  obstetric care of HCV-infected women, 409–410
Primary biliary cirrhosis, histology, 113
Primary sclerosing cholangitis, histology, 113
Prospective studies
  acute hepatitis C, 86–89
  chronic hepatitis C, 89–93
Proteins, HCV, 10–15

Q

Quantitative assays, linearity, 35–36
Quasispecies, 27–29
  compartmentalization, 32–33
  liver damage and, 33

R

Relapse, 219–220
Renal transplantation
  graft rejection, 341–342
  hepatitis C, 338–344
  outcomes and, 340–342
  immunosuppression, 342
Replication, 16–18, 29, 32
Retrospective studies, chronic hepatitis C, 93–96

Ribavirin, 203, 210
  in children, 398
  for posttransplant HCV disease, 277, 288
  side effects, 206–207
Ribavirin-interferon combination therapy, 203
  acute hepatitis C, 80
  in children, 398
  chronic hepatitis C, 210–219, 421–422
  cirrhosis, 257, 259, 278
  early discontinuation, 218–219
  genotypes and, 63–64
  history, 453
  HIV-HCV coinfection, 323–324
  mixed cryoglobulinemia, 304
  patients with renal disease, 338
  posttransplant HCV disease, 277, 288–289
  response rates, 212–218
  retreatment
    after relapse, 220–222
    of nonresponders, 224
  side effects, 206–207, 229–230
  trials of, 211
  twenty-four-week stop rule, 234
Ribozyme, as HCV treatment, 465
Rituals, HCV transmission and, 174, 190
RNA detection assays
  acute hepatitis C, 87
  antiviral therapy, 77–80
  qualitative, 38–40
  quantitative, 40–41

S

Schistosomiasis, hepatitis C and, 191
Scoring, 117–121
Screening
  blood donations, 42, 193
  global, 193
  of health care workers, 194
Scute, 445
Scutellaria baicalensis, 442
Sensitivity, of assay, 35
Seroconversion, acute hepatitis C, 87
Serological assays, 36–38
Serology, after renal transplantation, 343
Seropositivity, 26
Serotyping, 38
Sexual transmission
  hepatitis C, 175–176, 178, 190, 408

HIV-HCV coinfection, 317–318
Sheih-qing-wan, 430–431
Sho-saiko-to (TJ-9), 432–433, 442–443
Sialadenitis, hepatitis C and, 307
Silybum marianum, 429
Silymarin, 436–438
Skullcap, 442, 446
SNMC (Stronger Neominophagen C), 438–440
Sophora flavescens, 444
Sophora subprostrata, 444
Specificity, assay, 35
Staging, fibrosis, 89–90, 117, 120
Steatohepatitis, 113, 114
Steatosis, chronic hepatitis C, 111
Stronger Neominophagen C (SNMC), 438–440
Structural proteins
  humoral response to, 133
  target of anti-HCV drugs, 457–458
Superquant, 40
Syh-mo-yiin, 430–431
Syh-nih-sann, 430–431
Symphutkum officinale, 445
Synthetic HCV vaccines, 478–479

T

Tang-kuei, 445
Terminalia belerica, 431
Teucrium chamaedrys, 445
T helper cells, 148–151, 152, 155
Thymus extracts, 441–442
TJ-9 (sho-saiko-to), 432–433, 442–443
Traditional medicine. *See* Complementary and alternative medicine
Transmission
  hepatitis C, 189
    blood and blood products, 172–173, 189
    in children, 390–393
    cosmetic services, 174
    dialysis patients, 333
    health-care related procedures, 173–174
    injecting drug use, 171–172, 190, 393
    injections for medical purposes, 173–174, 189–190
    intrafamilial, 392–393
    intranasal cocaine use, 172
    mother-to-infant, 175, 190–

191, 318, 391–392,
406–408
occupational exposures, 174–
175
perinatal, 175, 190–191, 318,
391
pregnancy, 406–409
rituals, 174, 190, 194–195
sexual transmission, 175–
176, 178, 190, 408
to dialysis staff, 331–332
traditional medicine, 190,
194–195
unsafe injections, 173–174
HIV-HCV coinfection, 317–318
renal failure patients, 332–335
Treatment modes
anti-HCV immunotherapy,
461–464
antisense molecule, 464
antiviral. *See* Antiviral therapy;
Interferon monotherapy;
Ribavirin-interferon combination therapy
complementary and alternative
medicine, 426–446
gene therapy, 465
ribozyme, 465

U
Uroporphyrin, 353
Uroporphyrinogen decarboxylase
(UROD), 353–355

V
Vaccines. *See* HCV vaccines
Valerian, 445, 446
Viral load, 26–27
Viral markers, 25–37
in clinical research, 45–46
patient management and, 42–45
Viral persistence, 29, 32, 158–161
Viremia, 26–27
Virion, 17–18
Virology
molecular biology-based tests,
38–42
serological assays, 36–38
terms, 35–36
Viscum album, 445

W
Western medicine, complementary
medicine compared to, 428–
429
Wilson's disease, histology, 113

X
X-linked agammaglobulinemia
(XLA), hepatitis C and, 394

Y
Yutan, 443–444

Z
Zingiber officinale, 442
Zizyphus jujuba, 442